Theories of Counseling and Psychotherapy

Systems, Strategies, and Skills

Linda Seligman

Late Professor Emeritus, George Mason University

Lourie W. Reichenberg

Licensed Professional Counselor, Falls Church, Virginia

PEARSON

Original edition, entitled THEORIES OF COUNSELING AND PSYCHOTHERAPY: SYSTEMS, STRATEGIES, AND SKILLS, 4th Edition, by SELIGMAN, LINDA W.; REICHENBERG, LOURIE W., published by Pearson Education, Inc, publishing as Pearson, Copyright © 2014by Pearson Education, Inc.

Indian edition published byPearson India Education Services Pvt. Ltd. Copyright© 2016.

ISBN 978-93-325-5789-5

First Impression, 2016

Published by Pearson India Education Services Pvt.Ltd, CIN: U72200TN2005PTC057128.
Formerly known as TutorVista Global Pvt Ltd, licensees of Pearson Education in South Asia

Head Office: 7th Floor, knowledge Boulevard, A-8(A) Sector-62, Noida (U.P) 201309, India

Registered Office: Module G4, Ground Floor, Elnet Software City, TS -140, Block 2 & 9
Rajiv Gandhi Salai, Taramani, Chennai, TamilNadu600113.Fax: 080-30461003,
Phone: 080-30461060, www.pearson.co.in email id: companysecetary.India@pearson.com

Printed in India by Rahul Print O Pack

On December 24, 2007, my friend, colleague, and co-author, Linda Seligman, died. She once wrote "My work in this field has been a great source of fulfillment, education, and inspiration to me. I wish you the same experience!" With this fourth edition of Theories of Counseling and Psychotherapy, I have tried to maintain the same quality and high standards that Linda embraced. This text is dedicated to her memory.

Lourie W. Reichenberg
Falls Church, VA

PREFACE

This text was first published in 2001, and since that time it has been used by tens of thousands of students. I have made many changes to this fourth edition of *Theories of Counseling and Psychotherapy* based on developments in counseling and psychology and on feedback and reviews received from students and faculty who have used this text in their courses.

The basic structure of the text has been maintained, including the BETA format, descriptions of important treatment approaches, skill development sections, case studies, and exercises for large groups, small groups, and individuals. In addition, the discussions of relevant research, documenting the validity of each approach, have been expanded. Updated information is provided on all treatment approaches presented in the text, with considerably expanded information on many (see the "New to This Edition" section later in this preface).

ORGANIZATION OF THIS TEXT

This text organizes the major theories of counseling and psychotherapy into four broad categories: **B**ackground, **E**motions, **T**houghts, and **A**ctions. Each section in the BETA format reflects the emphasis of the underlying theories:

- ***Background:*** Sigmund Freud and classical psychoanalysis, Alfred Adler and individual psychology, post- and neo-Freudians, and brief psychodynamic therapy
- ***Emotions:*** Carl Rogers and person-centered therapy, existential therapy, Gestalt therapy, and newer approaches, including narrative, solution-focused, and feminist therapy
- ***Thoughts:*** Albert Ellis and rational emotive behavior therapy, and Aaron Beck and cognitive therapy
- ***Actions:*** behavior therapy, cognitive–behavioral therapy including acceptance and mindfulness approaches, and reality therapy.

Introductory chapters on each of these four areas help readers to understand the commonalities among theories in each group. Each chapter that presents a treatment system follows the same organization to facilitate comparison and ease of use, beginning with a brief overview of the approach and a biographical sketch of its developer, and then moving on to the theoretical concepts, goals, and strategies of each treatment modality. Particular attention is given to the application of each treatment system to people from diverse backgrounds. Finally, at the end of each chapter, skill development and other exercises allow students to apply the knowledge they have gained about each treatment modality. These exercises are:

- ***Skill development section:*** This section teaches one or more key skills associated with the treatment system under review.
- ***Case illustration with the Diaz family:*** Edie, her husband Roberto, and their daughter Ava appear throughout the text to illustrate how treatment approaches can be used with both genders, different ages, and different cultural backgrounds.
- ***Large-group exercises:*** These exercises are designed to facilitate discussion and a deeper understanding of each treatment approach.
- ***Small-group exercises:*** These exercises provide practice in essential skill development.
- ***Individual exercises:*** These exercises will help readers develop self-awareness and solidify learning.

Although this text focuses primarily on systems of counseling and psychotherapy that are designed for treatment of individuals, an overview of family systems theory is included in Chapter 18. Chapter 19 discusses the nature, strengths, and shortcomings of integrated and eclectic treatment systems. Although these two chapters consider a range of treatment approaches, their structure generally follows the format of the earlier chapters. Chapter 20 concludes with a synthesis of the major treatment systems, information on how clinicians select their preferred treatment approach, and a questionnaire to help readers identify which approach best reflects their beliefs and personal style.

Dr. Seligman has written two texts organized according to the BETA format that can be used as companion pieces to *Theories of Counseling and Psychotherapy*. The first text, *Fundamental Skills for Mental Health Professionals* (Pearson, 2009), focuses on technical skills rather than theories. It covers some of the same skills as *Theories of Counseling and Psychotherapy,* as well as additional technical skills necessary for clinical practice. All are covered in an in-depth and comprehensive way. The second text, *Conceptual Skills for Mental Health Professionals* (Pearson, 2009), teaches more advanced conceptual skills needed by clinicians, such as case conceptualization, multicultural competency, and dealing with client crises. Although these two texts are intended to stand alone, they can also be used in combination. Ideally, learners will first use *Theories of Counseling and Psychotherapy* to develop an understanding of the BETA format and the important treatment systems. In a subsequent course, they would use the *Fundamental Skills* and *Conceptual Skills* texts. Their familiarity with the BETA format and the treatment systems would facilitate their learning and accelerate their skill development.

NEW TO THIS EDITION

Based on reviewers' comments and professors who use the text in their graduate programs, significant changes have been made to this fourth edition. It was my intent to make the text practical and functional for both students as well as teachers.

Changes to Structure

- Chapters that introduce each section in the BETA format have been rewritten to provide students with an overview of the theories contained in that section. These section openers are intended to enhance students' understanding of behavior, emotions, thoughts, and actions while also providing a preview of the theories to be discussed in each section. In recognition of course length and what the reviewers report they actually use in the classroom, the Skill Development, Case Illustration, and Exercises sections have been removed from these introductory chapters. As a result, some of the more popular Skill Development sections have been moved to other chapters, while some have been eliminated.
- Part six, *Other Treatment Approaches,* has been renamed to more accurately reflect that these chapters are not a part of the BETA format. Chapter 18 is now *Family Systems Approaches,* Chapter 19 is *Integrative Therapies,* and Chapter 20 is *Solidifying Understanding of Treatment Systems*. This section of integrated treatment systems remains at the end of the text for a reason. Students should first read and learn about the main theories of psychotherapy and give consideration to which approach best suits their philosophy before beginning to cherry-pick techniques from different theoretical orientations. I recognize that most clinicians use integrative approaches, and that is addressed in Chapter 19, along with a discussion of points to consider when formulating a system.
- In keeping with the current focus on research-supported treatments, each chapter has been updated to include the latest research available. As can be expected, most of the new

research involves cognitive and cognitive–behavioral treatments (found in Chapters 12 through 16). Psychodynamic psychotherapy, experiential therapies, and interpersonal psychotherapy have also been the focus of new research and that is included in Chapters 2, 5, 6, 18, and 19.

- The common factors approach and support for the importance of an effective and sustained therapeutic alliance have been the focus of much newly published research. This information is integrated where relevant (usually in the discussion of the therapeutic alliance) throughout the text. Chapter 1, *Contexts of Effective Treatment,* includes an extended discussion, as does the chapter on theoretical integration.
- The fourth edition of this text brings a stronger multicultural focus. Beginning with Chapter 1, in which Hays's ADDRESSING acronym is explained, each theoretical chapter in the text includes a revised multicultural section intended to be more culturally sensitive.

Changes to Individual Chapters

- Reorganization of the constructivist theories (Chapter 11) now incorporates what had been a separate chapter on solution-focused therapy in the previous edition. The section on feminist therapy has been enlarged considerably.
- The chapter on post- and neo-Freudians (basically any psychodynamic theory except Adler) has always been tricky. The good news and the bad news are the same in that this chapter provides a comprehensive survey of post-Freudian psychodynamic theories. Some instructors love this, while some will leave it out of the syllabus because it contains too much information.
- A reorganization of Chapter 19 on integrative therapy includes enhanced consideration of Wachtel's cyclical psychodynamics and also the transtheoretical model of change.
- Clarification of the differences between cognitive and cognitive–behavioral therapy have been made throughout Chapters 12 through 16. With much overlap in treatments, and much controversy in the field about whether the newer acceptance- and mindfulness-based theories are truly cognitive, are a new wave of behavioral therapy, or are part of Eastern religious traditions and therefore spiritual, I decided to include them in Chapter 16. A complete reorganization of Chapters 15 and 16 to reduce overlap resulted in moving the history of behavioral therapy to the introductory chapter, and moving the discussion of planning and implementing behavior change to Chapter 16. More information on exposure-based treatments and CBT techniques was also added to Chapter 16, and the Skill Development section was thoroughly revised to include exposure-based treatment for a client with a hoarding problem. Additional enhancements to Chapter 16 include a discussion of mindfulness-based cognitive therapy.
- With the move of mindfulness-based and dialectical behavior therapies to Chapter 16, the decision was made to remove the chapter on emerging approaches. Although reviewers had found the section on transpersonal therapy to be interesting, they were inclined not to teach it in their courses due to the time constraints of a 15-week semester. Therefore, transpersonal approaches are not included in this edition.
- Resources and websites have been updated in every chapter as needed.

Many more changes and additions have been made in all chapters. More than 400 new references, most from the past 2 years, have been added. In many cases, this is new research that has been added to the application section of each chapter. In other cases, new references are the result of the chapter changes listed above.

These changes and additions result in a comprehensive analysis of more than 15 of the leading treatment systems in use today, with shorter discussions of nearly 50 more.

EFFECTIVE WAYS TO USE THIS TEXT

For many years I taught counseling theories, abnormal psychology, and other courses at a local university while also maintaining a private practice. Although very different experiences, I found working with students and working with clients to be equally rewarding both personally and professionally. Both experiences have also contributed broadly to my understanding of what professors want in a counseling theories text, and what students need to be able to put theoretical material into practice. I was always delighted at the end of a semester to hear a student say, "This is one of the psychology textbooks I'm going to keep!"

This text has been designed for flexibility and ease of use. Although each college and university has its own curriculum and required courses, this text can be adapted to almost any curriculum in counseling and psychology and also can be used for training and staff development. Here are a few suggestions for using the text:

1. The text is ideally suited for use in a two-semester or two-quarter course on theories and techniques of counseling and psychotherapy. Such a curriculum would provide students with an in-depth and comprehensive understanding of the fields of counseling and psychotherapy. The first three parts (11 chapters covering introductory material, treatment systems focused on backgrounds, and treatment systems focused on emotions) could be covered in the first semester, with the remaining three parts (focusing on cognitive, behavioral, and eclectic treatment approaches) covered in the second semester. If each class session covers one chapter, then any remaining classes can be used for role-playing and exams.

2. The entire text also could be covered in a one-semester course, particularly courses for doctoral and advanced master's degree students in which depth of knowledge is prized. The following illustrates one way to cover this text in a 15-week semester:

Week 1: Chapters 1 and 2—Contexts of Effective Treatment; Overview of Background-Focused Treatment Systems
Week 2: Chapter 3—Sigmund Freud and Classic Psychoanalysis
Week 3: Chapter 4—Alfred Adler and Individual Psychology
Week 4: Chapters 5 and 6—Post- and Neo-Freudians: Analytical Psychology, Ego Psychology, Object Relations, and Self Psychology; Brief Psychodynamic Therapy
Week 5: Chapters 7 and 8—Overview of Emotion-Focused Treatment Systems; Carl Rogers and Person-Centered Counseling
Week 6: Chapters 9 and 10—Existential Therapy; Gestalt Therapy
Week 7: Chapter 11—Emerging Approaches Emphasizing Emotions and Sensations
Week 8: Chapters 12 and 13—Overview of Thought-Focused Treatment Systems; Albert Ellis and Rational Emotive Behavior Therapy
Week 9: Chapter 14—Aaron Beck and Cognitive Therapy
Week 10: Chapters 15 and 16—Overview of Action-Focused Treatment Systems; Behavior Therapy and Cognitive–Behavioral Therapy
Week 11: Chapter 17—Reality Therapy
Week 12: Chapter 18—Family Systems Approaches
Week 13: Chapters 19—Integrative Therapies
Week 14: Chapter 20—Solidifying Understanding of Treatment Systems
Week 15: Conclusion, final examination

3. Chapters can easily and logically be selected and combined to create a course. For example, the following 15 selected chapters encompass the four types of clinical approaches in the BETA format (background, emotions, thoughts, actions) and constitute a one-semester course on established theories of counseling:

Chapter 1: Contexts of Effective Treatment
Chapter 3: Sigmund Freud and Classic Psychoanalysis
Chapter 4: Alfred Adler and Individual Psychology
Chapter 5: Post- and Neo-Freudians: Analytical Psychology, Ego Psychology, Object Relations, and Self Psychology
Chapter 8: Carl Rogers and Person-Centered Counseling
Chapter 9: Existential Therapy
Chapter 10: Gestalt Therapy
Chapter 11: Emerging Approaches Emphasizing Emotions and Sensations
Chapter 13: Albert Ellis and Rational Emotive Behavior Therapy
Chapter 14: Aaron Beck and Cognitive Therapy
Chapter 16: Behavior Therapy and Cognitive–Behavioral Therapy
Chapter 17: Reality Therapy
Chapter 18: Family Systems Approaches
Chapter 19: Integrative Therapies
Chapter 20: Solidifying Understanding of Treatment Systems

In a 15-week semester, one chapter could be covered per week, providing a comprehensive picture of the major treatment approaches.

4. A variety of short courses or seminars can be created from the contents of this text. For example, Part two could be used for a course on psychodynamic and psychoanalytic approaches to treatment; Part three for a course on process-experiential approaches in counseling and psychotherapy; Parts four and five could be combined for a comprehensive look at cognitive and behavioral treatment systems; and Part six for a course on eclectic and integrated approaches to treatment.

5. The Skill Development sections are designed to accompany the treatment system taught in that particular chapter. However, these sections can be used independently of the theoretical portions, perhaps taught in a subsequent semester following a course on theories of counseling and psychotherapy or used as part of a practicum or internship to facilitate skill development.

6. Like the Skill Development sections, the exercises are intended to accompany review of the treatment system in each chapter. However, they are designed to be used flexibly. Large-group exercises are appropriate for classroom discussion. Small-group exercises allow clusters of four learners to practice and improve their clinical skills with the benefit of peer feedback and support. Individual exercises offer people the opportunity to work alone and apply their learning to themselves, with their responses written in journals.

Faculty members, of course, can choose to use any or all of the exercises that accompany each chapter. Ideally, time should be allocated, either during or outside of class, for at least some of the large- and small-group exercises in each chapter. However, if time is limited, the individual exercises enable students to continue their learning and skill development outside of class. Although instructors may decide to review students' journals at the end of a course to determine whether they have completed the individual exercises, I encourage them not to grade or evaluate these journals so that students feel free to express themselves, try out new skills, and gain learning and self-awareness. Students should be told at the beginning of the course whether they will be required to share their journals in any way.

ACKNOWLEDGMENTS

I am grateful for the generosity of my family and friends who indulge me the isolation required to write these texts. This is my fourth jump down the rabbit hole, and I am always cognizant of the responsibilities others take on while I am single-mindedly absorbed in my work. I owe a special note of gratitude to Sumita Anand Changela, MA, for her research assistance over the summer, and for updating the application of the counseling theories to multicultural groups in many of this book's chapters.

I am indebted to Meredith Fossel, senior acquisitions editor at Pearson. Without her efforts this text would not have been published. Further thanks to her editorial assistant Krista Slavicek, to Don Laurila, production manager, and to Lorretta Palagi, copyeditor, for her astute editorial eye and sharp red pencil.

I would like to acknowledge and thank the reviewers for their helpful comments and suggestions to the fourth edition: Devika Dibya Choudhuri, Eastern Michigan University; LaRae M. Jome, University at Albany; Susan H. Packard, Edinboro University of Pennsylvania; and Timothy S. Vandergast, William Paterson University.

But above all, I would like to express my appreciation to my husband of 25 years, Neil Reichenberg, who shares my passion for words, as well as for our three young grandchildren: Izaak, Jaycee, and Orion.

ABOUT THE AUTHORS

Linda Seligman, PhD

Dr. Linda Seligman received a PhD in counseling psychology from Columbia University. Her primary research interests included diagnosis and treatment planning as well as counseling people with chronic and life-threatening illnesses. Dr. Seligman was a professor at George Mason University for 25 years. She served as co-director of the doctoral program in education, coordinator of the Counseling Development Program, associate chair of the School of Education, and head of the Community Agency Counseling Program. She was later named professor emerita. Dr. Seligman also served as associate at Johns Hopkins University and as a faculty member in counseling psychology at Walden University.

During her lifetime, Dr. Seligman authored 15 texts, including *Selecting Effective Treatment; Diagnosis and Treatment Planning in Counseling; Developmental Career Counseling and Assessment;* and *Promoting a Fighting Spirit: Psychotherapy for Cancer Patients, Survivors, and Their Families*. She also wrote more than 80 professional articles and text chapters. She lectured throughout the United States as well as internationally on diagnosis and treatment planning and was recognized for her expertise on that subject. In 1990, the American Mental Health Counselors Association (AMHCA) designated Dr. Seligman as Researcher of the Year. In 2007, AMHCA honored her with the title of Counselor Educator of the Year.

Lourie W. Reichenberg, MA, LPC

Lourie W. Reichenberg is a licensed professional counselor in private practice in Falls Church, Virginia. She also provides clinical supervision for therapists and interns at The Women's Center in Vienna, Virginia. She earned her master's degree in counseling psychology from Marymount University. She has taught crisis counseling, abnormal psychology, and counseling theories to graduate and undergraduate students.

She is currently on the executive committee of the Virginia Association of Clinical Counselors, and serves on the board of directors for the Northern Virginia Licensed Professional Counselors.

Reichenberg is a member of the CrisisLink LOSS team, which provides assistance in the community after a suicide has occurred. She served on the CrisisLink Board of Directors from 2003 to 2006, and is on the organization's Advisory Council. She is a past editor of the Northern Virginia Licensed Professional Counselors, and was the editor of the *Journal of the College and University Personnel Association* from 1988 to 1993. She coauthored *Selecting Effective Treatments* (2007, 2012) with Dr. Seligman, and has published many professional articles including a chapter on grief and loss in *Crisis Assessment, Intervention and Prevention* (Jackson-Cherry & Erford, 2010, 2013). She has edited more than 30 texts and monographs. Her primary interests include crisis counseling, grief and loss, and helping individuals, couples, and families cope with life transitions. She approaches her work as a therapist, educator, and community volunteer, from a humanistic, person-centered, and emotionally focused perspective, and incorporates mindfulness into her practice.

BRIEF CONTENTS

CONTENTS

CHAPTER 1

Contexts of Effective Treatment

Before we begin to consider specific theories of counseling and psychotherapy, we pave the way by providing some information on the history and development of these approaches. Treatment *is* effective and many factors have a strong relationship to treatment outcome. This chapter focuses on many of those factors, including the following:

- Characteristics of successful clients
- The therapeutic alliance
- The training, skills, and experience of effective clinicians
- Personal and professional characteristics of the clinician
- Culturally competent counseling
- Treatment setting
- Ethical guidelines and standards
- Role induction.

Later in this chapter, the Diaz family—Roberto, Edie, and Ava—are introduced. Then the Skill Development section focuses on a review of effective questioning and interviewing techniques that lead to productive intake assessments. The Exercises section includes activities that reinforce those skills. The use of minimal encouragers and the Exercises section focuses on questioning and interviewing for a productive intake assessment.

DEVELOPMENT OF THEORIES OF COUNSELING AND PSYCHOTHERAPY

Prior to the late 19th century, people had little understanding of emotional difficulties and mental disorders. Many people with severe symptoms were forcibly confined in institutions and exposed to largely ineffective treatments, while those with mild or moderate difficulties typically received no professional help.

The development of psychodynamic approaches to psychotherapy, spearheaded by the work of Sigmund Freud, led to the emergence of what has been called the first force of psychotherapy. Viewing past experiences as the source of people's present emotional difficulties and emphasizing unconscious processes and long-term treatment, psychodynamic approaches provided a solid foundation for the field of psychotherapy, but that approach had clear limitations.

The research and practice of B. F. Skinner as well as more modern theorists such as Albert Ellis, Aaron Beck, William Glasser, and Donald Meichenbaum led to the emergence of the second force: behavioral and cognitive theories and interventions. Behavioral treatment approaches, widely used in the 1970s, have been integrated with cognitive approaches, developed primarily in the 1980s, leading to the cognitive–behavioral approaches that received considerable attention and empirical support in the 1990s. Cognitive and behavioral treatment systems emphasize the influence of thoughts and actions on emotions. They use interventions that generally focus on the present and seek to minimize dysfunctional cognitions and behaviors while replacing them with more helpful and positive thoughts and actions.

Carl Rogers's innovative work emerged in the 1960s and led to the development of the third force, existential-humanistic psychotherapy. The work of Fritz Perls, Viktor Frankl, and others contributed to this force, which emphasizes the importance of emotions and sensations and of people taking charge of and finding meaning in their own lives. These approaches also drew attention to the importance of the therapeutic alliance.

Now, at the beginning of the 21st century, clinicians are entering the era of the fourth force. Elements of first-, second-, and third-force treatment approaches are integrated into a comprehensive and holistic effort to understand people as fully as possible. Clinicians' awareness and understanding of components of individual identity (such as gender, culture, age, race, and sexual orientation) facilitate development of positive therapeutic relationships and effective treatment plans. Becoming culturally competent, being an ally with clients, and being open to their multiple perspectives of themselves and their world are essential to today's clinicians. Networking and collaboration with other mental health professionals, providers of community resources, and important people in clients' lives are now viewed as integral to treatment. Theories of counseling and psychotherapy, as well as their implementation, have changed in response to the fourth force. New approaches such as narrative therapy, dialectics, and therapies that incorporate Eastern thought and philosophy provide powerful ways to understand people's experiences more fully and empower people to take an active role in changing their emotions, perceptions, and behavior.

UNDERSTANDING THEORIES OF COUNSELING AND PSYCHOTHERAPY

Theories of counseling and psychotherapy also have been referred to as treatment systems, treatment models, treatment approaches, theories of change, and other terms. In this text, these terms will be used interchangeably to refer to an integrated set of concepts that provides explanations for and descriptions of the following:

- Stages, patterns, and important factors in people's emotional development
- Healthy emotional development, as well as problematic or abnormal emotional development
- How to help people develop in positive ways and reduce symptoms that are distressing and/or cause impairment in functioning
- The role of the clinician and how that role contributes to treatment
- Strategies for putting the theory into practice (e.g., identifying and modifying cognitive distortions, reflecting feelings, developing a clear plan for behavioral change)
- Specific skills or interventions that can enhance implementation of the treatment approach (e.g., use of earliest recollections, analysis of dreams, diaphragmatic breathing)
- Information on people who are likely to benefit from this treatment approach; this information might include their ages, cultural background, symptoms, mental disorders, treatment settings, and other factors.

An effective theory is "clear, easily understood, and communicable . . . coherent and not contradictory . . . comprehensive, encompassing explanations for a wide variety of phenomena . . . explicit, generating research" (Hansen, Stevic, & Warner, 1986, p. 356). Effective theories are grounded in an understanding of human development. They provide a framework for gathering and organizing information and exploring personality. They present a theory of development and change that helps us understand people and their concerns. They provide steps and interventions that encourage learning and growth and that allow for evaluation of progress and modification of treatment plans if needed. They provide reassurance and direction. They lend themselves to development of testable hypotheses that can be investigated to determine the validity and usefulness of the approach and they promote further study and improvement of the treatment process.

Treatment approaches that have proven their value over time are theoretically "robust . . . reasonably well validated . . . and have clearly defined pragmatic roles in intervention practice" (Stuart, 1998, p. 7). Of course, treatments must be monitored to ensure clients are progressing and goals may be changed to align with changes in a client's circumstances (Lambert, 2010).

Treatment Is Effective

Not only is psychotherapy effective, but it is one of the most effective tools available for working with problems related to mental health. Across most mental disorders, the positive effect of psychotherapy is achieved in the first 10 to 20 sessions (Schnyder, 2009). Studies also indicate that the positive effects of psychotherapy last long after treatment has ended. In a landmark study, Martin Seligman (1995) found that 87% of people who reported feeling "very poor" and 92% of those who said they felt "fairly poor" before therapy showed clear improvement by the end of treatment. In addition, this study found that improvement was long lasting and was reflected in changes in presenting concerns as well as improvement in occupational, social, and personal domains. Long-term treatment was generally superior to short-term treatment, especially when treatment was terminated prematurely due to limitations in insurance coverage. This effectiveness study is so important because it was a naturalistic and realistic study, providing information on how treatment is actually performed. This means that it continued until people were satisfied with their progress or left treatment prematurely because they were not getting the help they wanted, could no longer afford treatment, or encountered other reasons to leave treatment. Treatment methods and schedules were not artificially controlled but, rather, allowed for self-correction to improve treatment, encompassed a wide range of specific and integrated treatment approaches, and often addressed multiple concerns.

Lambert and Cattani-Thompson's (1996) review of the literature focused primarily on structured and planned efficacy studies but drew conclusions similar to those of Seligman. They stated, "Counseling is effective. . . . The effects of counseling seem to be relatively lasting. These effects are attained in relatively brief time periods, with the percentage of clients who show substantial improvement increasing as the number of counseling sessions increases" (p. 601).

More recent publications echo and synthesize these positive findings (Leichsenring, 2009; Levy, Ablon, & Kachele, 2012). Approximately 75% to 80% of clients benefit significantly from counseling or psychotherapy (Lambert & Ogles, 2004). This improvement rate compares favorably to many medical procedures. These positive outcomes tend to endure.

Although differences in outcome among various forms of therapy are not strong, this does not detract from the importance of effectively using treatment approaches and strategies. Rather, treatment outcome depends on many factors including duration of treatment; therapeutic approaches and strategies; the client, the clinician, and their interaction; and social and environmental factors. Clinicians and researchers no longer ask whether psychotherapy is effective; that has been conclusively demonstrated. Nor do they ask which treatment modality works best. The so-called "brand wars" ended in a stalemate around the turn of the century. Now we know that most treatments work, reinforcing what Rosenzweig said in 1936, in what has become known as the Dodo bird verdict. At the end of Lewis Carroll's *Alice in Wonderland*, the Dodo bird announces, "Everybody has won, and all must have prizes." The evidence for the equality of all treatment systems has been increasing with the years (Robinson, Berman, & Neimeyer, 1990; Smith, Glass, & Miller, 1980; Wampold, Minami, Baskin, & Callen Tierney, 2002).

So, if all treatments are effective, the questions become more challenging and complex: What are the important ingredients of a successful therapeutic relationship? When is psychotherapy most likely to be effective? What are the characteristics of successful clinicians? What client traits, attitudes, and behaviors enhance treatment? How can these characteristics be fostered? What treatment models and strategies are most effective for specific problems? Which theories can be integrated to produce even greater effectiveness? What are some of the common factors that are inherent in all treatment modalities? These are only a few of the important questions that today's clinicians are asking that will be addressed in this text.

Common Factors

Although more than 400 forms of counseling and psychotherapy have been identified and described (Stricker & Gold, 2006), common factors, or a common set of variables, are at play in the different forms of therapy that make them all effective. Common factors implicit in most therapies include:

- A therapeutic relationship characterized by collaboration, trust, mutual investment in the therapeutic process, shared respect, genuineness, positive emotional feelings, and a holistic understanding of clients and their backgrounds and environments
- A safe, supportive, and healing context
- Goals and a sense of direction, preferably explicit but sometimes implicit
- A shared understanding between clinicians and clients about the nature of the problems and concerns to be addressed in treatment and the change processes that will be used to resolve them
- A credible treatment approach to address the client's symptoms
- Therapeutic learning, typically including feedback and corrective experiences
- The encouragement of clients' self-efficacy and problem-solving skills
- Improvement in clients' ability to identify, express constructively, and modify their emotions
- Improvement in clients' ability to identify, assess the validity of, and modify their thoughts
- Improvement in clients' ability to assess and change dysfunctional behaviors as well as acquire new and more effective behaviors that promote coping, impulse control, sound relationships, and good emotional and physical health.

Successful treatment is reflected in attitudinal shifts. People who expect to get better are more likely to get better. Therapists who instill hope and optimism, as well as feelings of mastery and self-efficacy, are more likely to promote treatment success (Anderson, Lunnen, & Ogles, 2010; Duncan, 2010; Seligman & Reichenberg, 2012). Clients are more likely to stay in therapy, and therefore benefit from the therapy, if attention is paid by the therapist to the creation and maintenance of a collaborative therapeutic relationship (Anderson, Ogles, Patterson, Lambert, & Vermeersch, 2009). More will be said about these important conditions later in this chapter.

Understanding Mental Health

Just as it is important for clinicians to be aware of the breadth of factors in positive change as a backdrop to studying systems and strategies of treatment, so is it useful for them to have a concept of mental health. Witmer and Sweeney (1992) advanced a holistic model for optimal health and functioning that delineates five important aspects of people's lives:

- ***Spirituality***—values, beliefs, ethics, purpose and direction, optimism, inner peace
- ***Self-regulation***—sense of worth, mastery of one's own life, spontaneity and emotional responsiveness, sense of humor, creativity, awareness of reality, physical health
- ***Work***—paid employment, volunteer experiences, child rearing, homemaking, and education that provide psychological, social, and other rewards
- ***Friendship***—positive interpersonal relationships and social supports that provide rewarding activities and interactions
- ***Love***—intimate, trusting, sharing, and cooperative long-term relationships

These five areas serve as a map of healthy functioning. More important, for purposes of this text, they delineate areas for assessment. Deficits in any of these five areas are likely to impair functioning, cause distress, require help, and be an appropriate focus for treatment. Knowledge of treatment systems, strategies, and skills enable clinicians to help their clients make changes that will move them toward healthy functioning.

Varieties of Theories of Counseling and Psychotherapy

This text reviews those systems of counseling and psychotherapy that should be part of the repertoire of today's clinicians. Whether clinicians describe themselves as integrative or eclectic (incorporating a variety of themes and techniques into their work), or affiliate with a particular theoretical model, the various treatment approaches all shed light on people's challenges and change processes and provide skills that promote emotional health. Clinicians no longer seek the one right theory but, rather, the concepts and skills they need to form a sound therapeutic alliance with clients and develop individualized treatment plans that are likely to ameliorate difficulties and improve growth and development.

But systems and strategies of counseling and psychotherapy are only part of the treatment process. Current research suggests that treatment approaches and interventions are just one factor in producing change. In a landmark study, Miller, Duncan, and Hubble (1997) found that clients attributed 40% of the change they experienced in treatment to *extratherapeutic factors* (including people's internal resources and events in their lives), 30% to the *therapist–client relationship,* 15% to particular *techniques and interventions,* and 15% percent to their *hope and expectation of positive change.*

Several important points emerge from this finding. First, clinicians may not be as powerful as they might think; clients' experiences and inner resources seem to be the most powerful factor in change. Consequently, clinicians must take the time to know and understand their clients, to grasp their perspectives on the world, to hear their stories, and to learn about their lives so that the clinicians can help them to make the most of those extratherapeutic factors. Second, the therapeutic alliance is of great importance. Promoting a positive relationship characterized by conditions and interactions that encourage desired changes can make a significant difference in the success of the treatment process. Observing that interventions represent only 15% of the factors contributing to change, readers may be tempted to ask, "Why, then, pay so much attention to learning treatment systems and strategies?" In reality, 60% or more of client change can be attributed to treatment approaches. In addition to the direct influence of the approach (15%), the skills and strategies of the clinician are largely responsible for the development of the therapeutic alliance (30% of the source of change) and for engendering hope and positive expectations in clients (15% of the source of change). Furthermore, counseling and psychotherapy can also make a difference in people's ability to make positive use of extratherapeutic factors such as support systems, community resources, and educational programs. Thus, treatment systems and strategies are important not only for their direct impact on symptoms and problems but also for their indirect impact on the treatment alliance as well as on client attitudes and behaviors associated with successful treatment.

CHARACTERISTICS OF SUCCESSFUL CLIENTS

"It is clients who make therapy work" (Bohart & Tallman, 2010, p. 94). Both the personal qualities and the backgrounds of clients help determine the success of their treatment. Clinicians can maximize the positive influence of these factors in three ways:

- First, they need to be aware of those client characteristics that are likely to correlate with therapeutic outcome. By understanding each client's strengths, resources, and capacity for self-agency, successful therapists work to promote a strengths-based perspective from the very beginning of the first session (Gassman & Grawe, 2006). Clients who perceive they are functioning well are more likely to transcend diagnoses or descriptions of pathology and less likely to end treatment prematurely (Duncan, Miller, Wampold, & Hubble, 2010).
- Second, therapists need to believe that clients are motivated and capable of change and use that belief to instill hope and optimism during the treatment process.

- Third, therapists should promote client involvement by providing an atmosphere in which clients feel safe discussing difficult feelings and trying out new ideas. By creating environments in which true collaboration takes place, clinicians can instill or develop in clients those qualities that are typically associated with a positive therapeutic outcome—feelings of shared warmth, affection, affirmation, and respect. Clients who identify with their clinicians also are more likely to have positive outcomes. The interaction of client and clinician makes a difference in clients' feelings of mutuality and their ability to identify with their clinician.

Role of the Client

Both pretreatment characteristics and those qualities that clients manifest in treatment have a strong impact on outcome. The following within-session client behaviors and attitudes play an important part in the treatment process.

MOTIVATION The term *motivation* is a broad one that clinicians use to describe a range of client behaviors associated with readiness for treatment and ability to engage productively in that process. Particularly important aspects of client motivation include engagement in and cooperation with treatment and a willingness to self-disclose, confront problems, put forth effort to change, and, if necessary, experience some temporary anxiety and discomfort in the hope of eventual benefit. Other signs of strong client motivation include low levels of defensiveness and a belief that treatment is necessary and important. Not surprisingly, self-referred clients are less likely to terminate treatment prematurely than are clients referred by others.

Motivational interviewing can have a profoundly positive impact on a client's readiness for treatment. Techniques developed by Miller and Rollnick (2002) help clients, particularly those with substance use disorders, eating disorders, and other behavior problems, prepare for, and make the most of, treatment.

POSITIVE BUT REALISTIC EXPECTATIONS FOR TREATMENT *Hope* or *optimism* is another essential element of treatment. Therapy and counseling are hard work for both clients and clinicians. For people to persist in that process and tolerate the increased anxiety it often causes, as well as the commitment of time and resources, they must believe that treatment has something positive to offer them and that, at the end of that process, they will be better off than they were before treatment.

People who have a clear and accurate understanding of psychotherapy and its strengths and limitations are more likely to have successful treatment outcomes. Pretreatment preparation of clients via role induction (discussed later in this chapter) can make a considerable difference in people's expectations for treatment and correspondingly in their commitment to treatment, willingness to self-disclose, and alliance with the clinician (Acosta, Yamamoto, Evans, & Skilbeck, 1983; Lawe, Horne, & Taylor, 1983). Similarly, effective engagement of the client in the very first session has been shown to make a positive contribution to successful treatment (Odell & Quinn, 1998).

FULL PARTICIPATION IN TREATMENT Clients who succeed in treatment freely present their concerns, collaborate with the clinician in a mutual endeavor, and take steps to improve their lives. They develop a problem-solving attitude and maintain positive expectations of change (Sexton & Whiston, 1991). They recognize that at least some of their difficulties come from within themselves and believe they have the power to improve their situation. They view the need for personal change as significant and can identify a specific problem (Lambert & Cattani-Thompson, 1996). According to Asay and Lambert (1999), "Clients who do better in psychotherapy and maintain treatment gains believe that the changes made in therapy were primarily a result of their own efforts" (p. 32). These people probably feel empowered as a result of their treatment successes and are optimistic that they can continue to make positive changes and choices, even after treatment has ended.

OTHER CHARACTERISTICS Some research has found a positive correlation among client intelligence, education, socioeconomic level, and initial symptoms of depression or anxiety with the likelihood of a positive outcome. Client gender and age seem unrelated to outcome.

Client and Clinician Diversity

We live in an increasingly diverse society. In 2012, more babies were born to minorities than were born to White parents (Tavernese, 2012). Minorities accounted for 92% of the total U.S. population growth in the decade from 2000 to 2010, calling into question the relevance of the term *minority*. Speaking about diversity and the complexity of human identity and experience, Laura Brown (2008) noted: "We are all diverse here" (p. 23). By the year 2050, fewer than half of the U.S. population will be of White European descent (Sue & Sue, 2008).

Clinicians need to be aware of how their clients' worldview (gender, age, and cultural ethnic, socioeconomic, religious, and family background) has shaped their experience of personal problems and their views of counseling as a way to address those problems. Counselors must also be culturally competent and able to respond appropriately to people whose cultural backgrounds differ from their own. To help people understand themselves and others in all of their "social locations" that are constructed in the context of social, interpersonal, and relational realities, Pamela Hays (2001, 2008) developed an easy to remember acronym, ADDRESSING:

A = age
D = disability (acquired)
D = disability (developmental)
R = religion and spirituality
E = ethnicity
S = socioeconomic status
S = sexual orientation
I = indigenous heritage
N = national origin
G = gender/sex.

Hays noted that the ADDRESSING acronym is a foundation on which to build, and not an all-inclusive model. Because of the richness of the model, every person, client and clinician alike, will have experience in a wide range of "locations" or what Brown (2008) refers to as "components of identification" (p. 24). Some may have experienced or expressed bias, while others may have internalized bias into their identities (Brown, 2008). Clearly, therapists have much to consider with the meeting of each new client.

Hays (2009) believes that knowing the history of a person's culture is as important as understanding the backgrounds of people in therapy. It is not just the cultural background that is important, but also the level of acculturation or identity development with which the client currently identifies.

The American Psychological Association (APA) *Guidelines on Multicultural Education, Training, Research, Practice and Organizational Change for Psychologists* (APA, 2003) provides definitions as well as practical strategies for addressing multiculturalism. The guidelines recommend that psychologists "strive to apply culturally-appropriate skills in clinical and other applied psychological practices" (APA, 2003, p. 377). Culturally competent practice involves the application of psychological skills that integrate a focus on the client based on his or her cultural context. For example, when working with a 67-year-old Hispanic woman who lives with her daughter and was recently diagnosed with Stage 4 ovarian cancer, a clinician making a culturally competent assessment would consider a number of factors including racism, fluency in English, changes in social status, spiritual or religious tradition, mobility, acculturation, generational history, family support, and community resources as they relate to the presenting problem.

Diversity comes in many forms, and guidelines that provide a frame of reference for working with lesbian, gay, bisexual, and transgendered (LGBT) clients are also available (APA, 2012). Clinicians must do more than just develop skills to assess and treat LGBT clients; they must also be cognizant of their own attitudes and values related to LGBT clients and their relationships.

Treatment can be more effective when culture is factored in (Schnyder, 2009). Rather than taking the perspective that some implied "norm" exists and that some people differ from that norm, it is more helpful for clinicians to recognize their own multiple social locations and consider them in relationship with their clients' multiple social locations. Even people who are similar in age, gender, and cultural background can have very dissimilar worldviews and may respond best to very different treatment approaches. Clinicians are reminded that we are all unique, and that no one individual can speak for an entire age group, gender, race, religion, or culture.

According to Schnyder (2009), culture is a "set of beliefs, attitudes, and value systems that derive from early stages of life through enculturation, and become an internal mode of regulating behavior, action, and emotion" (p. S127). Culture, then, is specific to the individual, and to be truly culturally competent, psychotherapy must take into account any culturally relevant components that impact the client's life. This includes not only those components that relate to the presenting problem, but also taking a culturally relevant history; learning how culture affects the client's meaning-making abilities, attitudes toward seeking help, and expectations about treatment; and then tailoring therapy to the client's individual needs. Culture is a dynamic concept that changes across generations as a result of the changing environment.

Asian Americans, for example, are a widely diverse group, counting as many as 30 different cultural backgrounds in their ranks. They are highly educated: 44% of Asian Americans have at least a bachelor's degree, compared with 24% of the total U.S. population. They embrace many different religions, including Christianity, Islam, Buddhism, Taoism, and Confucianism. Many are first-generation Americans, some are recent arrivals to this country, and still others come from families who have lived in the U.S. for generations. Like other groups, Asian Americans are very diverse.

It is not enough for therapists to understand their Asian clients' social locations, they must also understand Asian cultural values of emotional self-control, collectivism, conformity, achievement, humility, and respect for elders (Hall & Okazaki, 2002). In Asian culture, social roles are important, as are academic and career success and putting the family's needs above the individual. Enculturation, or adherence to one's culture of origin, is also important. Some elements of culture, such as food preferences or native language, may diminish over time or over generations, but values may remain (e.g., filial piety, emotional self-control).

Culture as it relates to counseling has been the subject of much recent research, especially in the areas of cultural competence and ethnic and racial socialization processes (Hall, 2010; Hughes et al., 2006). Cultural identity and level of acculturation are important in developing an effective therapeutic alliance. Sue and Sue (2008) identify three aspects of cultural competence:

1. Being aware, on the part of therapists, of their own cultural values and biases
2. Understanding the worldview of culturally diverse clients
3. Developing culturally appropriate interventions.

AWARENESS Therapists must not only be culturally aware, they must also look at their own biases, experiences, and lack of expertise. Culturally sensitive therapists:

- Value and respect differences
- Are aware of their own cultural heritage
- Feel comfortable with the differences among people
- Become aware of circumstances that may require referral to another therapist
- Acknowledge their own gender, racial, ethnic, or sexual biases.

UNDERSTANDING CLIENTS' WORLDVIEWS Therapists must be open to the worldview or social location of others. This does not mean that therapists must adopt their clients' worldviews but, rather, that the therapist is nonjudgmental, open, and willing to learn. Allowing clients to tell their stories without fear of being judged or challenged is encouraging to clients. To do this, therapists must have knowledge beyond their own cultures, be aware of culture-bound syndromes, and understand the concept of cultural relativism (Sue & Sue, 2008).

USING CULTURALLY APPROPRIATE INTERVENTIONS No one style of therapy or type of intervention is appropriate for all populations. To be most effective, therapy must be respectful of the person's "values, religious beliefs, worldviews, goals, and preferences" (APA Presidential Task Force on Evidence-Based Practice, 2006, p. 278). Family support and attitudes that strengthen interdependence are associated with decreased levels of psychological problems. Family support may even be protective against the development of schizophrenia. Family support may be less important or even viewed as negative in American culture in which autonomy is valued (Hall, 2010).

When shaping interventions, it is important for therapists to consider their clients' historical, cultural, and environmental experiences. Sue and Sue (2008) recommend counselors take a holistic approach, learn a variety of theories and techniques, and examine the traditional helping skills of various cultures. Counselors should also be aware that it might not be enough to offer interventions on the individual level; it may become necessary for a therapist to take action to effect systemic change at the organizational or institutional level, if programs, policies, and practices used by the organizations are oppressive to their clients.

THE THERAPEUTIC ALLIANCE

Fifty years of research indicates, with increasing clarity, that the strength of the therapeutic alliance is one of the most powerful predictors of client outcome regardless of the therapist's theoretical orientation (Norcross, 2010). Therefore, it is imperative that clinicians acquire a sound understanding of the elements of a positive therapeutic alliance, develop the skills and strategies they need to create successful working relationships with their clients, and be able to adapt their treatment style to individual clients to help them participate in and appreciate the value of the therapeutic alliance. They must also learn to attend to the alliance, to monitor the relationship, and to mend any ruptures as they occur.

Carl Rogers's person-centered counseling, discussed in greater detail in Part 3 of this book, emphasizes the importance of essential therapist characteristics that he believed would promote client self-esteem and self-efficacy. Rogers referred to these traits—empathy, unconditional positive regard, and congruence (or being genuine with a client)—as the necessary conditions in which change could occur.

It seems intuitive. A therapist should be competent, caring, warm, and trustworthy and have a good number of interpersonal skills. Five decades of empirical research continue to point to "the relationship" as the most important ingredient of change. As every human knows intuitively in his or her bones, it is "the nurture and comfort of the other human" (Norcross, 2010, p. 113) that makes therapy work. Although other variables are also at play, including specific interventions, the presence of the following essential conditions of the therapeutic relationship make it likely that those interventions will succeed.

EMPATHY Empathy is the clinician's ability to see the world through the client's eyes and to communicate that understanding so that the client feels heard and validated. A therapist's empathy helps clients feel that their therapists can relate to their experiences and are with them emotionally. Therapist empathy is strongly associated with positive change in clients and may be an even better predictor of treatment outcome than are treatment interventions. Indeed, empathy accounts for 9% of the variance in treatment outcomes (Elliott, Bohart, Watson, & Greenberg, 2011).

UNCONDITIONAL POSITIVE REGARD Unconditional positive regard is transmitted through emotional warmth, appropriate reassurance, the communication of confidence and interest in the client, and the use of therapeutic interventions that empower the client. It gives clients the message that they matter. Clinicians are nonjudgmental and "privilege the client's experience" (Norcross, 2010, p. 117) by recognizing that the client's experience always trumps the therapist's expertise. Clinicians who are warm and caring have a higher likelihood of a positive outcome than do those who are aggressive and confrontational (Lambert & Cattani-Thompson, 1996).

CONGRUENCE Being genuine with a client, or congruence, also contributes to the establishment of a positive therapeutic relationship. Clinicians who are genuine with clients give them clear, accurate, unambiguous, and honest, yet sensitive, messages. The clinician does not merely verbalize concern while counting the minutes until lunch. If clinicians believe clients are making harmful or self-destructive choices, they provide feedback and clarification and show clients possible ways to change, but they never coerce, attack, or humiliate clients.

As with other essential conditions of treatment, clinicians must be careful that they do not move beyond encouraging positive change into an authoritarian role in which they tell clients how they should be and make value judgments about the clients' thoughts, feelings, and actions. Occasionally, clients present a danger to themselves or others, and clinicians must intervene forcefully to prevent suicide or physical injury. However, under most circumstances, clinicians must honor their clients' right to decide what is best for them.

The essential conditions of psychotherapy are intertwined and build on each other. Consequently, empathy, unconditional positive regard, and congruence all facilitate the development of hope in clients as do support, encouragement, and affirmation (Odell & Quinn, 1998). In addition, the clinician's communication of direction and optimism, emphasis on the client's strengths, ability to address problematic client behaviors and attitudes, and building of a collaborative client–clinician relationship all can build the client's positive expectation of change (Miller, Hubble, Duncan, & Wampold, 2010).

Having a shared vision of the treatment process and its goals is another important element in the therapeutic alliance (Hill, 2009). If client and clinician view themselves as engaged in an important shared endeavor that is likely to be successful, have clear and mutually established goals in mind, and agree on the tasks and procedures that will be used to achieve those goals, their collaboration is likely to be smooth and efficient.

The treatment approaches discussed throughout this book provide clinicians with many skills and strategies that they can use to develop and enhance the all-important client–clinician relationship and thereby maximize the likelihood of a successful treatment outcome. Although the client–clinician relationship evolves over time and can improve throughout the treatment process,

Walborn (1996) concluded that a positive therapeutic alliance must develop by the fifth session if treatment is to be successful.

Guidelines for Building and Maintaining a Positive Therapeutic Alliance

Objective measures of the therapeutic alliance usually indicate that clinicians' and clients' perceptions of that relationship are congruent. However, this is not always the case. When clients' and clinicians' views of the therapeutic alliance differ, research suggests that clients' perceptions of the nature and quality of the therapeutic alliance make the difference in treatment effectiveness. Consequently, clinicians need to meet their own standards for a successful therapeutic alliance while also ensuring that clients have a positive view of that interaction. Clinicians should be attuned to their clients' verbal and nonverbal messages, ask them for feedback and reactions to their treatment, and address any barriers to the establishment of a positive alliance.

Division 29 of the American Psychological Association conducted meta-analytic reviews on the elements involved in effective therapeutic relationships. Norcross (2011) expanded on those findings. We have already discussed the major elements of empathy, unconditional positive regard, and congruence. Following are some additional procedures and interventions that can promote the development of a positive therapeutic alliance:

- Facilitate the client's efforts to begin treatment by establishing a collaborative relationship. Be sure that clinician and client have a shared understanding of goals and the process of treatment.
- Support the client's decision to seek treatment by discussing the importance of taking a first step and the courage that is involved in seeking help.
- Discuss the client's expectations for treatment, and encourage realistic hope for positive change. This can be accomplished by acknowledging the person's difficulties and discussing ways in which treatment usually can help with such concerns.
- Because clients who rate the alliance positively are more likely to stay in treatment and to achieve positive gains, any strains or ruptures that occur in the therapeutic relationship must be addressed and repaired. However, some recent research indicates that therapists are unlikely to know when their clients are unhappy with treatment or when a rupture has occurred. Therapists are encouraged, therefore, to monitor the relationship, to solicit clients' opinions on how treatment is going for them, and to discuss strains in the relationship before they become permanent tears (Safran, Muran, & Eubanks-Carter, 2011).
- Provide appropriate feedback about the client's behavior or the effect of that behavior. Feedback should be positive, or presented in a positive manner. Therapists can prepare the client to receive feedback, and should proceed carefully with clients who are depressed or who may process the feedback in a negative way.
- Self-disclosure or sharing a small piece of information about yourself, especially if it establishes a commonality between you and the client, can convey genuineness. Examples would be a brief mention of a visit you once made to the client's hometown or of the fact that you, too, had experienced the death of a sibling. Be careful, however, not to focus too much on yourself or share very personal material.
- Engage the client actively in the therapeutic process and begin to engender both a sense of empowerment in the client and confidence in the treatment. This can be accomplished by suggesting small, manageable, helpful steps or activities that the person can do between sessions.
- The therapist's own feelings toward the client must be managed if treatment is to be effective (Hayes, Gelso, & Hummel, 2011). Therapists can address and manage their own

countertransference reactions by using empathy, self-insight, managing their own anxiety, self-integration, and using their conceptualizing ability (Norcross, 2011). Those who need additional help should address the issue in supervision or seek their own therapy.

If a good alliance is formed between the therapist and the client, the client will experience the relationship as therapeutic regardless of which treatment approach is used. It goes without saying, that the therapist's degree of cultural competency is a necessary prerequisite to establishing a positive therapeutic alliance.

CLINICIAN SKILLS, TRAINING, AND EXPERIENCE

Skills, training, and experience make a difference in clinician effectiveness. Generally, "clinical expertise is used to integrate the best research evidence with clinical data in the context of the patient's characteristics and preferences to deliver services that have a high probability of achieving the goals of treatment" (APA Presidential Task Force on Evidence-Based Practice, 2006, p. 284). "The most effective clinicians are those who are able to improvise and switch strategies flexibly in the immediate clinical moment" (Douglas, 2008, p. 451). Inherent in this expertise is the clinician's ability to recognize the limits of his or her skills and knowledge and the ability to recognize biases that can impact clinical judgment.

Recent research has been moving toward a consensus on necessary skills and experiences. A review of the literature suggests that clinician training should include the following areas of preparation and competence (Norcross, 2010; Seligman, 2004)[1]:

- ***Appropriate Interpersonal Skills***—As already mentioned, successful therapists need to possess appropriate interpersonal skills and be "able to communicate a caring, respectful attitude that affirms a client's basic sense of worth" (Norcross, 2010, p. 123). Therapists must respond appropriately to challenging clients, such as those who express anger or those who are suicidal. They need to be able to separate their own feelings from those of the client, and must be skilled at developing and maintaining a collaborative relationship with the client (Anderson et al., 2009; Zuroff, Kelly, Leybman, Blatt, & Wampold, 2010).
- ***Professional Orientation, Identity, and Ethics***—Includes knowledge of the history of our profession, roles and functions of mental health professionals, relevant professional organizations and credentials, ethical and legal guidelines, and the use of technology to enhance one's professional roles.
- ***Social and Cultural Foundations of the Profession***—Includes cultural sensitivity, appreciation, knowledge, and competence; understanding of social problems and their causes and remedies; and skills in outreach, prevention, social change, advocacy, coalition building, and community organization and intervention.
- ***Human Growth and Development***—Includes knowledge of theories of individual development, family development, personality development, cognitive development, and sexual development; ability to distinguish between healthy and unhealthy growth and development; and ability to provide information on and facilitate healthy development.
- ***Lifestyle and Career Development***—Includes understanding of the economic and occupational arenas and their meaning to society, individuals, and families; knowledge of career development; and skill in using counseling, information, inventories, technology, and other resources to promote rewarding and healthy career development and decisions.

[1]Adapted from Seligman, L. (2004). *Diagnosis and treatment planning in counseling* (3rd ed.). New York: Plenum. Used by permission.

- ***Theories of Counseling and Psychotherapy***—Includes the ability to establish a positive therapeutic alliance; knowledge of a broad range of well-accepted treatment approaches and their use and implementation; ability to conduct effective interviews, formulate appropriate treatment goals, develop sound treatment plans, and help clients in crisis; and consultation skills.
- ***Group Counseling and Psychotherapy***—Includes understanding of group development and dynamics, the various types of groups, and leader and member roles and functions; understanding of dynamics of group cohesion; knowledge of effective approaches to group treatment; and awareness of the benefits, drawbacks, and appropriate use of these approaches.
- ***Assessment and Appraisal***—Includes knowledge of a broad range of assessment tools (e.g., inventories to assess personality, ability, career development) as well as their appropriate use; skills in presenting, planning, and integrating assessment into the treatment process; ability to conduct intake interviews, mental status examinations, and observations; understanding of statistical concepts relevant to assessment and of ways to demonstrate cultural competence in assessment; and awareness of when and how to make referrals for assessment.
- ***Research and Program Evaluation***—Includes knowledge of the importance of research and of statistical, technological, and other procedures essential to conducting sound research; skills in planning and conducting research; and understanding of relevant research studies and how to use them to enhance professional effectiveness.
- ***Diagnosis and Psychopathology***—Includes knowledge of the hallmarks of healthy and pathological personality and functioning; familiarity with the current edition of the *Diagnostic and Statistical Manual of Mental Disorders*; ability to formulate a case conceptualization and make an accurate multiaxial assessment; awareness of ways to assess and address dangerousness and risk in clients; and awareness of when clients should be referred for psychiatric, neurological, or other evaluations.

A study by Sexton (1995) indicated that, when clinicians rated the importance of their skills, two of the most important were knowledge of theories of counseling and psychotherapy and an understanding of intervention strategies used in individual treatment. These two competencies reflect the primary focus of this book. The skill rated as most important, understanding abnormal behavior, also has considerable relevance to using systems and strategies of counseling and psychotherapy successfully and will be discussed in Part 7 of this book.

The broad and extensive array of skills and competencies described in this chapter may seem daunting. However, novice clinicians already possess some of these abilities when they begin their training. Most of these skills are taught in graduate school, whereas others are developed when clinicians embark on their internships and postgraduate employment. In addition, these competencies develop and improve with experience.

PERSONAL AND PROFESSIONAL CHARACTERISTICS OF THE EFFECTIVE CLINICIAN

In a review of multiple treatment studies, Anderson and colleagues (2009) found that the facilitative interpersonal skills of the therapist account for much of the variability in treatment outcomes. In fact, they found that "many psychotherapies, as routinely practiced, are evidence-based when delivered by therapists who can offer high levels of interpersonal skills on a performance-based measure" (p. 767). As we have discussed, establishing a collaborative, client-centered relationship and the ability to address and repair any ruptures that occur in that relationship are the essential facilitative skills for a clinician. Anderson et al. and others recommend that counselor training programs and supervision emphasize the development of facilitative interpersonal skills for future therapists.

The literature also suggests personal and professional qualities in clinicians that contribute to treatment effectiveness. Many are the same qualities that most of us value in friends and colleagues. The profile of the effective clinician is, in many respects, comparable to a profile of an emotionally healthy person (Ackerman & Hilsenroth, 2003). Effective clinicians typically are:

- Characterized by strong interpersonal skills, including patience, warmth, caring, a sense of humor, and friendliness
- Genuine, sincere, and authentic; able to make appropriate self-disclosures, provide useful feedback, and acknowledge their mistakes and limitations
- Emotionally stable, mature, and responsible
- Well adjusted and fulfilled, self-aware, with positive and realistic self-esteem, good relationships, a sense of direction, and a rewarding lifestyle
- Able to acknowledge their mistakes and limitations
- Capable of high levels of thinking and conceptualizing
- In possession of good insight into themselves and others
- Aware of, sensitive to, and respectful of cultural characteristics and differences
- Engaged in and appreciative of the value of personal and professional growth and learning
- Ethical, objective, and fair
- Flexible and open to change and new experiences, willing to take reasonable risks
- Affirming and encouraging of others
- Clear and effective in both oral and written communications.

Barbanell (2006) suggested that many people become psychotherapists because they have a "propensity towards selflessness" (p. 11). At the same time, effective clinicians are likely to manifest emotional health and well-being as well as the ability to put their own needs aside at least temporarily so they can understand, support, and help others. Apparently, having personal difficulties in the past does not prohibit people from later becoming emotionally healthy and effective clinicians. In fact, the process of honestly looking at and bravely tackling their own issues and concerns may help people develop the positive traits often found in successful clinicians. Not surprisingly, the majority of mental health professionals (more than 75%) have participated in their own psychotherapy (Geller, Norcross, & Orlinksy, 2005).

Research has not clearly demonstrated that a particular age, gender, professional orientation, or background is associated with successful treatment outcomes. However, clients often express strong preferences for clinicians in a certain age group, of one gender or the other, or with a particular cultural or religious affiliation. For example, most women prefer a female therapist (Wintersteen, Mensinger, & Diamond, 2005). When clients have the type of clinician they prefer, they may have more confidence that treatment will help them, which may enhance the therapeutic alliance. Yet the research has not found improved outcomes or effectiveness when clients and clinicians are matched by gender (Cottone, Drucker, & Javier, 2003). More research is needed in the area of client–clinician matching.

THE IMPACT OF SETTING ON THE TREATMENT PROCESS

The setting in which treatment occurs is another important area that influences counseling and psychotherapy. Treatment programs typically limit the range of clients and problems they address. In addition, they may set guidelines for the number and frequency of sessions and even determine the treatment approach used. Counseling in a high school, for example, will differ greatly from psychotherapy in a private practice specializing in treating trauma survivors or in an inpatient program treating people with severe depression and psychotic symptoms.

Treatment settings also have a strong impact on client expectations. The person seeking help from a career counseling center will almost always have different expectations and concerns than a person contacting a community mental health center.

Clinicians must be aware of the guidelines and requirements of the setting in which they practice and also be knowledgeable about the typical clients seen for treatment in that setting. Of course, the clinician's primary goal is to provide people with the help they need. However, sometimes a referral is indicated to a treatment program that is more appropriate for a client's needs.

ETHICAL GUIDELINES AND STANDARDS

Each professional association for clinicians, including the American Psychological Association (APA, 2002) and the American Counseling Association (ACA, 2005), has its own set of ethical guidelines and standards. Familiarizing oneself with and abiding by those ethical standards is essential to sound clinical practice for many reasons, including the following (Seligman, 2004):

- Ethical standards give strength and credibility to the mental health professions.
- Ethical guidelines help clinicians make sound decisions.
- Providing clients with information on when clinicians can and cannot maintain confidentiality, as well as on other important ethical guidelines, affords clients safety and predictability and enables them to make informed choices about their treatment.
- Practicing in accord with established ethical standards can protect clinicians in the event of malpractice suits or other challenges to their competence.
- Demonstrated knowledge of relevant ethical and legal standards is required for licensure and certification as a counselor, psychologist, or social worker.

Clinicians are responsible not only for acting in ethical ways themselves but also for helping their colleagues to become aware of and adhere to these standards. Clinicians who believe a colleague is acting unethically should first discuss this matter with the colleague and provide any needed information. If clinicians believe that the colleague is still acting unethically, clinicians should consider reporting this matter to the appropriate licensing board and professional association.

Although a detailed discussion of the ethical standards for each of the mental health professions is beyond the scope of this book, an overview of these standards is presented here because of their importance and relevance to clinicians practicing counseling and psychotherapy. The ethical standards of the various mental health professions have far more similarities than differences. Underlying these guidelines are the following general ethical and moral principles (Corey, Corey, & Callanan, 2011; Herlihy & Corey, 2006):

- ***Autonomy***—Clinicians help people develop the skills and strengths they need to make wise choices for themselves. Inherent in this guideline is the mandate that clinicians understand, respect, and appreciate diversity.
- ***Nonmaleficence (Do No Harm) and Beneficence***—Clinicians should always keep in mind the importance of actively promoting the well-being of their clients and acting in the best interests of their clients.
- ***Justice***—Fairness is an essential ingredient of clinicians' professional relationships and interactions, whether they are with clients, colleagues, students, or others.
- ***Fidelity***—Clinicians "maintain their commitments to their profession and to their clients. They are reliable and responsible, nurture and sustain trust in their relationships, value and protect the therapeutic alliance, and are truthful and congruent in their communications" (Seligman, 2004, p. 356).

In addition to these general principles, the following ethical guidelines, with headings adapted from the ACA Code of Ethics (2005, p. 3), are among the most important:

- ***The Counseling Relationship***—As stated previously, clinicians always act in the best interests of their clients. They competently develop treatment plans and use approaches and interventions that are likely to be helpful. If they believe their services are no longer beneficial to a client, they refer that person to more appropriate sources of help. They avoid potentially harmful dual relationships (e.g., client and student, client and family member) and do not engage in sexual intimacies with current or former clients, following the guidelines of the clinicians' professional associations. They provide clients with written information about their services and charge fees that reflect common practice in their area. Respect for and appreciation of diversity and of people's rights and dignity is reflected in all their professional interactions.
- ***Confidentiality***—Clinicians inform clients about the clinicians' obligation to maintain confidentiality, as well as about exceptions to that guideline. Under most circumstances, they maintain their clients' confidentiality and take steps to ensure that their employees also follow this ethical guideline. When working with minors; people who present a danger to themselves or another person; or those who engage in abuse of children, elderly people, or people with disabilities, clinicians may need to break confidentiality but always do so with thought and care. Court orders and clients' requests also may require clinicians to disclose otherwise confidential information.
- ***Professional Responsibility***—Clinicians practice only within their areas of competence. They engage in professional development in order to maintain and improve their skills and are active in their professional associations. They have sound relationships with other professionals, make good use of consultation and collaboration, present themselves and their credentials accurately, and never exploit clients or employees.
- ***Evaluation, Assessment, and Interpretation***—Clinicians make knowledgeable, professional, and helpful use of diagnosis and assessment. They use strategies and tools that are within their range of competence and are appropriate for the client's needs. The selection, administration, scoring, and interpretation of inventories are established procedures that should be followed to reflect cultural competence.
- ***Teaching, Training, and Supervision***—Educators and supervisors maintain standards—similar to those of clinicians. They have clear policies and ensure that their students and supervisees are informed of those policies and procedures. Educators and supervisors provide clear and useful feedback on their performance, offer referrals for help with educational and emotional difficulties if needed, and have recourse available if students or supervisees believe that unfair or erroneous decisions were made about their professional development. Educators and supervisors ensure that their students and supervisees know and abide by the ethical guidelines for their profession.
- ***Research and Publication***—Writers and researchers in mental health fields also are subject to ethical guidelines. They must be sure not to harm research participants. They provide opportunity for voluntary consent whenever possible, make available to participants and colleagues clear information on their work, and follow guidelines for submission of manuscripts to professional journals. They appropriately acknowledge any help they received from colleagues and students.

ROLE INDUCTION

In general, clients who are informed of what to expect have a better understanding of treatment and their role in the process, seem more optimistic about making positive changes, and demonstrate greater willingness to self-disclose and talk about their concerns. *Role induction* is the process of orienting people to treatment so they are more likely to become successful clients who understand and can make good use of the therapeutic process. Role induction can help both client and clinician engage productively in a common endeavor and can contribute greatly to the efficiency and success of therapy.

Role induction typically entails discussing the following topics with clients early in the therapeutic relationship and ensuring that clients understand and are comfortable with the information that has been discussed:

- The nature of the treatment process
- How treatment promotes positive change
- The kinds of issues and concerns that usually respond well to counseling and psychotherapy
- The collaborative nature of the client–clinician relationship
- The roles and responsibilities of the clinician
- The roles and responsibilities of the client
- The importance of honesty and self-disclosure on the part of the client
- Ethical aspects of the therapeutic relationship, especially guidelines for maintaining and breaking confidentiality
- Ways to contact the clinician and what to do in the event of a client emergency
- Obtaining third-party payments (e.g., from managed care, health insurance)
- Clinician's fees and appointment schedules
- The kinds of changes people can realistically expect from treatment
- Risks inherent in treatment.

Role induction is typically discussed in the first session of treatment as part of the intake and assessment process. Following is an introduction to the Diaz family, who will be with us throughout the course of this book. A skill development review on questioning and interviewing and a sample intake assessment complete this chapter.

INTRODUCTION TO THE DIAZ FAMILY

Because this text promotes both theoretical understanding and skill development, extensive clinical examples are provided. The clients who will become most familiar to readers are the Diaz family, introduced here. We use a three-person family to illustrate the treatment approaches so that readers can become familiar with the application of interventions to both genders, to adults and children, and to people of different cultural groups. This family includes Edie Diaz, her husband Roberto, and their daughter Ava. Family members present a range of concerns. However, many avenues are available to help them improve their lives, as the case examples at the end of each chapter will illustrate. By studying these examples, readers will learn to apply the systems, strategies, and skills presented in the chapters.

Edie Diaz

Edie Diaz initiated the family's request for treatment. Now age 38, she is a White, Jewish woman. She was born in Brooklyn, New York, and spent her early years living with her biological parents and older sister. Her father was an accountant, and initially her mother stayed at home with the children. When Edie was 4 years old, her mother discovered that Edie's father was having an extramarital affair and insisted on a divorce. At that point, the father, who had been very close to Edie, withdrew from the family.

After her parents separated, Edie's mother found employment as a salesclerk in a department store to support her family and, with her two daughters, moved in with her parents. Edie's maternal grandparents cared for the children while their mother worked. The grandmother resented her caretaker role and was very critical of the children, especially Edie. The grandfather abused both Edie and her sister. Both grandparents are now deceased, but Edie has clear memories of the mistreatment she received and continues to experience strong resentment toward her grandparents.

When Edie was 10 years old, she was diagnosed with cancer. She had to undergo chemotherapy, which caused her to lose her hair and gain weight. Teasing from her classmates contributed to her already low self-esteem. However, a positive aspect of her illness was her increased involvement with her father. He visited her regularly in the hospital, brought her gifts, and gave her a sense of family once again. Edie and her father have continued to have contact and they currently see each other at least once a month.

Although Edie's prognosis for recovery from cancer was poor, she has been in good health since her treatment. However, her treatment raised questions about whether she could ever become pregnant and created a sense of anxiety and foreboding that never left her.

When Edie was 14, her mother remarried. Edie described her stepfather as physically and emotionally abusive. He yelled at the children, told them they were worthless, and frequently hit them. Edie dealt with this by avoiding her stepfather as much as possible. She was afraid to complain to her mother about the stepfather's behavior, thinking that her mother would become angry and punish her.

Edie continued to live with her mother and stepfather until she was 18. She had always been a good student and was able to earn a college scholarship. After college, she received a master's degree in library science and worked as a librarian until Ava's birth.

Edie had not dated much before she met Roberto. He had installed a computer system in the library where she worked and then asked Edie out for lunch. After dating for 6 months, Roberto proposed marriage, and Edie accepted. They were married when Edie was 24 and Roberto 28. Although their relationship was initially very close, with many shared interests and activities, their lengthy efforts to conceive a child had an adverse effect on the marriage. Finally, after a year of infertility treatments, Edie became pregnant and then gave birth to Ava. Despite subsequent fertility treatments, she has not been able to become pregnant a second time, a source of great sadness to her.

Edie reported marital and emotional difficulties since her initial efforts to become pregnant. When Ava was born, Edie left her job to care for her child. She missed her rewarding and successful career, but felt that she had to do everything in her power to safeguard her only child. Edie reported long-standing and increasing symptoms of sadness, loneliness, and discouragement. Since her marriage, she has gained more than 50 pounds and finds little joy or intimacy in her relationship with Roberto. Finally, last year when Ava was 9, Edie resumed work as a librarian. However, she is now experiencing strong feelings of self-doubt, guilt, and worry about Ava.

Edie has maintained contact with her mother and sister, as well as with her father. Her mother is still married to the stepfather who mistreated Edie. She finds it painful to be in his presence and never lets Ava spend time alone with him. Edie and her sister communicate frequently by e-mail but see little of each other because of geographic distance. Her sister has had a series of unrewarding relationships with men and now has an intimate relationship with a woman—her best relationship so far.

Roberto Diaz

Roberto's background is very different from Edie's. Roberto's grandparents and parents came to the United States from Puerto Rico. Roberto was born in New York City, the fifth of eight children. Although he always had frequent contact with both his mother and father, his parents separated when he was young. Nevertheless, he describes his family as warm and loving, always ready to help.

Roberto's neighborhood was rough, and he became involved with street gangs at an early age. His father taught him to defend himself with both fists and weapons. Because he was tall and stocky and had few fears, Roberto became a leader among his peers.

Roberto had little interest in school, preferring to teach himself. When he was 17, he left school to learn about computers. He received a GED as well as some specialized training in computers and now has a job he enjoys, installing Internet systems. He takes great pride in his abilities and his success in earning a good income for his family.

Roberto had two brief marriages and many relationships before he met Edie. He was impressed by her intelligence, stability, and caring and hoped that by marrying her he would find the committed and loving relationship he was seeking. He stated that, although he was very attached to his family, he was disheartened by Edie's long period of unhappiness. He reported that they were rarely intimate and no longer had a rewarding relationship. He told the therapist that he was "almost at the end of his rope" and that Edie had better make some changes fast if this marriage were to continue. At age 42, he was eager to get his life back on track.

Ava Diaz

Ava, age 10, is a tall girl who resembles her father both physically and temperamentally. She has recently been misbehaving at school, and her teacher describes her as a bully. A good student, Ava has excelled in English and history but seems to be losing interest in school. She has one close friend in the neighborhood but otherwise socializes with a wide variety of children.

Throughout this book, you will learn more about the Diaz family and their strengths and difficulties. You will also learn effective ways to help Edie, Roberto, and Ava, as well as your own clients.

SKILL DEVELOPMENT: QUESTIONING AND INTERVIEWING

This chapter reviews two important skills: asking questions and conducting an intake interview. Questions are used by all clinicians, regardless of their theoretical orientations. They use questions throughout the treatment process to elicit information and to promote client self-exploration, self-awareness, and self-expression.

Questions are especially important in eliciting background information and are the primary intervention used in conducting an intake interview. Many mental health agencies use a structured intake interview as a way to systematically gather information on clients. This helps clinicians to be consistent and thorough in the information they seek and increases the likelihood of obtaining information that is essential to understanding each client. Although counselors and psychotherapists in schools, private practices, and career counseling settings may not conduct formal intake interviews, those clinicians, too, can benefit from bearing in mind the topics that are usually covered in these interviews, although they might elicit that information from their clients in less structured ways.

Asking Helpful Questions

Questions are a powerful intervention. They can focus the treatment on core issues, and provide enough information to deepen the clinician's awareness and understanding. Questions can also exaggerate the power imbalance between clinician and client; lead people to feel judged, attacked, and demeaned; and turn a treatment session into an inquisition. Consider the following example of a client statement followed by four questions posed by clinicians:

CLIENT: I got a speeding ticket on my way to our session today.
INTERVENTION 1: What happened?
INTERVENTION 2: How did you feel about that?
INTERVENTION 3: Why did you do *that?*
INTERVENTION 4: How fast were you going?

Each of the four clinician interventions moves the session in a different direction, some more positive than others. The first two responses are likely to be helpful. Intervention 1 gives the client an opportunity to describe and process the incident, perhaps leading to recognition of difficulties with behavior and impulse control; and intervention 2 encourages exploration of feelings, perhaps leading to a discussion of emotions related to the client's treatment. Neither intervention is judgmental, and both give the client many possible ways in which to respond. Interventions 3 and 4, however, are unlikely to have a positive impact on the therapeutic process. The third question may be interpreted by the client as suggesting that he made poor choices and perhaps deserves punishment. The fourth question focuses on a specific piece of information. Although this information may be relevant to the discussion, asking immediately for the speed may suggest that it is the most important aspect of the incident. If, indeed, the person was going at a high speed, having to disclose that information to the clinician may be embarrassing and may even lead the client to withhold accurate information. Clearly, the nature and timing of a question are instrumental in both building rapport and achieving treatment goals.

PURPOSEFUL QUESTIONING When clinicians make an intervention or respond to clients, they consider the direction in which they want to move the session and the impact they want their words to have on the client. To beginning clinicians, having such a high level of awareness and direction may seem almost impossible. However, with training and experience, that sort of clinical thinking becomes rapid and almost automatic. Even new clinicians should be able to look at a transcript of a treatment session and discuss the probable intention and impact of an intervention.

When formulating questions, clinicians should consider:

- What information they want to elicit
- How that information will advance the therapeutic process
- What they want to focus on or emphasize with their question
- What tone they want to establish in the session.

OPEN AND CLOSED QUESTIONS Questions can be open or closed. An open question is usually designed to elicit narration, perhaps about the client's feelings, thoughts, behaviors, or experiences. Open questions encourage people to talk at greater length or depth than do closed questions and generally are more powerful and productive. Open questions are broad and give clients responsibility and flexibility in how they might respond. Open questions often begin with "how," "could," "what," and "why" but may have other openers. Interventions 1, 2, and 3 in the previous example are open questions, encouraging the person to respond with at least a few sentences. Clinicians rely much more on open rather than closed questions because they are more likely to promote client self-awareness and exploration.

Closed questions ask for a specific piece of information, often a fact, and invite a limited response of only a few words. Closed questions often begin with "who," "when," "where," "are," "do," and "is." Closed questions can make people feel like they are on the spot. Intervention 4 in the previous example is a closed question.

However, closed questions do have a place in counseling and psychotherapy. Questions such as "Do you have siblings?" "Would you like to schedule an appointment for next week?" and "Where were you born?" yield important information. In addition, closed questions can help narrow the focus of a session that is drifting or can help a confused or highly emotional client present clearer information. For example, the clinician might say, "It sounds like your experience of being robbed was terrifying and overwhelming. I'd like to get a better idea of what happened. When did you first realize you were being followed? . . . What did the thief say to you? . . . When did you decide to give him your money? . . . Who was the first person you told about the robbery?" Although focusing on emotions is generally helpful to clients, closed questions can help people who are overwhelmed and distraught to ground themselves in the facts before focusing on feelings.

PHRASING QUESTIONS As with most interventions, questions should be phrased so that they are clear, concise, and easily understood. They should encourage and empower, moving treatment toward its goals. In general, questions that begin with "what" and "how" promote exploration and are well received by clients, whereas questions that begin with "why" can sound negative and accusatory (as in intervention 3 on page 20).

Questions may end in a question mark or may be a statement that suggests a question, such as "Tell me more about the robbery." These implied or indirect questions should follow the same guidelines as direct questions.

PACING OF QUESTIONS An uninterrupted series of questions can have a negative impact on the treatment process. Like questions beginning with "why," this pattern can increase a person's defensiveness and exaggerate the clinician's power. Even in an initial or intake session, clinicians should not deliver a barrage of questions. Instead, other interventions, such as reflections of feeling and meaning (discussed later in this book), should be interspersed among or combined with the questions so that the session has the flow of a dialogue, preserving the collaborative nature of the treatment. The following example demonstrates how a series of questions can be softened by varying the nature of the questions and including other interventions:

CLIENT: Yesterday, I got so anxious, I thought I would pass out.

CLINICIAN: That must have been frightening to you. What seemed to trigger your anxiety?

CLIENT: I guess it was a telephone call I received.

CLINICIAN: Telephone call?

CLIENT: Yes, from my brother. We've been out of touch for years. And then he suddenly calls to invite me to his daughter's wedding.

CLINICIAN: That must have brought up all sorts of feelings.

CLIENT: You're right. I felt shocked and angry, but also relieved to hear from him. I hadn't even known if he was still alive.

CLINICIAN: A mix of positive and negative emotions! What thoughts did you have about the call?

SUBJECT MATTER OF QUESTIONS Of course, just as the format and the pacing of questions have an impact on the development of the therapeutic relationship, so does the content of the questions. Although no topics are unacceptable in counseling and psychotherapy, clinicians should introduce topics when they believe clients will be fairly comfortable discussing them. For example, initiating discussion of a client's history of abuse during the first 10 minutes of an initial session usually is unwise; discussing that information with the client after some rapport has developed, however, is probably essential to effective treatment.

Questions usually should be presented so that they do not cause great discomfort. Asking questions about areas that the client is reluctant to discuss, as well as about painful memories or other highly charged subjects, should be done with extreme caution.

Questions generally yield more useful information when they focus on the client rather than on people who are not involved in the treatment. For example, asking "What thoughts did you have when your mother left your father?" is likely to be more productive than "What was your mother's reason for leaving your father?" The first question keeps the focus on the client and encourages self-exploration, whereas the second shifts the focus away from the client and asks for mind reading. Exercises at the end of this chapter are designed to improve your questioning skills and give you an opportunity to apply some of the concepts covered in this section.

Conducting an Intake Interview and Assessment

An intake interview may be a formal process that precedes the referral of a client to another clinician, a structured interview that occurs during the first session or two of treatment, or simply the informal get-acquainted process that occurs during the early sessions of counseling. Intake or initial interviews differ greatly, depending on client, clinician, and context. For example, school counselors rarely conduct structured intake interviews but, rather, gradually acquire information about their students over many brief meetings. Intake interviewers in hospital emergency rooms generally focus on the present, assessing the urgency and dangerousness of a client's symptoms. In community mental health centers, structured and comprehensive intake interviews are the norm.

The primary purpose of a comprehensive intake interview is for clinicians to obtain enough information on clients' history, current situation, presenting concerns, and characteristics to conduct an assessment and formulate an accurate diagnosis and develop a treatment plan that is likely to succeed. Clinicians also need to assess whether clients are at risk of harming themselves or others. Because the intake interview occurs during the first few sessions of the therapeutic relationship, clinicians must also orient clients to treatment (which is accomplished through role induction, discussed earlier) and promote rapport and a collaborative therapeutic alliance.

Although clients may complete forms to provide some information, the intake process is primarily a dialogue between client and clinician. Questions are the major vehicle for eliciting information; as we have discussed, however, a barrage of questions is unlikely to be productive either in eliciting important personal material or developing rapport. Clinicians should follow the guidelines for formulating questions (presented in the previous section) when conducting an intake interview.

CONTENT OF THE INTAKE INTERVIEW A comprehensive intake interview and assessment generally covers the following topics, with questions, sequence of subjects, and depth of interview adapted to the client's age, concerns, motivation for help, and level of self-disclosure, as well as to the setting and the theoretical orientation of the clinician (Seligman, 2004):

- Demographic and identifying information, including age, relationship status, and living situation
- Presenting problems, including reasons for seeking help now, symptoms, onset and duration of difficulties, the impact of concerns on the person's lifestyle, and previous efforts to obtain help
- Prior and additional emotional difficulties
- Current life situation, including important relationships, occupational and educational activities, social and leisure activities, stressors, and sources of gratification
- Ethnic, cultural, religious, and socioeconomic information
- Family background, including information on the composition of family of origin and current families, relationships within the families, parenting styles, parental role models and messages, family values, family strengths and difficulties
- Developmental history
- Career and educational history
- Medical history, including significant past and current illnesses, medical treatments, and medications

- Health-related behaviors, including use of drugs and alcohol, exercise, diet, and overall self-care.

In addition, clients should have the opportunity to provide information that was not covered in the intake interview but that they view as important.

EXAMPLE OF AN INTAKE INTERVIEW

The following intake interview is with Edie Diaz. Edie sought counseling from a community mental health center. Her therapist is a woman, about 10 years older than Edie. Assume that Edie has already been provided with information about the nature of treatment and her role as a client.

When reading this transcript, pay particular attention to how questions are used in the interview. Look at whether they are open or closed and how they are integrated with other kinds of interventions. Think about what the therapist's intent might have been in asking each question. Also, compare the content of this interview with the list of topics usually covered in an intake interview. An initial interview may not cover all topics. Are important aspects of this client's life ignored? Should these areas have been discussed in this session, or are they better left for exploration after Edie and her therapist build some rapport? Consider whether some topics or questions were particularly fruitful, and whether others had a negative impact on the session. How would you have improved this intake interview?

THERAPIST: Edie, we've gone over the consent-to-treatment forms and talked about the counseling process. Do you have any further questions about that information?

EDIE: No, it all seems pretty clear.

THERAPIST: Well, feel free to ask any questions that come up during our work together.

EDIE: Thank you. I will.

THERAPIST: I can see from the forms you completed that you are 38 years old and live with your husband Roberto and your daughter Ava.

EDIE: Yes, that's right.

THERAPIST: What prompted you to seek some help at this time?

EDIE: A lot of things. It's hard to know where to begin.

THERAPIST: We can start almost anywhere, and probably one issue will lead us to talk about another. But often people have a specific concern in mind when they actually pick up the phone to make an appointment. I wonder if that happened for you?

EDIE: Well, yes, I guess it did. Ava will be ten in a few weeks, and she and I were planning her birthday party. After she went to bed, I started to think about when I was ten. That was such a hard time for me.

THERAPIST: I can see even thinking about it brings up strong feelings. What made that such a hard time for you?

EDIE: I was diagnosed with cancer when I was 10. It was awful. I had chemotherapy, lost all my hair, even my eyebrows, and gained lots of weight. Can you imagine what that's like for a child? I felt like such a freak. And everybody was acting like I was going to die. *Almost* everybody. . . .

THERAPIST: That must have been a terrible experience for you. Very frightening.

EDIE: Yes, it was. And I'm so afraid it's going to happen to Ava. She means the world to me. I couldn't stand it if she had to go through what I went through. And I still worry about my health too. The doctors told me years ago that I was cured, but it's hard for me to believe that.

THERAPIST: So not only are you worrying about Ava, who means so much to you, but also about yourself. . . . When you were talking about having had cancer, it sounded like someone came into your mind who had been optimistic about your prognosis.

EDIE: Yes, my father.

THERAPIST: How did that affect your experience with cancer?

EDIE: It made an enormous difference. It was the one good thing that came out of that whole mess. You see, my parents divorced when I was about four. My mother told me my father had been involved with another woman, so she divorced him and tried to keep me and my sister away from him. I didn't see much of him for about six years. Then, when I was diagnosed with cancer, he insisted on seeing me. We formed a relationship for the first time. He would take me out for ice cream and talk with me about what was happening to me. No one else would. He was there for me. And we've been close ever since.

THERAPIST: Sounds like you really value your relationship with him.

EDIE: I do. I wish Roberto and Ava could have that kind of bond.

THERAPIST: We'll certainly talk more about your experience with cancer, but maybe this is a good time to talk about your family. How do you perceive the relationship between Roberto and Ava?

EDIE: It's interesting because they look alike, both tall and big boned. They even have similar personalities, but they often conflict. Both of them are pretty headstrong. Roberto is really a workaholic. If he's not actually at work, he's glued to the computer, trying out some new piece of software or surfing the Net. He's good at his work and thrives on new challenges, but he almost feels like a visitor in our home.

THERAPIST: How does that affect you?

EDIE: I feel a real sense of loss. Roberto and I were so happy when we married. It felt like we couldn't be together enough. We would take walks and go dancing and go to the beach. Anything we did together was wonderful. And then gradually things changed.

THERAPIST: Changed?

EDIE: Yes, I guess it started when we decided to have a baby. That cursed cancer came into the picture again. The doctors told me that I probably couldn't become pregnant because of all the medical treatments I had. But I was determined. We saw every specialist I could find, and after many months of trying I did become pregnant with Ava. But all that took a toll on our marriage. Even sex went on a time schedule, trying to do everything we could to conceive. It was worth it to have Ava, but things have been difficult ever since.

THERAPIST: So, having Ava was a great joy for you, but it sounds like you had to pay quite a price.

EDIE: Yes, and then when we tried to have a second child, things got even worse. Years of trying. I guess we have given up on that now. Ava is wonderful, but I still wish I had a second child.

THERAPIST: I hear your sadness and longing.

EDIE: Yes.

THERAPIST: We'll want to talk more about those feelings, too. But I'd like to broaden the picture and talk about other parts of your life. What would a typical day be like for you?

EDIE: Not very exciting. I get up early, get dressed, wake Ava and Roberto, make breakfast, and help Ava get ready for school. After they both leave, if I don't have to go to work, I might clean the house, do some shopping, plan dinner, and then I make sure to be home when Ava gets back from school. If I have any extra time, I read or watch television. Last year I went back to work part-time. I'm employed as a librarian, working two days a week.

THERAPIST: How do you feel about the way you spend your time?

EDIE: It's all right. We have a beautiful home, and I want to be there for Ava. Lately I've started to think about working more hours, though. I loved being home with Ava, but I missed having a job and being in more contact with the world. I was out of work so long that I worried about learning the new library computer systems, but I've managed so far.

THERAPIST: So for now, your time is focused on caring for your family and working part-time. Let's look at some other aspects of your current life. In addition to your father, what contact do you have with other family members?

EDIE: I see my mother fairly often. She comes over at least once a week, usually after Ava comes home from school, so they can have some time together.

THERAPIST: What is your time with your mother like?

EDIE: We get along all right most of the time.

THERAPIST: I hear some mixed feelings there.

EDIE: I just can't respect the choices my mother made, and it makes me angry. My mother remarried when I was about fourteen. I don't like to say this about anyone, but I really hate my stepfather. I lived with him and my mother for four years, and I don't think he ever said a kind word to me. Any little thing I did wrong, like leave my schoolbooks on the table, he would yell at me and hit me. And he treated my mother that way too. Still does. I don't know why she stays with him.

THERAPIST: Sounds like you have a lot of anger at your stepfather. How do you handle those feelings?

EDIE: I try not to think about him much. I rarely see him and, of course, I won't let Ava be alone with him. But things still happen that make me angry. Last week, my mother was visiting, and we were going to take Ava shopping for a dress for her party. We were heading out the door when he calls, saying he doesn't have to work late after all, and my mother should come home and make dinner. And off she goes without a second thought.

THERAPIST: So you had some bad feelings about your relationship with your mother as well as anger at your stepfather. How do those feelings affect your relationship with your mother?

EDIE: I used to tell her how I felt. And when I was a teenager, I sure let her know how unhappy I was. But it didn't seem to make any difference to her, so I just gave up. She knows how I feel, but she won't change. It's a barrier between us.

THERAPIST: It sounds like you've found a way to maintain a relationship with your mother but you wish it could be better.

EDIE: Yes, I do.

THERAPIST: That might be another aspect of your life that we could work on.

EDIE: Yes, I'd like that.

THERAPIST: Besides your mother and father, I know you have an older sister. What is your relationship with her like?

EDIE: That's another relationship that has had problems over the years. We used to be very close when we were children. She's four years older than I am, and she would try to protect me from . . . things.

THERAPIST: Protect you?

EDIE: We had some problems with my grandparents, but I don't want to talk about that.

THERAPIST: That's up to you. Perhaps as we continue to work together, you will want to talk about that, but that's your decision. How do you and your sister get along now?

EDIE: We don't see each other much. She lives in Las Vegas, likes the fast track. Beth's had lots of problems with men, drugs, and gambling. I try to talk to her and have helped her out with money a couple of times. Actually, she has settled down some lately. She's living with a woman. . . . I guess she's a lesbian. At first I was real uncomfortable with that, but whenever I call her, she seems okay. This sounds like her best relationship yet.

THERAPIST: So there has been a sort of reversal in your relationship with your sister. When you were younger, she tried to protect you from some difficult situations, but as adults, you have tried to protect her.

EDIE: True, but neither of us was really able to protect the other one.

THERAPIST: You wish it had been different?

EDIE: Yes, I do. But Beth *is* doing better.

THERAPIST: And that must be a relief for you. I wonder what your own use of drugs and alcohol is like?

EDIE: No problems there for me. I had all the drugs I wanted when I had cancer. I never drank much, but I had to stop drinking for so long when I was trying to become pregnant that I just never started again.

THERAPIST: You've told me about your history of cancer, but what is your current medical condition like?

EDIE: The doctors say I'm doing well, though they think I might go into menopause early because of the chemotherapy. I have gained a lot of weight though, nearly fifty pounds since before I was pregnant. I feel tired a lot . . . maybe because of the extra weight.

THERAPIST: Tell me about your sleeping and eating.

EDIE: I have trouble falling asleep most nights, and then I'm tired for the rest of the day because I get up early. My eating isn't very good either. I try to make nutritious meals for my family, but I snack during the day . . . peanut butter, cookies, whatever is around. I know I should do something about my weight and get some exercise, but I've been saying that for years and haven't done anything. Maybe you can help me with that too.

THERAPIST: We can certainly talk about ways to address those concerns. There are a few more areas I want to cover before we finish our session today. I know you are employed as a librarian, but I'd like to hear more about your education and work.

EDIE: I was always a good student and enjoyed school. I guess it was an escape for me from all the problems at home. The only time when school got bad was during my cancer treatments; all the kids would tease me, and I hated to go to school. I was never very social or popular, and I guess I withdrew even more after that. But I still got good grades. My goal was to get a scholarship so I could go away to college. And I did! So I left home when I finished high school and went to the state university, majored in English. I like to read, so that major made sense to me. But after I graduated, I really didn't know what to do. I worked in sales for a while, but that was definitely not right for me. After a year or so, I decided to get my master's in library science. I borrowed some money from my dad and went to graduate school. I got a good job with the New York Public Library right after I got my degree, paid my father back for the loan, and was moving up in the system when Roberto and I got married. I guess my priorities shifted then. I focused more on my marriage and trying to become pregnant, but work was still rewarding for me. I felt like I had found my niche there.

THERAPIST: So your academic work and your job as a librarian have been great sources of success and pride to you.

EDIE: Well, you're putting it more strongly than I would, but I guess you're right. In some ways, I feel more content in the library than anywhere else I've ever been.

THERAPIST: So it also is a source of comfort for you. There is almost a spiritual quality to your talk about the library, and that makes me wonder about the place of religion and spirituality in your life.

EDIE: Formal religion doesn't mean much to me anymore. Both of my parents are Jewish, but we hardly ever went to synagogue, just on the high holidays. I never had any religious education either. I still put down Jewish on forms that ask for your religion, but I don't practice the religion. And Roberto isn't Jewish. His family is Catholic. They used to go to church, but he hasn't gone in years. I worry about Ava's lack of religious education, but she doesn't seem to miss it. I do talk to her about God, though. I think believing in God comforted me as a child, and I want her to have that feeling too. When she was little, I taught her prayers to say at bedtime, but I don't think she prays anymore. I gave you a long answer to your question, but I guess this is a part of my life that confuses me. I have always felt a connection to God, to a spiritual side of myself, but then I wonder if I'm being a hypocrite because I don't follow any organized religion. Maybe that's something we can talk about, too, but it's pretty far down on the list.

THERAPIST: Yes, we can get back to that. I'd like to hear some more about your childhood years. We've talked about your parents' divorce, your relationships with your sister and your parents, your stepfather, your treatment for cancer, and your enjoyment of most of your school years. What else stands out as important during those years?

EDIE: Not too much. My mother says I was precocious as a baby, walking and talking early. I had a few friends in the neighborhood, but I've always been kind of shy and was never very popular. I only dated three or four guys very briefly before I met Roberto. I guess I haven't told you about my grandparents, my mother's parents.

THERAPIST: What do you want to tell me about them?

EDIE: They took care of us when my mother went back to work after the divorce. I don't want to talk about them any more right now.

THERAPIST: All right. Let's put that topic on the shelf until you want to take it down. What other parts of your life might be important to talk about?

EDIE: I do want to mention my friend, Sandi. She lived near me and had her first child when I was pregnant with Ava. Our children played together, and we became good friends. Three years ago she moved to California. I really miss her, but we're still in touch by e-mail.

THERAPIST: So Sandi is another important person in your life, but here's another relationship that has involved loss. What else do you want to be sure to mention before we finish our session?

EDIE: I think that's about it. I didn't think I would have so much to say!

THERAPIST: Yes, you did cover a lot of ground. I can see that trying to get some help through counseling is really important to you and that you are already involved in that process. We'll get back to most of these topics again and probably also find some important areas we overlooked, but it's time to stop for today. How did you feel about our first session?

EDIE: I liked talking to you; I wasn't sure I would. Where do we go from here?

THERAPIST: Let's schedule another appointment and try to home in on some goals.

EXERCISES

General instructions about group and individual exercises appear in the preface to this book. Review that explanation before beginning these exercises.

Large-Group Exercises

1. Read the introduction to the Diaz family on pages 18–20. Edie and Roberto come from very different backgrounds. Edie grew up in a middle-class, White, Jewish family, living in the suburbs, whereas Roberto grew up in a lower middle-class, Roman Catholic Latino family,

living in an urban area. These differences in their backgrounds are likely to affect their expectations for and attitudes toward counseling. Discuss the following:

- How would you go about understanding and addressing the impact of Edie's and Roberto's background differences on their orientations toward treatment?
- In what ways might you individualize treatment for Edie and for Roberto in order to increase the likelihood of developing a positive therapeutic alliance with each of them?

2. The following exercises are designed to help you learn more about both asking questions and conducting an intake interview. In addition to working on these specific exercises, try to be more conscious of the questions you ask in your everyday activities, particularly when you meet a new person. Do you tend to ask open or closed questions? Are your questions just part of making conversation, or are you consciously trying to get to know the person you have met? Are you receiving the responses you want? If not, what might you do differently?

Now, read the following three client statements and the four clinician responses to each client statement. The client is a 42-year-old woman whose husband died recently. Consider the following aspects of each clinician response and then discuss which seems to be the best intervention in response to each client statement.

- Whether the question is open or closed
- The information you expect will be elicited by each question
- The focus of each question (e.g., the direction in which it moves the session)
- The tone of each question and the impact it is likely to have on the client.

Client Statement 1

CLIENT: It's been three months since my husband died and two months since I began counseling, but I miss him even more than I did right after his death.

COUNSELOR A: Why do you think that is?

COUNSELOR B: Do you think I am doing something wrong in counseling you?

COUNSELOR C: What prevents you from getting over his death?

COUNSELOR D: What feelings come up for you as you think about missing him?

Client Statement 2

CLIENT: Even though I miss George, I have gone back to work, and I'm concentrating fairly well.

COUNSELOR A: How are you managing to do that?

COUNSELOR B: How do you feel about that?

COUNSELOR C: Do you think you are ready to stop counseling now?

COUNSELOR D: Is your work still as demanding as it was?

Client Statement 3

CLIENT: I know I should get out and meet new people, but I just feel stuck.

COUNSELOR A: Where are you stuck?

COUNSELOR B: Did you sign up for the art class as we agreed?

COUNSELOR C: What has helped you when you have felt stuck before?

COUNSELOR D: Do you think you could be sabotaging your efforts to change?

Small-Group Exercises

Now that you have improved your ability to make good use of questions, try out that skill via an intake interview. Divide into groups of four people, and then break each of those groups into two dyads. Each pair should take a turn conducting an interview; one person should assume the role of the clinician, while the other becomes the client. Use the interview topics listed previously in this chapter to structure your interview. Record this interview to facilitate analysis and feedback.

When you are in the client role, think about a comfortable way to approach the intake process. You can assume a persona, making believe you are someone you know well and presenting information as that person might. Details can be changed to protect the person you are role-playing. You might also choose to talk about yourself if that feels comfortable. Like any client, keep in mind that you do not need to answer all of the clinician's questions, and it is your right to disclose as much or as little as you choose. However, because this is a learning experience, try to approach this exercise in a way that allows you to be a cooperative and collaborative client who will not present the clinician with too great a challenge. Allow approximately 20 minutes for the interview and 10 minutes for feedback.

While one pair is engaged in an intake interview, the other pair should observe and take notes, preparing to provide feedback. Remember to emphasize strengths when giving feedback. When identifying weaknesses in the role-play, be sure to suggest alternatives that might have been more successful. Feedback should cover the following topics:

- The overall tone of the interview
- How well important areas of information were covered in the interview
- The nature of the questions that were asked (open or closed, implied or direct)
- The focus of each question (e.g., the direction in which it moved the session)
- The tone of each question and the impact it had on the client
- The strengths of the interview
- Ways in which the interview might have been improved.

Individual Exercises

General instructions on individual exercises appear in the preface to this book. Review that explanation before beginning these exercises. Your responses should be written in your journal.

1. Previously in this chapter, we identified three essential characteristics of effective therapeutic relationships: empathy, unconditional positive regard, and congruence or genuineness. Therapists also instill hope in their clients. List each of these characteristics on a piece of paper. Then select at least one (but no more than three) that you believe is already a strength for you. For each, write out your rationale for believing you would be successful in transmitting that quality to a client. For example, you might perceive yourself as very empathic because you can easily engage people in conversations, and are a good listener who is not judgmental.

   For each of the items you did not select, write down one change you might make to maximize your ability to transmit that characteristic to clients. For example, you might try to communicate more unconditional positive regard to others by deliberately acknowledging positive statements they have made about themselves. To improve your ability to communicate hope, you might focus on making fewer judgmental statements and instead look for new possibilities.
2. List some of the important perspectives or viewpoints you would bring with you if you were a client. Write briefly about how you would like a clinician to adapt treatment to meet your needs. What can you learn from this about your own work as a clinician?

Summary

This chapter introduced the development of theories of counseling and psychotherapy, the elements of a useful theory, a model for mental health, and some of the treatment ingredients that facilitate positive change. The nature of a positive therapeutic alliance, client and clinician characteristics, the importance of cultural competence, and relevant ethical standards were also discussed. The Skill Development section provided a review of how to ask helpful questions and conduct an intake interview.

Recommended Readings

Duncan, B. L., Miller, S. D., Wampold, B. E., & Hubble, M.A. (Eds.). (2010). *Heart and soul of change in psychotherapy* (2nd ed.). Washington, DC: American Psychological Association.

Seligman, L., & Reichenberg, L. W. (2012). *Selecting effective treatments: A comprehensive, systematic guide to treating mental disorders* (4th ed.). Hoboken, NJ: Wiley.

Additional Sources of Information

http://www.counseling.org/Resources/CodeOfEthics/TP/Home/CT2.aspx—The American Counseling Association's most up-to-date Code of Ethics.

http://www.apa.org/ethics/code—The American Psychological Association's 2002 *Ethical Principles of Psychologists and Code of Conduct.*

http://www.multiculturalcounseling.org—Website for the Association for Multicultural Counseling and Development.

CHAPTER 2

Overview of Background-Focused Treatment Systems

This chapter focuses on the first of the four general types of treatment approaches discussed in this book by area of focal concern: background, emotions, thoughts, and actions (BETA). Background-focused treatment systems emphasize the importance of unresolved problems and issues in the client's past. Clinicians advocating these approaches believe that unless treatment facilitates healing of past wounds and relieves developmental blocks, people will continue to repeat harmful and dysfunctional patterns.

WHY FOCUS ON THE PAST IN TREATMENT?

Psychodynamic theorists believe that the roots of current problems lie in the past and that exploration and interpretation of past experiences are essential to alleviating current concerns. Whether or not readers share that point of view, some understanding of the past can shed light on the nature and dynamics of people's current concerns and provide a context for understanding them more fully. Repetitive patterns can be identified, as can possible precipitants of current and future difficulties. For example, the adolescent who was insolent to his teacher can be better understood by knowing whether he has long-standing difficulty with authority figures or whether this is an isolated and uncharacteristic incident.

People's presenting problems are not always their most significant concerns. Embarrassment, guilt, shame, distorted perceptions, limited self-awareness, or other factors can lead clients to focus initially on minor concerns while withholding information on more significant issues. An example is a young woman who sought help in dealing with the end of a recent relationship; history-taking during the intake and assessment process revealed a background of abuse by her father and brother, as well as a series of subsequent self-destructive relationships.

Diagnosis, using the *Diagnostic and Statistical Manual of Mental Disorders,* Fifth Edition (DSM-5; American Psychiatric Association, in press), is an important aspect of the clinician's role. Making an accurate diagnosis often depends on knowing the duration of a person's symptoms and whether and how often that person has experienced the same or other symptoms in the past. Taking a careful history is essential when making a diagnosis.

In this postmodern era of counseling and psychotherapy, most clinicians recognize the importance of taking a holistic approach to understanding their clients. This involves learning about people's development, their cultural and socioeconomic backgrounds, physical health, their families and other important relationships, their strengths and abilities, their dreams and goals, what gives their lives meaning, and other important aspects of their lives. Each person has a story to tell, and by listening to these stories and learning about people's lives, clinicians can see the world through their clients' eyes as much as possible. This can help clinicians to minimize their biases and preconceptions and truly know, appreciate, and respond to each person as a special individual.

In light of the many reasons why knowledge of clients' histories is essential to effective treatment, we strongly encourage all counselors and psychotherapists to engage in at least a cursory exploration of clients' pasts. How much time and attention the clinician devotes to this depends on the preferences of the clinician and the openness, concerns, and background of the client. Some readers may adopt a psychodynamic theoretical orientation and focus extensively on background, whereas others may prefer to integrate a discussion of background into another theoretical approach. Regardless of theoretical orientation, history-taking is an essential clinical tool.

To understand contemporary psychodynamic theory, we must first understand Freud's concepts of psychosexual drives, which he believed were innate and largely unconscious. These drives reveal themselves in sexual stages of childhood development (oral, anal, phallic, and latency). Freud's theory of life instinct, which gets its energy from the libido, and his later proposal of the death instinct (thanatos) to explain aggression and self-destructive behavior, were controversial in his time and still are today. But an understanding is necessary as a foundation on which to view his concepts of personality structure (id, ego, superego) and the important role of the unconscious. We will learn more about these topics in Chapter 3.

BASIC ASSUMPTIONS SHARED BY PSYCHODYNAMIC PSYCHOTHERAPY MODELS

Before we take a look at the evolution of psychodynamic psychotherapy from Freud's initial psychoanalysis to briefer forms of interpersonal and relational therapies more commonly used today, we must keep in mind that all of the treatment modalities under the psychodynamic umbrella share the following basic assumptions (Fonagy & Target, 2009):

1. ***Psychology Causation Underlies Behavior.*** The psychodynamic approach assumes that conscious or unconscious thoughts, feelings, and beliefs lie at the root of psychological problems and disorders.
2. ***The Unconscious Influences Us.*** Not all thoughts, feelings, and actions are conscious. An active unconscious mind exists in each of us, of which we might be completely unaware. The goal of psychodynamic treatment is to bring awareness to these unconscious thoughts that motivate behavior so that the person can act in a more conscious manner.
3. ***Interpersonal Relationships Are Internalized.*** Interpersonal relationships, especially early attachment figures, are internalized and contribute to expectations about relationships and views of the self. They also help shape the organization of personality.
4. ***Psychological Conflict Is Inevitable.*** Thoughts, feelings, and desires cause internal conflict and have the potential to undermine healthy development.
5. ***Everyone Develops Defense Mechanisms.*** Defense mechanisms exist to protect the ego and help reduce anxiety.
6. ***Complex Meanings Underlie Behaviors.*** Complex meanings are at the root of symptomatic behaviors. For example, an inability to be around people may be a reflection of inner feelings of shame. These feelings may be unconscious.
7. ***The Therapeutic Relationship Is Powerful.*** It is a generally accepted (and empirically validated) assumption that the therapeutic relationship is helpful.
8. ***A Developmental Perspective Is Assumed.*** Psychodynamic psychotherapists work from a developmental perspective. The background is important to understanding how and why problems have developed.

THE ROLE OF THE THERAPIST: TRANSFERENCE, COUNTERTRANSFERENCE, AND DISCLOSURE

A major change has occurred in the role of the therapist. No longer is the analyst aloof and anonymous, providing a blank slate for the analysand's projections. Rather, contemporary psychoanalysis assumes that therapists and clients each view the world through their own cultural lens, backgrounds, and biases. As a result, the therapist cannot be objective and neutral. Together, they collaborate in determining whether and what kind of treatment is appropriate and how it will be structured.

Most post-Freudian therapists make use of their countertransference feelings. During Freudian times a therapist's reactions toward a client were viewed as something to be avoided at all costs. The current view is that these feelings are a normal part of interpersonal relationships and can be used to enhance the relationship and deepen therapy. Ferenczi (1980) and others pointed out the mutuality of the therapeutic process and that both the client and the therapist are always influencing each other. Therapists who are in tune with their countertransference feelings can employ those feelings in the service of the therapy, helping clients to better understand themselves and their relationships.

"The practitioner's emotional response to the patient is one of the most important tools for therapeutic work" (Strean, 2001, p. 7). Attitudes about disclosing those feelings to clients have also changed over the years. During Freud's time it would have been considered a technical error. Contemporary psychodynamic theory takes a different approach and tends to address countertransference when issues arise. However, knowing what to disclose and when to disclose it is vitally important. Maroda (2010) warns that therapists must share their perceptions of the client in an appropriate manner, because such disclosure can have a positive or negative effect on the therapy. She provides the following overall guidelines:

- Disclosure always relates to the material at hand.
- It is an immediate and emotional reaction to the client.
- It is only done in the best interest of the client.
- Therapists do not share material from their own lives.
- The disclosure is not made to further the therapist's own agenda.
- It is never seductive.

When the therapist provides feedback in a judicious manner, the therapeutic alliance is strengthened, the client's self-esteem is increased, and the client is more likely to use the newfound knowledge outside of the session in his or her own relationships. This reparative learning has been termed a "corrective emotional experience." We will learn more about transference and countertransference in the coming chapters.

AN INTRODUCTION TO THEORETICAL MODELS OF PSYCHODYNAMIC PSYCHOTHERAPY

Although each of the different psychodynamic theories provides a comprehensive working model based on the assumptions listed earlier, no one theory provides an approach that suits everybody. Just as we grow and our lives change to meet new circumstances, so too do theories of psychology evolve and grow to meet the ever-changing (and challenging) needs of clients. Following is a brief introduction to the historical psychodynamic theories that will be the focus of Part 1 of this text. All have evolved during the past century since Sigmund Freud first laid the foundation.

Sigmund Freud and Classic Psychoanalysis

Classic psychoanalysis is the term used to describe traditional psychotherapy developed by Sigmund Freud more than 100 years ago. Although many theories of human development and psychotherapy have been advanced since Freud's time, he is generally regarded as the father of psychotherapy. His ideas and strategies continue to inform and contribute to treatment in the 21st century.

Classic psychoanalysis was developed by Freud in the early 1900s. The client was referred to as the *analysand*. She (a century ago most people who sought analysis were women) would lie on a couch, with Freud seated on a chair at the head of the couch outside the client's field of vision. Through the use of free association, recalling whatever came to mind including material from dreams, fantasies, projections, and transference feelings toward the therapist, the analysand would do the work of psychoanalysis, "to make the unconscious conscious" (Freud, 1957). It was not uncommon for analysis to continue in this manner, three to four times a week, for years.

Despite the broad applicability of Freudian psychoanalysis, some constraints limit the use and appropriateness of this approach. Few people have the time, financial resources, and inclination to engage in such intensive treatment. In addition, the slowly paced nature of the process; the relatively passive role of the client on the couch; and the emphasis on sexuality, early childhood, and the unconscious make the approach a poor choice for many people. Those in crisis, those who want to play a more active and equal role in their treatment, and those who are uncomfortable with or do not believe in Freud's focus on infantile sexuality are unlikely to respond well to psychoanalysis.

Indeed the numbers are limited. As of 2006, fewer than 5,000 people were reported to be in classical or traditional psychoanalysis (Adler, 2006). Despite the limited application of this form of psychoanalysis, schools to train analysts flourish in New York City, Washington, DC, and other large cities. Not only do people seek training in this approach, but clients seek psychoanalysis from these training facilities and also from psychoanalysts in independent practice. Few contemporary psychoanalysts, however, draw exclusively on the ideas of Freud. Rather, they use his ideas as the basis for their work but incorporate the ideas of his contemporaries (Adler and Jung) as well as more recent theorists in ego psychology, object relations, self psychology, and relational theory.

Freud's Contemporaries: Alfred Adler and Carl Jung

Alfred Adler and Carl Jung were Freud's colleagues early in their careers but ultimately developed their own theories. In 1902, Alfred Adler and Freud were charter members of the Wednesday afternoon psychoanalytic meetings that later became known as the Vienna Psycho-Analytical Society. Adler initially shared Freud's perspectives on human development and psychotherapy. However, as Adler's thinking evolved, he came to disagree with the emphasis Freud placed on biological and physiological determinants of psychological development. Adler believed that early childhood experiences played an integral part in future development, but he viewed Freud's concepts as too deterministic and limited. Adler eventually established his own theory of human development and psychotherapy, which he called *Individual Psychology*.

Adler developed a practical, teleological approach that replaced Freud's theory of sexual drives and libido with his belief in the goal-striving nature of people. For Adler, all behavior was purposeful and helped people to achieve their goals. People are not viewed as the victims of their biology or circumstances, but can choose to change both their goals and their behaviors. Social interest is an important concept in Adlerian therapy. These and many of Adler's other theories are practical and useful and in widespread use today, especially in working with families and children. Most Adlerian therapists incorporate lifestyle assessment, early childhood recollections, discussions of birth order, and other interventions into their work. We will learn more about Adler and his Individual Psychology in Chapter 4.

Carl Jung was another psychoanalyst who worked closely with Freud for a number of years and then split off to develop his own theory. Jung's theory of analytical psychology reflected his interest in philosophy, religion, and metaphysics, in addition to psychology. Jung, himself an intuitive, spiritual man, believed the unconscious mind was divided into two parts: the personal unconscious in which repressed memories, archetypes, and the shadow self are stored, and the collective unconscious, where archetypes, myths, and symbols from our evolutionary past reside. Jung's theoretical model was far more complicated than Freud's and evolved several times over the course of his life. Through the use of symbols, dream interpretation, rituals, and myth, Jung helped clients find deeper, spiritual meaning in their lives.

Jung's analytical psychology seems to be experiencing a rebirth in recent years, especially among people seeking a merger of spirituality, psychology, and philosophy. The literature shows a renewed interest in tracking the sacred, metaphysical and transpersonal topics, synchronicity, and the nature of the psyche in a connected universe. Jung's ideas also helped build the foundations of Alcoholics Anonymous and the Myers-Briggs Type Indicator. Fifty years after his death, Jung's personal journal and drawings were just recently made available to the public. Referred to as *The Red Book*, the document has caused quite a stir in analytical psychology. More will be said about this and other Jungian accomplishments in Chapter 5.

Ego Psychology, Object Relations, and Self Psychology

Although some clinicians still practice classic psychoanalysis, most of those who embrace the basic tenets of Freud's work have gravitated toward different theoretical models of psychodynamic psychotherapy. The difference between the approaches lies in their choice of which aspect of childhood development to emphasize (Sharf, 2012).

Whereas Sigmund Freud focused on inborn drives as determinants of personality development, his daughter, Anna Freud, who lived and worked with him until his death in London in 1939, focused more on the ego's needs to adapt to the environment developmentally. She focused on children's issues and took a structured, developmental approach to her work. Anna Freud was the first to identify a developmental aspect to anxiety.

Karen Horney, Erik Erikson, and others built on Freud's tripartite foundation (id, ego, superego) and focused on faulty ego development, rather than libidinal or sexual drives, as the cause of pathology. Thus they were referred to as "ego psychologists." Erikson in particular was concerned with the interplay of superego (societal norms) and biological drives in the development of identity across the life span. Erikson divided the life cycle into eight stages, with each stage having its own important life task to be mastered. In his 80s he started work on the ninth and final stage in his book, *The Life Cycle Completed* (Erikson, 1982). It was published posthumously.

Karen Horney was the first to challenge Freud's Oedipal complex from a woman's perspective. She and Helene Deutsch proposed drives inherent in females such as the drive toward motherhood and security. Horney emphasized the role of culture and environment in the developmental process, and how people often fall victim to what she referred to as the "tyranny of the shoulds"—the expectations that we and others put on ourselves. She wrote in 1937 that "the most important neurotic conflict is between a compulsive and indiscriminate desire to be the first under all circumstances and the simultaneous need to be loved by everybody" (Horney, 1937, p. 258).

In the 1980s and 1990s, the tide shifted away from instinctual drive theory, to a more developmental, relation-centered perspective that focused on the now classic research of John Bowlby and Mary Ainsworth related to early childhood attachment and the concept of the secure base (Ainsworth, Blehar, Waters, & Walls, 1978; Bowlby, 1978). Object relations theorists, for example, are more focused on the attachment between the early "objects" (or caregivers) and the young child. Early childhood attachment, they believe, is the springboard from which personality and future relationships are formed.

Relational theorists attend not only to the relationship between the client and others, but more specifically on the interrelationship between the client and clinician. Based on the work of Harry Stack Sullivan, an interpersonal relational framework arose in psychoanalysis. Stephen A. Mitchell (1988) was a leading proponent and author of relational psychoanalysis theory. The relational model also incorporates Bowlby's earlier work with attachment, the importance of subjective experience over objective knowledge, the relationship-seeking tendency of human nature, and the latest developmental and neurological evidence of the protective effect of positive relationships on the development of good mental health. Today, many psychodynamic psychotherapists follow the interpersonal relational model.

Beginning with publication of *The Analysis of the Self* in 1971, Heinz Kohut created the concept of self psychology. As did others before him, Kohut rejected Freud's drive theory, replacing it instead with an emphasis on the subjective experiences of the individual. Self psychology is developmental—beginning with the infant's first needs—and relational—recognizing the importance of social interactions or what Kohut refers to as *selfobject* experiences. These experiences with others provide the opportunity for growth across the life span. Through concepts such as selfobject experiences, which nurture the self and help to develop self-esteem; vicarious introspection, in which the therapist empathizes with and validates the client; and healthy narcissism, which helps the client to recognize and value his or her true self, Kohut's work has contributed greatly to our understanding of self, especially in the areas of personality disorders, narcissism, and the transferential relationship. Over the years, self psychology has had many adherents and some detractors.

More will be said about the impact of ego psychologists, object relations theorists, and self psychologists as we chart the evolution of psychoanalysis in Chapter 5.

Brief Psychodynamic Therapies

As the name implies, brief psychodynamic psychotherapy offers a time-limited, focused approach that respects the psychodynamic frame but may incorporate other cognitive, experiential, and behavioral interventions. At a time when managed care, insurance requirements, and other financial considerations require therapy to be focused, efficient, and effective, most psychodynamic psychotherapies practiced today fall under the brief model.

There is no doubt that all types of psychodynamic psychotherapies are effective in reducing symptoms, healing interpersonal relationships, and improving mental health. Empirical evidence supports the effectiveness of these approaches (Lazar, 2010; Norcross, 2011; Shedler, 2012). Meta-analytic reviews also indicate that longer term therapy not only helps, but imparts benefits that continue long after therapy has ended (Shedler, 2010).

THE FUTURE OF PSYCHODYNAMIC PSYCHOTHERAPY

All psychodynamic therapists work from a background-focused, Freudian perspective, but the theories continue to evolve, so they integrate other influences into their practices. Newer approaches in use today include mentalization, dialectic and schema theories, mindfulness and spiritual-based concepts, and therapies that emphasize a client's strengths and resilience rather than devolving into past experiences or unconscious instinctual drives. More will be said about these more integrated concepts in later chapters as we look at the integration of diverse psychological theories into the development of exciting new treatment modalities that provide therapists with flexibility and more autonomy in their choice of treatment modality.

Summary

This chapter has reviewed the importance of background in understanding people. It has provided an introduction into a sampling of approaches and theorists that reside under the psychodynamic umbrella including classic psychoanalysis (Sigmund Freud), Individual Psychology (Alfred Adler), analytical psychology (Carl Jung), and post-Freudian theories (ego psychology, object relations, and self psychology), and touched on the current use of brief, time-limited psychodynamic approaches. All of these approaches to psychotherapy are covered in greater detail in Chapters 3 through 6. Now we turn to Chapter 3 for a more in-depth look at the life and work of Sigmund Freud, a master at using past history to help people change in positive ways.

CHAPTER 3

Sigmund Freud and Classic Psychoanalysis

In 2006, on the 150th anniversary of Sigmund Freud's birth, the cover of *Newsweek* proclaimed "Freud Is Not Dead." The question of whether psychoanalysis, reflecting the ideas of Sigmund Freud, is obsolete has often been explored. However, even the frequent revisiting of this question testifies to the strength and influence of Freud's ideas. To wit, the American Psychological Association (2006) devoted a special edition of the journal *Psychoanalytic Psychology* to "The Relevance of Sigmund Freud for the 21st Century." Freud established the foundation for today's counseling and psychotherapy; he succeeded in bringing our knowledge of personality, human development, and psychological symptoms into everyday knowledge. Many of Freud's concepts, including the unconscious, the ego, and defense mechanisms, have become so widely accepted that we sometimes forget they began with Freud.

Freud's efforts required great courage; he disagreed radically with the thinking of his peers, withstood years of verbal and written attacks, and worked prodigiously to advance his ideas. Freud's contributions can be seen in all areas of psychological inquiry today. Transgenerational, biological, and evolutionary psychology—all have their roots in Freud's original scientific theories. Even though some of Freud's theories are no longer accepted, his legacy includes laying the groundwork for current theories of mental health.

SIGMUND FREUD

Sigmund Freud was born in Freiberg, Moravia, on May 6, 1856. His father was 40 years old, a widower with two sons, when he married his second wife, who was only 19 at the time. Freud was the couple's first child, born 2 years after his parents' marriage. As the firstborn and reportedly his mother's favorite (Jones, 1953), Freud had a special place in his family, although his mother gave birth to seven more children in the next 10 years. His father, a busy merchant with a commanding but gentle disposition, seems to have been a role model for his son. When Freud was 19 months old, his 8-month-old brother Julius died. Freud recalled early feelings of jealousy and resentment toward his brother and later reproached himself when his brother died. Memories such as these probably contributed to Freud's emphasis on the formative power of early childhood experiences.

Freud's family was Jewish, and this cultural and religious background affected him throughout his life. His Jewish heritage, with its emphasis on learning and family, contributed to Freud's appreciation for study, family history, and in-depth analysis. It also influenced his place of residence and his career choice, probably colored the reception his work received, and eventually led him to flee from Austria when Hitler came into power.

When Freud was a child, the ill treatment of Jews in many parts of Europe prompted his family to move to Vienna, Austria (at that time a relatively safe place for Jews), where he spent most of his life. Freud was a diligent student, studying at the University of Vienna between 1873 and 1881, when he completed medical school. Jones (1953) reported that career choices open to Jews in Vienna at that time included business, law, and medicine. Although Freud felt drawn to politics or social work, he chose medicine as the best available option. He was interested in learning about the mind and did his residency in neurology, beginning his medical career in theoretical medical work.

In 1884, Freud began studying and experimenting with cocaine as a tool to heighten mental powers (Mahoney, 1998). However, evidence of the negative impact of this substance on his colleagues dampened his enthusiasm for the drug.

Love had an important influence on Freud's career. He became engaged to Martha Bernays, daughter of the chief rabbi of Hamburg, in 1882. To earn enough money to marry and support a family, Freud took a position at a psychiatric clinic. Over their 4-year engagement, Freud wrote more than 900 letters to his wife-to-be, providing her with the details of his daily life.

Freud married Martha Bernays in 1886 and, about the same time, opened a private practice in neuropathology in Vienna. Growing up in a large family probably influenced him to have a large family himself and to value and feel comfortable with family around him. The couple had six children during the first 10 years of their marriage. Martha's sister, Minna, also was a part of the family, living with them from 1896 until her death in 1941, helping Martha and offering emotional support to Freud.

Freud's work and his family were the most important parts of his life. Jones (1955) speaks of the "unshakable devotion and a perfect harmony of understanding" (p. 386) between Freud and his wife and of Freud's efforts to raise his children in an atmosphere that would minimize anxiety, limitations, and criticism, and allow personalities to develop freely. Although he often saw 10 patients a day, Freud found time for his hobbies, especially collecting antiquities, reading biographies and other literature, studying mushrooms and rare wildflowers, and traveling. He was much affected by family joys and sorrows; his letters reflect the profound impact of the military involvement of his three sons, the capture of one during World War I, the death of his daughter Sophie in 1920, and the death of a grandson in 1923.

In that same year, Freud was diagnosed with cancer, probably related to the many cigars he smoked each day. During his remaining years, he had 33 operations on his jaw and palate, which prolonged his life but caused him considerable pain. In his later years, he wore a prosthesis in his mouth and wrote frequently of the severe discomfort caused by this apparatus and his many surgeries. Despite this, Freud continued to see patients and to write until the year of his death.

In March 1938, the Nazis invaded Austria. Although he was 82 years old and seriously ill, Freud decided that he must leave Austria. His daughter Anna and his son Martin had already been questioned by the Nazis, and the family members believed that they would not survive long in Vienna. Freud, his wife, and his daughter Anna left Vienna and went to England, where he was welcomed by friends. He tried to bring his four sisters with him. Unfortunately, they were not permitted to leave the country, and Freud was only allowed to leave money for their welfare. All four sisters died in concentration camps during the next 5 years.

Despite additional surgery in England, Freud's cancer was deemed incurable. Because he wanted to continue writing and seeing patients as long as possible, he put off taking the pain killers that might cloud his mind until 4 months before his death. He died on September 23, 1939, leaving a legacy that many of his followers have shaped into psychodynamic psychotherapy.

THE DEVELOPMENT OF PSYCHOANALYSIS

Freud's early work focused on the study of neurology. His research on the brain and spinal cord was his first notable contribution to the field. During the 1880s, he became interested in the work of Josef Breuer, a well-known physician in Vienna. Breuer used hypnosis and verbal expression to treat emotional disorders. His famous case of Anna O., a woman who experienced conversion symptoms (paralysis of limbs and disturbances of sight, eating, and speech) and dissociative symptoms in relation to the death of her father, captured Freud's attention. He became increasingly interested in psychological disorders and their treatment (Freud, 1938). He studied hypnosis with Charcot and investigated the use of electrotherapy, baths, and massage treatments for people with emotional difficulties. Although Freud sometimes used hypnosis, none of these other strategies seemed effective to him. Experimentation led him to initiate what he called the concentration technique, in which patients lay down with their eyes closed while Freud placed his hand on their foreheads and urged them to say whatever thoughts arose. He used questions to elicit material and promote self-exploration. This was an early version of modern psychotherapy. Although Freud later stopped touching his patients in this way because of its erotic possibilities, he continued to emphasize the importance of patient self-expression and free association.

Freud first used the term *psychoanalysis* in an 1896 paper. His writings during the 1890s reflected growing awareness of the importance of sexuality in people's lives. He initially believed that symptoms of hysteria and neurosis were due to childhood sexual experiences, perhaps traumatic sexual abuse such as seduction of the child by the father. A combination of difficulty in substantiating this idea and the negative reactions it elicited led Freud to change his ideas. He subsequently focused more on infantile sexuality and fantasies rather than actual sexual experiences as instrumental in determining emotional difficulties. In retrospect, Freud probably was wiser than even he knew. More than 100 years later, clinicians are now well aware of the high incidence of child sexual abuse. Probably at least some of his patients who described early sexual experiences to Freud did indeed have those experiences.

The combination of Freud's interest in understanding the human psyche and an effort to address difficulties he experienced in his own life led him to explore the meaning of his dreams and fantasies, as well as his childhood sexual feelings toward his mother and anger toward his father. His major work, "Interpretation of Dreams" (Freud, 1938), was completed in 1899 and advanced the powerful concepts that dreams reflect repressed wishes and that mental and physical processes are intertwined. Freud's ideas were largely ignored or rejected when the book was published. However, again he expressed ideas that ultimately gained widespread acceptance: the close connection between the mind and the body.

Despite the mixed reactions to his work, Freud moved forward to collaborate with colleagues who shared his viewpoints. In 1902, he suggested to Alfred Adler and several others that they meet to discuss Freud's work. This became the Vienna Psycho-Analytical Society, which met weekly at Freud's home. In 1910, Freud designated Carl Jung as president of the International Psychoanalytical Association. Adler and Jung eventually separated from the psychoanalytical association and went on to make their own important contributions to psychotherapy, as discussed in Chapters 4 and 5 of this text.

Growing international recognition of his work led to Freud's first visit to the United States in 1909, where he lectured at Clark University at the invitation of its president, Stanley Hall. Hall was a pioneer in experimental psychology and viewed Freud's work as a major contribution. *Five Lectures on Psycho-Analysis* was eventually published. These lectures were widely read and broadened awareness of Freud's work.

By this time, Freud had replaced hypnosis with free association in his work and encouraged analysts to experience their own analysis, a requirement still maintained by programs that train psychoanalysts. He also believed that patients needed to lie on a couch during treatment with the therapist out of view in order to relax them, facilitate self-expression, allow transference reactions to develop, and enable analysts to think freely without worrying about their nonverbal messages. Patients were told never to withhold any thoughts so that Freud could understand the unconscious, often reflected in sexually related fantasies stemming from early childhood experiences, that had produced symptoms.

Freud's writings during these years included not only his theoretical works but also lengthy case studies, reflecting his ideas. "Dora" (Decker, 1998) was the report of an 11-week analysis that Freud performed on an 18-year-old woman whose father was having an affair. Her father's lover befriended Dora, while the woman's husband made sexual advances toward Dora, creating a situation that would cause many people to have emotional difficulties. "Little Hans" (Freud, 1936) was Freud's analysis of a 5-year-old boy who would not leave his house because he feared being bitten by a horse. Freud conducted the analysis secondhand, meeting only with the boy's father, and enabled the father to help his son use Freud's insights into the boy's displacement of his fear of his father onto horses. Fourteen years later, the boy visited Freud to report that Freud had cured him of his phobia of horses. Other important cases include the so-called "Man with Rats," who had what Freud termed an obsessional neurosis characterized by doubts and compulsions as well as terrifying dreams involving rats. This 11-month analysis was also successful. Another patient, "Wolf Man," sought help from Freud when the patient was 23 years old and incapacitated by his compulsions. Freud believed this man may have witnessed parental intercourse as a child, exacerbating his ambivalent feelings toward his father. After 4 years of treatment, this patient, too, was free of serious symptoms.

By World War I, Freud saw 12 to 13 patients a day, each for 55 minutes with 5 minutes in between. His services were sought by the rich and famous. He reportedly cured the conductor Bruno Walter of partial paralysis of his right arm in six sessions and required only four sessions to relieve composer Gustav Mahler of a problem with impotence by exploring its psychodynamic origins (Jones, 1957).

Freud's interests broadened during the war years. He became interested in what was then called shell shock or traumatic neurosis, symptoms that developed after exposure to war experiences. The primary treatment for this disorder had been electrical stimulation of the skin and muscles. According to Freud, psychoanalysis, not electricity, was the proper treatment for this disorder, which he believed reflected an emotional conflict between the desire to escape and the need to honor one's sense of duty. Freud's thinking paved the way for our modern understanding of posttraumatic stress disorder.

Freud also became interested in understanding homosexuality, writing, "homosexuality is assuredly no advantage, but it is nothing to be ashamed of, no vice, no degradation, it cannot be classified as an illness" (Jones, 1957, p. 195). Here, too, Freud's ideas were very advanced—not until the 1970s did the American Psychiatric Association and the American Psychological Association officially determine that homosexuality is not a mental disorder. Freud was less astute in his understanding of women, a controversial aspect of his theory. This is discussed in detail later in this chapter.

Freud continued to broaden his interests in his later writings, which addressed not only the human psyche but also art, religion, anthropology, sociology, biology, and literature. He placed greater emphasis on context and society and acknowledged the important ways in which they both reflected and shaped human development. He expanded his definition of the unconscious, viewing it as containing more than repressed material, and also broadened his definition of sexuality, describing it as a great source of energy. In addition, Freud also expressed approval of "lay analysts"—people such as his daughter Anna Freud, who had been trained in analysis and had themselves been analyzed, but had not received an MD degree. We may think of these lay analysts as the forerunners of today's nonmedical clinicians: the psychologists, counselors, social workers, and psychiatric nurses who are the primary providers of psychotherapy.

IMPORTANT THEORETICAL CONCEPTS

Freud began his work as a theoretician, and it is through his comprehensive theory of personality that he has made his major contributions. This section reviews the most important aspects of his theory, including his concepts of human nature, the three structures of the personality, how personality develops, levels of consciousness, dreams and the unconscious, and defense mechanisms. Freud's ideas, like those of many of the theorists discussed in this book, have great depth and complexity and this book can only provide an overview of those ideas. Readers are strongly encouraged to read more about all of these theorists.

View of Human Nature

Freud placed great emphasis on the influence of biology and of early childhood experiences. He believed that, because of their biology, people go through predictable stages of psychosocial development and must struggle to find a balance between their strong sexual drives and their need to behave in socially acceptable ways. According to Freud, biological processes are mediated by early patterns of attachment, as well as by how people negotiate the stages of development.

Freud also recognized the importance of context. For example, he viewed people as seeking to win love and approval by acting in ways that reflected the dictates of their families and societies. This perspective is compatible with current thinking on diversity and multiculturalism.

Freud has been criticized for taking a deterministic stance, emphasizing irrational and instinctual forces in shaping people. Certainly, he viewed those forces as important, but perhaps the essential message in his work is that people need not be the victims of biology. Rather, we can use psychotherapy and other sources of help and personal growth to gain insight, lessen the power of the unconscious, and free ourselves to make conscious and healthy choices. Understanding early development, as well as the pressures of the libido and the superego, and strengthening our egos can enable us to lead the sorts of lives and have the types of relationships that we desire. Freud himself achieved much both personally and professionally, apparently reflecting his own success in balancing the competing pressures inside him.

Personality Structure

According to Freud, the personality is comprised of three systems: the id, the superego, and the ego. These structures often overlap and intertwine and are not discrete entities, although each has distinctive properties. Keep in mind that Freud's concept of the id (the biological component), the ego (the psychological component), and the superego (the social component) is simply a sort of map designed to clarify the nature of the personality. Just as states and countries are separated by artificial boundaries, so are these structures of the personality separated into artificial constructs. In reality, they operate together as the internal forces that form our personalities. However, using this theoretical structure can facilitate understanding of strengths and areas of difficulties in a personality.

THE ID The *id* is the first system of the personality. Present at birth, it encompasses all of the inherited systems, including the instincts, and is largely unconscious. The id derives its energy from bodily processes and is in close touch with the needs and messages of the body, seeking to satisfy them when possible. The id is subjective and emotional and, in its pure form, is not moderated by the external world. Simply put, the id wants what it wants when it wants it. The id, like the infant in which it originates, is intolerant of tension, pain, and discomfort and seeks to avoid them by pursuing pleasure and gratification (the pleasure principle). It is demanding and its needs, rather than logic, morality, or the constraints of society, determine the direction of its wants.

The id has two important strategies for obtaining pleasure: reflex actions and primary process. Reflex actions include automatic processes, such as coughing and blinking, that reduce tensions, especially those of a biological nature such as a tickle in the throat or a speck in the eye. The primary process strategy is more complex; it allows people to form a mental image of a remedy for their discomfort, a wish fulfillment. Freud believed that dreams served this function, offering a wish-fulfillment image. Although the image may assuage some of the discomfort, it also can cause frustration in failing to resolve the problem. It is the ego, discussed later in this section, that helps people truly find wish fulfillment and reduce discomfort in realistic ways.

Freud believed that people have both life instincts and death or destructive instincts. Life instincts, reflecting the needs of the id, lead us to pursue pleasure and avoid pain. The *libido,* present at birth, is an important aspect of the life instinct. This was originally defined by Freud as sexual desire, but its meaning has been broadened over the years to refer to energy and vitality, a zest for life. A desire for sexual fulfillment is only one facet of the life instinct, but it is an essential one because it leads people to procreate and continue the human race. The death instinct (*thanatos*) and the life instinct (*eros*) are in opposition to each other, much like good and evil. According to Freud, the death instinct has its origins in aggression and other destructive forces. Freud's concept of a death instinct, or a "death drive," was a longing to return to the state of nonexistence that we experienced before we were born (Higdon, 2012). The idea was controversial in his time, and has not received much support over the years. Even so, self-defeating behaviors, repeating painful patterns, self-inflicted wounds, and death wishes are all internalized aggression, which indicates masochism and self-loathing. If the energy created by the death instinct is directed outward, it results in violence and aggression. Based on Freud's definition of a death instinct, it appears that at least for some people, there is a drive toward self-destruction.

In *Civilization and Its Discontents* (1930), Freud explains the dualistic model in terms of civilization. The life instinct strives to unite people, families, and nations, whereas the death instinct results in an opposite pull of destruction. He writes, "This struggle is what all life essentially consists of . . ." (p. 122). Freud believed that human aggression is innate, but it can be channeled into nondestructive activities (sports, power, positive energy). The death instinct is Freud's attempt to explain the human tendency toward destruction that overrides the pleasure principle. Recognizing the possible presence of this force can help us to understand human behavior, particularly the compulsion to repeat, which results in the development of patterns of behavior.

THE SUPEREGO The *superego* can be thought of as the opposite of the id. The superego is a sort of rigid conscience that internalizes the rules and guidelines of a person's world. Messages from parents, teachers, and society as well as racial, cultural, and national traditions are important contributors to the development of a person's superego. The moral code of the superego is perfectionistic, diligently discriminating between good and bad, right and wrong. The formation of the superego allows self-control to take the place of parental control. When people follow the idealistic dictates of their superego, they typically feel proud and righteous but may sacrifice pleasure and gratification. On the other hand, when they ignore the superego, shame, guilt, and anxiety may result. The superego serves an essential function in curtailing the drives of the id; but like the id, the superego is too controlling and extreme in its directives.

THE EGO The *ego,* like the superego, becomes differentiated from the id as the child develops, although energy from the id provides the power for both the ego and the superego. The ego is not present at birth but evolves as the baby realizes its separateness from the mother.

The ego is aware of both the pressures of the id and the constraints of the superego and seeks to moderate both while still meeting their needs. The ego has been described as "the mental agent of rational and self-conscious selfhood" (Brunner, 1998, p. 83). It is a mediator and organizer. Guided by the reality principle or reality testing, the ego has considerable power; it can effect changes in the environment, postpone or suppress instinctual demands, and encourage sound moral judgment and flexibility. Using logic, intelligence, objectivity, and awareness of external reality, a healthy ego considers, modifies, and integrates both internal and external pressures on a person; decides when and how the person should respond to those demands; and identifies wise choices and behaviors that promote self-preservation.

Stages of Development

Freud believed that people develop according to predictable stages, with those occurring during the first 5 years of life being the most important. The importance of inborn drives during those early years is a major factor in determining later personality development.

THE ORAL STAGE The *oral stage* makes up the first year or so of a child's life. The mouth is the most important zone of the body for the infant, with sucking and eating providing the nurturance that will sustain the child's life during the oral-incorporative phase. Biting is a way for the child to express aggression during the subsequent oral-aggressive period. The mouth also becomes the child's first erotic zone. Freud believed that developmental problems at this point could later manifest themselves in symbolic and sublimated forms through symptoms such as gullibility (swallowing anything), overeating, and argumentativeness (oral aggressiveness).

THE ANAL STAGE Freud termed the second stage of development, between the ages of 18 and 36 months, the *anal stage* because of the importance of toilet training and the process of elimination during those years. In this second stage, the focus of gratification shifts from the oral functions to the social pleasure of impressing the parents and the physical pleasure of emptying the bowels. According to psychoanalytic theory, parents who use punitive and restrictive means to develop children's bowel and bladder control are likely to promote stingy, compulsive, controlling, and withholding characteristics in their children; those who reward and praise their children lavishly for appropriate elimination are likely to foster creativity. Feelings about the body and its functions also are shaped during these years. Understanding the relationships between children's bodily functions and their subsequent personality development can help define healthy parenting as well as provide insight into emotional difficulties that may stem from early developmental problems.

THE PHALLIC STAGE The third stage, between ages 3 and 5, is known as the *phallic stage*. According to Freud, this complex stage is strongly related to our adult sexual relationships. During these years, feelings of pleasure become associated with the genitals, and masturbation and sexual fantasies develop.

Freud believed that at this age children harbor unconscious sexual desires for the parent of the other gender along with an unconscious wish to eliminate the parent of the same gender, perceived as standing in the way of the child's desires. In boys, this is termed the *Oedipus complex*, referring to a man who, according to the literature of ancient Greece, unknowingly married his mother. According to Freud, fear of retribution from the father causes boys to develop castration anxiety, which, in turn, allows them to repress their desire for their mother and resolve their feelings appropriately through identification with the father.

In girls, the parallel situation is referred to as the *Electra complex*, named after a woman in Greek literature who had strong feelings of love and devotion toward her father. Freud hypothesized that the female equivalent of castration anxiety is penis envy, in which girls become jealous and resentful because of their lack of a penis. He believed that girls, like boys, typically resolve this phase by identifying with their same-gender parent.

Contemporary psychoanalysts acknowledge the possibility that a girl may experience penis envy but also believe that a boy may have womb or breast envy. However, they downplay the importance of both patterns, viewing them as only one of many internal and external experiences that may be important in children's development. In addition, although Freud saw many parallels between the ways in which both boys and girls passed through this stage, many modern theorists now emphasize that, for both genders, the mother is typically the first love and source of nurturance. Mothers are, of course, the same gender as their daughters but not as their sons. Most girls, then, must shift the primary source of their attachment from women to men while most boys do not make this shift, probably an important difference in their development of love and attachments.

Many aspects of emotional development evolve during the phallic years, including self-esteem and self-image, sexuality, need for love and approval, feelings toward authority figures, and sense of initiative.

THE LATENCY STAGE Freud viewed the time between ages 5 and 11 as a relatively quiet period in a child's sexual development; therefore, he called these years the *latency stage*. Sexual drives become less important, while social interests increase. Children turn outward, form relationships, progress through school, and develop rewarding hobbies and activities. Emotional development focuses on their ability to take on and succeed in new challenges and endeavors and to set and achieve realistic goals. Children who negotiate this stage successfully typically develop feelings of empowerment and have initiative, whereas those who cannot deal with the demands of this stage may experience low self-esteem.

THE GENITAL STAGE The final stage in Freud's model is the *genital stage,* which follows the latency stage and continues throughout the life span. During this stage, adolescents and adults solidify their personal identities, develop caring and altruistic feelings toward others, establish positive loving and sexual relationships, and progress in successful careers. Each stage builds on and integrates the growth and learning of the previous stage and ideally results in the development of an emotionally healthy adult.

Levels of Consciousness

Most people have few, if any, memories of times before the age of 3 or 4. In addition, we all have had experiences we either cannot recall at all or that only come into awareness when something reminds us of them, triggering their recall. What has happened to those memories?

According to Freud, we have three levels of consciousness: the conscious, the preconscious, and the unconscious. The *conscious* is material in awareness, always available to us. The *preconscious* holds information that may not be part of current awareness but which can be readily accessed. This material may be benign, such as the memory of a person we knew years ago but do not think of until we see her again in the grocery store; or it may be aversive, such as the memory of a car accident that returns to us each time we hear the screech of car brakes applied in a hurry. The *unconscious* holds memories that are highly charged, including repressed drives and impulses (such as a child's sexual feelings toward a parent) and recollections of experiences that may be too painful or unacceptable to be allowed into the conscious or preconscious. Freud believed that the unconscious held many times more memories than were in the preconscious or the conscious. Psychoanalysis can bring memories from the unconscious into the conscious. However, without benefit of therapy, those memories may either remain in the unconscious or emerge into consciousness in symbolic or distorted ways, perhaps via dreams or symptoms.

Dreams and Other Reflections of the Unconscious

Freud believed that dreams, symptoms, and errors all reflect the unconscious and its fantasies. His writings, "Psychopathology of Everyday Life" (1938) and "The Interpretation of Dreams" (1938), discuss in depth the process by which the unconscious is revealed. Freud believed that all dreams are meaningful and that dream analysis may be the most important way to understand people. He viewed dreams as fulfilling wishes or impulses that could not be allowed into awareness, providing a vehicle for working through disturbing thoughts and feelings. Although people may recall the manifest content of dreams, the defenses of the ego displace and condense the underlying significance of a dream so that it is disguised. Unconscious events and emotions may be represented in dreams by items or experiences that seem unimportant but may nevertheless cause anxiety because of their latent meaning.

For Freud, errors, omissions, slips, and poorly performed tasks also had latent meaning, and the term *Freudian slip* has come to mean a misstatement that reveals an unconscious wish or feeling. For example, a man who was attracted to his next-door neighbor, a woman called Lou, left her a note about a package that had been delivered to him by mistake. However, he addressed the note to "Dear Love" rather than "Dear Lou."

Defense Mechanisms

Many of us have experienced frequent and painful episodes of anxiety. According to Freud, people have an innate drive toward reduction of tension and anxiety. Freud was particularly interested in what he labeled *signal anxiety,* the anxiety that results from a conflict between internal wishes or drives and constraints that come from either internalized prohibitions or external reality. He believed that signal anxiety would automatically trigger ego defense mechanisms, usually learned during early childhood and developed as a way of dealing with inner conflict, anxiety, pain, shame, sorrow, and other negative emotions.

Everyone has defenses. Some are healthy, mature defenses that promote adjustment and enable people to transform undesirable wishes into ones that can be fulfilled. For example, sublimation is a defense mechanism that can change a self-destructive sexual desire into the drive to create a work of art. On the other hand, some defenses distort reality and interfere with efforts to build relationships. An example is splitting, in which people view themselves and others as being either all good or all bad and vacillate from idealization to devaluation of themselves and others. Which defense mechanism people use at a particular time depends on their level of development and the degree of anxiety they are experiencing.

The literature identifies and describes more than 40 defense mechanisms. These have been categorized in various ways including the following:

- ***Primary vs. Secondary Defense Mechanisms***—Primary or fundamental defense mechanisms include repression and denial, which keep unacceptable thoughts or impulses from consciousness. Secondary defense mechanisms are outgrowths of the primary ones; examples are projection, sublimation, and reaction formation.
- ***Relationship to Developmental Stage***—Defense mechanisms associated with the oral stage include primitive defenses such as denial and distortion. Regression, undoing, and reaction formation are some of the defense mechanisms linked to the anal stage. Most sophisticated defense mechanisms are associated with later stages of development. For example, intellectualization has been associated with the phallic stage, and sublimation with the latency stage.
- ***Psychotic vs. Neurotic Defenses***—Psychotic defenses are most likely to be evident in children, in dreams, and in people with psychotic disorders. Examples include distortion, denial, and delusional projection, all of which reflect a loss of contact with reality. Neurotic defenses are far more common, although they, too, are typically associated with emotional difficulties. Among these defenses are rationalization, intellectualization, and displacement.
- ***Immature vs. Healthy Defenses***—Immature defenses are common in adolescents as well as in people with mood, personality, and impulse control disorders. Included in this group are such defenses as projection, splitting, and acting out. On the other hand, examples of healthy defenses are humor, altruism, sublimation, and conscious suppression.

The following is a list of some of the most common defense mechanisms, along with brief definitions (American Psychiatric Association, 2000):

Healthy, Adaptive Defense Mechanisms

- ***Affiliation***—turning to others for help and support, but retaining responsibility for one's own difficulties
- ***Altruism***—deriving satisfaction from investing heavily in helping others

- ***Anticipation***—reducing anxiety by considering the probable consequences of future events and finding ways to address them effectively
- ***Humor***—focusing on the amusing aspects of situations
- ***Sublimation***—redirecting potentially harmful emotions or impulses into socially acceptable ones
- ***Suppression***—intentionally avoiding paying attention to nonproductive and troubling issues, experiences, and emotions.

Immature or Potentially Maladaptive Defense Mechanisms

- ***Acting Out***—exhibiting negative behaviors rather than using thoughts or emotions to deal with a situation
- ***Avoidance***—refusing to deal with troubling situations or experiences
- ***Denial***—refusing to acknowledge an aspect of reality that is evident to others
- ***Displacement***—transferring strong feelings from the situation in which they originated to a less threatening situation (e.g., expressing anger toward one's dog rather than one's supervisor)
- ***Dissociation***—temporarily disconnecting from a situation via memory loss or loss of awareness
- ***Help-rejecting Complaining***—constantly complaining and requesting help, which is then rejected when offered
- ***Idealization***—exaggerating the positive and ignoring the negative aspects of a person or situation
- ***Identification***—modeling oneself after another person in order to gain approval
- ***Intellectualization***—avoiding emotions by focusing on thoughts and abstractions
- ***Isolation***—disconnecting thoughts and emotions
- ***Passive aggression***—expressing anger and hostility in indirect ways (e.g., "accidentally" breaking a person's heirloom vase)
- ***Projection***—attributing one's own unacceptable thoughts, emotions, or actions to another
- ***Rationalization***—justifying one's choices in self-serving but invalid ways
- ***Reaction Formation***—replacing unacceptable thoughts and emotions with their opposite to overcompensate
- ***Regression***—reverting to a lower developmental level in thoughts, emotions, and behavior
- ***Repression***—relegating disturbing thoughts and feelings to the unconscious rather than dealing with them effectively
- ***Resistance***—blocking memories, insights, or avenues to positive change
- ***Somatization***—channeling conflicts into physical symptoms
- ***Splitting***—perceiving the self and others as either all good or all bad
- ***Undoing***—negating or invalidating unacceptable thoughts, emotions, or actions.

The study of people's use of defense mechanisms is a fruitful line of inquiry today and provides insight into ways in which clinicians can help people cope with anxiety and other emotional difficulties. Research suggests that the construct of defense mechanisms is relevant across cultures and religions (Tori & Bilmes, 2002).

TREATMENT USING CLASSIC PSYCHOANALYSIS

Extensive supervision and training are required to master the rich array of treatment strategies associated with classic psychoanalysis. This text presents an overview of these strategies, but readers should bear in mind that additional training is needed before they can be used skillfully.

Goals of Psychoanalysis

The overall goal of psychoanalysis is to achieve equilibrium between the id and the superego. The ego must be strong enough to handle the demands of living, "and not be overwhelmed by guilt, shame, or nervous anxiety" (Austad, 2009, p. 69). It is through the process of working through that the ego is transformed. Specific treatment objectives include the following:

- Improving the ego's conscious and mature control over irrational and harmful impulses and instincts
- Enriching the nature and variety of the ego defense mechanisms so that they are more effective, mature, and adaptable
- Encouraging development of perspectives that are grounded in an accurate and clear assessment of reality and that promote adjustment
- Developing a capacity for healthy and rewarding intimate relationships along with the ability to express oneself in rewarding ways
- Reducing the perfectionism, rigidity, and punitiveness of the superego.

Freud's writings offer a rich array of approaches to achieving these goals.

Therapeutic Alliance

Psychoanalysis, as performed by Freud as well as by contemporary therapists, usually is a long-term, intensive process. People are typically seen for treatment from two to five times a week for 3 to 5 years. Freud advocated having the patient lie on a couch while the therapist sat in a chair positioned behind the patient's head so the therapist could not be observed during the session. This was designed to both relax and reduce distractions for the patient and to allow the therapist to remain as anonymous as possible. Therapist neutrality is important in fostering the development of transference.

Although clients do most of the talking in psychoanalysis, therapists actively guide the sessions in meaningful directions and promote the uncovering of repressed material. They can be described as listening with a third ear attuned to underlying meanings, symbols, contradictions, and important omissions that may point the way to unlocking the unconscious. Questions, interpretations, and free association are common interventions that psychoanalysts use in their work.

Transference and Countertransference

In transference the client projects onto the therapist characteristics of another person, usually a parent, and reacts to the therapist as though he or she really does possess those characteristics. Transference involves a distortion or misperception of the therapist and is not a direct response to the way the therapist actually is. The unobserved and neutral psychoanalyst is more likely to elicit transference reactions than is a therapist who engages in self-disclosure and interacts more actively with clients.

Transference can be positive, negative, or mixed. For example, a client may project onto the therapist the seductive but loving traits of his mother (mixed), the angry and rejecting attitude of his father (negative), or the warm and nurturing characteristics of his grandmother (positive). Freud saw the establishment of transference as a key component of successful treatment. Processing clients' working through of the transference is an important source of personal growth.

Three stages are involved in the lengthy process of working through a transference. Once the transference develops, it is further established and explored in order to elicit repressed material. Gradually, the original dysfunctional pattern reemerges, now in terms of the transference to the therapist. Finally, the origins of the transference are understood and resolved, strengthening the ego and freeing the client to relate to others in healthier ways.

In classical psychoanalysis, countertransference, the clinician's feelings about the client, was to be avoided. Clearly, therapists were instructed not to respond to a client's transferential feelings of love, as in the case of Anna O., a client who developed an erotic transference to Freud's colleague, Breuer (Freud, 1915, 1925). Freud wrote that clients can experience both positive (erotic or love) transference and negative (angry or hostile) transference as a result of the therapeutic process, and clinicians should recognize the distinction between the client's transference and their own reactions to the client, which spring from the clinician's unresolved issues. Clinicians should not assume that they are too skilled or insightful to develop countertransference reactions, but should carefully monitor any strong emotional reactions they have to clients for the possibility of countertransference. The importance of clinicians having an awareness of their reactions is one of the primary reasons personal analysis is a required part of training in psychoanalysis.

Today, many psychoanalytic and other theoretical orientations pay attention to countertransference, as a therapist's natural response to a client. Countertransference is used to help the therapist understand the client and help provide a corrective emotional experience. In all forms of therapy, the therapist must be aware of countertransferential feelings toward the client and avoid inappropriate reactions. Therapists learn to seek consultation, supervision, or personal psychotherapy if necessary, as part of a lifelong process of screening their own countertransferential feelings. Therapeutic use of countertransference will be discussed in greater detail in Chapter 5.

Free Association

Freud used many approaches to access repressed material, including analysis of dreams and transference as well as free association. The process of free association reflects the most important rule of psychoanalysis: People should say whatever comes into their minds without censoring or judging. Free association is the automatic linking of one thought to another, which we all experience. We may hear a song that reminds us of the dance we attended when we first heard it, reminding us of our date for the dance, reminding us of the rage a parent expressed when we returned home after curfew, reminding us of the beatings we received from that parent, reminding us of our repressed impulse to attack the parent. A song, then, through a chain of association, can bring up strong feelings of anxiety because of its link to emotions that we have been unable to accept and process successfully. Freud encouraged free association in his patients to facilitate their recall of past material and release intense feelings. Blocks in the chain of association are another source of information about repressed material.

Abreaction

Although Freud placed primary emphasis on uncovering repressed material, he also recognized the importance of emotions, discussed in depth in Part 3 of this book. He believed that affect needs to accompany the recall of past material in order for people to successfully understand and work through the importance that material has for them. To facilitate this link between emotions and the recall of repressed information, Freud often encouraged abreaction in his patients. Abreaction entails recalling a painful experience that had been repressed, working through that painful experience and the conflicts it created by reliving in memory the experience and its associated emotions, analyzing that experience, and achieving an emotional release as the culmination of that process. This technique is used today not only in psychoanalytic treatment but also in other treatment approaches that help people cope with strong emotional reactions to past events.

Interpretation and Analysis

The most fundamental techniques in Freudian psychotherapy are analysis and interpretation, and they are designed to promote awareness and insight. Whether his focus was on dreams, slips, transference, free association, or symptoms, the tools of analysis and interpretation enabled Freud to bring unconscious material into consciousness. Once this had occurred, people could gain insight into and work through previously repressed material and make connections between that material and their present difficulties, resulting in positive change.

Analysis is the process of thoroughly exploring and understanding the unconscious representations in the material people present in treatment. For example, in analyzing a dream, Freud would explore with the client the meaning of each item in the dream. The person would be encouraged to free-associate to the dream, to talk about both the emotions reflected in the dream and those experienced upon awakening and recalling the dream, and to discuss events in the recent past that might have triggered the dream. Emphasis would be on the wish fulfillment represented by the dream and on suggestions of repressed, unacceptable sexual or other urges.

Interpretation is the process of elucidating the unconscious meaning of the symbols in material that clients present and of linking those new insights to their present concerns and blocks. Cognitively and emotionally working through material previously housed in the unconscious enables people to understand the influence the past has had on them and to use the mature defenses and strategies of the ego to make choices that are wiser and freer of the negative impact of unconscious material.

APPLICATION AND CURRENT USE OF FREUDIAN PSYCHOANALYSIS

Freud himself recognized that his approach was only suitable for a limited group of people. In light of the length and depth of the psychoanalytic process, readers might be tempted to conclude that it is designed for only those people with severe mental disorders. In fact, the opposite is true.

Application to Diagnostic Groups

During Freud's time, mental disorders were categorized into two broad groups: psychoses and neuroses. *Psychoses* involve a loss of contact with reality, a significant disturbance in a person's ability to accurately perceive and interpret both internal and external experiences. Because they are likely to be experiencing delusions, hallucinations, and other perceptual distortions, people with psychoses and severe mental illnesses cannot engage in the sort of self-examination that is required in psychoanalysis. They are unlikely to benefit from this mode of treatment.

People with *neuroses,* on the other hand, experience disorders of thoughts, emotions, and behaviors that interfere with their capacity for healthy functioning. Although their defenses and difficulties may lead to some confusion and misunderstanding about the meaning of their experiences, they have a capacity to form relationships, can engage in productive analysis, and can distinguish dreams and fantasies from reality. In Freud's time, six major neuroses had been identified (Stafford-Clark, 1965):

1. Hysteria, now known as conversion disorder, involving a loss or disturbance of the senses or motor ability such as blindness or paralysis without medical cause
2. Anxiety states, including phobias and generalized anxiety disorders, both involving unreasonable fears
3. Obsessional disorders, now called obsessive-compulsive disorders, involving anxiety as well as repetitive thoughts and behaviors
4. Depression, especially the melancholic (nonreactive) type

5. Paranoid attitudes, comparable to today's paranoid personality disorder, involving pervasive suspiciousness, hypersensitivity, and sometimes jealousy
6. Sexual perversions, now called paraphilias.

Freud divided the neuroses into two categories: transference neuroses, which involved a conflict between the id and the ego; and narcissistic neuroses, involving a conflict between the superego and the ego. He believed that only transference neuroses (including the first four in the previous list) were treatable by psychoanalysis, although today most psychoanalysts view all nonpsychotic disorders as potentially treatable by psychoanalysis.

Application to Multicultural Groups

Many reasons exist for questioning the appropriateness of using traditional psychoanalysis with clients from a collectivist background. Psychoanalysis encourages anonymity in the therapist, and it seems to view the importance of self-satisfaction and individual development as greater than that of social and family involvement and dedication. With its emphasis on talk, analysis, and uncovering, psychoanalysis is a very Western or Eurocentric approach. A classical psychoanalytic approach may not be well accepted by people from other backgrounds and cultures and is generally not well accepted by people with strong spiritual or religious beliefs or by those from a collectivist societal context in which interdependence and group cohesion are valued. However, contemporary psychoanalysis, as influenced by relational psychoanalysis, indicates a shift from the fundamental two-person psychology to a social constructivist understanding of human relationships, which allows for more open dialogues about the spiritual lives of the patient.

In recent years, articles such as that of Tummala-Narra (2009) have explored spirituality and religion as part of identity formation from a contemporary psychoanalytic perspective, since both psychoanalysis and spirituality share the goal of a search for particular aspects of one's identity. In addition, from a collectivist viewpoint, Kakar (2006), a trained psychoanalyst of Indian descent, suggests that therapists can convey a cultural openness with their clients. Being aware of assumptions underlying the culture into which the therapist was born and the culture into which the therapist has been professionally trained can increase multicultural sensitivity. Practitioners of contemporary psychoanalysis recognize that people are a product of their life experiences and that the cultural background of the client and of the clinician must be taken into consideration.

Current Use of Freudian Psychoanalysis

Traditional psychoanalysis seems best suited to treatment of people with at least moderate ego strength who have already achieved some success and satisfaction in life via relationships and occupational and leisure activities. Such people are in reasonable contact with reality and, on the surface, may seem to lead normal lives and to be fairly functional. In fact, however, these people are significantly impaired by long-standing symptoms such as depression, anxiety, and sexual or physical symptoms without any identified medical cause. Their lives may be constricted, they may have repeated failures in relationships or work that are caused by their own self-destructive behaviors, they may have pervasive and harmful personality patterns, and they may not have succeeded in ameliorating their difficulties.

EVALUATION OF FREUDIAN PSYCHOANALYSIS

The continued attention to Freud's ideas reflects the important and enduring contributions of his work. Freud provided a solid foundation for future theorists who elaborated and expanded on his theories. Their contributions will be discussed in the remaining chapters in Part 2 of this text.

Limitations

Psychoanalysis does have limitations, many of which stem from its lengthy and costly format. In addition, the approach is not designed to help people with urgent concerns, may not pay adequate attention to multicultural dimensions, and says little about developing healthy adult lifestyles.

Unfortunately, despite his admission that his understanding of women was limited, Freud advanced some erroneous and harmful ideas about women. Because they typically are children's primary caregivers, he blamed mothers, and largely exonerated fathers, for their children's emotional distress (Enns, 1993). He distinguished between vaginal orgasm (experienced during intercourse) and clitoral orgasm and stated that vaginal orgasms reflected sexual maturity in women (Matlin, 1996). He suggested that women experience penis envy that can be at least partially resolved by giving birth. Freud seemed to view men as emotionally healthier than women (Bradley, 2007), whom he viewed as suffering from greater narcissism, masochism, shame, and envy. Even in the 1920s opposition erupted to Freud's explanation of female sexuality (Mitchell & Black, 1995). Many believed Freud had adopted a phallo-centric view and minimized the importance of female organs. Freud's theory on female sexuality considers women to be "essentially castrated men" (Moore, 2007, p. 321). Freud acknowledged that "in general our insight into the developmental processes in girls is unsatisfactory, incomplete, and vague" (p. 321). Freud's ideas of penis envy, castration anxiety, and the Oedipal complex "placed the possession of the phallus as the core of adult masculine identity" (Bradley, 2007, p. 67).

Dispelling these mistaken beliefs took many years and probably did harm to women. We now know that taking a holistic and family systems approach is essential in understanding the causes of children's distress; that only one type of orgasm exists, no matter how it is achieved; that any envy that girls and women experience toward males can stem from many factors including preferential treatment that they perceive males as receiving; and that men are not healthier overall than women. Indeed, Freud was guilty of observational bias, using the ". . . male life form as the norm" and trying "to fashion women out of a masculine cloth" (Gilligan, 1993, p. 6). Karen Horney (1950), one of the first female psychoanalysts, was also the first woman to challenge Freud's views publically. She dismissed the Oedipal conflict and suggested instead that it was really young boys who were jealous of women's ability to give birth. Horney, and the concept of womb envy, will be discussed in more depth in Chapter 5.

Reading about Freud's misconceptions about women may bring up feelings of anger, and you may tend to dismiss his entire theory. However, keep in mind that these misconceptions represent only a small fraction of Freud's ideas and that Freud lived in an era when women and their roles were very different from those of today. Freud always valued women, including his wife; his daughter Anna, who will be discussed later in this book; and his female patients, colleagues, and supporters. His later work advanced a more contemporary view of women, perceiving them as more personal and emotional in their decisions than men are and as having a more flexible superego.

The research substantiating the value of classic psychoanalysis is limited, partly because the lengthy and intense nature of the treatment means that each analyst works with only a small number of people and that each treatment process is unique. Some contend that psychoanalysis can never demonstrate its value because it does not lend itself to empirical research. However, there is a growing body of evidence for the effectiveness of long-term approaches in general, and psychodynamic approaches in particular. Shedler (2010) cites several studies in which clients who participated in long-term psychotherapy (50 to 150 sessions) not only improved, but continued to improve over time.

Long-term psychodynamic psychotherapies have been found to be effective in the treatment of borderline personality disorder (Levy, Wasserman, Scott, & Yeomans, 2012) and panic disorder (Levy & Ablon, 2012). A study by Cogan (2007) found that therapeutic goals such as symptom reduction, being able to work and love, and being "content in the face of life's challenges" (p. 206) made the difference between those who benefited from psychoanalysis and those who did not.

Fonagy and Target (2009) point out consistency between Freud's model of the unconscious and recent neurobiological research that indicates the conscious mind is just the tip of the iceberg and that most thoughts, feelings, and experiences are unconscious and out of awareness. Human consciousness does not understand or even know the underlying causes of maladaptive behavior. A developmental perspective of psychopathology appears to be correct. Longitudinal studies indicate that three-quarters of adults with mental disorders had diagnosable symptoms in childhood (Kim-Cohen et al., 2003).

Empirical evidence *is* available to support the efficacy of newer psychodynamic treatments that are based on psychoanalytic concepts (Shedler, 2010, 2012). These newer treatment approaches are of briefer duration and require fewer sessions than classic psychoanalysis. More will be said about contemporary psychodynamic theories in the following chapters.

Strengths and Contributions

Probably Freud's most important contribution is the profound impact his thinking had on our understanding of personality development. Most of us acknowledge the importance of childhood experiences, understand the major role that sexuality plays in development, recognize the powerful influence of parent figures in our lives, assume that dreams and slips are often meaningful, accept the existence of the unconscious, and acknowledge that internal conflicts commonly occur within the three structures of our personalities. We also recognize the healing power of the therapeutic relationship, believe that talk therapy can be a powerful vehicle for promoting positive change, and are optimistic that treatment can help most people to lead more productive and rewarding lives. Whether or not we agree with the psychoanalytic model of treatment or with an emphasis on infantile sexuality, Freud's profound contributions to our understanding of psychological development and knowledge of psychotherapy are undeniable. Although few readers will go on to become psychoanalysts, all will find that their conceptions of mental health and mental illness and their approaches to treatment are colored by their knowledge of Freudian psychoanalysis.

SKILL DEVELOPMENT: ANALYZING THE COUNTERTRANSFERENCE

Most of the chapters in this book provide a practical skill development section as well as a case illustration to demonstrate the application of the theory. We use the story of the Diaz family—Edie, Roberto, and their daughter Ava—who were introduced in Chapter 1, to illustrate the use of countertransference in psychodynamic psychotherapy. As noted in this chapter, Freud coined the concept of countertransference and considered it to be the therapists' transference of material from their own lives onto the client. Today, with the onset of more relational therapies, and the growing amount of research on both attachment and the therapeutic process, most psychodynamic psychotherapists use a broader definition of countertransference that includes the "normal" or expected responses of the therapist to the client.

Countertransference is a clinically meaningful experience that can provide the therapist with insight into the client's interpersonal dynamics and the reactions that others have to him or her. Psychodynamic psychotherapists who monitor their own countertransference feelings can often use this information in the service of the therapy, because it provides a rich source of clinical information about the client.

SKILL DEVELOPMENT: THE USE OF COUNTERTRANSFERENCE

Read the following excerpt from a session between Edie and her counselor. Think about the therapeutic relationship, the therapist's self-disclosure of countertransferential material, and how the disclosure might benefit or harm the therapeutic process. Notice what the clinician chooses to share, and what she holds back. The next exercise will give you the opportunity to discuss your observations.

Dialogue Demonstrating use of Countertransference

EDIE: I'm sorry I was late. I might have to leave early, also.

CLINICIAN: Is there a problem?

EDIE: No, I just have a lot of things going on.

CLINICIAN: Okay. Well, let's get started then.

EDIE: Things are so busy right now. Roberto and I are just like two ships passing. We really don't talk much anymore, and when we do it's about Ava. You know, arranging who's picking her up after school, or making sure she's eaten lunch, that type of thing.

CLINICIAN: So you feel like you and Roberto are drifting apart?

EDIE: I don't know if we were ever close to begin with. He's always on the computer. I told you he's a workaholic. I almost feel like he's abandoning me for his computer.

CLINICIAN: Abandoning is a pretty strong word.

EDIE: What would you call it? I'm married, but I'm home alone every night. I mean, he's there, but he's in the basement on his computer. I feel like he's left me for another woman, except his "woman" is his computer.

CLINICIAN: You sound pretty upset. Can you think of any other times when you've felt this way.

EDIE: (thinks for a minute) Umm . . . right after my parents separated. They'd been arguing a lot and I was only five when my dad finally left, but I remember feeling so abandoned (starts to cry softly). He just left me. How could he do that? He just walked out of my life one day and I didn't see him for six years. Every birthday, every holiday, I would get all hopeful the night before, anticipating that he would call the next day. But nothing. As the years went by, I just got used to it. Looking back now, at myself as a little girl, I think about Ava at that age. It was so devastating to me. To not be wanted by my father . . . I know how much I went through to have Ava, and leaving her is something I would never consider doing. I just don't know how my father could do that to me.

CLINICIAN: What were you feeling?

EDIE: Alone . . . abandoned . . . angry.

CLINICIAN: Like you feel now, when Roberto goes down to the computer room?

EDIE: Wow, yeah. That's exactly how I feel. Like he's leaving me. I get so angry at him.

CLINICIAN: But he's downstairs.

EDIE: Yeah . . . (thinking).

CLINICIAN: I wonder if the strong reaction you have when Roberto "abandons" you to the computer is related to the feelings you had as a little girl when your father left.

EDIE: Yeah, like I'm that little girl sitting on the sofa just waiting for him to come back.

CLINICIAN: Your father? Or Roberto?

EDIE: (gives a little laugh). Either. Both. I guess it's the same reaction, but I just realized that at least Roberto's working. It's not like he's out with another woman, or looking at porn or anything. He's actually working to make more money at his job, so he can provide more for us.

CLINICIAN: It doesn't sound like he's abandoning you.

EDIE: No. No, he's really not. I never thought of it that way before. He's really just trying to get ahead financially. Do you think this could be because of my dad walking out when I was five that I just think everyone is going to abandon me?

CLINICIAN: I'd be curious to know if there are other times you've felt that way.

EDIE: Well (smiling sheepishly). Actually, today before I came here. I wasn't really too busy this morning. I was late because I couldn't decide if I wanted to come here today. I didn't know if I could trust you, to tell my story to. I was afraid you'd be like that other therapist who canceled on me. That's why I said I might have to leave early. But I don't want to leave. I just realized something about myself. I guess I get really mad at people when I feel like they're abandoning me.

CLINICIAN: And what does your anger do?

EDIE: What do you mean?

CLINICIAN: When you get angry, how do people react? Do they get closer to you, or further apart.

EDIE: Oh, further apart. Nobody wants to be around me when I'm angry.

CLINICIAN: So your anger serves a purpose.

EDIE: I guess so. I guess it keeps people away from me.

CLINICIAN: And then you don't have to get close to them.

EDIE: Or feel vulnerable. It's kind of a vicious circle, isn't it? I want to be closer to Roberto, but when he gets on the computer at night to do work, I feel abandoned, so I get angry at him. Then he doesn't want to be around me, so he comes to bed late, and we don't talk.

CLINICIAN: Well, you've got a lot to think about this week.

In psychodynamic therapy, the "work" of the session is in helping the person work through childhood issues and feelings that might have been adaptive at that time (i.e., Edie getting angry at her father protected her from becoming depressed and overly sad), but that are not working now or are not truly applicable to the current situation. For instance, Roberto's workaholism, while distressing to Edie, is not a sign that he is abandoning her. Quite the contrary, he is working harder to support her and Ava. But Edie is reacting as if she were still 4 years old. The clinician gently suggests an interpretation, and because Edie was open to it, this allowed a dialogue that provided insight into how her past relationships were affecting her current relationship, including the here and now of her feelings toward the therapist.

Exercise

1. Discuss the dialogue you just read. Consider the following dimensions of this clinician's intervention: timing, purpose, content, impact on the client–clinician relationship, overall effectiveness. What would you have done differently to improve this intervention? Now imagine what the effect on Edie would have been if the clinician had chosen not to disclose her countertransferential feelings. Would Edie have benefited? Why or why not? How might it have impacted the therapeutic relationship if the therapist had remained silent? How would Edie have changed in her relationship with Roberto?
2. Sometimes the use of countertransference may be almost inseparable from the clinician's work as a therapist. In the above scenario, the therapist was actively working to help Edie recognize the differences between her childhood feelings and those she had as an adult. What if Edie's relationship with Roberto had been harmful? Would the therapist still have proceeded? How directive should the therapist be?

EXERCISES

Large-Group Exercises

1. Make a critical assessment of Freud's theory. What do you think of the underlying concepts (the unconscious, id, ego, superego, defense mechanisms)? What positive (or negative) contributions did Freud make to the field? What, if anything, is lacking in his theory? How does long-term psychoanalysis fit in with today's world?
2. Critique Freud's drive theory. Do you agree that all instincts are either life instincts (basic survival, pleasure, reproduction, love) or death instincts (self-destructive behaviors, masochism, aggression, violence). Do you think his ideas are applicable today?
3. Review the list of ego defense mechanisms provided earlier in this chapter. Identify two or three defense mechanisms that you believe would characterize Edie's way of coping with anxiety. Identify two or three defense mechanisms that you believe would characterize Roberto's way of coping with anxiety. Be sure to provide a rationale for your conclusions.

Small-Group Exercises

Form into your groups of two dyads. Each dyad should take a turn conducting an interview on early childhood experiences, with one person in the dyad being the interviewer, the other the interviewee. Spend 10 to 15 minutes asking your partner about his or her recollections of any or all of the following:

- Being fed by a caregiver
- Being toilet trained
- Developing an identification with the same-sex parent or caregiver
- Early experiences of independence and taking initiative.

After each role-play, group members should give the interviewer some feedback, using the guidelines given in the preface. Feedback should include (but not be limited) to (1) use of questions, (2) ability to elicit information, (3) client–clinician rapport, and (4) eye contact and other nonverbal behaviors.

Be sure to take care of yourself during this exercise and during all exercises in this book. You can choose what you do or do not want to reveal about your early childhood experiences. If you find strong emotions or troubling memories coming up for you, be cautious about sharing them. Remember that this is an exercise, not a counseling session. If any exercises are very troubling for you, consider the possibility that counseling might help you better understand and handle those feelings.

Individual Exercises

1. Now that you have an understanding of the three structures of the personality—the id, the superego, and the ego—you can be more aware of the dynamics of some of your inner conflicts. Write briefly about a time when you experienced a conflict between your id and your superego and how you resolved that conflict.
2. We all make mistakes, make slips, and forget commitments. Try to be more conscious of these processes in your own life for the next week. Each time you notice one of these errors, think about whether it is a random occurrence or whether it might reflect a wish or another psychological process.

Summary

This chapter reviewed psychoanalytic theory and strategies as developed by Sigmund Freud. It also provided information about Freud's background and on the development of his concepts, which form the foundation for modern conceptions of psychological development, mental health, and the treatment of mental disorders. Freud's theory is based on instincts—all instincts are either life or death drives—eros, thanatos, and libido. It emphasizes the three structures of the personality (id, superego, and ego), the five stages of psychosexual development (oral, anal, phallic, latency, and genital), defense mechanisms, and levels of consciousness (unconscious, preconscious, and conscious). Treatment focuses on promoting insight by analysis of dreams and other clues to the unconscious; interpretation, working through, and abreaction; and the analysis of transference and countertransference.

Recommended Readings

Freud, S. (1938). *The basic writings of Sigmund Freud* (A. A. Brill, Trans.). New York, NY: Modern Library.

Higdon, J. (2012). *Psychodynamic theory for therapeutic practice* (2nd ed.) New York, NY: Palgrave Macmillan.

Jones, E. (1953, 1955, 1957). *The life and works of Sigmund Freud* (3 vols.). New York, NY: Basic Books.

Roth, M. S. (Ed.) (1998). *Freud: Conflict and culture.* New York, NY: Alfred A. Knopf.

Stafford-Clark, D. (1965). *What Freud really said.* New York, NY: Schocken.

Additional Sources of Information

http://www.apsa.org—Website of the American Psychoanalytic Association (a good resource for information on training in psychoanalysis) and the *Journal of the American Psychoanalytic Association.*

http://www.psychoanalysis.org.uk/ijpa—Website of the International Journal of Psychoanalysis.

http://www.ipa.org.uk—Website of the International Psychoanalytical Association, which is based in England.

http://www.psychoanalysis.org—The New York Psychoanalytic Society and Institute publishes the *Journal of Clinical Psychoanalysis.*

CHAPTER 4

Alfred Adler and Individual Psychology

Alfred Adler moved away from Freud's sphere of influence to focus on psychosocial rather than psychosexual underpinnings of human behavior. Adler called his own theory of human development *Individual Psychology*, to reflect the unique beliefs and skills that each person develops from early childhood and that serve as a reference for their attitudes, behaviors, and private view of self, others, and society.

Adler's ideas are compatible with current thinking about mental health. Adlerian therapy pays considerable attention to social context, family dynamics, and child rearing. This approach is phenomenological, empowering, and oriented toward both present and future. As a result, Adler's ideas are currently viewed as an important approach to psychotherapy, especially for clinicians working with children and their families.

ALFRED ADLER

Alfred Adler was born on February 7, 1870, in Vienna, Austria, the third of six children. His father, Leopold Adler, was a merchant. Alfred Adler had a difficult childhood. When he was 3 years old, a brother died in the bed they shared (Orgler, 1963). Adler himself was prone to accidents and illnesses. Twice he was run over in the streets; he had pneumonia, suffered from rickets and poor eyesight, and was sickly and delicate. Because of his medical problems, Adler was pampered, especially by his mother. However, when his younger brother was born, Adler felt dethroned as his mother shifted her attention from him to her new baby. This led Adler to transfer his attention to his father and to his peers, from whom he learned "courage, comradeliness, and social interest" (Orgler, 1963, p. 3). Adler's subsequent interest in birth order, inferiority, and parental overprotectiveness may have originated in his own childhood experiences.

Adler was initially not a good student; a teacher suggested that Adler's father apprentice his son to a shoemaker rather than encourage his academic pursuits. However, Adler subsequently became a strong student, demonstrating in his own life that people can change their goals and their lives. From childhood on, Adler was interested in psychology and social issues. Even in his first professional position (as an eye specialist) after he completed medical school, Adler was interested in the total person; he sought to understand the connection between mental and physical processes and their impact on people's work and social lives. Adler found his next position as a general physician more rewarding because it meshed with his beliefs. However, he was troubled by feelings of helplessness when treating people with terminal illnesses. This led Adler to another career change; he entered the field of neurology while continuing to study psychology and social science in an effort to understand people more fully.

Adler's insights into personality development brought him recognition in his field and probably helped capture Freud's attention. In 1902, Freud wrote to Adler and several other leaders in the fields of neurology and psychology, suggesting they meet to discuss his work. This led to Adler's involvement in the Vienna Psycho-Analytical Society.

Descriptions of Adler's personal style are mixed. Orgler's (1963) research suggests that Adler was warm and friendly, whereas Jones (1955), Freud's biographer, described Adler as "morose, cantankerous, contentious, and sulky" (p. 130). Perhaps these descriptions reflect aspects of Adler's personality as well as his displeasure with Freud's belief that sexual impulses are basic determinants of psychological development.

This rift finally led Adler to separate himself from the Psycho-Analytical Society, where he had achieved power and leadership, to form the Society for Individual Psychology. His work for the rest of his life had the goals of deepening his understanding of people and finding better ways to help them. Adler's strong social interest prompted him to write and speak on child rearing and educational practices; establish child guidance clinics in the Viennese public schools; and initiate programs to train teachers, social workers, physicians, and other professionals in ways to promote children's mental health. Using live demonstrations and writing books for the general public, he made his ideas and techniques accessible to a wide audience, which was important to him. His wife Raissa, described as a "strong feminist and political activist," was an ardent supporter of Adler's social activism (Sherman & Nwaorgu, 2002, p. 181). Beginning in the 1920s, Adler traveled frequently to the United States, where he generated considerable interest in his ideas. His tireless involvement in his work continued until his death. On May 28, 1937, while preparing for a lecture in Scotland, he died of a heart attack.

THE DEVELOPMENT OF INDIVIDUAL PSYCHOLOGY

Adler's professional development falls roughly into four time periods. The first phase of his career followed his completion of medical school. Neither his initial work as a physician nor his subsequent work in neurological research seemed right for him, although he made contributions in both areas. His great interest was the mind rather than the body.

When he joined forces with Freud to further the field of psychoanalysis, Adler entered the second phase and seemed, at least temporarily, to have found his place. His focus finally was on promoting healthy emotional development. However, before long, he felt stifled by the apparent rigidity of some of Freud's beliefs and his limited interest in the whole person.

Adler's disengagement from Freud signaled the third period in his professional development. This freed Adler to move forward with his own ideas. According to Ansbacher and Ansbacher (1956), Adler replaced "biological, external, objective causal explanation with psychological, internal, subjective causal explanation" (p. 9). He replaced the concept of the sexual drive and the libido with the drive to gain power, superiority, and become a fully functioning adult. The goal of Adler's Individual Psychology was to comprehend and help the unique individual, a departure from what he perceived as Freud's overgeneralized ideas.

A final stage in Adler's career came after his service as a psychiatrist in World War I. Seeing the bonds among soldiers during their war experiences convinced him that the drive toward social interest was even stronger than the drive for superiority and power. He proposed that people's basic motivation is "an innate predisposition for social interest" (Grey, 1998, p. 8) and viewed people as driven primarily by needs for significance, self-worth, and social involvement. Adler's thinking moved in directions that are compatible with what many now view as the fundamental purpose of therapy: to help people feel empowered and self-actualized and build rewarding social involvement and relationships.

IMPORTANT THEORETICAL CONCEPTS

Adler's theories, like Freud's, have considerable depth and richness. Adler's concepts emphasize the unity and uniqueness of each individual. He believed that understanding people grew from knowledge of their goals and drives, their family constellations, their private logic, their social contexts, and their styles of life. According to Adler, people are not victims of biology or circumstance but can choose to change both their goals and their behaviors. Adler shared Freud's belief that much of what determines the direction of people's lives is unconscious and needs to be analyzed to bring their goals and lifestyles into conscious awareness.

View of Human Nature

Adler, like Freud, acknowledged the importance of the first 5 years of life in influencing people's future development. However, Adler's view was less deterministic. He believed that biological and physiological factors provided probabilities for future growth but that "the self, with creative power as part of its inner nature, is the important intervening variable" (Ansbacher & Ansbacher, 1956, p. 179).

For Adler, those characteristics of the person that were determined by heredity and early upbringing were less important than what the person made of them. He believed that behavior is purposeful and goal directed, and that we can channel our behavior in ways that promote growth. Adler believed that what matters to people is developing and working to achieve meaningful and rewarding goals, along with a lifestyle that leads to a positive sense of ourselves, connectedness to other people and our communities, and satisfying work (Adler, 1963a).

The Importance of Feelings of Inferiority

Striving to achieve superiority is an important element of Adlerian theory. Not to be superior over others, but to achieve mastery in one's own life and to overcome feelings of inferiority, becomes a goal as strong as Freud's drive theory, and Carl Rogers's theory of self-actualization. Adler (1963b) believed that feelings of inferiority during the early childhood years have a great impact on development. Nearly all children experience these feelings, perceiving themselves as small and powerless in relation to their parents and older siblings. How young children are treated and how they deal with their feelings of inferiority are important in shaping them. It is through mastering an issue, through the attainment of superiority, that one achieves a sense of accomplishment. Human beings create their own internalized goals and then strive to meet them. Through effort, improvement, success, and completion, they live up to their own high standards. Every person has an internalized ideal self they are trying to live up to. This striving for superiority is an attempt to overcome feelings of inferiority.

Adler developed this theory after his own struggle to overcome multiple childhood illnesses. He believed children who succeed in reducing their feelings of difference and inferiority by building their strengths and abilities, making wise and creative choices, and striving in healthy ways toward growth and power are likely to develop in positive ways. On the other hand, children who are pampered or neglected and whose efforts toward empowerment are thwarted are far less likely to experience positive growth and development. Adler believed that pampered children often grow up expecting others to care for them and so do not develop their own resources, while neglected children may become discouraged and hopeless when their efforts to overcome an inferior role are ignored or rejected.

Individual efforts to overcome inferiority can have an impact on a person's overall lifestyle. For instance, a child who cannot compete in sports with his older brother who is physically stronger and more mature, may choose instead to stay home and study, ultimately surpassing his brother in academic ability. Similarly, a middle child who cannot keep up with her popular and successful older sister may elect instead to drop out, look at alternative lifestyles, and become the leader of a Wiccan community. It is through the attainment of superiority, regardless of venue, that one achieves mastery, achievement, and life satisfaction.

Family Constellation and Birth Order

Adler paid considerable attention to other early influences on development including family constellations and birth order. This is in keeping with Adler's emphasis on the social nature of human problems. He believed that, through an examination of the family constellation, we can understand people's lifestyles. Conversely, by understanding their outlooks on life, we can understand the roles people have in their families (Dreikurs, 1973).

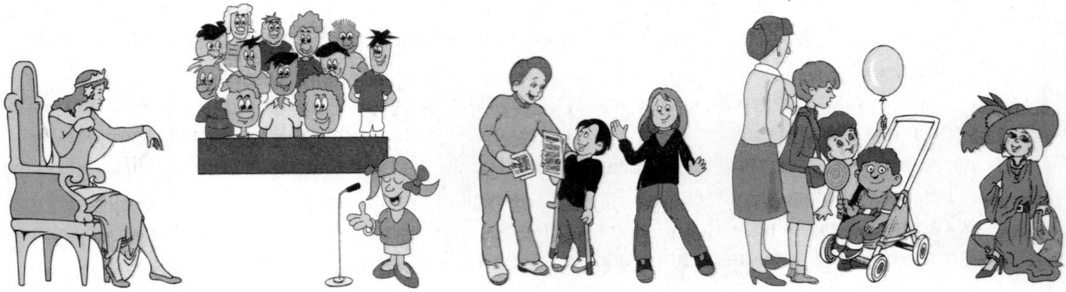

FIGURE 4.1 Birth Order Examples.

A person's family constellation includes the composition of the family, each person's roles, and the reciprocal transactions that a person has, during the early formative years, with siblings and parents. The child is not a passive recipient of these transactions; rather, children influence how parents and siblings respond to them. Each child comes to play a role in the family that is determined by the interactions and transactions within that family (Adler, 1963b).

Children are affected by both their similarities to and differences from their families. According to Adler, siblings who are most different from us influence us most. That difference gives us the opportunity to compare and contrast ourselves with others, see new possibilities, and rethink the choices and roles we have taken on in our own lives.

Birth order is another aspect of families that, according to Adler (1963b), has a profound impact on development. Five psychological positions in the family, described by Adler, and characteristics believed to be associated with each position (see Figure 4.1) are as follows:

1. *Oldest children* tend to be the most intelligent and achieving of the five groups. Their verbal skills are especially strong. Firstborns, who initially grow up in a family of adults, tend to be dependable, well organized, and responsible. They generally are well behaved and cooperative, conforming to societal expectations and being fairly traditional. Their many strengths often help them attain positions of leadership.

While firstborns are the only child in the family, they tend to be the center of attention and sometimes are spoiled. However, when siblings are born, oldest children tend to feel dethroned and may feel threatened, angry, fearful, and jealous in response to losing their special role as only child. Dealing successfully with the birth of a sibling can help firstborns to become more affiliative and self-confident. Laird and Shelton (2006) found that in later years a significant number of firstborns had developed substance abuse problems, which they related to loss of attention and the need to oversee their younger siblings.

2. The *second child* feels pressure to catch up and compete with the oldest child. Because second-born children usually realize they cannot outdo the successes the firstborn has already achieved, they gravitate toward endeavors in which the older sibling is either unskilled or uninterested. A common pattern is for a firstborn to excel in a traditional area such as English or mathematics and for the second-born to seek success in a more creative and less conventional area such as singing or drawing and to emphasize social rather than academic success. The more successful the firstborn, the more likely it is that the second-born will move in directions opposite to those of the typically well-behaved and achievement-oriented firstborn. Second-born children tend to be more caring, friendly, and expressive than their older siblings.

3. The *middle child* is often the second child and is likely to manifest many of the strengths of the second-born. However, some middle children feel squeezed between older children who have already found their place and younger children who seem to receive more love and attention. Middle children sometimes have difficulty finding a way to become special and can become discouraged, viewing themselves as unloved and neglected. This pattern is usually less evident in large families where two or more children share the role of middle child but is particularly likely in families with only three children. With encouragement and positive parenting, however, middle children often become well adjusted, friendly, creative, and ambitious, prizing their individual strengths.

4. *Youngest children* encounter three common pitfalls: They may be pampered and spoiled by the rest of the family, they may feel a need to go at top speed at all times just to keep up with their older siblings, and they may become discouraged about competing with their brothers and sisters. Decisions may be made for them, and they may not need to take on much responsibility for themselves or others. Adler expressed concern that these children would experience strong feelings of inferiority. However, last-born children also can acquire considerable power in the family and thrive on the special attention they receive. They often become adventurous, easygoing, empathic, sociable, and innovative. They typically pursue interests that are all their own to avoid competition with siblings. Their most likely ally is the oldest, who also has feelings of being different.

5. *Only children* have much in common with both firstborn and last-born children. They seek achievement like firstborns and usually enjoy being the center of attention like the youngest. They may become pampered and spoiled, focusing only on their own needs, but also may integrate the achievement orientation of the firstborn with the creativity of later-born children. Because other family members are all adults, these children typically mature early and learn to cooperate and deal well with adults. However, if their parents are insecure, only children may adopt parental worries and insecurities.

Research has validated many of Adler's assumptions about the impact of birth order on personality, but some discrepant results suggest the importance of caution when drawing conclusions about the connections between personality and birth order (Grey, 1998; Herrera, Zajonc, Wieczorkowska, & Cichomski, 2003; Lombardi, 1996; Parker, 1998). Variables within families can have a complex impact on these patterns. For example, when twins are born, families tend to treat one child as older than the other, artificially determining their birth order. When a firstborn is a girl or is impaired in some way, families may inadvertently promote the second child into the position of firstborn. High expectations will be held for that child, while the firstborn will be treated like a second-born. Large families may operate as though they have more than one group of children, with each group having a child who functions as the oldest, one who functions as the youngest, and children in the middle. This is especially likely in families in which many years separate groups of children. In addition, the way in which children respond to their positions will have an impact on their personalities and behaviors.

Clinicians should not stereotype people according to birth order. At the same time, exploring birth order and the influence it has on the development of an individual's personality can facilitate understanding of that person. Inventories such as the White-Campbell Psychological Birth Order Inventory (White, Campbell, & Steward, 1995) can facilitate accurate assessment of the impact birth order has had on a person.

Research on birth order has found a definite relationship between place in the family and some events that occur in life. Younger siblings, for instance, are more likely to engage in riskier behaviors than are firstborns (Sulloway & Zweigenhaft, 2010); middle children score higher in maladaptive perfectionism. Career choice and lifestyle themes, as measured by the BASIS-A Inventory, have also been found to be correlated with birth order (Ashby, LoCicero, & Kenny, 2003; Gfroerer, Gfroerer, & Curlette, 2003; Laird & Shelton, 2006; Rule & Bishop, 2005). All tend to support Adler's theory that a person's lifestyle is related to his or her place within the family.

Lifestyle

The composition and interactions of people's families exert the major influence on the development of their lifestyle, another important concept in Adler's theory. Grey (1998) views lifestyle as the most fundamental of Adler's concepts, describing it as "the sum total of all the individual's attitudes and aspirations, a striving which leads him in the direction toward his goal of believing he has significance in the eyes of others" (p. 37). Lifestyle is "the creative and created self" (Sherman & Nwaorgu, 2002, p. 183).

Similar to the personality or the self, lifestyle encompasses four ingredients: (1) the person's subjective worldview, including beliefs about the self and others, values, inner narratives, expectations, and attitudes; (2) goals; (3) behavioral strategies that the person uses to achieve goals and negotiate the life journey; and (4) the outcomes or consequences of those behaviors. Lifestyle can be assessed informally via exploration of these four areas or can be explored through the use of an inventory.

Lifestyle, then, is the unique way in which each of us seeks to find our place in the world, to overcome feelings of inferiority, and to achieve our goals. These goals nearly always involve achievement of significance, superiority, competence, and mastery. Each person has an image, usually unconscious, of what life will be like when those goals have been reached. Adler called this "fictional finalism" and believed that this goal is firmly established between the ages of 6 and 8 and remains constant throughout a person's life. Dreikurs (1973), who contributed greatly to Adler's work, described our private logic as the inner rationale we use for justifying our lifestyle and the way to achieve our goals.

Private Logic

Private logic is another of Adler's major constructs. Private logic, our beliefs about ourselves and our place in the world, is subjective and based on lifestyle. Adler quotes Seneca's admonition that everything depends on the view you take of it. Thus, private logic, no matter how faulty, provides a life pattern or "law of movement" that begins in childhood and provides a compass by which to live. If the idea is wrong, it will eventually be confronted by reality. The need (for superiority, for power, or to be aversive) does not change, rather the person's worldview or personal logic will contrive to drive his or her thinking and behavior (Adler, 1998).

Because we are part of a larger social system and must learn to interact with that system, we develop our own set of rules to help us to overcome our feelings of inferiority and achieve our goals. Consider, for example, a 4-year-old boy who does not want to put on his shoes, despite his mother's request to do so. The child evaluates the situation and knows he must cooperate with his mother and put on the shoes. But how can he do this without caving in to his mother's wishes and feeling inferior? Using his private logic, he comes up with a solution and tells his mother to close her eyes. His private logic is telling him that if she closes her eyes and does not see him putting on the shoes, she will not have gained the upper hand, and he will not feel inferior for having lost the battle.

Private logic is unique to each person—and is not always logical! Those who lack social interest can become disconnected from society, experience anxiety about group interactions, and fear rejection. These feelings of inferiority can cause a self-focus that leads to neurosis, psychosis, addictions, and an inability to cope in the world. In the case of the psychopath, we can see the result of erroneous private logic in uncooperativeness, social isolation or withdrawal, and antisocial personality.

The goal in Adlerian therapy is to understand a person's private logic to help the person better understand where his or her beliefs get in the way of daily functioning, to lessen the faulty thinking of private logic, and to help people change its framework to see things in a more healthy way. Private logic is unique and feelings of superiority or fear of inferiority are meaningful only to the individual. The person is responsible for how he or she achieves the three tasks of life (work, love, and social interest; discussed below) and it is social interest that is the key component of developing a healthy lifestyle (Manaster, 2009).

Goals

Adler viewed the healthy, well-functioning adult as a person who is independent, emotionally and physically self-reliant, useful and productive, and able to cooperate with others for both personal and social benefit. Through psychotherapy and education, Adler sought to help people realize that feelings of pain and inadequacy are caused not by others but by their own faulty logic and the behaviors and attitudes that stem from that logic. By enabling people to become aware of their faulty logic; to establish healthy, realistic, and rewarding goals; and to align their lifestyles, their thinking, and their behavior with those goals, therapists can help people overcome their feelings of inferiority, dependency, and inordinate fears of failure. They can then develop the self-confidence and social interest that people need to achieve a healthier adjustment and a more rewarding lifestyle.

These concepts can be applied to Edie Diaz, the woman discussed throughout this book. Edie developed a guiding self-ideal, early in life, of being wife and mother in a caring and supportive family. Her short- and long-range goals all focused on that ideal as did many elements of her lifestyle. However, the abuse and neglect she experienced during childhood have made it difficult for her to overcome her feelings of inferiority; she does not know how to realize her goals, to become part of a family and community, and to appreciate herself. She is working, in counseling, to develop an effective private logic and lifestyle and to align her lifestyle with her self-ideal.

Social Interest

Adler had a clear idea of emotional health. He distinguished between well-adjusted and maladjusted people on the basis of their goals and their lifestyles. People who are well adjusted have a private logic that reflects common sense as well as social interest; they perceive themselves as part of a community and appreciate individual differences. Those who are maladjusted focus only on their own needs and fail to recognize the importance of their social context and the needs of others.

This idea reflects Adler's (1963a) belief that development can be explained primarily by psychosocial connections rather than psychosexual drives. He believed that people are, by nature, social beings interested in belonging to a group and desiring to solve the problems of their society. Through awareness that we are part of the human community, as well as through the development of social interest, our feelings of inferiority, alienation, and anxiety diminish; and we develop feelings of belonging and happiness. We no longer view ourselves as alone, seeking to diminish others to advance ourselves. Instead, we recognize that the goods and ills in our society all have an impact on us and that we can best achieve our own goals of significance and competence by contributing to the greater good. Adler's emphasis on social connectedness is very timely and congruent given the importance to clinicians of developing multicultural competence and appreciating diversity.

People's social interest is best reflected in their accomplishment of what Adler viewed as the three life tasks: occupation, love, and social interest (Adler, 1938). Social interest can be assessed by how successfully people are able to negotiate relationships, the degree of closeness they maintain in those relationships, and their connectedness and contributions to society. Although Freud acknowledged the importance of love and work, Adler (1938) added social interest, which he defined as "living in the fellowship, co-operation, humanity, or even the super ego" (p. 86), to the important areas of life. Although Adler viewed early childhood experiences as important in determining the nature of our social interest, he believed that social interest could be taught and developed in later life, conveying optimism not only for the individual but also for our society.

Phenomenological Perspective

Another viewpoint compatible with current thinking on human development and change is Adler's emphasis on a person's perception of reality, not what actually is or what others perceive. For Adler, the internal and subjective were more important than the external and objective. His theory can be thought of as *phenomenological,* meaning that he focused on a person's inner reality, the way that person perceived the world. Adler saw each person as a unique individual and believed that only by understanding that person's perceptions of the world, private logic, lifestyle, and goals can we really make sense of and know that person. This is the essence of Adler's Individual Psychology.

TREATMENT USING INDIVIDUAL PSYCHOLOGY

Adler's theory is an optimistic, growth oriented, and educational one. Adler believed that people could change their goals and lifestyles in order to achieve happier and more fulfilled lives. His ideas have endured because they draw on the important concepts of Freudian psychoanalysis; incorporate many elements of modern cognitive, behavioral, and humanistic treatment approaches; and add their own valuable and useful ideas. They also appeal to common sense.

Therapeutic Alliance

Adler departed from the ideas of Freud in his conception of the client–clinician relationship. Adler emphasized the importance of a cooperative interaction that involves establishment of shared goals as well as mutual trust and respect. This view is consistent with the aims of his treatment; he sought to foster responsibility and social interest and saw the establishment of a therapeutic relationship in which client and clinician collaborated to achieve goals they had formulated together as important in promoting client growth.

Clinicians following Adler's approach have a complex role that calls for the application of a broad range of skills. These clinicians are educators, fostering social interest and teaching people ways to modify their lifestyles, behaviors, and goals. They are analysts who identify faulty logic and assumptions. They explore and interpret the meaning and impact of clients' birth order, dreams, early recollections, and drives. They are role models, demonstrating ways to think clearly, search for meaning, collaborate with others, and establish and reach meaningful goals. And they are supportive and encouraging, urging clients to take risks and helping them accept their own mistakes and imperfections.

Thoughts and behaviors, as well as background, are primary targets of the Adlerian clinicians' efforts. Private logic, lifestyle, and the guiding self-ideal all stem from heredity and early experiences. Helping people understand these constructs can enable them to challenge and modify their beliefs and develop new and more rewarding goals, a modified lifestyle, and constructive and positive social interest and behaviors.

Stages of Treatment

Although they often merge and overlap, four treatment phases can be identified in Adler's model: (1) establishment of a collaborative therapeutic relationship and a shared view of the treatment goals; (2) assessment, analysis, and understanding of the person and the problem; (3) encouragement of change through interpretation; and (4) reorientation by turning insight into action and focusing on assets rather than weaknesses (Carlson, Watts, & Maniacci, 2006; Day, 2008).

PHASE 1: ESTABLISHING THE THERAPEUTIC RELATIONSHIP AND SETTING GOALS Adler was ahead of his time in emphasizing the importance of a positive therapeutic relationship. He advocated many of the approaches later described by Carl Rogers to build that relationship (see Chapter 8). Adler believed in the importance of true caring and involvement, the use of empathy, and both verbal and nonverbal techniques of listening to overcome the feelings of inferiority and fear that many clients bring with them into treatment. Initial questions explore clients' expectations for treatment, their views of their problems, how they have tried to improve their lives, and what has led them to seek treatment at the present time.

Encouragement is an essential component of this initial phase of treatment and is used throughout treatment to counter clients' discouragement. Sweeney (2009) described seven actions that can be used in counseling as well as in other relationships to provide encouragement:

- Focus on what people are doing rather than evaluate their performance. Asking "What did you do to pass all of your courses?" is more encouraging than "Did you get the best grades in your class?"
- Focus on the present more than the past or the future.
- Focus on behavior rather than the person. "Your careful driving really helped you deal with the sudden snowstorm" is more encouraging than "You're a great driver."
- Focus on the effort rather than the outcome. "Sounds like you really feel good about developing your skating skills" is more encouraging than "Sounds like your skills are almost good enough to make the team."
- Focus on motivation from within (intrinsic) rather than from the outside (extrinsic). "You must have felt a great sense of satisfaction, knowing that all your studying resulted in success on the bar exam" is more encouraging than "You finally passed the bar. Now you'll get that raise."
- Focus on what is being learned rather than the lack of learning. "What did you learn from this challenging relationship?" is more encouraging than "You really need to make better choices in your friends."
- Focus on what is positive rather than what is negative. "So the odds are on your side" is more encouraging than "So the physician said there is a forty percent chance that your disease will recur."

Counseling and psychotherapy offer clinicians many opportunities to encourage clients and to show them genuine caring and concern. A telephone call to a client in crisis, a note to a client in the hospital, sharing an article on home buying with a client who is purchasing a first home are all appropriate ways for clinicians to form partnerships with clients and provide support and encouragement.

As client and clinician build a collaborative, democratic, and trusting relationship, they can work together to formulate a clear statement of the problem, as well as meaningful and realistic goals. They also can discuss and negotiate agreement on the structure of the treatment process and the guidelines and procedures for their work.

PHASE 2: ASSESSMENT, ANALYSIS, AND UNDERSTANDING OF THE PERSON AND THE PROBLEM A distinctive feature of Adlerian therapy is the focus on in-depth assessment. For the first time in psychoanalysis, the importance of the family constellation on the individual's functioning was considered, along with birth order and earliest childhood recollections. Both the initial interview and the lifestyle interview provide detailed information about the client's current level of functioning and background leading up to the current distress (Carlson et al., 2006). In the initial interview, or what Adler (1956) referred to as "the general diagnosis," the clinician conducts a general assessment of six key domains: identifying information, background, current level of functioning, presenting problem, expectations for treatment, and summary. The goals of this phase of treatment are understanding clients' family background, lifestyles, private logic, and goals, and identifying self-destructive behaviors and faulty logic.

Lifestyle assessment. The more in-depth lifestyle assessment is one of the characteristic features of Adlerian theory and practice. The Life Style Interview (see Figure 4.2) is a semistructured

Following is an abbreviated list of the types of information that might be asked by an Adlerian therapist in a Life Style Interview to elicit background information and developmental influences impacting the style of life (Carlson et al., 2006). The first nine sections are related to the family constellation; the tenth section gathers early childhood recollections.
I. *Sibling Relationships.* Names and ages of siblings (in order of birth); relationship (as a child) with siblings; sibling behavior toward client; current relationship
II. *Physical Development.* Health; childhood growth
III. *School Experience.* Grades; relationship with teachers; attitudes toward school
IV. *Meanings Given to Life.* Religious beliefs; childhood fears, dreams, ambitions. If you could have changed anything from childhood what would you have changed?
V. *Sexual Development.* Attitudes toward sexuality, masturbation; questions of sexual abuse or sex play
VI. *Social Development.* Friendships (depth and breadth)
VII. *Parental Influences.* Childhood relationship with each parent described individually; how each handled conflict; showed affection; any preferential treatment
VIII. *Influence of Neighborhood and Community During Early Development.* Socioeconomic; cultural factors; role of family in the community
IX. *Other Influences and Role Models.* Any other role models or significant relationships in the child's life
X. *Collection of Early Recollections.* Early memories, before age 10

FIGURE 4.2 Sample Outline of the Life Style Interview.

process that takes place over three consecutive sessions and consists of 10 sections (Carlson et al., 2006). The first 9 sections are referred to as the family constellation interview, which solicits information from early childhood through adolescence. The final section gathers early childhood recollections. Focusing primarily on how people have addressed the tasks of love, work, and friendship, clinicians seek a holistic understanding of their clients and comprehension of their goals and private logic.

Particularly important are assessing people's levels of satisfaction with themselves, their relationships, and their lives and looking for examples of faulty logic. Structured guidelines are available to help clinicians conduct comprehensive and informative lifestyle assessments. Among these are *Understanding Life-Style: The Psycho-Clarity Process* (Powers & Griffith, 1987), the *Individual Psychology Client Workbook* (Powers & Griffith, 1986), the *BASIS-A Interpretive Manual* (Kern, Wheeler, & Curlette, 1997), and the *Manual for Life Style Assessment* (Shulman & Mosak, 1988). The lifestyle assessment has become a popular tool for therapists in many areas of counseling. Fisher and Fisher (2002) adapted the assessment for use with chemically dependent clients. Adler's complete assessment for children can be found in *Social Interest: A Challenge to Mankind* (Adler, 1938, pp. 218–225).

Family constellation and birth order. An understanding of the impact of the family constellation on a person comes from both objective and subjective sources. Objective information includes people's birth order, the number of children in the family, the gender of each child, the number of years between the births of each child, and any special circumstances such as the death of a child or the presence of a physical or intellectual disability in any of the children. Subjective information includes people's perceptions of themselves as children, how their parents felt about and treated each child, clients' relationships with their parents and siblings, ways in which they resembled and differed from their siblings, and patterns of rivalry and cooperation within the family. Additional information on birth order was presented earlier in this chapter.

Dreams. Adler used dreams as a vehicle for promoting self-awareness. De-emphasizing symbolism, Adler viewed dreams as providing important information on lifestyle and current concerns. He believed that both past and current dreams were useful sources of information, with recurrent dreams and recurrent themes within dreams being particularly important. The key to understanding dreams, according to Adler, is the emotion they create and their usefulness in solving current life problems.

Earliest recollections. Adler viewed people's earliest recollections as important sources of information on their current lifestyles. According to Adler (1931), whether memories are recalled accurately is unimportant. Rather, he believed that people only retained early memories that were consistent with their views of themselves. Consequently, what mattered were people's reports of their memories.

Adlerian therapists usually elicit at least three early memories so that they can identify recurrent themes and patterns. Once the memories have been elicited and written down, each memory is explored with the client. The clinician usually asks about the age when the person believes the recalled events occurred and the thoughts and emotions associated with the recollections. The client's role in the memories are explored, because his or her relationships and interactions with other people in the memories are believed to reflect the person's lifestyle. More information on analyzing earliest recollections is provided in the skill development section of this chapter.

Priorities and ways of behaving. People's behaviors also provide a rich and endless source of information about their lifestyles. Inquiring in detail about a person's behavior over a period of time or looking at a series of choices and actions can reveal consistent and repetitive behavioral patterns that reflect lifestyle. Adler and his associates (Adler, 1956; Mosak, 1971) identified the following common lifestyles, reflected in ways in which people orient themselves toward the world:

- Ruling and dominating others
- Avoiding interpersonal and other challenges
- Pleasing and seeking approval from others
- Controlling and managing
- Depending on others and needing to be cared for
- Pursuing superiority and perfection
- Seeking achievement
- Being a martyr or victim
- Seeking comfort
- Promoting social welfare and progress

Summarizing findings. After an extensive process of exploration, assessment, and analysis, clinicians formulate hypotheses about the nature of clients' lifestyles as well as the faulty assumptions and self-destructive thoughts and behaviors that interfere with their efforts to achieve their goals. This information is presented to clients for discussion and revision, paving the way for the third phase of treatment.

PHASE 3: REEDUCATION, INSIGHT, AND INTERPRETATION Phase 3 can be especially difficult for clinicians because they need to be both encouraging and challenging. While remaining supportive, they use interpretation and confrontation to help people gain awareness of their lifestyles, recognize the covert reasons behind their behaviors, appreciate the negative consequences of those behaviors, and move toward positive change. Several strategies help clinicians remain caring through this phase of treatment:

- They focus on the present rather than the past.
- They are more concerned with consequences than with unconscious motivation.
- They present their interpretations in ways that are likely to be accepted by clients.

Rather than being dogmatic or authoritarian, clinicians state interpretations as guesses or hunches. They might say, "I have a hunch that you threw your brother's hat in the sewer because you wanted more attention from your parents" or "I wonder if you have refused to set a more realistic sale price for your house because the house represents part of your ideal self." With gentle interpretations such as these, clinicians seek to educate clients and to promote self-awareness, insight, and discussion rather than to persuade clients to agree with them.

Clinicians continue to play an active role during this phase of treatment, presenting alternate possibilities, providing information, and helping people weigh their options and make decisions. Emphasis is on beliefs, attitudes, and perceptions because, according to Adler (1998), it is only by cognitive means and social interest that behavioral change will occur.

PHASE 4: REORIENTATION, REINFORCEMENT, TERMINATION, AND FOLLOW-UP Once clients have gained some insight and modified their distorted beliefs, they are ready to reorient their lives and initiate new ideas and patterns of behaviors. Clients now view their lives from different perspectives and can make more rewarding choices. Clinicians foster this outcome by helping people become full participants in their social system, shift their roles and interactions, and take positive actions to achieve their revised goals. Throughout, clinicians model and nurture optimism and flexibility; they support clients in developing the courage to be imperfect and take on rewarding challenges.

The reorientation and change phase can be divided into four parts (Sweeney, 2009):

1. Clients clarify their goals and determine whether they are realistic.
2. Common sense and clear thinking are applied to clients' feelings, beliefs, and goals. Although clients are reminded that their choices are their own, clinicians help them use common sense to evaluate and, if necessary, modify their thinking.
3. New learning is applied to the clients' lives.
4. Any barriers to progress are addressed and removed.

This final phase of treatment enables people to solidify the gains they have made and move forward with their lives in healthier and more fulfilling ways. Clinicians continue to provide education, teach skills, and make interpretations. However, their primary role is reinforcing positive changes. Clients and clinicians collaborate in evaluating progress, strengthening social interest and healthy and rewarding beliefs, and planning future steps toward goal attainment. Together, they determine when the client is ready to complete treatment and agree on follow-up procedures to ensure that clients stay on track and continue their positive growth and forward movement.

Interventions

Adler's Individual Psychology offers a wide range of creative and useful interventions. Many have already been discussed in this chapter, such as the use of earliest recollections and analysis of family constellation and birth order. Additional interventions include the following:

- *Catching oneself* encourages people to be more conscious of their repetitive faulty goals and thoughts. Clinicians facilitate this by identifying warning signs of difficulties and encouraging clients to view them as stop signs that remind them to pause and redirect themselves. This concrete approach helps people develop self-awareness and monitor themselves without being self-critical. For example, a man who often lost his temper and became inappropriately angry recognized that his whole body became tense before he exploded. He was taught to identify signs of physical tension, view them as stop signs, and use deep breathing as a quick and effective way to diffuse his anger.
- *Pushing the button* is designed to help people become more aware of the control they can have over their emotions, rather than allowing their emotions to control them. Clinicians encourage people to alternately imagine pleasant and unpleasant experiences, observe the emotions that accompany each image, and recognize that they can determine which button to push. A young woman who frequently consumed too much alcohol at social events imagined the pride she took in remaining sober (pleasant experience) as well as the embarrassment and physical discomfort she felt after becoming intoxicated (unpleasant experience). Vivid images of these two contrasting experiences helped her abstain from alcohol (push the healthy button).
- In *spitting in the client's soup,* clinicians identify the underlying motivations behind clients' self-defeating behaviors and then spoil their imagined payoff by making it unappealing. This is illustrated in the following dialog:

  THERAPIST: Let's schedule another appointment and try to hone in on some goals.

  CLIENT: I feel so awful that Dana broke up with me, I've thought about killing myself.

  CLINICIAN: I guess you want to make her feel guilty. But if you kill yourself, you won't be around to see how she's feeling . . . or go to college or buy that car you were talking about. You'll just be lying in the ground.

In addition to these specific techniques associated with Adlerian therapy, clinicians who follow this theoretical model also use many other techniques. Some of these, including encouragement, interpretation, and use of questions, have been discussed previously in this book. Others include the following:

- *Immediacy* focuses the session on the interaction between the client and the clinician; often it is a mirror of the client's interactions outside of the session. For example, a client accused a clinician of disliking him when the clinician provided information on parenting that differed from the client's style of parenting. The clinician helped the client see that when people disagreed with him, he viewed it as evidence that they disliked him.
- *Prescribing the symptom* (also called paradoxical intention) asks the client to magnify the problem behavior; for example, a clinician might tell a person who has trouble sleeping not to go to sleep at night. The goal of prescribing the symptom is to help the person realize the problem behavior, become aware of the consequences to the behavior, and recognize that it is within his or her control to change it. Oftentimes, the exaggeration seems silly or humorous. Clearly this intervention should not be used if the symptom poses a danger to the client such as self-harming behaviors, drinking, or suicide.
- *Confrontation* involves pointing out discrepancies in the material that clients present. For example, a counselor might say, "Help me understand your decision to spend five thousand dollars on a necklace when you've told me that you're concerned about being able to make the down payment on the house you want to buy."
- *Task assignments* are used throughout the treatment process. Client and clinician agree that the client will engage in a planned activity such as observing and listing times when she feels angry or exercising three times a week. Not only do the specific tasks advance the treatment, but the process of coming to an agreement on tasks, making a commitment to complete them, and planning and executing the tasks can promote feelings of competence and responsibility.
- *Humor, silence, advice,* and *reflection of feeling* are other techniques in the repertoire of the Adlerian psychotherapist. The many types of interventions associated with this treatment approach offer clinicians many avenues to build rapport with their clients, promote insight and self-awareness, and encourage positive change.

APPLICATION AND CURRENT USE OF INDIVIDUAL PSYCHOLOGY

Adler's model of Individual Psychology is used with a broad range of situations and clients. Not only is it used for treatment of children, individuals, couples, families, and groups, it also is used in career development, education, training, supervision, consultation, and organizational development.

Application to Assessment

Adlerian theory, with its emphasis on understanding lifestyle and private logic, lends itself to the development of tools to facilitate assessment. Many useful inventories have been developed to aid clinicians in implementing this theory. Wickers (1988) developed the Misbehavior Reaction Checklist to help teachers and parents understand the purpose of a child's misbehavior. Several tools are useful in lifestyle assessments. For example, the Kern Lifestyle Scale (Kern, 1992) and the Basic Adlerian Scales for Interpersonal Success–Adult Form (BASIS-A; Kern et al., 1997) are self-scoring instruments designed to obtain lifestyle information and promote self-awareness in career, personal, and relationship counseling as well as in business settings. These and many other inventories, audiotapes, booklets, and other materials based on Adler's ideas, are published by CMTI Press (http://www.cmtipress.com). All enhance the work of the Adlerian clinician.

Application to Diagnostic Groups

Most of the common problems and mental disorders seen in counseling and psychotherapy are amenable to treatment via Adlerian therapy. According to Sherman and Nwaorgu (2002), this approach addresses a broad spectrum of problems from individual "mistakes that lead to negative life styles to a whole breadth of social problems such as racial conflict . . . discrimination, war, poverty, drugs, issues of democracy, and inadequate parenting. Conceptualized in this way, everyone has a problem, and this remains part of the human condition" (p. 192).

The literature documents the use of this approach with "all the major categories of psychopathology" (Sherman & Nwaorgu, 2002, p. 193). Certainly, this approach seems useful with people who have mood, anxiety, or personality disorders; people with these disorders typically engage in thoughts and behaviors that are ineffectual and unrewarding and that reflect an excessive focus on their own needs rather than their place in society and their family. Most of these clients are capable of engaging in the self-examination, self-awareness, and learning that are integral to the Adlerian approach.

The literature also provides many examples, techniques, and descriptions of the use of Individual Psychology. Morrison (2009), for example, found it to be useful to people having dysfunctional responses to traumatic experiences. People with low self-esteem and social and relationship concerns also seem likely to benefit from Adlerian therapy. Children with behavioral problems and those who have been traumatized are well suited to treatment with Adlerian play therapy (Morrison, 2009). Dreikurs applied Adlerian principles to his work with children and Dinkmeyer's work with Systematic Training for Effective Parenting (STEP) evolved from Adlerian theory. Terms such as natural consequences and "I" messages are now a part of the language of parenting (Sweeney, 2009). More will be said about Adlerian family therapy in the chapter on family systems later in this book.

People with drug and alcohol problems, criminal behavior, and other impulse control disorders can be understood and helped through Adler's model. The problem is reframed from a disease or pathological focus to a social focus: They are failing to meet their needs for power and belonging in positive ways (Adler, 1979; Gladding, 2010; Rule & Bishop, 2005). Adlerian theory is compatible with Alcoholics Anonymous and other 12-step programs and can be empowering (Carroll, 1999).

Although people with psychotic disorders may not be able to engage in the kind of self-examination that Adlerian therapy requires, they can be better understood through Adler's ideas and helped to overcome resistance so they can optimize treatment and medication management (Sperry, 2006). Individual Psychology can help make sense of the loss of contact with reality experienced by people with psychotic disorders and suggest useful ways to help them.

Application to Multicultural Groups

Individual Psychology not only has much that would appeal to a diverse and multicultural population, but it actively seeks to address problems of discrimination and disenfranchisement. According to Sherman and Nwaorgu (2002), "Adlerians take seriously social discrimination based on ethnicity, gender, poverty, religion, and education level as issues for consideration in the treatment of clients" (p. 193).

Counselors who use an Adlerian approach are familiar with the dichotomy of inferiority and superiority. Acknowledging, understanding, and actively challenging feelings of inferiority or stigmatization with clients who feel disenfranchised may be particularly helpful. The emphasis on culture (broadly defined to include age, developmental or acquired disability, ethnicity, religion or spirituality, socioeconomic status, sexual orientation, indigenous heritage, national origin, and gender), social interest, and the family constellation, as well as the importance of collaboration, has wide appeal. According to Adler, prejudice, racism, and gender discrimination grow out of misguided efforts to gain superiority by degrading others. True self-esteem comes not from oppressing others but from working cooperatively to contribute to the common good, empowering ourselves as well as others, and facing life's challenges together.

Adlerian psychotherapy provides a positive model for working with all populations. The Adlerian process is respectful of diversity and addresses issues of racial, gender, and cultural inequity among others. Adler's approach focuses on a constructivist model that works flexibly and collaboratively with individuals and their families. According to Carlson and colleagues (2006, p. 32), the Adlerian research literature is replete with a wide range of multicultural issues including gender, religion and spirituality, racism, sexual orientation, culture, ethnicity, and social equality.

Adlerian therapy, with its focus on positive strengths and encouragement, can also be effective with a wide range of populations, including children with ADHD, oppositional defiant disorder, and at-risk youth (Day, 2008; Sapp, 2006). Adler's focus on community and social interest is consistent with the values of clients who come from more collectivist societies such as the Middle East, Asian countries, and Latin America. Religion and spirituality are also consistent with Adlerian theory, which considers religion to be a part of social interest (Carlson & Englar-Carlson, 2008).

Adler's approach has particular relevance to people with disabilities. He wrote of the feelings of discouragement and inferiority and the efforts toward compensation that often emerge in people with developmental or acquired disabilities. His understanding of this dynamic, as well as his emphasis on understanding maladjustment and promoting healthy empowerment, responsibility, and realistic self-esteem, should be helpful in treatment of people who are having difficulty coping with physical and mental challenges (Livneh & Antonak, 2005; Livneh & Sherwood, 1991). Of course, clinicians should be cautious not to overgeneralize and assume that all people with disabilities experience feelings of inferiority.

A logical extension of Adler's insights into people with disabilities is to people with other potential challenges in their lives, such as recent immigrants, people who grow up in one-parent homes, those who experience poverty or abuse, and those who feel disenfranchised for any reason. Counselors should be aware of social exclusions of groups of people, whether ethnic and racial groups; gay, lesbian, bisexual, transgendered, and questioning groups; women; people with disabilities; or others (Lee, 2007). Adler's understanding of the connection between early experiences and the development of lifestyles and goals provides insight into ways in which people with difficult backgrounds cope with their lives, as well as ways to help and empower them.

Although Adler's theories seem compatible with multicultural competence, clinicians still must exercise caution when using Individual Psychology. Adler's approach in its traditional form involves an extensive gathering of history and background information that may be seen as intrusive by people of Asian backgrounds who may prefer to proceed slowly and establish trust before revealing too much information. The in-depth, lengthy process might also not be well suited to people in crisis who are focused on more immediate concerns, and those who have little interest in lengthy self-analysis. His emphasis on individual responsibility and power as well as his exploration of early recollections also may be incompatible with the thinking of some people from non-Western cultures. Consequently, the approach may need to be adapted to such clients.

EVALUATION OF INDIVIDUAL PSYCHOLOGY

The strengths in Adler's treatment system far outnumber its shortcomings and weaknesses. Although developed nearly a century ago, his ideas seem remarkably timely and relevant today.

Limitations

Like other approaches focused on background, Adlerian therapy suffers from a dearth of empirical research. The research literature in general supports the "central constructs of Adlerian psychological theory" (Carlson et al., 2006, p. 36). For example, some empirical validation of Adler's ideas on the impact of birth order has been done (Rule & Comer, 2005; Sulloway, 1995). A study of the Adlerian Life Style Inventory to assess the lifestyles of Native American women residing on reservations provided some support for the broad usefulness of a lifestyle assessment (Roberts, Harper, Caldwell, & Decora, 2003). However, more empirical research is needed to fully support the growing importance of Individual Psychology.

In addition, many of Adler's concepts such as fictional finalism and superiority are not well defined and risk oversimplification. Adlerian therapy understands and gives credence to underlying psychological and societal impacts on pathology, but fails to account for biological or genetic influences. We now know the impact of genetics on anxiety and mood disorders, schizophrenia, and other conditions, and recognize that biopsychosocial factors interact in the development of many conditions. Adler has also been called overly optimistic in his belief that social interest is innate. Empirical research has yet to document that idea.

Strengths and Contributions

Adler's contributions, not only to the current practice of psychotherapy, but also to the thinking of some of the other leaders in our field, is enormous. Rollo May, Viktor Frankl, Carl Rogers, and Abraham Maslow all acknowledged their debt to Adler, leading Albert Ellis to predict that even more than Freud, "Adler is probably the true father of modern psychotherapy" (Watts, 2003, p. 1). The development of cognitive therapy, reality therapy, person-centered counseling, Gestalt, existentialist, constructivist, and social justice approaches to treatment has been influenced by Adler's ideas (Rule & Bishop, 2005). Whether or not clinicians describe themselves as followers of Adler's approach, nearly all counseling and psychotherapy now reflects some of his concepts, including:

- The focus on social justice
- The impact of early experiences and family constellation on current functioning
- The importance of taking a holistic approach that considers mind, body, and spirit
- The need to view people in their family, social, and cultural contexts
- The recognition that thinking influences emotions and behavior
- The emphasis on strengths, optimism, encouragement, empowerment, and support
- The relevance of lifestyle and goals
- The need to identify, understand the purpose of, and modify repetitive self-defeating behaviors
- The importance of a collaborative therapeutic alliance
- The benefits of having a therapist and client with realistic and mutually agreed-on goals
- The recognition that having problems and differences is a normal part of life and that these can be viewed as opportunities for growth rather than as pathology
- The view of therapy as an educational and growth-promoting process as well as a remedial one.

Individual Psychology can easily and effectively be combined with many contemporary treatment approaches. Its emphasis on beliefs and behavior is compatible with cognitive-behavioral therapy, rational emotive behavior therapy, and reality therapy. Adlerian lifestyle assessment has much in common with narrative therapy's emphasis on stories that provide the structure of life. Of course, the attention to early memories and childhood experiences is psychoanalytic in origin, whereas the emphasis on the therapeutic alliance reflects elements of humanistic approaches.

Many of Adler's ideas have become more important than ever in light of some of the pervasive problems in our society today. Our growing awareness of the enduring harm that can result from childhood trauma has focused attention on the significance to adults of their early childhood experiences and memories. Adler's call for social equality of women, respect for cultural and religious diversity, and an end to marginalization of minority groups (Carlson et al., 2006) still needs attention in our society. His emphasis on responsibility, resilience, character building, and social interest seems especially relevant in light of the many acts of bullying, torture, and violence in our society. The importance of fathers and of sibling relationships is another area of current attention. Probably of greatest importance are Adler's emphasis on respect for individual differences and the importance of each of us becoming a contributing part of a larger social system.

SKILL DEVELOPMENT: ANALYZING EARLIEST RECOLLECTIONS

Eliciting and analyzing people's earliest recollections can provide understanding of their lifestyles and how they view the world. The following four-step procedure, followed by examples, will help you learn to use early recollections in treatment. Exercises later in this chapter give you the opportunity to practice these skills.

1. ***Eliciting the recollections.*** Begin by inviting people to think back to their childhood, as early as they can remember, and describe at least three incidents that they recall. They should come up with experiences that included them and that they actually remember clearly rather than family stories or pictures they have seen. The clinician should write down each recollection as it is described.
2. ***Processing each memory.*** Ask about the person's feelings during the memory; discuss any actions or movements in the memory, especially transactions between the client and others; ask what part of the memory seems most vivid or important; and ask what meaning the memory has for the teller.
3. ***Analyzing the memories.*** Looking particularly for commonalities among the three or more recollections, consider the role of the client in the memories, the emotions associated with the memories, who else is present and how they are interacting with the client, the nature of the situations recalled, and the way in which the client responded to the events and interactions in the memories.
4. ***Interpretation and application.*** Develop a hypothesis or hunch, based on the common themes and patterns in the recollections, as to what these memories disclose about the person's goals and lifestyle. Present this hypothesis to the client for discussion and clarification.

Consider the following three recollections provided by a 27-year-old single woman:

Recollection 1: I remember being in my bed. It was very dark and I felt afraid. I was crying. Then my father came into the room. He picked me up and held me. He said something like, "What's the matter? Everything is all right now."

Recollection 2: I was in a department store. Somehow I got separated from my mother. I looked around, and I couldn't see her. I didn't know what to do, and I started to scream. This man came over, a salesperson or a manager in the store. He took me into a little room—an office, I guess—and he said he would help me find my mommy. He asked my name and then I heard something about a lost child over the loudspeaker. The man gave me some candy and kept talking to me. It seemed like a long time, but finally my mother came. She was crying too. I was so happy to see her.

Recollection 3: I was riding a tricycle, and I fell down. Nobody was around to help me. My knee was bleeding. I was crying and hurt, but nobody came. Finally, a neighbor heard me. He came out to see what the problem was, and then he called my mother. I felt better as soon as there was somebody to help me.

Analysis: In all three recollections, the woman is scared and perceives herself as needing help. Through crying, she is able to let others know that she needs help but is not able to otherwise help herself. In all three instances, she is rescued by caring men. They reassure her and provide the help she needs. Although her mother subsequently provides help in two of the memories, it is the men who are there when the child really needs help. Discussion revealed that this woman often felt fearful and doubted her own ability to move ahead in her career and cope with her life. She had been engaged twice and was eager to marry, but both times her fiancés had broken the engagement, telling her that she was too needy and dependent. The woman became aware that, although she was a successful teacher, she expected to get into trouble in some way and was hoping to be rescued from the demands of her career by marriage. At the same time, she indicated that she didn't trust people very much, especially women, and that she often felt overwhelmed by the day-to-day demands of her life. By assuming a needy and helpless role, she was actually undermining her relationships but believed that the way to find a man to rescue her was to become as needy as possible: the child crying loudly for help. This information played an important part in her treatment.

CASE ILLUSTRATION

Ava, age 10, is Edie and Roberto's daughter. The family's counselor decided to have some individual sessions with Ava to get to know her and her role in the family better and to develop a positive relationship with her. In addition, both Edie and Roberto expressed concerns about Ava's behavior. They described her as always being willful and independent, with these problems worsening in recent months. They reported that Ava is disobedient, both at home and at school, and that her teacher told them that some of the children do not want to play with her because she is "bossy." In addition, Ava's grades have been declining.

Ava was willing to meet with the counselor for an individual session. Ava was quite open and started off the session by describing how much she enjoyed seeing the cartoon version of the movie *Tarzan.* She had been particularly impressed by Tarzan's ability to swing through the trees, overcome the "bad guys," and help all of the animals. Ava also talked about some of her concerns related to her family. She described her mother as "crying a lot and moping around," while her father worked long hours and "just yells about everything." She also reported a dream that she compared to *Alice's Adventures in Wonderland* in which her mother was getting smaller while Ava was getting larger. As Ava talked, the counselor began to formulate hypotheses about Ava's lifestyle, her goals, and the reasons for her misbehavior.

Toward the end of the session, the counselor asked Ava to describe three early recollections:

Recollection 1: Ava recalled that when she was about 4 years old she became afraid of spiders. Once, while taking a walk with her father, she noticed a spider on her shoe and became upset. Her father brushed the spider off and squashed it. Ava was so impressed by this that she began squashing every bug she saw until her mother discouraged this.

Recollection 2: Another memory from a year or so later involved an incident when the mother of her friend Lori took Ava and Lori swimming. When Ava got out of the car, she swung her car door into another car and chipped the paint. The person sitting in the car complained to Lori's mother, but she just told him "not to make a big deal out of nothing" and took the children into the pool.

Recollection 3: The last memory involved a fight between her parents when Ava was in kindergarten. Her mother had burned the meatloaf that was to be served for dinner. When Roberto arrived home, he yelled at Edie for being careless. Edie began to cry, but Roberto just went into the other room and ordered pizza. Ava remembered thinking that the pizza was much better than the meatloaf would have been.

In all three memories, Ava's initial role is observer. Although her own behavior is a factor in the first two memories, what she recalled most sharply were the actions of the adults who used strength and anger to gain power and control. In the last two memories, other people's feelings are disregarded. Roberto and the friend's mother seem admirable to Ava while her own mother is viewed as weak.

These memories confirmed many of the counselor's hypotheses. Ava's misbehavior seemed to be a misguided attempt to gain power. She wanted to be in charge and wanted other people to stop controlling her. Her recollections suggest that she believes the way to obtain power is to become dominating, telling other people what to do as she has observed her father and others do. Her mother, who has a very different style, is devalued in Ava's mind because she seems to lack power. This has carried over to Ava's loss of interest in school, which her mother highly values. Ava's behavior is harming her relationships with both her peers and her parents.

Future sessions will involve both play therapy and talking to help Ava recognize her self-destructive efforts to obtain power and to change both her private logic and her repertoire of behaviors so that she finds more rewarding ways to gain power. Discussion would include exploration of Ava's roles and relationships with family members, basic messages and coping behaviors she learned as a child, her current lifestyle, and whether her beliefs and behavior are helping her to achieve the central goals of her life. This information also will be used in sessions with Roberto and Edie to help them parent Ava more effectively.

EXERCISES

Large-Group Exercises

1. Ask for two or three volunteers from the class who are willing to share their earliest recollections. Taking one person at a time, list that person's memories on the board and then process and analyze them according to the guidelines in the Skill Development section. Encourage the person with the memories to play an active part in the analysis. Discuss the relationship of the patterns that emerge from the recollections to the person's lifestyle.
2. Refer to the history of Roberto as presented in previous chapters. Ask for two volunteers—one to play Roberto and one to serve as the interviewer. The person assuming the role of Roberto should feel free to be creative and add information as long as it is consistent with

what is already known about Roberto. Engage in a role-played interview that will shed light on Roberto's lifestyle. The interviewer might ask about family constellation and birth order; earliest recollections, successes, and disappointments both in childhood and as an adult; goals and values; and social involvement and relationships. After the role-play, discuss the interview and try to identify Roberto's private logic, goals, priorities, and lifestyle. Allow at least 45 minutes for this exercise.

3. Divide the participants into four groups based on their birth order. Groups should be formed for oldest, youngest, middle, and only children. Have each group meet for 15 to 20 minutes and discuss the following questions:

- What are the common characteristics of people with your birth order?
- What important differences emerged among the people in your group?
- What are common misconceptions or stereotypes about people in your birth position?
- What preconceptions do you have about the characteristics of people in the other three birth order positions?

Each group should select a spokesperson who will present the group's conclusions to the class as a whole.

Small-Group Exercises

1. In a previous chapter, you gained experience in conducting interviews and using open questions. You build on those skills in this exercise. Form into your groups of four people, but this time change partners so you are interviewing someone you have not interviewed before. Spend about 15 minutes conducting an interview with that person, focusing particularly on the following four areas:

- Childhood behavior and misbehavior
- Family constellation
- Important values and goals
- Ways in which the person has sought to achieve those goals.

Next the interviewer should lead the interviewee in a discussion of the patterns that emerged. Remember to be encouraging and to help your partner feel comfortable.

At the conclusion of each role-play, spend 5 to 10 minutes providing feedback to the person in the interviewer role on the following aspects of the exercise:

- Therapeutic alliance
- Use of open questions
- Ability to elicit relevant information on the four topics
- Use of encouragement

2. In groups of four, discuss memories of times when you misbehaved as a child. Help each other determine whether the motive of the misbehavior was power, attention, revenge, or display of inadequacy. Then discuss helpful responses that your teachers or parents might have made to your misbehavior.

Individual Exercises

1. List at least three of your earliest memories. Process and analyze them according to the guidelines in the Skill Development section. What patterns emerge? What sorts of goals and lifestyle do they suggest? How does this information relate to your image of yourself? Write your memories and responses to these questions in your journal.
2. Identify a challenge you are facing that you are not sure you can handle successfully. Imagine yourself capable of dealing with that challenge. Be sure the image of yourself is clear and vivid in your mind. Now think about how the person reflected by this image of yourself would handle the challenge. As you address this issue in your life, act as if you are that image of yourself and keep reminding yourself that you can handle the situation. After you have made some progress, monitor your success. Think about how well this technique is working and how you might improve on this intervention. Write a summary of this experience in your journal.

Summary

Adler's Individual Psychology has made an important contribution to counseling and psychology and continues to be widely practiced. "The beauty of Individual Psychology is its flexibility" (Watts, 2000, p. 26). Adler's model is useful with a broad range of people and difficulties. His emphasis on encouragement and logic rather than pathology, power and importance rather than sexuality, and family and society rather than the unconscious are appealing and contribute to people's empowerment. Many of Adler's concepts, including goals, private logic, priorities, and lifestyle, provide a useful framework for understanding people. In addition, the interventions and tools that have grown out of his model help clinicians use his ideas to assess, educate, and encourage change in their clients.

Many opportunities exist for further education on Adler's work. The North American Society of Adlerian Psychology, the International Association for Individual Psychology, and the Rudolf Dreikurs Institute all hold annual conventions. Ongoing training can be obtained at Bowie State University in Bowie, Maryland, as well as the Alfred Adler Institutes in many cities, including Boca Raton, Florida; Chicago; and New York City. Information on these programs can be obtained from the North American Society of Adlerian Psychology.

Recommended Readings

Adler, A. (1938). *Social interest: A challenge to mankind* (J. Linton & R. Vaughan, Trans.). London, UK: Faber and Faber.

Adler, A. (1963). *The practice and theory of individual psychology.* Paterson, NJ: Littlefield, Adams.

Carlson, J., & Maniacci, M. P. (2011). *Alfred Adler revisited.* New York, NY: Routledge.

Dreikurs, R., & Soltz, V. (1964). *Children: The challenge.* New York, NY: Meredith.

Grey, L. (1998). *Alfred Adler, the forgotten prophet: A vision for the 21st century.* Westport, CT: Praeger.

Hoffman, E. (1994). *The drive for self: Alfred Adler and the founding of individual psychology.* Reading, MA: Addison-Wesley.

Journal of Individual Psychology: The Journal of Adlerian Theory, Research, and Practice, http://www.utexas.edu/utpress/journals/jip.html

Stein, H. T. (2007). Adler's legacy: Past, present and future. *Journal of Individual Psychology, 63*, 205–213.

Sweeney, T. J. (2009). *Adlerian counseling: A practitioner's approach* (5th ed.). Philadelphia, PA: Taylor & Francis.

Additional Sources of Information

http://www.alfredadler.org—Website for the North American Society of Adlerian Psychology.

http://www.alfredadler.edu/resources/adlerianlinks.htm—Resources for Adlerian therapists.

http://www.iaipwebsite.org—Website for the International Association of Individual Psychology (IAIP).

http://www.alfredadler-ny.org—Website for the Alfred Adler Institute of New York. Includes information on training and resources.

CHAPTER 5

Post- and Neo-Freudians: Analytical Psychology, Ego Psychology, Object Relations, and Self Psychology

One of Freud's greatest contributions was his ability to attract to his ideas people who were themselves brilliant and innovative thinkers with a deep interest in human development and psychology. Carl Jung, like Alfred Adler, was a close colleague of Freud and was strongly influenced by his concepts. Jung, however, disagreed with Freud on several major theoretical concepts and went on to develop his own innovative ideas. Jung and Adler were not the only analysts to develop alternatives to strict psychoanalytic orthodoxy. Anna Freud, the youngest daughter of Sigmund Freud who, according to Hergenhahn (2009), became "the spokesperson for psychoanalysis" (p. 565) after her father died, and a pioneer in child psychology, extended his theories into child analysis, education, and parenting. At the same time, Melanie Klein began developing her own views on analysis with children, and Karen Horney, another follower of psychoanalysis, disagreed with Freud's theory that anatomy is destiny and suggested instead that men envy the woman's capacity for motherhood. Within Horney's work are the first seeds of feminist theory.

Each of these important people was among the first to propose alternatives to psychoanalytic orthodoxy. These Freudian revisionists, men and women who initially accepted the tenets of Freudian psychoanalysis, were followed by Harry Stack Sullivan, John Bowlby, Heinz Kohut, and others who moved forward to develop their own influential ideas. These post-Freudians can be loosely categorized into the following four groups:

- ***Analytical psychologists***—Carl Jung
- ***Ego psychologists***—Karen Horney, Harry Stack Sullivan, and Anna Freud
- ***Object relations theorists***—Melanie Klein, John Bowlby, Harry Stack Sullivan, Stephen Mitchell, and others
- ***Self psychologists***—Heinz Kohut and others

We turn now to a brief look at each of these theorists. The Skill Development section later in the chapter introduces interpretation, a technique associated with the psychoanalytical theories.

CARL JUNG AND ANALYTICAL PSYCHOLOGY

Carl Jung was once a close colleague of Freud. However, Jung's ideas, like those of many important theoreticians, went through several phases during the 60 years of his professional life, and evolved into an individual theory of his own.

Biography of Carl Jung

Carl Gustav Jung was born on July 26, 1875, in Kesswil, Switzerland. His father was a minister descended from a long line of clergy associated with the Swiss Reformed Church. Jung was apparently a lonely and introverted child who began experiencing terrifying dreams at an early age (Ewen, 1993; Jung, 1963).

Jung's impressions of his parents had a great impact on his thinking, as his work reflects. His father disappointed Jung because of the father's inability to fully experience his faith; Jung placed great emphasis on the experience of spirituality and viewed that as an important part of our inner world (Schwartz, 1995). Just as his father seemed paradoxical (the minister who was a disbeliever), so did his mother, a woman who followed socially accepted and often repressive standards in her outward behavior but had a different and almost clairvoyant inner self.

From adolescence, Jung was an avid reader who studied philosophy, anthropology, the occult, and parapsychology on his own. Sedgwick (2001) described Jung as ". . . a thinking and intuitive kind of person, with a near-visionary capacity and proclivity for mystical experience" (pp. 20–21). Jung attended medical school at the University of Basel where he initially specialized in internal medicine, but subsequently shifted his focus to psychiatry.

An important turning point occurred for Jung in 1907 when he defended Freud against an attack by a professor at the University of Heidelberg (Kelly, 1990). This led Freud to welcome Jung as his disciple and eventually as his successor, not recognizing the important differences in their ideas (Jones, 1955). The two worked closely for 6 years. During that time, Jung accompanied Freud to lecture at Clark University in the United States. However, in 1913, Jung resigned as both president and member of the International Psychoanalytical Association because of his conviction that delusions and hallucinations frequently reflected universal archetypes rather than repressed memories.

Jung was a prolific theorist and writer throughout his life, with his work filling 18 volumes. Nevertheless, throughout his career, he had many periods in which he questioned himself and sought to resolve his doubts by immersing himself in his unconscious, using vehicles such as sand play, dialogues with figures in his dreams, and art to develop his understanding of the unconscious. Jung worked productively in his later years (Ewen, 1993). His work reflects his belief that the years from midlife on are the time when creativity and personality integration are at their height. Jung died on June 6, 1961, at the age of 85, having lived long enough to witness the considerable impact of his work.

Development of Jung's Theories

Jung gained renown early in his career because of his writings on mental disorders, especially *The Psychology of Dementia Praecox* (Jung, 1907/1960). During the early years of his collaboration with Freud, Jung's writings focused primarily on his experimental studies of word association, memory, and physiological responses to emotional changes. The publication of *Symbols of Transformation* (Jung, 1912/1956) led to the end of his association with Freud and marked a shift in his writings.

During the subsequent 20 years, Jung's work continued to address many of the concepts that had grown out of psychoanalysis, notably analytical psychology, the ego, the conscious, and the unconscious. However, his view of these concepts was quite different from Freud's. Jung also wrote about art, literature, and culture during these years.

The focus of his writing shifted again during the last 25 years of his life. His work became increasingly spiritual, and he developed many of the constructs that make his work unique, including archetypes, the collective unconscious, anima and animus, and the shadow. (All will be discussed later in the chapter.)

During his later years, Jung not only continued his writing but maintained a psychotherapy practice and lectured throughout the world. He received many honors and considerable professional recognition. His work continues on at the International Association for Analytical Psychology, founded in Zurich in 1966 as a training and accreditation center for Jungian analysts.

Important Theoretical Concepts

Jung's theory, known as analytical psychology, rests on his concept of the psyche. His concept of psychotherapy, in turn, focuses on helping people integrate and make conscious aspects of the psyche or personality.

THE COMPONENTS OF THE PSYCHE Jung's concept of the psyche is much more complex than that of Freud. Figure 5.1 offers a simplified picture of Jung's conception of the psyche.

THE CONSCIOUS MIND According to Jung, psychic functioning includes three levels: the conscious mind, the collective unconscious, and the personal unconscious. Jung believed as did Freud that the conscious mind was only a small fraction of the psyche, including the ego, the persona, two attitudes, and four functions.

Conscious Mind

Ego

Persona

Two Attitudes (Extraversion and Introversion)

Four Functions (Thinking, Feeling, Sensation, Intuition)

Unconscious Mind

Collective Unconscious	**Personal Unconscious**
Archetypes	Repressed or Forgotten Memories
Self	Complexes
Anima/Animus	Archetypes
Shadow	Shadow
Other Images, Myths, Symbols	

FIGURE 5.1 Jung's Conception of the Psyche.

The ego. The ego is the center of the conscious mind. The ego gives us our sense of the world and our reality. It therefore exerts considerable influence over our transactions with our environment. It is formed of perceptions, memories, thoughts, and feelings that are within our awareness and give us a sense of identity. The development of the ego, along with our bodily sensations, allows us to differentiate ourselves from others. Although the ego is relatively weak in relation to other parts of the psyche, it can protect itself by consigning threatening material to the personal unconscious through the process of repression. In this way, it connects and integrates the conscious and unconscious levels of personality.

The persona. The persona is the idealized side of ourselves that we show to the outside world, the face of the collective psyche. This mask or protective facade conceals our problems and sorrows but enables us to function well in society, deal with other people, and pursue our daily needs and activities. Our persona may change in an effort to adapt to social situations and is affected by the group or person we are with at a particular time. The persona is a sort of compromise. It is inauthentic in that it usually does not reflect our true thoughts and emotions, which might not be socially acceptable. At the same time, it usually captures enough of who we are and what we need to make us comfortable with it.

Attitudes and functions. The two attitudes are *extraversion* and *introversion*. The four functions include *thinking* and its opposite, *feeling; sensation* and its opposite, *intuition*. People tend to interact with the world through one of the four functions, termed their primary or superior function. Its opposite function is the least developed, inferior function and is most problematic. For example, if someone's primary or superior function were thinking, this would guide most of his or her decisions. Its opposite, feeling, would probably not be well developed and the person would have difficulty giving emotions much weight in their decisions. Opposites in the personality provide psychic energy and, in the well-functioning person, are in balance. The attitudes and functions form the basis for the Myers-Briggs Type Indicator (discussed further on pages 92 and 97).

THE UNCONSCIOUS MIND Freud and Jung agreed on the nature of the unconscious up to a point. Both believed that it was a large and powerful part of the psyche and contained repressed material. However, Jung presented a more complex and potentially positive view of the unconscious, viewing it as a source of creativity and spiritual and emotional growth, as well as of confusion and symptoms. The unconscious includes fantasies, knowledge and learning, memories of experiences and relationships, and subjective reactions to events and people (Sedgwick, 2001). According to Jung, these are housed in the personal unconscious and the collective unconscious, the two levels of the unconscious mind. The personal unconscious reflects the history of the individual while the collective unconscious "pertains to world history . . . to the evolutionary history" of the human mind (Sedgwick, 2001, p. 32).

The collective unconscious. The collective unconscious has been described as the storehouse of latent memory traces inherited from the past that predispose people to react to the world in certain ways. The collective unconscious transcends individual experience and reflects "the cumulative experiences of humans throughout their entire evolutionary past" (Hergenhahn, 2009, p. 556). Fear of the dark and fear of snakes are examples of reactions that Jung believed originated in the collective unconscious, reflecting archaic remains.

The collective unconscious also includes a wealth of myths, images, and symbols of which *archetypes* are especially important examples. Archetypes are unconscious universal energies that result from repeated human experience and predispose people to view the world and organize their perceptions in particular ways. Archetypes are innate and have been transmitted through cultures and generations. Archetypes appear in dreams and fantasies, often through symbols, and influence how we think, feel, and behave throughout our lives. Jung wrote extensively about certain well-developed archetypes.

The Self. The Self, a central archetype, is the regulating center of the personality, integrating and balancing the needs and messages of the conscious, the personal unconscious, and the collective unconscious. Primarily located in the collective unconscious, the Self can emerge through dreams, symbols, perceptions, and images. It rarely emerges before the second half of our lives and is reflected in our spiritual and philosophical attitudes. The Self gives the personality unity, equilibrium, and stability (Jung, 1953, 1960). It is the goal of personality development, approached but rarely reached.

Anima/animus. The anima is the psychological feminine component in a man, whereas the animus is the psychological masculine component in a woman (Schwartz, 1995). The anima and animus are archetypes that have evolved from generations of experience. They have two functions: They are a part of the Self and are also projected onto others. These archetypes influence how we feel about and present the masculine and feminine sides of ourselves. The anima and animus also shape our relationships, especially with the other gender.

The shadow. The shadow originates in ancestral archetypes but can be manifested in both the collective and the personal unconscious. It is our dark side that we do not wish to acknowledge, so we attempt to hide it from ourselves and others. The shadow includes morally objectionable traits and instincts and has the potential to create thoughts, feelings, and actions that are socially unacceptable, shameful, and evil. At the same time, the shadow's unrestrained and primitive nature is a wellspring of energy, creativity, and vitality. The shadow is, in a sense, the opposite of the persona. The persona seeks social acceptance and approval, while the shadow embraces the socially undesirable.

The personal unconscious. The personal unconscious is unique to each individual and forms over that person's lifetime. It includes memories of thoughts, feelings, and experiences that were forgotten or repressed; have lost their intensity and importance over time; or never had enough energic charge to enter consciousness.

Images from the personal unconscious can be triggered by daily stimuli. For example, a view of a child riding on a pony can bring back a long forgotten image of oneself as a young child being led around a ring on a pony. Memories that have merely been forgotten or deposited in the personal unconscious because of their lack of importance may be recalled clearly or in fragments when something triggers their entry into consciousness. Repressed material, however, will generally emerge from the personal unconscious in incomplete or disguised forms, via dreams or symbols.

Complexes. Complexes are dynamic structures of the personality, located in the personal unconscious. They have an archetype at their core that has attracted a related and emotionally charged collection of feelings, thoughts, perceptions, and memories. Complexes have an impact on our daily lives but, because they are located in the unconscious, are generally out of our awareness. Complexes that have been discussed extensively in the literature include the Oedipus complex and the mother complex.

CONCEPT OF HUMAN DEVELOPMENT Jung envisioned people's lives as divided into two periods. During the first half of life, we find our place and accomplish the basic tasks of developing values and interests, finding a partner, and making career choices. During the second half of life, with our foundation in place, we progress toward individuation. The search for individuation is a lifelong process in which a person becomes "a psychological individual, that is, a separate indivisibility or whole" (Jung, 1953, p. 383). As part of the process, the whole personality develops. We gain greater access to the unconscious and our latent potentials; we move toward a state of greater balance, harmony, and equilibrium; and we clarify who we are in relation to others. We become more our own person and less a reflection of the ways in which we have been programmed throughout our lives. During the second half of life, the Self evolves, the persona is weakened, the shadow is better integrated and understood, and archetypes emerge that empower us. Our values shift from materialism, sexuality, and procreation to spiritual, social, and cultural values. Our visions of our purpose and the meaning of our lives become clearer.

Jung's theory of development is an optimistic one, emphasizing growth that can accelerate throughout the life span. Part of the appeal of his ideas rests in his positive view of human development in the second half of life. The link between Jung's theories and existentialism is evident in his emphasis on finding meaning in our lives.

BALANCE AND POLARITIES To Jung, life consists of opposites—polarities—with their balance determining the psychological health and development of the person. He viewed extremes as harmful because they prevent the opposite construct from being realized and gaining satisfactory expression. A consequence of imbalance is the tendency of any extreme emotion to turn into its opposite over time. For example, idealizing, unrealistic love can be transformed into hatred if the love object fails to live up to the ideal image.

People have inborn self-regulating systems that govern energy flow and help maintain balance. These include the principle of equivalence, which states that energy lost in one system will reappear in another system, with the sum total of energy remaining constant; and the principle of entropy, in which the libido (defined broadly by Jung as total psychic energy) tends to flow from a more intense to a less intense component to prevent the overload of energy in any one area. Self-regulation is also facilitated by transcendent functions, which allow us to make the transition from one dimension of our personalities to another (Kelly, 1990).

DIMENSIONS OF PERSONALITY Jung attributed individual differences in personality to two dimensions: (1) the typical ways in which people take in and understand internal and external stimuli, and (2) the characteristic directions of their libidos (Jung, 1921/1971).

The four functions. Four functions determine how people process internal and external stimuli:

1. *Thinking.* People whose thinking function is dominant react cognitively and intellectually, seeking to interpret and understand a stimulus.
2. *Feeling.* The feeling function is the opposite of the thinking function. People whose feeling function is primary react emotionally, focusing on pleasure, dislike, anger, and other emotions raised by a stimulus.
3. *Sensation.* Sensation involves receiving and identifying physical stimuli through the senses and relaying them to consciousness. People who have sensation as their dominant function look at the facts and the substance of a stimulus, seeking concrete evidence of its meaning and value.
4. *Intuition.* Intuition is the opposite of sensation. People whose intuition is their dominant function rely on hunches about where a stimulus has come from, where it is going, and what the possibilities are to determine their reactions and decisions related to the stimulus.

Each person has a dominant or superior function that organizes experiences and perceptions as well as an inferior function that is closer to the unconscious. We have the least control over the inferior function, which causes us the most discomfort. Having balance or access to all functions can enable people to operate fully in a range of situations.

One role of the unconscious is to compensate for the dominance of the superior function by encouraging the opposite tendencies. A personality that remains overly one sided despite efforts of the unconscious benefits from psychotherapy to restore balance.

The two attitudes. The second determinant of personality is the libido's (or energy's) direction of movement. For each person, energy moves primarily in one of the two following ways:

1. *Extraversion.* People in whom this attitude dominates direct their energy toward the outside world; they tend to be outgoing and adapt easily to external change. They are energized by social and interpersonal situations rather than by solitude.
2. *Introversion.* This is the opposite of extraversion. People in whom introversion dominates are most comfortable channeling their libido inward. Although they may have good social skills, they tend to be introspective and replenish their energy by being alone. Crowds of people exhaust them.

Each of the four functions of the first dimension can be paired with each of the two attitudes of the second dimension, making eight possible personality types (e.g., thinking and introversion, thinking and extraversion, feeling and extraversion). The functions and attitudes may sound familiar because they form the basis for the Myers-Briggs Type Indicator (discussed later in the chapter).

Treatment Using Jungian Analytical Psychology

Like Freudian psychoanalysts, Jungian analysts view treatment as a lengthy and intensive process. Ideally, people are seen at least twice a week, usually with client and clinician facing one another (Schwartz, 1995).

GOALS OF PSYCHOTHERAPY Jungian analysis is deep and intensive, encouraging the emergence and understanding of material from both the personal and the collective unconscious. Regression facilitates access to the unconscious and is followed by progression, as the painful and unacceptable elements of the unconscious are made conscious, acceptable, and meaningful. This ultimately leads to resolution of inner conflicts, greater balance and integration in the person, individuation, growth in creativity and energy, and the expansion of spiritual feelings. Jung does not seek to bring people happiness but, rather, to enable them to cope with the inevitable pain and suffering of life and to find a balance between joy and sorrow.

Jungian treatment typically has four stages (Ewen, 1993):

1. ***Catharsis and emotional cleansing.*** Strong emotions are discharged while the therapeutic alliance forms. People begin to understand their pasts but do not need to relive them; Jung saw the reliving of past traumas as undesirable. Rather, catharsis and an understanding of both past and present allow people to ameliorate their present difficulties without increasing their pain.

2. ***Elucidation.*** The meaning of symptoms, the anima and animus, the shadow, and the person's current life situation and difficulties are clarified. In addition, people work through the childhood origins of their emotional difficulties, as well as their immature and unrealistic thoughts and fantasies. Transference and countertransference are explored and analyzed; Jung believed that both can inform and guide treatment.

3. ***Education.*** Education can help remedy any gaps in development or maturation that have resulted from maladjustment or imbalances. During this stage, the clinician is supportive and encouraging, helping people take risks to improve their lives. Many people stop treatment at this point, but some continue on to the fourth stage.

4. ***Transformation.*** This occurs when people have achieved an in-depth access to the collective unconscious and the archetypes. Transformation facilitates an ego–Self dialogue, leading to further emergence of the Self and greater balance. This in turn promotes individuation and self-realization (Dehing, 1992).

THERAPEUTIC ALLIANCE Jungian analysts take an active part in the treatment process. They are not only analysts but also educators and collaborators in the therapeutic endeavor. Through interventions (discussed in the next section), clinicians promote awareness and analysis of the unconscious, usually beginning with the recognition of the anima and the animus as well as the personal unconscious and the shadow. With awareness, these elements of the personality can become integrated and their impact on the person better understood and modified, leading to greater social awareness and personal transformation.

Jung placed great emphasis on the person of the clinician, not only as a transference object but as an individual. He believed that both client and clinician have an unconscious influence on each other that can facilitate treatment. Therapy, for Jung, was a reciprocal process in which both client and therapist experienced healing and growth, with each participant benefiting from the positive changes in the other. So that the emotional growth of the clinician did not create a barrier to treatment, Jung insisted that every clinician following his treatment approach undergo personal analysis.

Jung also emphasized the special atmosphere of the psychotherapy process. Viewing it as a sort of sacred place, he thought of psychotherapy itself as archetypal, providing healing, comfort, and guidance (Sedgwick, 2001). Jung moved psychotherapy away from the Freudian theory of drives and toward a more relational view (Colman, 2011).

INTERVENTIONS Jungian psychotherapy begins by focusing on the conscious, building a therapeutic alliance, and laying the groundwork for safe and productive exploration of the unconscious. Once that groundwork has been established, Jungian analysts use a range of techniques to provide access to the contents of the unconscious. Initially, the threshold of consciousness is lowered, permitting the unconscious to emerge through the client's material, including dreams, images, fantasies, and symbols. When contents of the unconscious are brought into consciousness, they are explored, clarified, interpreted, and ultimately understood. Then the material can be integrated into the overall psyche of the person and further meaning found until the integration feels complete and natural and the person can instinctively use the knowledge from the unconscious.

Other than the following interventions and an exploration of the person's personality in terms of the four functions and two attitudes, Jung's theory does not devote much attention to techniques. In this approach, the material for analysis (dreams, visions, fantasies, and perceptions) is provides the broad focus, rather than the tools used to explore the material.

Use of symbols. Jung's model of the psyche rests on his concepts of the Self and the archetypes (Goodman, 2010). Therefore, Jungian work stresses the capacity to think symbolically and see the underlying dynamics and patterns driving clients' thoughts, feelings, and actions. These patterns may appear in symbolic and indirect forms in people's dreams, symptoms, fantasies, and other material. Clinicians' ability to understand this psychological subtext can be enhanced by knowledge of the wide range of symbols found in myths, fairy tales, art, literature, and religions, which are our cultural storehouses. Even the therapeutic frame can become a space for symbolic meaning (Colman, 2011).

Dream interpretation. Jung (1964) saw dreams as providing easiest access to the unconscious and viewed them as reflecting people's inner lives as well as their unconscious responses. Jung took a broader view of dreams than did Freud; Jung believed they not only represented wishes and fears but also fantasies, memories, experiences, visions, truths, and more. Jungian dream interpretation involves retelling the recalled dream; describing its impact on consciousness; exploring events that may have triggered the dream; investigating the dream's objective and subjective content for archetypal images and symbols of the unconscious; and assimilating the dream into consciousness, having made sense of it.

Word association tests. In word association tests, the clinician reads single words, one at a time, to the client, who replies with the first word that comes into mind. Unusual responses, repeated responses, hesitations, and physiological changes such as flushing and visible tension all provide clues to the presence of complexes and other unconscious material. Associations also are used to explore the meaning of dreams.

Rituals. Jung recognized the importance of religious and secular rituals such as confirmations, weddings, and retirement celebrations in facilitating people's growth and passage from one phase of life to another, although he was skeptical about the value of rigid and entrenched rituals (Al-Krenawi, 1999). Jung sometimes incorporated rites and rituals into therapy and some modern Jungian analysts have embraced this intervention. Incorporating rich and meaningful interventions into Jungian analysis can enhance that process and increase its individual and cultural relevance and impact.

Application of Jungian Analytical Psychology

Jung conceptualized his work as having broad application. However, in determining the application of Jungian analysis, we must consider several factors including typical people whom Jung treated, Jung's writings on the application of his theory, and how his approach is used today.

APPLICATION TO CLIENTS AND DIAGNOSTIC GROUPS Jung's typical patients were sophisticated and relatively well-functioning people who sought greater self-awareness and self-realization. Most were in mid-life or older and craved a deeper meaning in their lives. Some had tried other treatment approaches without success and consulted Jung in the hope that his ideas and strategies would be more meaningful and effective. According to Sedgwick (2001), "Jung's approaches were encouraging to those seeking and creating deeper, sometimes uniquely spiritual meaning in their lives, and their Jungian paths sometimes involved direct transpersonal experience through introspection and imagination" (p. 23).

It is the growth-promoting aspects of this approach that are particularly compelling. Jungian analytical psychology is most appropriately thought of as a method for achieving personal growth and self-awareness for people who feel unfulfilled. This approach, then, seems best suited for people who already are fairly healthy but who believe that greater access to their spiritual dimension as well as greater understanding of their unconscious can bring them more integrated, balanced, and fulfilling lives.

APPLICATION TO MULTICULTURAL GROUPS Jung's concepts offer an alternative to conventional therapy that may be more compatible with the spiritual and cultural beliefs and behaviors of many multicultural clients. Jung's attention to spirituality and universal symbols is likely to have relevance to people from a broad range of cultures. Al-Krenawi (1999) views the flexible use of rituals as another element of Jungian analysis that gives this approach multicultural relevance. According to Al-Krenawi, "The accepted therapeutic use of ritual, its freedom from stigma and its legitimacy as a healing device in traditional cultures can help circumvent their members' suspicion of insight-oriented 'talking therapy.' . . . The use of rituals may reduce the novelty of Western therapy by connecting it to the clients' values and beliefs" (p. 11). The use of rituals also casts the therapist in a role resembling that of the traditional healer and this, too, may promote acceptance of this approach. Its emphasis on social context and its view of dreams and archetypes from cultural perspectives are other ingredients that enhance the multicultural relevance of Jungian analysis.

Sand tray therapy, in which a selection of miniature objects (buildings, people, animals, etc.) is made available for a person to use in a sand tray, helps people access their emotions nonverbally. It provides a safe environment in which repressed issues can be explored. Sweeney and Homeyer (2010) found that Latino children, Chinese children, those from the inner city, and even menopausal women and gay men all benefited from the experience. One drawback, however, is the degree of specialized training that is necessary prior to its use.

Current Use of Jungian Analytical Psychology

Despite its long-term in-depth orientation, Jungian analysis continues to have a loyal following among clinicians. A reenergized interest in spirituality in recent years has fueled renewed interest in Jungian analysis. An interest in the melding of spirituality, religion, and psychology has resulted in a wealth of books on topics such as tracking the sacred, the metaphysical, the shadow self, dream analysis, synchronicity, and archetypes of good and evil (Cambray, 2009; Dourley, 2008; Haule, 2010; Schoen, 2009; Stein, 2010; Tacey, 2009.) Recent advances in neuroscience, which seem to indicate that the quest for spirituality or religious experience may have a biological basis (Saroglou, 2012), have also contributed to a renewed interest in Jung's ideas. Jungian analysis continues to increase in popularity.

Evaluation of Jungian Analytical Psychology

Evaluating Jungian analytical psychology is difficult for several reasons. Jung's concepts are complex, ill defined, and sometimes seem contradictory. His treatment approach entails few specific interventions and is presented in broad and global terms. Similarly, the outcomes that Jung views as desirable involve such elusive constructs as self-realization and balance and rarely address amelioration of specific symptoms. Jung's ideas fail to meet the criteria for a useful, sound, and testable theory. Consequently, any discussion of limitations, strengths, and contributions must have as a backdrop the serious shortcomings of Jung's theory.

LIMITATIONS Despite growing attention to his ideas, Jung's work has not been empirically validated (Hill, Schottenbauer, Lui, Spangler, & Sim, 2008). His writing is dense and challenging, complicated by specialized terminology. His treatment approach is a lengthy one that pays little attention to immediate crises. Jung does not offer much in the way of readily accessible tools and techniques, and the practice of Jungian analysis requires extensive training and supervision. Although proponents of this approach attest to its positive impact, the literature provides little in the way of either empirical research or case studies that offer clear and replicable treatment steps and procedures. These shortcomings suggest that clinicians drawn to Jungian analysis should give careful thought to their decision.

STRENGTHS AND CONTRIBUTIONS Despite the esoteric nature of his theory, Jung's work has contributed to the thinking of the existentialists, the humanists, the Gestalt therapists, and others and can be integrated with these and many other approaches. His belief in synchronicity, the idea that nothing happens without having meaning and purpose, is reflected in the thinking of many transpersonal clinicians (Colman, 2011). Jung's awareness that people have a strong need for meaning in their lives and his emphasis on spirituality and the universality of people's images and experiences are very much in keeping with current psychological thought.

Current practice reflects several applications of Jung's work. The Myers-Briggs Type Indicator, a widely used personality inventory, is based on Jung's ideas. His concept of the collective unconscious places our lives in a broad context and further contributes to the meaning and historical continuity of our lives. His belief in spirituality as part of a healthy lifestyle found a home in the early creation of Alcoholics Anonymous. In a discussion on the spiritual underpinnings of addiction recovery, White and Kurtz (2008) wrote: "Jung brought an affirmation of the limits of professional assistance in recovery from alcoholism, and he added professional legitimacy to the transformative power of the spiritual experience" (p. 40). Jung's indirect influence on the creation of Alcoholics Anonymous, through its founder Bill Wilson, has been illuminated in numerous books and articles (Finlay, 2000; Forcehimes, 2004; Schoen, 2009).

Several writers and theorists have drawn on Jung's ideas in their work. Joseph Campbell, an author and mythologist best known for *The Power of Myth* and *The Hero with a Thousand Faces,* was influenced by Jung's work, particularly his writings on archetypes. Campbell focused his attention on myths, stating that myths embody the eternal essence of life and are about identity and the unrealized parts of the self (Ellwood, 1999). The influence of Campbell's writings about the mythological hero are reportedly evident in the *Star Wars* films. Another important and timely concept advanced by Campbell is the spiritual unity of culture and myths.

Although Jung has a relatively small group of devoted followers, his work has not been embraced by most clinicians except in their use of the Myers-Briggs Type Indicator (see "The MBTI" box). However, many people have manifested interest in his concepts of symbols, archetypes, and synchronicity as people increasingly recognize the importance of spirituality in their lives. The publication of *Liber Novus: The "Red Book" of C. G. Jung* (Shamdasani, 2009) 50 years after Jung's death invigorated analytical and depth psychologists if not all of psychotherapy (Stein, 2010). The "Red Book" is Jung's diary and sketchbook account of his life from 1913 to 1930, a period when he refined his theories of archetypes and the collective unconscious. The thought-provoking nature of his work and the originality and depth of his concepts continue to lead people to become Jungian analysts and to read Jung's works.

The MBTI

Because of the extensive training required to successfully understand and practice Jung's approach, and because it does not offer many tools to the typical clinician, we have chosen to illustrate what is probably the best known contribution of Jung's work to modern therapy: the Myers-Briggs Type Indicator (MBTI) (Myers, McCaulley, Quenk, & Hammer, 1998). Based on Jung's concept of psychological functions and attitudes, the MBTI was initially developed by Katharine Briggs and her daughter Isabel Briggs Myers. One of the most widely used personality inventories, it has an extensive range of uses and is especially appropriate for people who are emotionally healthy or have only mild difficulties. The MBTI is helpful in promoting personal growth, self-awareness, leadership skills, team building, and career development and in enhancing interpersonal skills (Seligman & Reichenberg, 2012). It is used with individuals, in couples counseling, and in work settings.

This inventory yields scores on four bipolar dimensions: introversion-extraversion, sensing-intuition, thinking-feeling, and judging-perceiving. Combinations of these scores yield 16 personality types. A children's version of the MBTI, the Murphy-Meisgeier Type Indicator for Children, is available for those in grades 2 through 8. All preferences on these inventories are considered equally desirable; the inventory is not designed to diagnose pathology but rather to promote self-awareness. The definitions of the first six dimensions are discussed on pages 91–92 of this chapter. The remaining two, judging and perceiving, can be defined as follows:

- **Judging**—People whose personality profile reflects a strong judging component tend to value planning, organization, order, and security. They may have a high need for achievement and generally are viewed as responsible and hardworking.
- **Perceiving**—People with high perceiving scores prefer to be spontaneous and flexible so that they can take advantage of opportunities. They tend to be casual and resourceful and typically make last-minute decisions rather than long-range plans.

For example, imagine that Roberto and Edie Diaz had both completed the MBTI as a way of increasing their self-awareness as well as their understanding of their interactions and the strengths and weaknesses in their marriage. Edie's MBTI type was ISFJ (introversion, sensing, feeling, judging), whereas Roberto's was ESTJ (extraversion, sensing, thinking, judging). His thinking score was especially strong, whereas Edie's feeling score was her highest. A large gap was evident between Edie's introversion score and Roberto's extraversion score as well as between her feeling score and his thinking score.

Each of the MBTI types reflects potential strengths as well as potential weaknesses. People with an MBTI type of ISFJ (like Edie) tend to be caring, sensitive, quiet, practical, and conscientious (Myers, 1998). If they feel unappreciated, they can become resentful and complaining. They may have difficulty asserting themselves and maintaining objectivity.

On the other hand, people with an MBTI type of ESTJ (like Roberto) tend to be decisive and self-confident, outgoing, and concerned with outcome rather than process. They can be impatient, overbearing, and insensitive to the feelings of others.

An examination of Edie's and Roberto's MBTI types sheds light on their difficulties. Roberto tends to devalue Edie's feelings, particularly because, with her strong introversion, she has difficulty articulating her feelings directly. On the other hand, Edie tends to devalue Roberto's need for socialization and results, and accuses him of being shallow and uncaring. Because both share sensing and judging preferences, they tend to have difficulty with spontaneity, flexibility, and change, and are likely to spend too much time on work and chores, neglecting the pleasurable side of their lives. At the same time, they both value organization and planning as well as concrete information.

Exploration of some of their similarities and differences helped the couple identify ways to make positive changes. For example, Roberto agreed to work on his tendency to be critical of Edie and Ava, and Edie agreed to work on articulating her feelings and needs more clearly. Both recognized the importance of having more fun as a couple and as a family.

THE EGO PSYCHOLOGISTS

Linking the ego psychologists is a shift away from Freud's emphasis on the drives and the id to a focus on the development of the ego. Most of these theorists took a broader perspective than did Freud, focusing on development over the life span, and emphasizing the importance of both the self-image and relationships. Beyond that, these theorists differed considerably and those differences sometimes led to rifts in the profession.

Karen Horney

Karen Horney initially believed in the ideas of Freud. However, as her clinical experience grew, she developed her own ideas, which laid the groundwork for important concepts of human development and psychotherapy.

BIOGRAPHY OF KAREN HORNEY Karen Danielson was born in Hamburg, Germany, on September 16, 1885. She always planned to be a doctor, even at a time when no German universities were admitting women to medical school (Eckardt, 2005). She received her medical degree from the University of Berlin, trained as a psychoanalyst, and began a practice in 1919. Her own analysis was with Karl Abraham and Hans Sachs, leaders in their field. In 1909, she married Oskar Horney and they subsequently had three daughters.

Karen Horney broke ground for women in psychoanalysis. She was a founding member, and the first woman teacher, at the Berlin Psychoanalytic Institute (Day, 2008). Between 1923 and 1935, she wrote a series of papers that critically examined the relevance of Freud's theories to women, challenging biological determinism and considering a more holistic approach that included culture, social, and interpersonal factors in the formation of personality. During the 1960s, these papers were embraced by proponents of the feminist movement because of their enlightened view of women (Gilman, 2001).

In 1932, Horney moved to the United States to become the assistant director of the newly established Chicago Institute for Psychoanalysis and subsequently became involved with the New York Psychoanalytic Institute. A complicated person who elicited strong and often conflicting reactions from others, Horney directly challenged Freud's work in her book *New Ways in Psychoanalysis* (1939), which apparently led to her disqualification as instructor and analyst at the New York Psychoanalytic Institute (Day, 2008). In response, she resigned from the institute and formed the American Institute for Psychoanalysis. Horney served as dean of this organization, which is still in existence.

Karen Horney died of cancer on December 4, 1952, shortly after her return from a trip to Japan where she had studied Zen Buddhism. She left a substantial body of work reflecting her broad and timely interest in topics such as women's development, parental and societal influences on children, and the causes of anxiety.

KAREN HORNEY'S THEORIES Horney's early works presented an analysis of Freud's theories with her own revisions. This ultimately evolved into her mature work, which explored human nature and development in both men and women and paid particular attention to culture.

Human nature and self-realization. Horney's view of human nature is positive and optimistic, more consistent with humanistic theorists than with Freud's ideas. She suggested that the purpose of life was actualization of the real self, the repository of the healthy conscience and values that promoted the best interests of all humanity (Paris, 1994). Self-realization involved developing one's innate capacities, emotions, and interests. Horney believed that people who achieve self-realization are self-aware, responsible, and able to make sound judgments. They seek healthy relationships and care about the welfare of others while maintaining their own integrity.

According to Horney, our potential for growth and self-actualization is present at birth and extends across the life span (Danielian, 2010). Children whose environments are nurturing and harmonious, promoting their healthy development, move toward self-realization. However, children raised in aversive environments, especially those that do not provide security, are likely to develop in unhealthy directions. They may develop unrealistic and idealized self-images rather than fulfilling their inherent potential.

Neurosis and basic anxiety. The drive for security, according to Horney, is a more powerful force than either the sexual or the aggressive drive. She believed that hostile, threatening, and unfriendly environments compound children's natural insecurity and lead them to develop a basic anxiety, including feelings of helplessness, isolation, and anger. This, in turn, leads to neurotic conflicts involving a repressed and apparently insoluble dilemma (Horney, 1945). For example, a person might want close relationships yet believe that people are untrustworthy. Neurotic conflicts are expressed indirectly through characteristics such as inconsistency, indecisiveness, fear of change, shyness, sadistic and vindictive behavior, and unexplained fatigue.

Horney (1945) believed that, in an effort to cope with their conflicts, people gravitate toward one of three styles of relating to others:

1. *Moving toward people* involves seeking safety through the protection of others, becoming compliant and self-effacing to please others, blaming ourselves for our interpersonal difficulties, and suppressing our own needs.
2. *Moving against people* is characterized by seeking mastery and domination over others, externalizing blame, being arrogant and vindictive, caring only about ourselves, exploiting and manipulating others, and feeling superior.
3. *Moving away from people* is reflected by avoidance of interpersonal contact, withdrawal and detachment, feelings of differentness, pursuit of self-sufficiency, numbing of emotions, and disregard of rules and restrictions.

Extreme versions of these styles are maladaptive because they restrict growth, lead to poor interpersonal relationships, and may lead to increased risk of physical illness (Horney, 1945). Emotionally healthy people do not need to use exaggerated and inflexible styles of relating to others but deal with the world in balanced and integrated ways that promote positive self-esteem, rewarding relationships, and personal development.

Selves and self-image. Horney believed that people have four competing selves (Paris, 1994):

1. The real self, which has potential for growth
2. The idealized self
3. The despised self, which results from recognizing that we fall short of the idealized self
4. The actual self, all we are at a given time.

The more self-actualizing we are, the more congruent are the real self, the idealized self, and the actual self.

For people without good self-esteem and a sense of wholeness, the idealized image typically dominates. Designed to enhance feelings of worth and provide a sense of identity, the idealized self-image may form the basis for intense striving or actually lead people to feelings of self-contempt because of their failure to live up to this image.

Although efforts to achieve the idealized self-image inevitably fail, people develop strong guidelines about what they must do in their efforts to reach this goal. Horney spoke of the "tyranny of the shoulds" (Horney, 1950; Hergenhahn & Olson, 2007), designed to make us over into our idealized selves. Horney (1950) described four patterns of "shoulds":

- Self-effacing people believe they should be grateful, humble, trusting, and giving.
- Arrogant-vindictive people believe they should be in charge and independent, attack before being attacked, and distrust others.
- Narcissistic people think they should be supremely competent, admired by all, and accept no limitations.
- Detached people believe they should not need other people or expect anything out of life.

Female development. Horney paid considerable attention to the development of girls and women. She couldn't understand Freud's focus on penis envy and believed it to be more of a metaphor for power—women do envy the freedom and power that men have. Horney believed it was equally possible that men experienced womb envy, since the goal of life is self-actualization and productivity, which women achieve naturally through giving birth. Men, she believed, compensate for their inability to give birth by directing their energy and productivity into work and careers (Horney, 1939).

Horney also spoke out against Freud's male bias. She proposed instead that the causes of anxiety and neurosis were the same for women as they are for men and that change could be effected by empowering women and modifying their social roles.

Impact of culture and society. Horney emphasized the role of culture and environment in shaping personality, as well as the importance of understanding people in context. She believed that people's innate characteristics were not fixed but were possibilities shaped through reciprocal interaction with their environments. But culture can change. Horney saw anxiety as less a result of sexual conflict and more a result of conflicts in American society such as competition versus love of humankind and autonomy versus rules and laws. "The most important neurotic conflict is between a compulsive and indiscriminate desire to be the first under all circumstances and the simultaneous need to be loved by everybody" (Horney, 1937, p. 258). Mental health, then, for Horney is defined not as adaptation, but as a centering experience between the dualities.

Horney's psychotherapy. Horney's system of psychotherapy is an optimistic one. She believed that through treatment people can resolve deeply repressed inner conflicts and free their innate constructive forces to grow and develop. She suggested that, with help, people could give up their idealized images and find satisfaction in seeking actualization of their real selves (Hergenhahn & Olson, 2007).

Horney viewed the clinician's role as helping people become aware of their conflicts without being overwhelmed by them (Rossano, 1996), facilitating both emotional and intellectual insight, and reawakening a person's capacity for self-realization and joy. To accomplish this, the clinician works collaboratively with the client. Techniques of free association, analysis of dreams, countertransference and transference, empathy, and education are important in both recovering the past and unraveling the personality structure. Emotional awareness and psychological growth are a two-way process, impacting the therapist and client both. Character splits, projective identification, and repetition compulsion frame the intersubjective space from which the real self emerges (Cohen, 2010). Horney's approach also pays considerable attention to exploring the cultural, social, and family context and life situation of the client.

CURRENT STATUS Horney's (1950) emphasis on unpacking cultural and interpersonal factors, what she referred to as "deep culture," and the development of nonlinear systemic connections that are inconsistent with the unconscious assumptions of mainstream Western scientific thought confounded many of her colleagues, but seem to be consistent with today's postmodern, constructivist belief in the fluidity of subjective and objective reality (Bertolino, 2010; Danielian, 2010). In addition, many of her concepts, such as the tyranny of the shoulds, self-actualization, the idealized self-image, basic anxiety, and neurotic styles of relating to the world, influenced the development of humanistic psychology and continue to facilitate our understanding of people.

Her belief that neglectful parenting results in the creation of children with emotional problems and that parents should be educated in how to raise children with genuine love and affection have been borne out by the research. This emphasis on early healthy relationships with parents helped set the stage for the relational model of psychoanalysis.

Harry Stack Sullivan

Harry Stack Sullivan is considered one of the most influential figures in psychoanalysis. He was the first to emphasize the importance of interpersonal relationships in the development of personality, and he identified the important role anxiety plays in motivating human behavior. Although his ideas, like those of the others in this chapter, draw heavily on Freud's, his emphasis on relationships and concern with the relevance of psychoanalysis led him to develop concepts and approaches that reflect fast-paced, interactive American society more than European culture (Mitchell, 1986). His important contribution to the development of future generations of interpersonal and relational therapists should not be overlooked.

BIOGRAPHY OF HARRY STACK SULLIVAN Harry Stack Sullivan was born on February 21, 1892, in rural Norwich, New York, the only child of a Catholic family living in a Protestant community. He experienced many personal difficulties, culminating in what he viewed as a schizophrenic episode during his freshman year in college (Ewen, 1993). He recovered and went on to receive his medical degree in 1917 from Valparaiso University of Indiana. After serving in the medical corps during World War I, he worked in government and psychiatric hospitals including St. Elizabeth's in Washington, DC, and Shepard Pratt in Baltimore where he focused on treatment of people with schizophrenia. This had a great influence on his theories.

In 1931, Sullivan moved to New York to further his training in psychoanalysis and to establish a successful practice, modifying traditional analysis according to his own ideas. He served as president of the William Alanson White Foundation, founded the still-thriving Washington School of Psychiatry, and initiated the journal *Psychiatry*. Because his ideas were new and controversial, many psychoanalysts felt they needed to choose whether to align themselves with Sullivan or Freud. Sullivan died on January 14, 1949. Although his writings fill seven volumes, most of them were published posthumously.

HARRY STACK SULLIVAN'S THEORIES Sullivan valued the contributions of Freud but disagreed with him in fundamental ways. For Sullivan, Freud's drive theory based on sexual and aggressive instincts was too inflexible, too quick to theorize without supporting data, and too prone to overlook the importance of relationships. Sullivan focused on clients' current behaviors and interactions (Teyber & McClure, 2011). Sullivan developed his own school of psychoanalysis—called Interpersonal Psychoanalysis—to address these shortcomings and communicate his own ideas.

Interpersonal relationships. Sullivan's theory can be thought of as a drive theory, with the search for relatedness being people's primary drive. Intimacy, according to Sullivan, is as strong an interpersonal drive as sexual desire. Both can bring people together in powerful unions that relieve anxiety and provide gratification. Intimacy occurs when people feel that the welfare of another individual is as important to them as their own well-being.

Sullivan believed that relationships proceed according to what he called the *principle of reciprocal emotions* in which the reciprocity of behaviors and attitudes determines the course of the relationship. He viewed pathology as resulting from unhealthy relationships (Sullivan, 1953). Excessive maternal anxiety, loneliness, failure to find satisfactory childhood friendships, and other relationship problems can impair self-esteem and the development of healthy relationships in adulthood.

Anxiety, tension, security, and euphoria. According to Sullivan, anxiety is "the central motivating force in human behavior" (Teyber & McClure, 2011, p. 9). Anxiety, caused primarily by disturbances in relationships, creates tension that disrupts equilibrium (Williams, 1994). Anxiety propels people to seek security in order to minimize tension and create feelings of safety, comfort, and self-esteem. For Sullivan, safe relationships are people's primary source of security. A lack of security leads to anxiety, which contributes to the development of pathology (Fonagy & Target, 2009).

Personality development. Sullivan viewed the personality as the result of myriad strategies the person developed in childhood to avoid or reduce anxiety and maintain equilibrium and a sense of well-being. These coping skills were learned through the parent–child relationship and were adaptive at that time. However, patterns of behavior developed, and as the child grew and matured, he or she overgeneralized the patterns to other relationships inappropriately (Teyber & McClure, 2011).

STRATEGIES OF PSYCHOTHERAPY Sullivan believed that all psychological dysfunction resulted from faulty interpersonal processes. Consequently, he focused his treatment on correcting people's harmful perceptions through the interpersonal process of psychotherapy (Strean, 1994). The relationship of the client and the clinician is a primary component of his approach and helped the client to have "a corrective emotional experience."

According to Sullivan (1953), clinicians should have a sincere desire to help, great respect and empathy for their clients, and a strong interest in them. Clinicians should ensure that sessions progress well, that meaningful work takes place, and that clients keep their anxiety at manageable levels.

Awareness is one of the primary goals of Interpersonal Psychoanalysis. Sullivan believed that if people have a good understanding of their interpersonal relationships and the reciprocal processes in those relationships, they can lead reasonably satisfying lives. Developing that awareness involves examination of clients' life histories from varying viewpoints, so that clinicians and clients can reach a consensus. This brings thoughts and feelings to the surface and facilitates clear thinking as well as new insights, perceptions, experiences, and ways of relating. In other words, "The goal is for the patient to abandon sick dynamisms and to substitute healthy ones in their place" (Chapman, 1978, p. 101).

Sullivan placed emphasis on drawing conclusions based on solid data and observations, and this is reflected in his use of consensus to determine meaning. Achieving consensual validation was necessary to reduce what he called *parataxic distortion,* occurring when people's perceptions and actions are colored and distorted by their unhealthy early childhood relationships and their private logic and images (Sullivan, 1947). Treatment helps people explore these distortions, especially those that are reflected in the client–clinician interaction, so that they can shift from parataxic to syntaxic modes of perceiving that are less influenced by early childhood experiences.

Many aspects of Sullivan's theory are innovative and contemporary and later joined with object relations and John Bowlby's work on attachment theory. He stressed the importance of the therapeutic alliance and viewed therapy as a learning process. He believed that his task was to remove obstacles so that people could realize their natural tendencies toward health, and he emphasized the importance of nonverbal communication. In addition, Sullivan paid attention to cultural background and differences, avoided giving advice, and recognized that brief therapy and flexible treatment schedules could be beneficial. He advocated short and simple interpretations and believed that clinicians should thoroughly understand what they were doing and what their goal was—in effect, plan the treatment (Shainess, 1978). According to Sullivan, when people's views of themselves were consistent with the consensually validated viewpoints that had evolved during their sessions, treatment was complete and people could now use their own resources to pursue more rewarding lives (Levenson, 1992).

CURRENT STATUS Sullivan's work has had an impact on ego psychology, self psychology, phenomenological approaches, interpersonal and relational psychotherapy, family systems therapy, and others. He maintained a deep respect for the uniqueness and power of the individual and for the limitations of psychotherapy. De-emphasizing the importance of dreams, free association, the libido, and transference in treatment, he focused instead on real-life interactions, behaviors, and interpersonal relationships, all of which are important in treatment today.

Anna Freud

Anna Freud, daughter of Sigmund Freud, was her father's colleague, travel companion, secretary, and later his caregiver (Coles, 1992). She was also an innovative theorist and clinician who focused on child development and analysis and the ego defense mechanisms. Her study of the impact of trauma on children is particularly relevant today.

BIOGRAPHY OF ANNA FREUD Anna Freud was born on December 3, 1895, the youngest of Sigmund Freud's six children and the only one to become a psychoanalyst. She first worked as a teacher but quickly shifted her interest to psychoanalysis. In 1922, she qualified to become a psychoanalyst. Current ethical standards were not in place when Anna Freud began to practice; for example, she was psychoanalyzed by her father for 4 years, and she treated the children of family friends (Young-Bruehl, 2008).

Initially, Anna Freud focused her practice on adults. However, her involvement in teaching, rescue work with children and families during World War I, and care of her nephew after her sister's death led her to focus on treating children and adolescents. Anna Freud believed in direct observation and assessment of children, the need to understand child development, and the importance of social interest, as well as the necessity of working with both healthy and troubled children. She combined these interests when she established an experimental nursery designed to serve Vienna's poorest families and provide a vehicle for study of the second year of life and the initial separation of the child from the mother (Sayers, 1991). Freud continued her work in London, where she opened a nursery for children who had been orphaned or separated from their families during World War II. Subsequently, she developed the Hampstead Child Therapy Clinic (now the Anna Freud Centre) for both research and treatment.

Although Freud's training was primarily experiential rather than academic, she wrote numerous books on subjects such as family law and the impact of war on children. Her most important book may be *The Ego and the Mechanisms of Defense* (Freud, 1946), an 80th birthday present for her father.

During her long life, Anna Freud witnessed the growing influence and importance of her own work as well as her father's. She died in London on October 9, 1982.

ANNA FREUD'S THEORIES Anna Freud's areas of specialization were child development and the ego defenses. Because she did not believe that traditional analysis was effective with young children, she emphasized a supportive and educational approach rather than an analytical one.

Child development. Developmental thinking was fundamental to Freud's work. She believed that children mature along a basic trajectory—from the infant's dependency on the mother to the adult's emotional self-reliance. Periods of imbalance or regression can signal problems in maturation, although Freud saw adolescent turmoil as normal, usually requiring time rather than psychotherapy.

The strengthening of the ego so that it gradually gains control over the id allows children to mature from primary process, instinctual, id-governed behavior to the secondary process, ego-driven behaviors and experiences of adults. Freud believed that the role of the mother, especially during the second half of the child's first year of life, is critical in ego development. She asserted that the presence of a constant maternal object and a reciprocal mother–infant relationship were essential for development of the child's healthy capacity for attachment. Thus, Freud suggested that orphaned or displaced children should reside with relatives or foster families rather than in institutions and that hospitalized children should be allowed to have a parent stay with them.

Child psychoanalysis. Freud conceived of child psychoanalysis as a method of understanding and asking questions, leading to the emergence of the child's inner experiences and internal world (Mayes & Cohen, 1996). She recognized that children rarely have an active wish for treatment. Rather, they cooperate with treatment primarily for three reasons (Freud, 1965):

1. They trust and believe in an adult whom they perceive as helpful and interested.
2. They wish to please the clinician.
3. They view the clinician as a sort of understanding and safe parent.

These attitudes needed to be nurtured in order to address children's reluctance to engage in treatment.

Freud viewed child analysis as different from adult analysis in important respects. She believed that children often cannot benefit from direct interpretation but can gain more from the use of stories about toys or other children. She recognized that behavior that appears maladaptive might reflect a child's best effort to cope with environmental stressors. In addition, what might be resistance in an adult may be a developmentally appropriate response in a child. The clinician has to take an active role to facilitate children's self-expression and to clarify the connection between their symptoms and the content of sessions. Freud's treatment of children usually focused on current life events rather than transference and repressed material.

Role of environment. Anna Freud believed that clinicians must pay attention to children's environments. She emphasized the need to establish a treatment alliance with the child's parents and to understand the child's social and family situation.

Freud believed that analysis should be used primarily to treat internal and internalized conflicts, not problems due essentially to external causes (Mayes & Cohen, 1996; Sayers, 1991). Freud saw the impact of environmental factors on children who had been separated from their parents during World War II. She had great compassion for these children and sought to help them, but did not view analysis as the best treatment for such externally caused difficulties. According to Freud, efforts to change the environment, as well as supportive interventions, were often more appropriate to facilitate development and address the aftereffects of external events such as inadequate parenting and environmental traumas.

Assessment. Freud believed strongly in the assessment of both emotionally healthy and troubled children as a way of identifying the hallmarks of age-appropriate development. She maintained a flexible concept of healthy development, recognizing that individual variations and fluctuations in development were often normal. She sought to obtain a balanced picture of children's development, focusing on areas of positive growth and adjustment as well as areas of impairment. To enhance her work, Freud developed several tools and assessment procedures, including the Diagnostic or Metapsychological Profile and the Hampstead Psychoanalytic Index, which systematized the process of gathering information on children's development (Sandler, 1996).

Ego defenses. One of Freud's major contributions was her comprehensive description of ego defense mechanisms (Sandler & Freud, 1985). She believed that people used defense mechanisms to cope with anxiety stimulated by either unacceptable drives from the id or harmful threats and commands from the superego. Freud shifted the emphasis of her approach from the drives to the ego defenses, which, according to Gabbard (2005), "anticipated the movement of psychoanalysis and dynamic psychiatry away from neurotic symptom formation and toward character pathology" (p. 22).

Strategies of intervention. Although Freud's work has particular relevance to the treatment of young people, she believed that psychoanalysis of adults could be enhanced by understanding and reconstructing childhood developmental issues (Coles, 1992). Consequently, her work has meaning for all clinicians.

Freud's concept of therapy emphasized several perspectives that are compatible with treatment today. She believed in the importance of the therapeutic alliance, saying, "To be in contact is so important, and to interpret does not always mean to be in contact" (Freud, 1983, p. 119). She advocated an optimistic and holistic perspective: "In treatment, you work with the healthy side of the child and you work with the ill side—you don't only work with the ill side, but you trust that the healthy side will come to your assistance, although it may not be there or it may not be strong enough" (p. 125). She emphasized the importance of clinician flexibility, letting treatment follow the needs of the child and perhaps suggesting a game to reduce a child's anxiety.

CURRENT STATUS Anna Freud's moderate and realistic stance led to her great influence in the field of child analysis; even today, her methods are widely used in the Western world and continue to be consistent with current thinking about childhood development, assessment, and treatment (Lerner, 2008).

Anna Freud has left a legacy of childhood developmental analysis, expanded ego defense mechanisms, and recommendations on child care policy. According to Lerner (2008), she was among the first to view childhood pathology in terms of developmental evolution, and to recognize "that the profile among trajectories (lines) in development determined the risk of pathology for the developing child" (p. 132). The implications are important for clinicians who should focus not only on etiology and development of symptoms, but on providing developmentally appropriate help to get the child back on the course of normal development (Freud, 1965). Furthermore, "Her innovative thinking and active collaboration in child care and health and in education and the law, in addition to her extraordinary capacity to be practical in providing care for children caught up in 'experiments' of nature and man-made catastrophes were brilliant applications of psychoanalytic theory in the service of children and their parents" (Solnit, 1997, p. 7).

Anna Freud's ideas and writings have left their mark. Her writings on child rearing include *Beyond the Best Interests of the Child* (Goldstein, Freud, & Solnit, 1973) and *Before the Best Interests of the Child* (Goldstein, Freud, & Solnit, 1979); those on the impact of war on children include *War and Children* (Freud & Burlingham, 1943) and *Infants Without Families* (Freud & Burlingham, 1944). Also important are her pioneering works on child and adolescent analysis and development; her emphasis on health and on the ego and its defenses; her belief that all people dealing with children must have practical as well as theoretical training; and her appreciation of the importance of the therapeutic alliance, healthy early attachment, the family system, and context.

Anna Freud's ideas also paved the way for other theorists and clinicians to focus on the bond between the child and the parent. Particularly important is research on attachment theory, increasingly acknowledged as a key variable in human development. The object relations theorists, including John Bowlby and his important work on attachment theory (Bowlby, 1978; Greenberg & Mitchell, 1983), are discussed next.

OBJECT RELATIONS THEORISTS

Although object relations theory may seem complicated, it offers clinicians many useful tools and concepts. In general, object relations theorists attend to the past by exploring people's early childhood relationships and attend to the present through the development of the client–clinician relationship. Observing what is occurring in that interaction can give clinicians information about what clients have experienced in past relationships, while an understanding of the past can shed light on present interactions.

Overview of Object Relations Theory

The central concept of object relations theory is that adult personality characteristics depend on the nature of people's early relationships, particularly the relationship the child has with the mother or primary caregiver. According to this theory, the infant is driven to attach to an "object," defined not as another person but as the internal mental structure that the infant forms of that person through introjection. This internal mental structure or representation is based on both actual and fantasized experiences that involved an investment of emotions and energy. The mother usually is the first internal object, but others evolve over time.

As the infant forms these introjections, feelings will inevitably arise that the infant cannot tolerate. Anger toward the mother is one of these feelings. Because experiencing these feelings might jeopardize the child's emotional gratification and safety, the child splits off and represses these unacceptable emotions. These are dealt with via projective identification, in which the split-off parts of the self are projected onto another person with whom the self can then identify.

In healthy infant development, where consistent and nurturing parenting has been provided throughout the child's life, the infant becomes able to reclaim the unacceptable feelings at about 8 months of age as he or she begins to individuate and separate from the caregiver. The infant then can accept the notion that the self and the caregiver each have both positive and negative emotions. Object relations theory sees the early mother (or primary caretaker) and child experience as the template for relationship patterns that follow. For these theorists, then, the critical events that shape people's lives occur not at 5 or 6 years, but at 5 or 6 months.

IMPACT OF INTERNALIZED OBJECTS ON RELATIONSHIPS These internal representations affect people's later sense of themselves as well as their perceptions of and capacity for forming external relationships. Object relations theorists believe that symptoms such as anxiety, depression, and impaired relationships reflect the nature of people's problems with object relations and corresponding threats to their sense of self.

INTERVENTION STRATEGIES Freudian psychoanalysis forms the backdrop for object relations therapists. Many of their approaches stem from his school of thought, and their work typically entails long-term and intensive analysis. However, changes in emphasis, application, and technique distinguish object relations therapists from classic Freudian analysts. In addition, significant differences of opinion characterize the object relations theorists discussed later in this chapter. The British

Psychoanalytic Group responded to these differences by dividing their curriculum into the *A* group (Freudian) and the *B* group (Kleinian). Winnicott began the *C* group, which saw value in both of the other groups. Object relations theorists were also divided according to national lines. For example, the British group (including Klein, Fairbairn, and Winnicott) emphasized transference and countertransference, whereas the American group (including Mahler and Kernberg) was more interested in ego functioning and adaptation (Scharff & Scharff, 2005).

Projective identification. All three groups viewed the process of projective identification, along with its exploration and analysis, as an essential treatment ingredient. Projective identification should be distinguished from transference. In transference, the clinician is viewed inaccurately as having characteristics of significant people in the client's early life; for example, the clinician may be seen as an angry and judgmental parent. In projective identification, a part of the internalized object or the self is projected onto the therapist. The internal object relationship is then recreated in the client–clinician relationship, where it can be reworked to allow modification of the internalized object (Scharff & Scharff, 2005). Being receptive to a client's projective identification is the first step in being able to uncover overwhelming feelings of rage and despair and, ultimately, contain them (Sweet, 2010).

Therapeutic alliance. Establishing a positive therapeutic alliance is much more important to object relations theorists than it was to classic psychoanalysts. Just as an important element in the mother's role is to provide nurturing and care, so are those elements perceived as important in the therapeutic process. According to object relations theory, clinicians should deliberately introduce these and other elements into therapy to facilitate transference and projective identification. In a sense, the therapist becomes a good-enough mother, providing a holding environment for people who may never have had adequate parenting. Affective exchanges between clinician and client bring the internal object relationships into the here and now, allow the client to reexperience those relationships, and promote insight and change.

Resistance. Resistance in clients is viewed as reflecting a rigid transference, growing out of the client's strong need for a particular type of object relationship. Resistance leads to the client's inability to relate to the clinician in ways that are flexible and reflective of present relationships. Resistance is a way for people to keep painful emotions and fantasies buried in the unconscious to protect the self from the threat these pose. Clinicians can reduce resistance by acknowledging and accepting clients' internal worlds and by being patient, consistent, safe, and available.

Countertransference. Understanding countertransference as well as transference and projective identification is important in object relations theory. Countertransference is viewed as inevitable in the interaction between the client and the therapist and is a source of important clues regarding the nature of the transference relationship (Greenberg & Mitchell, 1983). In understanding and dealing with their countertransference reactions, clinicians should be clear about whether those reactions stem largely from interactions with a client or from the clinicians' own issues and experiences. W. R. D. Fairbairn, a Scottish psychiatrist who practiced psychoanalysis in the 1930s, has been credited by many as the father of relational theory as it is practiced today, and also for emphasizing interpretation of the transference process (Celani, 2010; Grotstein & Rinsley, 1994; Scharff & Scharff, 2005).

Assessment. The clinician, in collaboration with the client, assesses the person's development; unconscious patterns; internalized object relationships; and underlying anxieties, defenses, and projective identifications. A thorough assessment is necessary to pave the way for well-timed and accurate interpretations that will make a difference.

Interpretation. Interpretation is a primary route to change. Through analysis and interpretation of transference, projective identification and countertransference, past and present experiences, and the manifestations of the unconscious, people work through their internalized and unconscious emotions and relationships. *Working through* is the process of obtaining clarification and resolution of projective identification patterns by experiencing them over and over at progressively higher levels of development. Kaner and Prelinger (2005) posited that "working through may well constitute the main work of therapy" (p. 275). Rather than a linear process, it is more like a dance between therapist and client. The more "repetitions are worked through, reworked, strengthened and confirmed, the more will be the therapeutic gains" (p. 275). This enables people to develop the capacity to transcend old patterns and have genuine emotional contact with others. When this is accomplished, and when people can have loving relationships, cooperate with and perceive others accurately, have empathy and concern for others, and manage their own stress, they are ready for their analysis to terminate.

The Object Relations Theorists

Many names are associated with the development of object relations theory. This section offers an overview of the backgrounds and ideas of some of the most important, including Melanie Klein and John Bowlby. Others who contributed to the development of object relations theory include W. R. D. Fairbairn, D. W. Winnicott, Otto Kernberg, Margaret Mahler, and Ivan Boszormenyi-Nagy.

MELANIE KLEIN Melanie Klein is regarded as the mother of object relations theory (Cashdan, 1988). Her work as an analyst grew out of her fascination with Sigmund Freud's work and her own experience in analysis. Like Anna Freud, Klein focused her work on treating children. After practicing in Budapest and Berlin, she relocated to England where she wrote and practiced until her death in 1960 (Greenberg & Mitchell, 1983).

Klein was a transitional figure who shifted the focus of psychoanalysis away from Sigmund Freud's drive theory and toward the importance of early relationships. Although her failure to successfully integrate drive theory and object relations theory probably explains why most of her ideas are not currently accepted, she contributed several important concepts to psychoanalysis.

Klein suggested that when a child is 3 to 6 months of age, the infant develops the capacity to internalize objects and integrate fragmented perceptions of the caregiver. Klein believed that these mechanisms, as well as introjection, splitting, projection, and projective identification, were used by infants to avoid fears of death and their own destructive impulses. Internalized objects color people's later relationships. Fantasies and anxieties stemming from people's internal object world form the basis for their later moods, behaviors, and self-images. The roots of modern object relations theory are evident in this concept.

According to Mitchell (1993), Klein "saw aggression as central in the formation of psychic structure beginning early in life and continuing throughout" (p. 155). Building on Freud's drive theory, Klein believed that all of life is a movement between the forces of the life instinct (*eros*) and the opposite death instinct (*thanatos*). As a result, Klein postulated people have two fundamental positions: paranoid-schizoid, which arises from thanatos, and depressive, which is related to the eros position. The *paranoid-schizoid* position stems from infants' natural fearfulness or paranoia. In an attempt to ward off danger, infants separate good objects and feelings from bad objects and feelings. Klein termed this pattern *splitting,* referring to splits in the ego as well as in the conceptual and emotional organization of the self. In the paranoid-schizoid position, people's emotional focus is on aggression and other-directed destructiveness, manifested through envy and grandiosity, and characterized by defenses such as splitting and projective identification. Splitting is currently viewed as a defense, common among people with borderline personality disorders, in which they view themselves, others, and their life experience in extremes—as either all good or all bad.

The *depressive* position reflects people's concern that images of and connections with the internalized objects are threatened by internal conflicts. The depressive position is characterized by the defense of regression; people in this position focus on emotions such as love, understanding, empathy, and reparation of the internalized object.

How these positions are manifested vary throughout a person's life. Mature people primarily manifest the depressive position, which is never fully overcome (Lubbe, 2011; Scharff & Scharff, 2005). Less healthy people are likely to turn their aggression against themselves through the use of self-harming behaviors, eating disorders, addictions, and suicide (Sweet, 2010; Waska, 2010). Recent research reinforces Klein's theory that depression and destructive and physically aggressive tendencies are evidenced in early childhood and may wax and wane at different times across the life span and that adult pathology can more often than not be foreshadowed to early stages of childhood (Fonagy & Target, 2009; Lubbe, 2011).

Klein also believed that play in children is comparable to free association in adults, reflecting unconscious material. This viewpoint is now well accepted in child psychoanalysis. Klein's merger of classic Freudian analysis with object relations theory continues to be popular in England, where it is one of the major schools of psychoanalysis. It is also taught in the United States at the Psychoanalytic Center of California.

JOHN BOWLBY John Bowlby is currently one of the best-known object relations theorists because of his development of attachment theory. Bowlby hypothesized the existence of a universal human need to form close emotional bonds (Fonagy & Target, 2009). Child and caregiver form a system in which the attachment behaviors of the infant (e.g., smiling, clinging) are ideally reciprocated by adult attachment behaviors (e.g., touching, soothing, feeding). This provides security and emotional regulation. Bowlby (1988) believed that a strong causal relationship existed between children's attachment to their parents and their later capacity to form affectional bonds and experience positive emotional development. The main variable in this connection is the extent to which children's parents provide them with a secure base that allows for growth and exploration.

Bowlby's clinical approach reflected his emphasis on attachment. He believed that, like a good parent, clinicians need to respect and encourage clients' desire to explore the world and make their own decisions. According to Bowlby (1988), therapists applying attachment theory provide the following conditions:

- A secure base from which people can explore painful and unhappy aspects of their lives
- Help and encouragement with this exploratory process, facilitating people's efforts to understand the connections between patterns in their current relationships and those in unconscious and internalized images
- Encouragement for people to consider whether and how their current perceptions, expectations, emotions, and actions may be the products of childhood experiences and messages, especially those connected to their parents
- A therapeutic alliance that can be analyzed and understood in light of clients' new insights and information
- Help in assessing the appropriateness, accuracy, and helpfulness of people's models of themselves and others.

Bowlby believed that the essence of treatment was to help people understand the nature and development of representational models of attachment figures that were governing their perceptions, expectations, and actions and, if indicated, to help them modify those in light of more recent experience (Bowlby, 1978).

Bowlby's ideas have provided the basis for many articles and research studies supporting and extending his concept of attachment to include experiences across the life span. For example, in a study of adult romantic relationships, Hazan and Shaver (1987) found a correlation between attachment style and patterns in current relationships. Research showed that children with a history of secure attachment are more likely than those without this sort of attachment to manifest many positive personal characteristics including resilience, self-reliance, empathy, social interest, and ability to form close intimate relationships. Attachment relationships also figure prominently in transgenerational transmission of deprivation; secure adults are more likely to have children who grow up and form their own secure attachments.

Mary Ainsworth (Ainsworth, Blehar, Waters, & Walls, 1978) conducted what is probably the most important and best-known research based on Bowlby's concepts. Ainsworth and her colleagues created what they termed the "strange situation" in which infants were observed before, during, and after a brief period of time in which they were separated from their caregivers and left with a stranger in an unfamiliar environment. The infants' responses were classified into the following four categories:

1. *Secure.* Children demonstrated curiosity and comfort in the presence of their caregiver, became anxious and distressed in the presence of the stranger, and sought and accepted comfort when the caregiver returned, soon resuming exploration.
2. *Anxious/avoidant.* These children were less anxious with the stranger, did not seek comfort from the caregiver, and did not seem to prefer the caregiver over the stranger. These children probably had experiences in which the caregiver did not help them regulate their emotions; consequently, they overregulate emotions and avoid troubling situations.
3. *Anxious/resistant.* Children in this group engaged in little exploration, were highly distressed during the separation, but had difficulty accepting comfort from the caregiver and continued to manifest anxiety or anger.
4. *Disorganized/disoriented.* Children in this group manifested confusing and undirected behavior such as head banging and a wish to escape, even after the caregiver had returned. Ainsworth suggested that the caregivers of these children had evoked both fear and comfort. A history of neglect or abuse often is associated with this pattern.

With the findings of Ainsworth and her colleagues as a basis, researchers have developed the Adult Attachment Interview, a structured clinical instrument designed to elicit narratives of childhood attachment relationships. Scoring classifies respondents as secure/autonomous, insecure/dismissing, insecure/preoccupied, or unresolved in terms of their attachments as adults (George, Kaplan, & Main, 1996).

Attachment Theory Across the Life Span

Hazan and Shaver (1987) found a correlation between attachment style and patterns in current relationships. Children with a history of secure attachment are more likely than those without this sort of attachment to manifest many positive personal characteristics including resilience, self-reliance, empathy, social interest, and ability to form close intimate relationships. Securely attached adults exhibit more energy, friendliness, and emotional stability (Conradi & de Jonge, 2009; Surcinelli, Rossi, Montebarocci, & Baldaro, 2010).

Bowlby indicated that the attachment system remains active across the life span. Since the 1980s, many assessment tools, including individual and family questionnaires and structured interviews, have been developed to assess the type and quality of adult attachment (Bartholomew

& Horowitz, 1991; George et al., 1996). Empirical studies of adult attachment have found distributions roughly equivalent to attachment patterns in infants: 55% securely attached, 25% avoidant, and 20% anxious (Levy, Ellison, Scott, & Bernecker, 2011). Early attachment-related trauma increases the risk for anxiety disorders not only in childhood, but in adolescence and on into adulthood (Bateman & Fonagy, 2012; Green et al., 2010). Contemporary neuroscience is just beginning to understand the intergenerational transmission of anxiety as well as the protection (or risk) that early attachment relationships offer against the development of psychopathology across the life span (Fonagy & Luyten, 2009; Nolte, Guiney, Fonagy, Mayes, & Luyten, 2011).

Additional research on adult attachment style has found it to be an important measure of the quality of a person's relationships (e.g., romantic relationships, friendships, parenting style), as well as identifying excessive dependency, borderline traits, and attachment anxiety. In general, secure attachment in adulthood is characterized by better mental health, whereas insecure attachment is associated with negative thinking and a corresponding increase in depression and anxiety (Surcinelli et al., 2010). Adults who have an anxious-avoidant attachment style have the highest depression scores of any of the four types, and those who feel insecurely attached and have negative thinking are more vulnerable to developing psychopathology.

Research has also verified Bowlby's belief that the therapist and the therapeutic relationship can provide a secure base from which clients can explore new experiences (Bowlby, 1988; Farber & Metzger, 2009; Goodman, 2010; Levy et al., 2011). In other words, the therapist can become an attachment figure.

New research indicates that attachment style may be relevant in psychotherapy outcomes. Specifically, some studies have suggested that securely attached clients have better outcomes than those with insecure attachment (Obegi & Berant, 2009). A meta-analytic review of 14 studies found that the client's attachment style contributed almost as much to treatment outcome as the therapeutic alliance (Levy et al., 2011). The authors conclude that adult attachment style is so important it should be a part of the initial assessment process with new clients. Awareness of a client's attachment style can contribute in meaningful ways to developing and maintaining the alliance, directing therapy, and providing positive therapeutic outcomes. Goodman (2010) warns, however, that no amount of assessment or manualized treatment can take the place of a therapist's own intuition and ability to adjust his or her style to the needs of the client and thereby provide a corrective emotional experience.

Current Status of Object Relations Theory

Object relations theories have made many important contributions to counseling and psychotherapy and remain important to these professions. Research by Bowlby (1978, 1988) and others has affirmed object relations theorists' emphasis on the child's attachment to the caregiver. Many believe that attachment problems in Western society are becoming more prevalent because of the high divorce rate, high stress in our daily lives, and demanding and busy schedules that make parents less able to meet children's attachment needs. This, in turn, has been implicated as a factor in the growing rates of youth violence and family instability. Cult and gang membership can be understood from an object relations perspective as a way of exploiting the universal need for attachment and belonging (Salande & Perkins, 2011).

Other contributions of object relations theory to contemporary counseling and psychotherapy include:

- The link it established between developmental theory and psychoanalytic practice
- The emphasis it placed on ensuring that the therapeutic situation is a safe place, a holding environment, and a place of containment that enables people to meet the challenges of emotional growth without being engulfed by troubling emotions
- The recognition of the importance of both countertransference and transference, the person of the therapist, the therapeutic alliance, and attention to the here-and-now clinical situation.

Object relations theory has become the dominant theoretical perspective within psychodynamic psychotherapy today and continues to evolve, with particular interest and research being conducted on the effects of attachment across the life span. Stephen A. Mitchell, a clinical psychologist and psychoanalyst, was a leading proponent of an integrative, relational perspective that shifted the focus away from classical Freudian drive theory toward the importance of human attachment plus relationships (Willock, 2001). In their book, *Freud and Beyond* (1996), Mitchell and Margaret Black clarified and organized post-Freudian theories into one cohesive text. Mitchell founded the International Association for Relational Psychology and published numerous books on the subject (*Can Love Last?,* 2003; *Relationality: From Attachment to Intersubjectivity,* 2000) before his untimely death from a heart attack, at the age of 54.

Similarly building on attachment theory, Greenberg and Johnson (1988; Johnson & Whiffen, 2005) integrated Bowlby's attachment theory with humanistic person-centered therapy in the creation of emotion-focused therapy. Their work, which provides a structure and process for understanding the importance of relationships and the connection between people, is particularly effective in work with people who have difficulty with emotion regulation, and as a theoretical orientation for work with couples (Johnson, 2004; Greenberg & Goldman, 2008). More will be said about Susan Johnson's emotion-focused couples therapy in the chapter on family therapy (Chapter 18).

Object relations therapy is being used with individuals, couples, and families; in play therapy, art therapy, and group therapy; and for treatment of substance misuse, anorexia nervosa, personality disorders (especially borderline and histrionic personality disorders), and even psychosis (Celani, 2010; Scharff & Scharff, 2005).

Attachment theory, unlike other psychoanalytic theories, is based on research, not just case studies. As research continues to shed light on the importance of early childhood attachments on the development of the self and the quality of later attachments across a person's lifetime, the work of John Bowlby and others will continue to influence positively the direction in which all forms of psychotherapy evolve.

HEINZ KOHUT AND SELF PSYCHOLOGY

Unlike object relations, in which the internalized relationships are at the center of development, self psychology places the self at the center. Heinz Kohut, who developed a theory of self psychology, was a classical Freudian psychoanalyst who believed a person's sense of self was deeply influenced by early caregivers. Children who do not receive adequate nurturing develop an impaired sense of self, which becomes the basis of much pathology. Kohut's emphasis on empathy, self-image, current experience, and the importance of taking a holistic view of people, as well as his groundbreaking work on narcissism, made essential contributions to counseling and psychotherapy.

Biography of Heinz Kohut

Born in Vienna, Austria, in 1913, Kohut was an only child. He completed medical school in Vienna in 1938 just 4 days before Kristallnacht turned his world upside down. He emigrated to England the following year. In 1940, Kohut and his mother Else moved to Chicago (Strozier, 2001). After a brief psychoanalysis, Kohut focused his work on psychiatry and neurology. He completed his residency at the University of Chicago and became a U.S. citizen in 1945. In 1948, he married Betty Meyer, a social worker.

During the 1950s, Kohut established a successful clinical practice, which provided the basis for his ideas. He has been described as meticulous but playful; he had the ability to invest himself heavily in his work as a clinician, teacher, researcher, writer, and leader in his field but also to set limits and to enjoy the moment (Strozier, 2001). Until 1965, Kohut was a spokesperson for Freudian psychoanalysis. However, his ideas about narcissism and his book *The Analysis of the Self* (1971) created a rift between him and other leading analysts of his time. This, coupled with his mother's development of paranoid delusions and her death in 1972, led him to engage in additional self-analysis and creative thought and writing. Kohut died in 1981, leaving behind a considerable body of work.

Kohut's Theories

Kohut considered the self to be the nucleus of the individual that regulates self-esteem, organizes experiences, and gives meaning to life (Strozier, 2001).

THE SELF Kohut emphasized the importance of establishing meaningful goals and of the attachment of young children to their parents. He conceived of the self as evolving out of this relationship. For Kohut, the observable self was the focus of analysis rather than Freud's ego, id, and superego (Cocks, 1994). Kohut believed that a strong self allows us to tolerate and successfully handle successes and failures, while a deficient self is developmentally frozen and prone to fragmentation (Gabbard, 2005; Kohut & Wolf, 1978). He described the self structure, which begins at 18 months of age, as having three self object needs (Goldstein, 2001):

1. The need for confirmation, validation, and mirroring responses from others
2. The need to internalize an idealized *selfobject*, which provides nurturing and helps the child learn to self-soothe
3. The need for a twin or alter ego, which seeks mutuality and equality in relationships with others as well as sharing of values and preferences.

Kohut's concept of the selfobject is broader than the internalized object discussed by the object relations theorists. They referred primarily to children's internalization of their image of the mother, whereas Kohut used *selfobject* as a generic term for our intrapsychic experiences of others, our mental representations of them experienced as part of the self or in service of the self. Selfobjects are needed throughout our lives. These internalized images constantly change and mature to provide us with a sense of ourselves, self-esteem, soothing, and validation, and to meet our needs for mirroring, idealizing, and twinship (Goldstein, 2001). Maturation and emotional health are reflected by our ability to use more appropriate and growth-promoting selfobjects.

VIEW OF PEOPLE Self psychology is based not on efforts to contain the drives but on understanding and promoting people's development in the context of a responsive environment so that they can achieve their positive potentials (Lachmann & Beebe, 1995). For Kohut, feelings of sexuality and aggression, appropriately moderated, are part of our normal development and integral parts of ourselves, not the primary source of our difficulties.

According to Kohut (1982), traditional psychoanalysis views a person with emotional difficulties as the "guilty man"—a person trapped in a conflict between the drives of the id and the constraints of the superego. Instead, Kohut speaks of the "tragic man," "attempting, and never quite succeeding, to realize the program laid down in his depth during the span of his life," his failures overshadowing his successes (p. 402). Kohut viewed the tragic man as typically the product of an unempathic mother and an absent father. A representation of both men and women with emotional difficulties, the tragic man has the potential for growth, joy, adjustment, and fulfillment but consistently fails to reach that potential (Cocks, 1994).

Empathy, providing affirmation and mirroring, is essential to development of the healthy self. Initially, children need empathy from their parents to promote the development of children's psychological strengths (Lerner, 2008). However, people later seek empathy from others. Empathy is an essential ingredient of the therapeutic relationship. This thinking reflects Kohut's emphasis on the present—what he called the *experience near* (as distinguished from the *experience far,* which refers to the id, ego, and superego and to early childhood experiences). Kohut believed that, although past experiences have a profound impact on our development, it is the present or here-and-now experiences that lead to their resolution.

NARCISSISM AND OTHER CLINICAL SYNDROMES Kohut perceived narcissism, one of the central concepts of his later work, as existing on a continuum. Healthy narcissism allows people to value themselves and their needs and to have self-confidence. Pathological narcissism often results when healthy development of a cohesive self is blocked. Unhealthy narcissism involves an unstable self-concept, grandiose fantasies of self-importance, a sense of entitlement, and an inability to think of others as anything but need-gratifying objects. Pathological narcissism can be reflected in a broad range of symptoms, including depression, anxiety, hypochondriasis, misuse of drugs, acting out, and dysfunctional sexual experiences, as well as fragmentation of the self and lack of a zest for life (Wolf, 1994). Kohut believed that this sort of narcissism was at the root of many people's emotional difficulties and that it could be modified through treatment.

Kohut also identified clinical syndromes that he often saw in treatment, including the fragmented self, the overstimulated self, the overburdened self, and the understimulated self (Lerner, 2008). In addition, he described some character or personality types, including the mirror hungry, ideal hungry, alter-ego hungry, contact shunning, and merger hungry. Kohut linked these syndromes and character types to particular early experiences and symptoms and suggested treatment strategies for each. This information is useful in helping clinicians understand personality disorders and other long-standing and pervasive unhealthy patterns that clients manifest, and facilitates efforts to treat these challenging disorders.

Intervention Strategies

In self psychology, treatment focuses on a client's subjective experiences and meanings, enabling the clinician to enter the client's world. From that vantage point, clinicians address the condition of the self, including symptoms, developmental deficits, intrapsychic conflicts, and relational and behavioral difficulties. The ultimate goal is development of a healthy and cohesive self.

EMPATHY Kohut viewed empathy (which he labeled vicarious introspection) as essential to effective treatment. Self psychology theorists believe that clinicians should take a nurturing role; emphasize active and open listening; and provide acceptance, understanding, and explanations or interpretations to facilitate the unfolding of the client's subjective world. Clinicians constantly reflect the essence of what clients have said, and clients' confirmation or rejection of these reflections allows clinicians to truly understand clients' inner reality.

Clinicians practicing self psychology avoid judging and view even narcissistic needs as developmentally understandable rather than immature and self-centered. Resistance and symptoms are viewed as efforts to protect the vulnerable self and maintain some internal cohesion. Clinicians' obvious interest in clients and their valuing of clients' words increase client investment in treatment and encourage disclosure of painful and unacceptable material.

TRANSFERENCE Clinicians' empathy for clients is used as a way to facilitate the development of transference. In an idealizing selfobject transference, the vulnerable client perceives the clinician as a source of strength and safety who is able to respond to unmet developmental needs, including mirroring, idealizing, and twinship (Lerner, 2008). Clients' needs reflect those that were frustrated in the course of development, and the transference is viewed as a reactivation of the selfobject experience. Empathy allows clinicians to contain and rebuild the early selfobject reflected in the transference relationship. Techniques such as *optimal frustration* and *optimal responsiveness* allow clients to change their internalizations, incorporating the skills provided by the clinician, so that clients develop an inner sense of self-competence that allows them to deal successfully with frustrations and nurture themselves. Kohut discusses this process in *The Restoration of the Self* (1977) and *How Does Analysis Cure?* (1984).

Current Status of Self Psychology

Since his death in 1981, Kohut's concepts have been expanded on and substantiated through empirical research on infant development (Lachmann & Beebe, 1995). In addition, his work also has gained in influence because of our increasing attention to personality disorders. Kohut's work also has demonstrated its value in treating depression and anxiety, eating disorders (Bachar, 1998), and the impact of abuse (Hirschman, 1997). In addition, self psychology seems to have value in treating people with psychoses and borderline personality disorders, although the approach needs to be adapted to treatment of people with these disorders.

Although research on the application of self psychology to a diverse client population is limited, some studies suggest that this approach has broad relevance and application. Elliott, Uswatte, Lewis, and Palmatier (2000), for example, studied Kohut's idea that optimal adjustment during life transitions depended on people's capacity for pursuing meaningful goals and achieving a stable sense of self. They found that people's adjustment to and acceptance of recent disabilities, as well as their subjective well-being and life satisfaction, were indeed related to meaningful goal orientation and sense of self. Kim (2002) found that, among male Korean immigrants, their concepts of God and their religious leaders provided them mirroring, idealing, and twinship selfobjects. In another study, Lesser (2000) found that group therapy based on self psychology promoted helpful self-awareness in women. Although more research is needed, these and other recent studies suggest that, when used with flexibility, self psychology is appropriate for use with most populations.

Kohut's emphasis on the importance of the client–clinician collaboration, his understanding of narcissism and the role it often plays in emotional disorders, and his phenomenological perspective, emphasizing people's subjective reality, are important contributions to the practice of depth psychotherapy and also to the development of humanistic approaches to counseling and psychotherapy. Kohut provides a way of understanding and helping people that is analytical in nature but at the same time consistent with the current clinical emphasis on early attachments; subjective reality; and the importance of promoting resilience, optimism, and empowerment in clients. Kohut's view of the tragic man captures the pitfalls of our ambitious and hurried society and enhances the timeliness of his theory.

SKILL DEVELOPMENT: INTERPRETATION

Interpretation is one of the fundamental skills of psychoanalysis and is employed by all of the clinicians discussed in this chapter. Interpretations provide people with an alternative frame of reference for viewing a problem or situation. Interpretations can link a current reaction that may appear unimportant to a past experience that has considerable depth and significance, thereby providing clients new understanding and routes to change.

Interpretations often reflect insights that clinicians have into clients' motives and behaviors that may not yet be in clients' awareness. For that reason, practitioners must deliver interpretations with great care. Ideally, questioning and information-giving can be used to help clients make their own interpretations. Timing is another critical variable in effective interpretations; they should be presented when people are ready to accept and understand them. Clinicians also should be clear about what they hope to accomplish in making an interpretation. Although it may enhance clinicians' self-esteem to realize that they are insightful and have drawn important connections between pieces of information that clients have presented, interpretations, of course, should never be self-serving or primarily for the purpose of demonstrating the clinician's skills. Rather, they should be used to move clients forward in positive ways such as helping them gain insights that will enhance their self-esteem, empower them, help them make better choices, facilitate their efforts to manage and change their emotions, and improve their interpersonal and other behaviors. Finally, presentation of interpretations should never create an adversarial situation in which clinician and client are in conflict or engaged in a debate about who is right. Generally, interpretations are most successful if they are presented tentatively as information for clients to think about and discuss. If interpretations are not meaningful to clients, they should have the right to reject them without being made to feel as though they are cowardly, unintelligent, or fearful of change. Using language carefully and thoughtfully can contribute to the successful delivery of interpretations.

CASE ILLUSTRATION

Consider the following dialogue between Roberto and his counselor. Think about the strengths and weaknesses in the dialogue and what you can learn from it about the use of interpretations. Notice the clinician's efforts to deliver interpretations in ways that are meaningful and acceptable to Roberto. The exercises in the next section will give you an opportunity to analyze this dialogue.

Dialogue Demonstrating Use of Interpretation

ROBERTO: I just don't understand what's wrong with Edie. She has a wonderful daughter and husband. Why can't she be contented?

CLINICIAN: I wonder how Edie's role compares with the one your mother took when she had young children?

ROBERTO: Oh, my mother was very different from Edie. She devoted her whole life to her children. Me especially. I think I'm her favorite. She was so happy with her family. I don't understand why Edie doesn't feel that way.

CLINICIAN: So the nurturing you received from your own mother and the joy she took in her role as mother make it especially hard for you to understand Edie.

ROBERTO: Yes, I guess that's true. But Edie loves Ava, and she's so sad that we can't have more children. Shouldn't she feel happy that she has a home and family?

CLINICIAN: I can understand that this would puzzle you and maybe even make you angry sometimes because Edie doesn't seem to be the kind of mother you think she should be.

ROBERTO: Yes, I guess I don't want to admit that to Edie, but I suppose she senses my anger. I'm trying to help her find herself, and I realize that times have changed and not all women feel like my mother did, but it still bothers me sometimes. I want Ava to have the best possible mother . . . like I did.

CLINICIAN: I can hear you really struggling with a conflict inside yourself. On the one hand, you want to help Edie figure out what would make her happy; but on the other hand, you are concerned that it might keep Ava from having the good mothering you had.

ROBERTO: Yes, that's really it.

CLINICIAN: Could it also be that sometimes you feel angry and almost deprived because Edie is not giving you the caring that your mother taught you to expect from a woman?

ROBERTO: Well . . . I don't know. . . . I mean, I'm a grown man; I don't need anybody to mother me anymore. I can take care of myself.

CLINICIAN: You have become very self-sufficient. Yet sometimes most of us still feel that little child inside us who wants a loving mother to ease our fears and tell us how special we are.

ROBERTO: Isn't there something wrong with a grown man having those feelings?

CLINICIAN: I don't think so, especially if we can recognize those feelings and use them in ways that help us.

ROBERTO: Well, I guess I do feel that way sometimes. Every once in a while I get this feeling like I'm a scared kid, like I just skinned my knee, and I want somebody to tell me it's all right. But that's a fantasy; there's nobody to wipe my eyes and wash my knee and make everything all right. And my problems now go way beyond a skinned knee.

CLINICIAN: It sounds like it's hard for you to let yourself talk about those feelings and even to have those feelings. But from what you're saying, they are there sometimes, and maybe they have an impact on your relationship with Edie and your expectations of her.

ROBERTO: You may have something there. I never thought about any connection between my feelings toward Edie and the kind of mother I have. What can I do about that?

EXERCISES

Large-Group Exercises

1. Discuss the dialogue you just read. Consider the following dimensions of the delivery of the dialogue: content, language, purpose, timing, impact on client–clinician relationship, how large a part the client played in the interpretation process, and overall effectiveness. Consider ways in which the dialogue might have been improved.
2. Consider what you know about Roberto's history from this dialogue as well as from information provided in previous chapters. Select one of the theoretical approaches described in this chapter that might provide understanding of Roberto's development, his current difficulties, and ways to help him. Discuss the application of that approach to Roberto, being sure to link past and present and generate ideas for his treatment.

3. Have each student list what he or she perceives as the three greatest contributions of the theories presented in this chapter as well as the three concepts that seem least acceptable. List these on the board, identifying areas of agreement among students. Discuss the thinking behind the choices.

Small-Group Exercises

1. Consider Jung's dimensions of personality, including the four functions and two attitudes. (You may take the Jung Typology Test online or complete the MBTI, but it is not necessary for this discussion.) Discuss with your group partner your understanding of your dimensions and how it reflects or is inconsistent with what you already know about yourself. After each interpretation, both participants and observers should provide feedback to the interviewer and the interviewee. Feedback should focus on but not be limited to the following areas:
   - Use of open questions
   - Clarity of information presented
   - Adequacy of opportunity for the interviewee to react to the information.
2. Divide into your groups of four students. One dyad should assume the roles of clinician and client, with the client being Edie or Ava. Do a 10-minute role-play in which the client discusses her early relationships with her parents and her current social and self-esteem difficulties. Using information already available about Edie and Ava, the clinician should make at least two interpretations, linking the past and the present. The two observers should take notes on the effectiveness of the interpretations and of the role-play as a whole. Then the four group members should discuss the nature, language, timing, purpose, and impact of the interpretations, focusing particularly on how they might be improved.

Individual Exercises

1. Think about your relationships with your parents. What kind of parents do you think they were when you were very young? You may be particularly likely to have some insights into this if you observed them while parenting your younger siblings or if you completed the exercise on early recollections in Chapter 4. Write a paragraph in your journal in which you discuss ways in which the parenting you received as a young child might be affecting your current expectations and behaviors in relationships.
2. Consider Jung's theory of the unconscious mind (pages 88–90). The persona is the representation of ourselves that we are most likely to present to other people. It seeks social acceptance and approval. In contrast, the shadow is the least acceptable part of ourselves; it generally reflects negative qualities and a dark side that we hide from ourselves and others due to its unacceptable nature. Think about the persona you project. What image of yourself do you present to other people? Then think about your shadow. Determining the nature of the shadow can be difficult, especially for ourselves. However, we have several places to look for information on our shadows. Because the characteristics of our shadows are so unacceptable to us, they are the characteristics we are most likely to find objectionable in others and even to project onto people who do not possess them. Our own areas of moral weakness, difficulties in adaptation, and socially unacceptable behavior provide other clues to the nature of our shadows. Comprehending our shadows takes effort, but the reward can be the ability to channel the obsessive and powerful attributes of the shadow into expanded energy and creativity. Take a look at your shadow side. Write about your observations about your persona and your experiences finding your shadow in your journal.

Summary

This chapter reviewed four schools of psychoanalytic thought that evolved after Freud: analytical psychology, ego psychology, object relations theory, and self psychology. All of the theorists discussed in this chapter initially embraced the ideas of Sigmund Freud, but later developed their own ideas. Carl Jung called attention to the innate patterns and images that influence psychological development, the importance of spirituality in our lives, our need for wholeness and balance, and the levels of the unconscious. As a clinician and educator, Jung sought to help people find knowledge, meaning, and fulfillment, as well as individuation and self-realization by developing and accessing awareness of their psyches. Other theorists de-emphasized the role of drives in human development and placed considerable emphasis on the ego or self and on early parent–child relationships and attachment. Most believed that children internalize images of their parents and that those images have a significant impact on the children's sense of themselves and their subsequent relationships. Although most of these theorists continued to view the transference relationship as important, they also believed in the collaboration of clinician and client and advocated the use of empathy, acceptance, and other affective and humanistic interventions to enhance treatment. Nearly all of these theorists continue to be read and studied. Their influence has been great, not only on psychoanalysis but on other theories that will be discussed in this book.

Recommended Readings

Carl Jung

Galanter, M., & Kaskutas, L. A. (Eds.). (2008). *Recent developments in alcoholism, Vol. 18: Research on Alcoholics Anonymous and spirituality in addiction recovery.* Totowa, NJ: Humana Press.

Journal of Analytical Psychology.

Jung, C. G. (1961). *Memories, dreams, reflections.* New York, NY: Pantheon.

Jung, C. G. (1964). *Man and his symbols.* Garden City, NY: Doubleday.

Shamdasani, S. (2011). *C.G. Jung: A biography in books.* New York, NY: W. W. Norton.

Karen Horney

Paris, B. J. (1994). *Karen Horney: A psychoanalyst's search for self understanding.* New Haven, CT: Yale University Press.

Harry Stack Sullivan

Chapman, A. H. (1978). *The treatment techniques of Harry Stack Sullivan.* New York, NY: Brunner/Mazel.

Grey, A. L. (1988). Sullivan's contributions to psychoanalysis: An overview. *Contemporary Psychoanalysis, 24,* 548–576.

Anna Freud

Sandler, A. (1996). The psychoanalytic legacy of Anna Freud. *Psychoanalytic Study of the Child, 51,* 270–284.

Young-Bruehl, E. (2008). *Anna Freud: A biography.* New Haven, CT: Yale University Press.

Object Relations Theorists

Cashdan, S. (1988). *Object relations therapy: Using the relationship.* New York, NY: Norton.

Celani, D. P. (2010). *Fairbairn's object relations theory in the clinical setting.* New York, NY: Columbia University Press.

Lubbe, T. (2011). *Object relations in depression: A return to theory.* New York, NY: Routledge.

Mitchell, S. A., & Black, M. J. (1995). *Freud and beyond: A history of modern psychoanalytic thought.* New York, NY: Basic Books.

Scharff, J. S., & Scharff, D. E. (2005). *The primer of object relations* (2nd ed.). Northvale, NJ: Aronson.

Strozier, C. B. (2001). *The making of a psychoanalyst.* New York, NY: Farrar, Strauss and Giroux.

Heinz Kohut and Self Psychology

Lachmann, F. M. (1993). Self psychology: Origins and overview. *British Journal of Psychotherapy, 10,* 226–231.

Livingston, M., & Livingston, L. (2000). Sustained empathic focus and the clinical application of self-psychological theory in group psychotherapy. *International Journal of Group Psychotherapy, 56,* 67–85.

Other References

Gabbard, G. O. (Ed.) (2009). *Textbook of psychotherapeutic treatments*. Washington, DC: American Psychiatric Publishing.

Hillman, J. (1996). *The soul's code: In search of character and calling*. New York, NY: Random House.

Sayers, J. (1991). *Mothers of psychoanalysis: Helene Deutsch, Karen Horney, Anna Freud, Melanie Klein*. New York, NY: Norton.

Additional Sources of Information

Specialized training in Jung's analytical psychology can be obtained from institutes and societies throughout the world, including the C. G. Jung Institutes in New York City, Los Angeles, and Chicago. Jungian seminars are conducted by the C. G. Jung Foundation, http://www.cgjungny.org. Additional relevant websites include:

http://www.cgjungpage.org—This website includes information on Jung and his theories, resources, and articles.

http://www.jungchicago.org—This website for the C.G. Jung Institute of Chicago includes information about relevant publications as well as services and training opportunities provided by the Institute.

http://www.jungplatform.com—A website that offers training and educational programs on Jungian themes in psychology.

http://www.annafreudcentre.org—A web page created by the London-based Anna Freud Center, which seeks to educate others about Anna Freud's work.

http://www.sonoma.edu/users/d/daniels/objectrelations.html—More information on object relations therapy.

http//www.theipi.org—Website of the International Psychotherapy Institute in Washington, D.C.

http://www.johnbowlby.com—Information on attachment theory and on John Bowlby and Mary Ainsworth.

http://www.psychologyoftheself.com—Website of the International Association for Psychoanalytic Self Psychology, including an e-journal.

http://www.iarpp.net—Website of the International Association for Relational Psychoanalysis and Psychotherapy. Includes a newsletter, journal, and online forum for members.

CHAPTER 6

Brief Psychodynamic Therapy

The final theory to be discussed in Part 2 is brief psychodynamic therapy (BPT). Like all of the theories reviewed in this part of the book, BPT is anchored in Freudian psychoanalysis. In fact, Freud himself often did brief therapy of 1 year or less. BPT also has been influenced by Anna Freud's ego psychology, developmental psychology, object relations theories, Kohut's self psychology, Sullivan's interpersonal theories, and family systems concepts (Strupp, 1992).

Compared to traditional psychoanalysis, BPT is much more compatible with today's clinical emphasis on the establishment of specific goals, efficiency of treatment, and an interactive and often reparative client–clinician relationship. Although brief therapy is not always brief, it is time limited, taking place in 6 to 50 sessions. Empirical research indicates that most significant changes occur in the first 8 sessions (Lambert, Bergin, & Garfield, 2004). BPT focuses on a specific crisis or problem, establishes circumscribed goals, and uses a broad and flexible array of interventions. What makes this approach psychodynamic is the assumption that a person's focal problem reflects or repeats earlier issues in that person's family of origin. Clinicians who practice BPT believe that, by addressing in treatment both the current focal conflict and its origins, people's presenting concerns can be resolved and they can improve their ability to deal with similar issues in the future.

BPT is an important treatment approach that is widely used. In a survey of members of the American Psychological Association, 25% identified their theoretical orientation as psychodynamic, the most popular orientation after eclectic. In addition, extensive research supports the value of BPT in treating a broad range of people and mental disorders. All therapists do some form of therapy that is brief, whether planned or not (Levenson, 2010). Of course, this approach is not appropriate for all people or problems; and many practitioners of brief psychodynamic therapy carefully assess people to determine suitability for treatment by BPT.

THE DEVELOPMENT OF BRIEF PSYCHODYNAMIC THERAPY

Several names are associated with the early development of BPT including Sándor Ferenczi and Franz Alexander. Ferenczi, from Budapest, was one of Freud's followers. However, Ferenczi objected to the passive stance assumed by traditional psychoanalysts and sought a more active, efficient approach to treatment. He encouraged clients to face their fears, advocated a narrower focus of clinical attention, and believed that clinicians should assume an active role in the treatment process.

Alexander, practicing at the Chicago Institute of Psychoanalysis in the 1940s, viewed therapy as providing a corrective emotional experience designed to promote new learning in which the person could relive an old conflict and, because the therapist's attitude is different than the parental or interpersonal response, the client could intellectually understand and experientially feel the irrationality underlying the emotional reaction (Alexander & French, 1946). Clients could relive the old conflict but with a new ending. Alexander stated that it is this correction of a neurotic pattern that forms the basis of therapeutic change. Rather than seeking to elicit transference, he suggested that clinicians behave in ways opposite to those likely to provoke transference. This could provide people with an experience designed to heal rather than reopen old wounds. Alexander later wrote of the need for flexibility in treatment, of choosing the best techniques suited to the situation, and of the therapist taking a more directive stance. He experimented with short-term treatment that focused on current life problems, and believed that treatment should enable people to apply what they learned to their lives outside therapy.

Many names are associated with contemporary applications of BPT, including:

- David Malan (Tavistock system of short-term dynamic psychotherapy)
- Lester Luborsky (time-limited dynamic supportive-expressive psychotherapy)
- James Mann (time-limited psychotherapy)
- Hans Strupp and Hanna Levenson (time-limited dynamic psychotherapy)
- Gerald Klerman (interpersonal psychotherapy).

We will consider the distinguishing features and contributions of some of these clinicians and their approaches later in the chapter, after we have reviewed the commonalities of BPT. However, the names of these approaches in themselves reflect their nature. They are brief, intensive, and active and pay considerable attention to emotions and relationships.

IMPORTANT THEORETICAL CONCEPTS

Although BPT can be effective, it differs from classic psychoanalysis in some important ways:

- Specific client features have a positive effect on treatment outcomes.
- BPT is relatively brief, having a time limit or a specific termination date, or having the number of sessions fixed at the start of therapy. Treatment is rarely longer than 1 year with treatment typically taking 12 to 20 sessions (Presbury, Echterling, & McKee, 2008).
- The focus is on specific intrapsychic conflicts identified early in treatment.
- Goals are established to clarify treatment priorities.
- The clinician is active and sometimes challenging, using interpretation but discouraging regression. Client and clinician sit face to face to promote interaction in a reality-based relationship that de-emphasizes transference but promotes a corrective emotional experience.
- Termination, with its issues of loss, separation, and ending, receives considerable attention.

Underlying Theory

According to BPT, emotional difficulties often result from people's inability to deal successfully with unacceptable feelings or impulses. When their ego defenses fail to mediate between their drives and the demands of external reality to suppress or modify unacceptable feelings, problematic anxiety arises. Clinicians using BPT believe that early interactions and intrapsychic experiences form enduring patterns in the mind and that these patterns show up in current difficulties, which typically reflect a repetition of early childhood issues (Alexander & French, 1946).

For example, a woman might find herself frequently attracted to married men who either reject her or take advantage of her. This may re-create her early relationship with her father, who was both seductive and rejecting, and her own inability to move beyond that relationship. Her ego defenses have been unsuccessful in mediating between her drive toward an intimate relationship with her father and the social unacceptability of such a relationship. Because these feelings have not been suppressed or modified in positive ways, the woman is caught in a conflict. She sabotages her efforts to find a rewarding relationship and is unhappy and frustrated about this pattern, but she is unable to alter her impulses so that she can establish a healthy relationship with an appropriate partner.

According to most BPT approaches, by strengthening the ego so that it can control self-destructive impulses, helping people gain insight and resolve conflicts, and using the therapeutic relationship to teach effective ways of relating to others, clinicians can help clients break out of their repetitive dysfunctional patterns and grow in healthy ways. Important ingredients for change include emotional release, a corrective emotional experience with the clinician, and acquisition of greater insight. As people succeed in connecting with their clinicians, expressing their emotions, and understanding themselves better, energy that has been bound up in defensive and self-protective maneuvers is now freed to enable them to move forward.

Selection of Appropriate Clients

The following qualities have been found to contribute to a person's suitability for short-term psychodynamic psychotherapy (Leichsenring, 2009):

1. High quality of object relations (presence of at least one good relationship in the past or present)
2. Realistic expectations
3. Presentation of a circumscribed chief complaint, understandable through BPT
4. Motivation toward change and growth, not just motivation toward symptom relief
5. Absence of a personality disorder.

The Process of BPT

Messer and Warren (1995) and others identified two triads that are important areas of focus in BPT. The first, the *triangle of insights* (also known as the *impulse–defense triad*), includes current and recent relationships, past real or imagined relationships (especially parents and siblings), and the relationship with the clinician. The second, the *triangle of conflict,* includes impulses and emotions, the anxiety and guilt associated with impulses, and the defenses used to reduce anxiety that arises from impulses. Exploration of these triads, leading to insight into their nature, can promote new learning and positive changes in people's lives.

Phases of BPT

Sifneos (1979a) identified five phases of treatment that are typical of most models of BPT:

1. ***Client–therapist encounter.*** Client and clinician develop rapport and build a therapeutic alliance. They identify a feasible and mutually agreeable focus of treatment, an emotional problem that is related to the client's core difficulties. The clinician begins to develop a psychodynamic formulation to explain the difficulty, generally reflected in repetitive dysfunctional relational patterns stemming from childhood. Client and clinician might prepare a written statement of goals and probable accomplishments through treatment.
2. ***Early treatment.*** This phase emphasizes the importance of reality in BPT. Clients' positive transference reactions are confronted to curtail regression, while clients are encouraged to distinguish magical and wishful thinking from reality.
3. ***Height of treatment.*** The primary thrust of this phase is to link present problems to the past. Although the past is explored in BPT, it is only examined in relation to the current focal problem. Anger and anxiety toward the clinician are common during this phase, leading to manifestations of resistance. Transference may be explored, when resistance is evident, to facilitate understanding of clients' discomfort and reduce their resistance. More commonly, the therapeutic relationship will be a source of information on dysfunctional relational patterns and a venue for trying out new ways of interaction. Clients are encouraged to make increasing use of new ways to solve problems.
4. ***Evidence of change.*** Clients become able to generalize and apply what they have learned through treatment. Positive changes may be noted including symptom reduction, improved problem solving, and enhanced interpersonal skills and relationships.
5. ***Termination.*** Initial goals have been sufficiently met for client and clinician to determine that treatment should end. Efforts are not made to expand goals or to effect significant personality

change; clinicians remain aware of the limitations of treatment. Attention is paid to addressing issues of loss and separation as treatment ends. Clients are congratulated on their efforts and accomplishments, and treatment is brought to a close with clients' awareness of work they can continue on their own.

TREATMENT USING BRIEF PSYCHODYNAMIC THERAPY

Brief psychodynamic therapy is not associated with a broad range of distinctive techniques, rather it is an attitude the therapist embraces. It draws heavily on analysis, interpretation, and other strategies associated with classical analysis. Practitioners of BPT also make extensive use of strategies associated with other treatment models such as narrative therapy, cognitive therapy, emotion-focused therapy, and motivational interviewing (Presbury et al., 2008). However, some generalizations can be made about approaches associated with BPT.

Goals

BPT seeks to resolve presenting problems and promote overall growth. Specific goals typically target the resolution of a focal conflict such as independence versus dependence, activity versus passivity, positive versus diminished self-esteem, and resolved versus unresolved grief. Growth-related goals include promoting understanding and change in people's inner experiences, increasing positive feelings toward the self, and facilitating application of learning so people can live their lives more successfully (Strupp, 1992). In addition, clinicians seek to give people the insight and tools they need to continue exploration of their conflicts and their interpersonal contexts in order to address them more effectively.

Therapeutic Alliance

Strupp (1992) said of BPT, "What may be the most therapeutic is the patient's experience of the therapist as a significant other whose feelings, attitudes, and values are *introjected,* thus effecting *corrections* of the patient's experience with significant others in his or her early life" (p. 25). Formation of a positive relationship with the clinician can help people to reexperience and handle successfully experiences they did not handle well in the past, thereby enabling them to change maladaptive patterns. The corrective experience of the therapeutic alliance can enable them to compensate for deficits in their early childhood relationships and form healthier relationships in the present. In addition, internalization of the clinicians' attitudes and behaviors toward them can help clients treat themselves more positively. A great deal of responsibility rests on the clinician in this model; consequently, personal therapy is recommended for those who practice BPT.

Although BPT acknowledges that transference and countertransference responses may need to be addressed in treatment, traditional interpretations of transference, focused on childhood attachment issues, are used sparingly. When transference and countertransference do occur, these theorists generally think of those processes in new ways. According to Levenson (2003), ". . . transference is not considered a distortion but rather the patient's plausible perceptions of the therapist's behavior and intent, and countertransference does not indicate a failure on the part of the therapist but rather represents his or her natural reactions to the pushes and pulls from interacting with the patient" (p. 305). The goal of exploring transference is not insight into early childhood attachment experiences, but providing a corrective emotional experience. Rather than encouraging transference responses, clinicians "resist the pull to respond to the client's interpersonal orientation in a complementary manner, so as not to reinforce the client's rigid way of approaching relationships" (Bernier & Dozier, 2002, p. 39). Instead, clinicians actively use client behaviors and reactions to the therapist as a way to increase clients' awareness of their habitual dysfunctional relationship patterns and promote more effective relationship skills.

Clinicians should also be skilled in empathic listening, caring and compassion, and understanding—the necessary and sufficient conditions espoused by Carl Rogers (see Chapter 8). As discussed previously, the creation of a positive therapeutic alliance is one of the most potent predictors of treatment outcome. This holds true whether the client is a child or an adult. Developing rapport and a strong therapeutic alliance are fundamental to a clinician's moving forward in the BPT model to establish an active and collaborative role in the client's treatment.

SPECIFIC MODELS OF BPT

Many names are associated with the development of BPT. Describing all varieties of BPT is beyond the scope of this chapter. However, we present expanded information on two approaches, interpersonal psychotherapy, developed by Gerald Klerman and his associates, and time-limited dynamic psychotherapy, developed by Hans Strupp and recently enhanced by the work of Hanna Levenson.

Klerman's Interpersonal Psychotherapy

It is difficult to determine where to categorize interpersonal psychotherapy (IPT). It is a medical model framed in Adolph Meyer's (1957) psychobiological approach to mental illness, and informed by the interpersonal work of Harry Stack Sullivan (1953, 1970). It is not really a psychodynamic approach, nor is it a humanistic approach. Some would argue that its lack of underlying theory of personality indicates that it is not a full-fledged approach at all. But there is no doubt that this time-limited approach is effective and growing in popularity worldwide, especially in places where it offers an alternative to costly medication in the treatment of psychological disorders.

IPT was initially developed by Gerald Klerman and colleagues in the 1970s in New Haven, Connecticut, as part of a collaborative research program on depression (Verdeli & Weissman, 2011). Influenced by Sullivan's ideas, IPT emphasizes social and interpersonal experiences. It recognizes the importance of the unconscious and of early childhood interactions but gives more attention to current relationships and patterns, social roles, and coping skills.

According to IPT, the death of a parent, or any other disruption in the relationship between a child and her or his primary caregiver, can increase vulnerability to depression as an adult. Once the vulnerability to depression has been established, stressful interpersonal experiences in adulthood can lead to the onset or recurrence of depression. IPT postulates that strong social bonds reduce the likelihood of depression.

IPT is a focused, time-limited approach in which client and clinician typically meet for 14 to 18 weekly sessions. Treatment focus is on (1) interpersonal deficits (social roles and interactions among people), (2) role expectations and disputes, and (3) role transitions, or (4) grief (Weissman, Markowitz, & Klerman, 2007). Treatment seeks to identify a focal concern, ameliorate symptoms, and improve interpersonal functions.

Treatment via IPT includes three phases:

1. ***Initial sessions.*** Treatment objectives of phase 1 include assessment of symptoms and identification of one or two focal concerns linked to the symptoms such as grief, interpersonal conflicts, role transitions, or interpersonal deficits. In addition, clinicians explain IPT and help clients recognize that their symptoms represent a disorder that can be ameliorated through treatment.
2. ***Intermediate phase.*** The focus of this phase is on the problem or interpersonal difficulty identified in phase 1. Goals are established and strategies are used to achieve those goals. IPT

encourages use of a variety of strategies including support, questions to elicit emotion and content, interpretation, identification of patterns, advice giving, education, clarification, feedback on communication, teaching of decision-making skills, behavior-change techniques, role-playing, and use of the therapeutic relationship. Although clinicians play an active role, clients are encouraged to take as much responsibility as possible for their treatment.

3. ***Termination phase.*** Termination is planned and carefully processed, beginning at least two to four sessions before the conclusion of treatment. Client's feelings of anger, sadness, loss, and grief are accepted and discussed. Clinicians give clients the message that they are now capable of handling these feelings and moving ahead in their lives.

Research has given considerable support to IPT, which was originally designed for the treatment of depression, but has since been found to be helpful in the treatment of a number of other conditions including bipolar disorder in conjunction with medication management (Frank, 2005), specific types of depression (peripartum, in conjunction with medical illnesses, with elderly clients, in the Hispanic population), bulimia and other eating disorders, post-traumatic stress disorder (PTSD) and social anxiety disorder, and conflicts in interpersonal relationships (Markowitz & Weissman, 2012; Mufson, Dorta, Moreau, & Weissman, 2011; Rafaeli & Markowitz, 2011).

IPT provides a time-limited, manualized treatment approach for working with all ages from adolescents to older adults, and in a variety of settings (Weissman et al., 2007). Many professionals, especially those just starting out, like this approach because it recognizes the role of relationships in people's lives and provides a prescribed course of treatment that is concise and easy to follow.

Time-Limited Dynamic Psychotherapy

Hans Strupp, working with his colleagues at Vanderbilt University, drew heavily on both object relations theory and the work of Harry Stack Sullivan in formulating time-limited dynamic psychotherapy (TLDP). Hanna Levenson expanded on and clarified the nature of TLDP. According to Levenson (2003), "TLDP is an interpersonal, time-sensitive approach for patients with chronic, pervasive, dysfunctional ways of relating to others" (p. 301). These clients typically have personality disorders, reflecting patterns of dependency, negativism, or externalization of blame, along with long-standing interpersonal difficulties. Research on the use of TLDP to treat people diagnosed with personality disorders indicated that 60% achieved positive outcomes after an average of 14 sessions. TLDP is not appropriate, however, for people who have cognitive processing problems, those with psychosis, neurological or substance abuse, or those whose behavior requires constant case management or support (Levenson, 2010).

The primary goal of TLDP is to change patterns of interpersonal interactions that probably stem from childhood relationships with caregivers. The therapeutic relationship is the primary vehicle for change. According to TLDP, clients interact with their clinicians in the same ways they have interacted with others throughout their lives. By identifying these persistent and problematic ways of relating and helping clients develop both understanding and new ways of interacting through the corrective emotional experience of the therapeutic alliance, clinicians help people improve their relationships (Najavits & Strupp, 1994; Strupp, 1992).

Countertransference is viewed as a "form of interpersonal empathy" (Levenson, 2010 , p. 25) during which the therapist is used to re-create the faulty dynamics of the person needing therapy. Using meta-communication, the therapist helps clients recognize their patterns of relationship behavior, acknowledge the role they play in the relationship problem, and change. Initially, treatment concentrates on present relationship patterns, but it shifts to exploring early origins of difficulties once current patterns have been identified and understood (Levenson, Butler, Powers, & Beitman, 2002). Once these have been clarified, clinicians help their clients to understand that, although their patterns of relating may have been adaptive at one time, they are no longer helpful to them. This paves the way for revision in interpersonal patterns, as well as development of new skills.

The role of the clinician is exploratory and positive. The quality of the therapeutic alliance in this approach is strongly related to outcome; therapists who are perceived as warm, affirming, and protective of their clients have more positive outcomes. Assessment must be rapid and interventions prompt; verbal contracts are sometimes set that delineate the length, breadth, and scope of therapy. Success outcomes may be spelled out with emphasis on strengths and resilience. Cognitive behavioral and other intervention strategies may also be integrated into the TLDP therapist's work (Levenson, 2010).

Integrative, attachment-based, and experiential, TLDP focuses on resilience, not pathology. Because TLDP is flexible and is designed to treat clients in a short time frame, it is ideal for group work with short-term psychiatric inpatients where clients may participate in as few as one session before discharge. Its focus on the here and now and maladaptive interpersonal patterns can help inpatients who are severely depressed and who experience acting out behavior relative to psychosis or mania to recognize their inappropriate thoughts and behaviors and teach them to use words and communications that are appropriate (Weiss, 2010).

The many other models of BPT are too numerous to discuss in detail here. Interested readers are encouraged to research them on their own. Summers and Barber (2009) have identified the following as the traditional brief dynamic psychotherapies on which newer models are based:

- ***Davanloo's intensive short-term dynamic psychotherapy*** (Davanloo, 1979, 1980).
- ***Luborsky's time-limited dynamic supportive-expressive psychotherapy*** (Luborsky, 1984; Messer & Warren, 1995)
- ***Malan's Tavistock system of short-term dynamic psychotherapy*** (Demos & Prout, 1993)
- ***Mann's time-limited psychotherapy*** (Demos & Prout, 1993)
- ***Sifneos's short-term anxiety-provoking therapy*** (Sifneos, 1979b, 1984).

APPLICATION AND CURRENT USE OF BRIEF PSYCHODYNAMIC THERAPY

Brief psychodynamic therapy is a major approach to treatment that is in widespread use in one form or another. BPT has many strengths. It is a flexible approach that is active and optimistic (Levenson, 2003). It encourages integration of treatment strategies from other theoretical perspectives. It is a brief, efficient, and effective treatment approach, meeting both client needs for rapid symptom relief and the requirements of managed care. Much is known about its use in treating various mental disorders but knowledge about its multicultural application is still limited.

Application to Diagnostic Groups

BPT is a sound treatment approach for many disorders. Research has substantiated its value in treating PTSD and other trauma-related disorders, grief, substance use disorders, physical complaints of psychological origin, bulimia, childhood psychosis, all types of mood disorders, and borderline personality disorder (Levy, Wasserman, Scott, & Yeomans, 2012; Seligman & Reichenberg, 2012). Of course, not all approaches to BPT are effective in treating all of these disorders. Matching of client to type of BPT should increase the likelihood of effective treatments. Time-limited dynamic psychotherapy, for example, is directed particularly at people with chronic and pervasive interpersonal difficulties, whereas interpersonal psychotherapy is especially effective in the treatment of depression.

BPT is not suitable for all people or all disorders. However, because BPT is a flexible approach that focuses on improving relationships, BPT can be a helpful adjunct to medication and other treatment approaches for people with psychotic disorders, bipolar disorders, and severe personality and substance use disorders. Treatment can be appropriate in individual as well as group settings.

Application to Multicultural Groups

BPT is currently being used with people of all ages. The literature has described its use with children, adolescents, elderly people, and other adults (Hinrichsen & Clougherty, 2006).

Some research is available across cultures. One study of Asian American students (Wong, Kim, Zane, Kim, & Huang, 2003), for example, found that those with low Caucasian identity and strong independent self-concepts found cognitive therapy more credible than BPT. Cultural variables, as well as self-image, then, seem to play a role in people's acceptance of BPT.

Given that BPT is an explicitly time-limited and focused therapy, it would seem difficult to fully comprehend a client's cultural context, which includes daily life, myths, folklore, literature, language, and family interactions. Getting to this level of understanding of an individual's background is time intensive and, therefore, may not be congruent with the time-sensitive nature of BPT. In addition, techniques such as exploration of childhood experiences, probing, confrontation of maladaptive patterns, and interpretation may be uncomfortable for people from some cultures. One approach that may provide clinicians with an emotional understanding of clients from their cultural context is to have clients express their feelings about an experience initially in their primary language and then translate those feelings into English (Kakar, 2006). This often reveals feelings, memories, symbols, and variations in affect expressed through associational links, reducing the impersonal tone that often results from reporting significant experiences, and allowing for a more accurate interpretation for the therapist and better understanding of the client.

Although not yet as fully accepted as other forms of therapy for people from non-Western cultures, BPT has been found to be as effective as cognitive–behavioral therapy in treating anxiety, depression, eating disorders, and some personality disorders (Lewis, Dennerstein, & Gibbs, 2008).

Overall Application

Clinicians should keep in mind the selection criteria listed previously in this chapter when deciding whether to use BPT with a client. Particularly suitable for BPT are people who are intelligent, insightful, interested in increasing their self-awareness, and open to change. Good candidates for BPT also have mature defenses, a focal complaint that is central to their concerns, and a history of at least one close, positive relationship (Horowitz et al., 2001). In other words, people who are relatively healthy and well functioning seem to respond particularly well to this approach. Binder (2004) adds that the client's expectation of improvement in therapy can enhance the development of a strong therapeutic alliance and reflect "a facet of his or her relating style" (p. 61) that works toward enhancing outcomes.

EVALUATION OF BPT

BPT is a treatment approach that is growing in importance through both practice and research. It has many strengths as well as some limitations.

Limitations

Some concerns and criticisms have been voiced about BPT. BPT's sometimes confrontational and authoritarian nature and its emphasis on early childhood issues can elicit anger, dependency, and even regression. Its short-term nature can result in a superficial sort of treatment that ameliorates symptoms but does not sufficiently address underlying personality patterns that adversely impact interpersonal functioning (Binder, 2004).

Levenson and Strupp (1999) found that the training usually provided on BPT does not seem to be adequate. They observed that therapists often have difficulty grasping the brief therapy paradigm that requires setting specific and circumscribed goals, adhering to the focal concern, and quickly developing a therapeutic alliance. Levenson (2010) recommends increased training opportunities, including the use of treatment manuals, especially for those with limited experience. Directive and specific feedback can be achieved through the use of videotaped sessions accompanied by anchored instruction. Attention to clinicians' relational skills, specifically emotion-tracking and empathy, should also be included.

Risks also are inherent in the process of interpretation as used in BPT. Hoglend (2003) found that infrequent use of transference interpretation was more effective than extensive use of these interpretations and that accuracy of interpretation also was positively associated with treatment outcome.

Strengths and Contributions

The theorists who developed BPT have made an important contribution through their efforts to build on the strengths of Freudian psychoanalysis and enhance that model through approaches that make it more efficient, more acceptable to many people, and more compatible with today's emphasis on brief treatment and on relationships.

One of the greatest contributions of BPT is the strong commitment of its proponents to research in order to improve and determine the value of this approach. Recent evidence indicates that a substantial research base supports the efficacy of a brief psychodynamic approach. In the past decade, no fewer than eight meta-analytical reviews seem to indicate that psychodynamic treatments have an effect size similar to those reported for cognitive–behavioral therapy, and therapeutic gains are maintained and even increase after therapy has ended (Rabung & Leichsenring, 2012; Shedler, 2012). In addition, brief therapy saves time and money; is suitable for people in crisis as well as for people with interpersonal problems, career concerns, or difficult decisions to make; and alleviates disorders of mood and anxiety.

The development of BPT continues. Integration of BPT with other treatment modalities is being pursued. The approach is being refined to treat specific groups of disorders. Tailoring the application of this rich and flexible approach should enhance its value and application even further over time. As we have seen, the research evidence indicates that many people benefit from brief psychodynamic therapy and BPT has become one of the most widely used treatment approaches of the 21st century.

SKILL DEVELOPMENT: IDENTIFYING A FOCAL CONCERN

Identifying a focal concern is important in BPT. This strategy also can improve effectiveness and clarify the direction of other approaches to treatment. The focal issue in BPT usually reflects dysfunctional interpersonal interactions and patterns that occur repeatedly in a person's life. These patterns are often linked to early childhood experiences, especially formative aspects of people's lives such as their early childhood attachment to and separation from their primary caregivers.

Whether or not clinicians seek an early childhood origin for focal concerns, analysis of present interactions can provide understanding of the dysfunctional patterns these concerns perpetuate. Luborsky and Mark (1991) sought to identify what they called the core conflictual relationship theme (CCRT), their version of the focal concern, by listening for patterns in three key areas: "the patient's wishes from the other person, the other person's actual or expected responses, and how the patient responds" (p. 119). By eliciting examples of relationship difficulties and examining these three areas for similarities, clinicians can make a tentative formulation about the nature of people's focal interpersonal concerns. This can be shared with clients, modified if necessary, and written down as a statement of the focus of treatment.

The following example illustrates the identification of a focal concern or CCRT for Julie, a divorced woman with a 5-year-old son named Danny. Julie sought counseling for interpersonal problems, especially in relationships with her parents, her ex-husband, and her boyfriend. Julie complained that these people did not really seem to care about her and treated her unfairly. When she was asked for examples of her relationship difficulties, Julie produced the following, with accompanying analysis according to the three key areas identified by Luborsky and Mark (1991):

1. ***Example 1: Asking my parents for financial help.***
   - ***What I wish for from the other person:*** I had worked up a detailed budget of my monthly expenses. It took me a long time to do that. It clearly showed that I needed at least $1,000 more a month. I wanted my parents to provide that.
   - ***The actual or expected response:*** Although I thought my parents would make up the difference between what I got from my ex and what my expenses were, instead they said I should get a part-time job. All they agreed to do is pay for after-school child care and gas for my car until I found a job.
   - ***My reaction:*** I feel really hurt and angry. I don't know if I can manage a job and a child. My parents don't understand how hard it is to be a single parent, and they don't seem to care. They had it easy. They always had each other and never had to struggle like this. If I didn't need them to baby-sit so I could take a break every once in a while, I wouldn't even let them see Danny. Then they would feel sorry.
2. ***Example 2: Telling Danny to clean up his room before bedtime.***
   - ***What I wish for from the other person:*** I think he should just do it. You know that T-shirt that says, "Because I'm the mom." Well, that's what I want. I tell him to clean up his room, and he should do it.
   - ***The actual or expected response:*** Oh no, not Danny; he always has to give me a hard time. I think he's putting things away; and then as soon as I leave his room to make a phone call or something, he's playing with his toys.
   - ***My reaction:*** Who does he think I am? His maid? I've sacrificed a lot for that kid, and the least he can do is obey me. So I yelled at him and gave him a time-out.
3. ***Example 3: Learning that before the divorce my husband loaned his brother some money without discussing it with me.***
   - ***What I wish for from the other person:*** I said to my husband, "Where are your priorities? Your own family needs money, and you lend it to your brother so he can start another business that will fail." I wanted him to see he had made a mistake and that he should try to get the money back.
   - ***The actual or expected response:*** Well, I didn't know if he would really ask for the money back, but at the very least I thought he would see he was wrong and promise not to do it again. No way! He just said, "I didn't tell you because I knew what you would say, and I really wanted to help my brother."

- ***My reaction:*** I knew what really happened. He wanted his parents to think he was so great. He was more concerned with pleasing them than with helping us. I was really mad, so I took some money out of the checking account and bought an expensive dress. Then when he asked me about it, I said, "You think you can do whatever you want with our money. Well, so can I."

Although more information should be obtained to conclusively establish the presence of patterns, these three examples provide enough information to allow the development of a hypothesis about Julie's focal conflict or CCRT. These examples suggest that, on one level, Julie views herself as special and deserving of treatment that reflects her specialness. When people do not treat her as special, particularly when she asks for something and is refused, she becomes angry and even punitive. Conflict arises because, under the surface, she seems to have considerable self-doubt. She questions her ability to be both a parent and an employee, perceives her husband as valuing his parents' opinions more than hers, and even feels powerless in her role as mother. Behind her unrealistic demands and expectations is a woman who needs others to reassure her of her importance. Not surprisingly, as a young child, Julie apparently received little affirmation and affection from her parents. The primary way in which she got attention was by throwing a temper tantrum, paralleling her current behavior. In addition, Julie's transference relationship with her clinician reflected her need for special treatment to counteract her doubts. She requested telephone conversations between sessions as well as reduced fees.

Analysis of Julie's CCRT and the similarities in the triad of her current relationships, her past relationships, and her transference to the clinician all shed light on patterns related to her focal relationship concern. Once these patterns have been understood and worked through, Julie might be able to make changes that will improve her relationships and help her feel better about herself.

CASE ILLUSTRATION

The following dialogue between Roberto and his counselor illustrates several aspects of brief psychodynamic therapy:

- The stance of the therapist as supportive but also confrontational, analytical, and educational
- The clinician's efforts to identify a focal conflict reflecting dysfunctional relationship patterns
- Recognition of commonalities among Roberto's past relationships, his present relationships, and his relationship with the clinician

CLINICIAN: Roberto, you look very upset.

ROBERTO: Yes, I am. Edie and I had another one of those fights. I give her everything she wants. . . . I don't know what more I can do.

CLINICIAN: Tell me about what happened.

ROBERTO: We were having a birthday party for Ava. Edie's family and my family were coming for dinner, and Edie had been cooking all day. I had asked her the day before what I could do to help, and I did everything she told me. I went to the jeweler to pick up the gift Edie had ordered, I got the wine and some of the groceries, I even vacuumed the house. So that morning I sat down to read my e-mail, and next thing I know she's standing there screaming at me: "I do all the work around here. Who do you think you are? Glued to your computer as usual." Yada, yada, yada. So I said to her, "Look, just give me 15 minutes to finish this, and then I'll come down." Not good enough for her. She goes off again. So I just left before I really lost it.

CLINICIAN: Sounds like you felt angry that she expected you to do even more than you had already done and wouldn't give you a few minutes for yourself.

ROBERTO: Yeah, e-mail is part of my work. If I don't take care of that, no job, no money.

CLINICIAN: So Edie's behavior doesn't make sense to you. This reminds me of our discussion of how much your mother expected of you and how unreasonable it seemed.

ROBERTO: Yeah, I can see that. I would be trying to get my homework done and the younger kids would be screaming, and she'd say, "Roberto, would you feed the baby and then take your brothers out to play so I can get something done around here?" What about me? When was I going to get my homework done? Yeah, I didn't like that either, but I just did it.

CLINICIAN: So in both cases, you were doing a lot to help a woman, but it felt like there was no time for your needs.

ROBERTO: Yeah, I'm always supposed to be the strong one. Roberto, fix this, do that, pay this bill. And I do it. But when is it my turn?

CLINICIAN: Yet in a way, it must feel good to be the strong one. I wonder if you might give people the message that you can handle anything because you enjoy having them see you as very capable?

ROBERTO: I guess so. It's like I'm strong and they're weak and they really need me. But then it gets to be too much.

CLINICIAN: Perhaps we saw a similar pattern in our work together. A couple of times when the phone rang here, you said, "Go ahead, doc, get the phone. It's okay." And when I was sick for a few weeks and had to cancel our sessions and I asked you how you felt about it, you said that it was fine; but I noticed that you seemed irritated and less open in the next few sessions. It seems hard for you to acknowledge that you have any needs, but you do; and they can build up and come out in ways that hurt you and other people.

ROBERTO: Well, everybody has needs, but I've always been able to take care of myself.

CLINICIAN: Yes, you have been very self-sufficient and take great pride in that. But maybe sometimes your need to be strong backfires and hurts you and those you care about.

ROBERTO: That could be right, but I don't want to turn into a wimp. I like who I am. Are you telling me to be different?

CLINICIAN: I'm certainly not telling you to be a wimp! I don't think you could do that if you tried. But, you know, sometimes part of being strong is recognizing that we can't do everything ourselves and letting other people know what we need.

ROBERTO: That's a new way to think about things. How could I have handled the problems around Ava's party differently?

At this point in the session, Roberto has gained insight into patterns that have shown up in old relationships, current relationships, and his relationship with his clinician. He has information to help him view his need to be strong in a different light. He is now ready to explore these patterns further and to consider ways to make some shifts that allow him to maintain his image of himself as a strong caretaker but also will help him articulate his own needs appropriately. Accomplishing this should lead to more mutuality in his relationships and enable him to avoid the anger and frustration he experiences when his needs are ignored for too long.

EXERCISES

Large-Group Exercises

1. Conduct a group interview of Edie. One participant should assume the role of Edie and should sit or stand in front of the class. Each student should then have the opportunity to ask Edie one or two questions. The goal of the interview should be an identification of Edie's focal conflict or CCRT. After the round-robin interview has been completed, analyze the information elicited from Edie, focusing on the following:
   - The *triangle of insights (impulse–defense triad),* including current and recent relationships, past real or imagined relationships, and the transference relationship
   - The *triangle of conflict,* including the aim or impulse, the injunction or threat that makes the aim dangerous or unacceptable, and the defense used to reduce the anxiety arising from the impulse
   - The *focal conflict.*
2. Consider the criteria described in this chapter that indicate whether a person is likely to be a good candidate for BPT. Apply them to Edie to determine whether she would be appropriate for treatment via this model.

Small-Group Exercises

Divide into your groups composed of two dyads. Role-play a 15- to 20-minute interview designed to identify your partner's focal conflict or issue. At the end of each role-play, all four participants should engage in identifying the repeated patterns that emerged and defining the focal issue. Take time to provide feedback to the interviewers about the following:

- Ability to elicit a focal conflict
- Interactions between client and clinician
- Use of open questions and other intervention strategies
- Strengths of the role-play and suggestions for improvement.

Individual Exercises

1. In this chapter, you learned to identify a core conflictual relationship theme (CCRT). Identify and list three important interactions you have had with others, at least one of which occurred at least 5 years ago. Next, examine the patterns used in the Skill Development section's example of Julie. Analyze your interactions in a similar way. For each, consider the following:
   - What you wish for from the other person
   - The actual or expected response
   - Your reaction.

   Now try to identify common patterns among these three areas and develop a written hypothesis about the nature of your CCRT.

2. Brief, time-limited treatment has elicited much debate among mental health professionals. If you were to enter counseling, would you prefer open-ended, extended treatment or brief, time-limited treatment? Write about what you think your treatment would be like in each case, highlighting benefits and limitations you would expect with each type.

Summary

Brief psychodynamic therapy, derived from traditional Freudian psychoanalysis, grew out of the work of Alexander, Ferenczi, and others, who found that length and depth of analysis were not clearly correlated with amount and stability of gains (Horowitz et al., 2001). The time period for BPT is typically much shorter than that for traditional analysis. It often has a fixed time limit and centers on a focal concern or core relationship pattern that is linked to the person's symptoms. Although clinicians practicing BPT assume that early childhood experiences, especially attachment to and separation from caregivers, are related to current relationship issues and do pay attention to transference, their primary focus is on the therapeutic alliance, present relationships, and ways to help people lead more rewarding lives. Goals are clear and circumscribed; clinicians are active and flexible; and strategies are designed not only to promote insight but also to elicit feelings, promote new learning, and change behavior. Research supports the value of this approach in treating a broad range of mild to moderately severe difficulties, notably depression.

Recommended Readings

Berzoff, J., Flanagan, L. M., Hertz, P., & Basham, K. (2011). *Inside out and outside in: Psychodynamic clinical theory and psychopathology in contemporary multicultural contexts* (3rd ed.). Lanham, MD: Rowman & Littlefield.

Goldfried, M. R. (2004). Integrating integratively-oriented brief psychotherapy. *Journal of Psychotherapy Integration, 14,* 93–105.

Messer, S. B., & Warren, S. (1995). *Models of brief psychodynamic therapy.* New York, NY: Guilford.

Presbury, J. H., Echterling, L. G., & McKee, J. E. (2008). *Beyond brief counseling and therapy: An integrative approach* (2nd ed.). Upper Saddle River, NJ: Pearson Education.

Teyber, E., & McClure, F. H. (2011). *Interpersonal process in therapy: An integrative model* (6th ed.). Belmont, CA: Thomson/Brooks Cole.

Weissman, M. M., Markowitz, J., & Klerman, G. L. (2007). *Clinician's quick guide to interpersonal therapy.* New York, NY: Oxford University Press.

Additional Sources of Information

http://www.interpersonalpsychotherapy.org—The website of the International Society for Interpersonal Psychotherapy, which offers training and certification, an annual conference, and access to IPT groups worldwide.

http://hannalevenson.com/institute.html—Levenson Institute for Training in Brief Therapy.

CHAPTER 7

Overview of Emotion-Focused Treatment Systems

In the preface to this book, you learned about the BETA model, which reflects the four important areas of focus in counseling and psychotherapy (background, emotions, thoughts, actions) and provides the structure of this text. Part 2 focused on treatment approaches that emphasize the importance of background. Although those approaches do not ignore clients' emotions, they are viewed primarily as a route to identifying long-standing patterns stemming from early attachments.

Part 3 of this book focuses on treatment approaches that emphasize emotions. This introductory chapter provides an overview of humanistic, or emotion-focused, psychotherapies as well as a survey of emotions and their characteristics. The information in this chapter will introduce you to some of the skills that are essential in helping clients identify and understand their emotions and also learn how to self-soothe and how to manage their emotions.

More than anyone else, Carl Rogers is associated with theories of counseling and psychotherapy that emphasize emotions. As much a way of being as a treatment approach, Rogers's person-centered counseling was built on a strong humanistic base. Humanism views people as capable and autonomous, with the ability to resolve their difficulties, realize their potential, and change their lives in positive ways. The person-centered clinician seeks to build a relationship with clients that will promote a deeper self-understanding, enable them to become more authentic and actualized, and empower them to use their strengths and flourish.

Humanistic therapies changed the way psychotherapy had been conducted. Up until that time, psychoanalysis, with its focus on the unconscious, and behavioral therapy, which focused on stimulus and response, were the only methods in widespread practice. In both methodologies, the therapist was traditionally seen as the expert. Carl Rogers revolutionized psychology and focused on the client as the expert on his or her own life. Rogers (1961) wrote: "It is the client who knows what hurts, what directions to go, what problems are crucial, what experiences have been deeply buried" (pp. 11–12).

DIMENSIONS OF HUMANISTIC TREATMENT SYSTEMS

The humanistic treatment systems presented in Part 3 not only pay particular attention to emotions and sensations but also are experiential; they view as important what people have observed, encountered, and experienced. These approaches are phenomenological because of the importance they ascribe to how people view themselves and their world. Now we look at each of the core concepts of humanistic therapy in more detail.

Humanism

Theories that focus on emotions rather than background or cognitions, including client-centered, existential, Gestalt, and emotion-focused therapy, are considered to be humanistic. They share the following common beliefs:

- The person should be viewed holistically.
- Each person has an innate self-actualization tendency.
- Humans have free will and are able to make choices.
- Because humans have free will and choice, they also have responsibility for those choices.

Humanistic theories emphasize the positive nature of human beings, which "far overshadows any emphasis on dysfunction or psychopathology" (Seeman, 2008, p. 39). Since Rogers's time, research on the impact of stress and emotions on health, the development of positive psychology, and the growth of Eastern-influenced and transpersonal theories have all focused on optimal functioning. Compared to Freud's complicated theory of drives and the unconscious, humanistic theories seem rather simple. Humanists generally assume only one drive—the inate need to self actualize.

Self-Actualizing Tendency

Implicit in all humanistic theories is a strong belief in the dignity and worth of each individual. Practitioners believe that people must be appreciated and accepted for themselves, not shaped to fit a mold. They believe that people have a right to their own thoughts and opinions, should be free to construct their own lives, and are fundamentally good and trustworthy. They believe in the human potential—in the inherent tendency of people to develop in positive ways that enhance and maintain themselves as well as humanity (Cain, 2008). Carl Rogers was one of the founders of the human potential movement and the creator of the encounter group model, which encourages group actualization.

Self-actualization is a calling to be, or to become, the best person that we can be. Emotion-focused and humanistic therapies are by their nature more open to spiritual and transpersonal experiences. A client is considered to be a "spiritual being on a spiritual path, even though they may not be aware of it yet" (Rowan, 1998, p. 45).

Phenomenological Perspective

Humanistic therapies also share a phenomenological way of viewing the world. There is no objective reality, rather each person has his or her unique perception of the world. That perception determines the person's beliefs, behaviors, emotions, and relationships. "The organism reacts to the field as it is experienced and perceived. This perceptual field is, for the individual, reality" (Rogers, 1951, p. 483).

Humanistic therapists believe in basic equality in the client–clinician relationship. No longer is the person coming for treatment referred to as a "patient," a medical term used in psychoanalysis. Instead they are client and clinician, a team, working together to help the client with their problems, not seeking a cure. Carl Rogers first made this very important move away from medical terminology, and toward empowering the person to work toward finding his or her own solutions to life's problems.

Holistic

Most of the humanistic psychotherapies consider the whole person. Just as the mind cannot be contemplated without the brain, neither can the person be helped without considering cognitive, emotional, physical, and spiritual issues. Gestalt therapy and focusing techniques are the most focused on bodily sensations and what Gendlin (1996) refers to as "felt sense." Most humanistic therapists value emotions and experience over thought processes. The theories that will be discussed in Part 3 of this book integrate mind, body, and spirit. Some theories, especially Gestalt and postmodern theories, also look at the individual within the broader context of society, culture, and other figure/ground perspectives.

Active

Compared with psychodynamic approaches, humanistic psychotherapies are active. Therapists take an active interest in their clients. They are responsive, authentic, and real, engaging with the client and being affected by the universal truths of the client's story. Gestalt is the most active of the humanistic therapies, transactional analysis the most directive, and Rogers's client-centered therapy the least active or directive. Overall, there is a shared "felt sense" in the humanistic therapies that is "spontaneous—vital—energetic—contactual—present—improvising—active—embodied—personal—concrete—open—and sensuous" (Totton, 2010, p. 20).

Focus on Emotions

Theories that focus on emotions consider emotion to be crucial to the experiencing and understanding of the self. Emotions can be both innately adaptive (helping the client to make sense of and respond to the environment) or maladaptive (Damasio, 1994). The goal of working with emotion in therapy is to help clients become more proficient at accessing, identifying, understanding, and regulating their emotions so they can live more fully. Emotions, both adaptive and maladaptive, are brought to life in the safe environment of the therapy session. Emotional schemas are identified and maladaptive emotions are brought into consciousness so they can be understood and transformed into new emotional experiences reflecting new self-narratives and meanings that incorporate a more resilient, self-actualized, and authentic sense of self (Pos, Greenberg, & Elliott, 2008).

AN INTRODUCTION TO THEORETICAL MODELS OF HUMANISTIC PSYCHOTHERAPIES

Carl Rogers and Person-Centered Counseling

Carl Rogers made emotions an important focus of treatment; we consider his theory, person-centered counseling, in Chapter 8. "Virtually all therapists today are Rogerian in style, no matter what their clinical or theoretical orientation" (*Psychotherapy Networker,* 2007, p. 26) largely because they subscribe to Rogers's belief in the core conditions of empathy, unconditional positive regard, and congruence as necessary ingredients in the development of a positive therapeutic alliance. Clients who perceive their clinicians as empathic, caring, and credible and who feel understood by them are likely to progress in treatment, whereas those who have a negative perception of their clinicians, whether or not that perception is grounded in reality, are less likely to make progress.

Existential Psychotherapy

Since the beginning of time people have grappled with what it means to be alive. At the heart of existential thought are the burning questions—why are we here? What happens when we die? And how do we best live our lives between the two bookends of birth and death? Viktor Frankl, a psychiatrist and survivor of Nazi concentration camps, resisted Freud's conceptualization of human behavior. He believed that people who had a reason to live could withstand almost anything that came their way. Frankl developed Logotherapy, which helps people find meaning in the midst of challenging and sometimes seemingly impossible circumstances. More a philosophical attitude about how to conduct therapy, rather than an actual system of psychotherapy, existential therapy, as developed by Viktor Frankl, Rollo May, James Bugental, and others, provides a different perspective on life. Through the four dimensions of spiritual, personal, social, and physical ways of being in the world, the purpose is to "gain insight into the unavoidable paradoxes that life presents and to gain strength from that knowledge (van Deurzen, 2002, p. xiv). All counselors will eventually confront issues of an existential nature, both in their own lives and in sessions with their clients. Chapter 9 will provide an overview of the existential approach to psychotherapy.

Gestalt Therapy

Gestalt therapy encompasses many of the concepts of both existential therapy and person-centered counseling. It emphasizes the importance of the therapeutic alliance and is phenomenological, experiential, humanistic, and optimistic. Promoting awareness through experience in the here and now is the goal of Gestalt therapy. As people become more aware, they reconnect with parts of themselves they may have been cut off from. This new awareness promotes growth and change. We consider Fritz Perls's approach to Gestalt therapy in Chapter 10, along with information on its integration with transactional analysis.

Constructivist Approaches: Narrative, Solution-Focused, and Feminist Therapy

Chapter 11 introduces the postmodern constructivist approaches of narrative, solution-focused, and feminist therapy. These treatment approaches are considered to be postmodern because they reject a linear cause-and-effect model of reality and instead look at the person in the context of his or her social and cultural environment. A collaborative client–clinician relationship, empowerment of the client, and use of the social network are essential. Familiarizing ourselves with these emerging approaches enriches our work as clinicians, helps us deal more productively with our clients' feelings, and contributes to our understanding of new directions in counseling and psychotherapy.

Now we take a deeper look at the dimensions of emotions, including their expression as influenced by age, gender, and cultural considerations

THE IMPORTANCE OF EMOTIONS IN COUNSELING AND PSYCHOTHERAPY

The most common disorders treated in both inpatient and outpatient mental health settings are mood disorders, primarily those characterized by depression. People typically seek treatment because they have feelings that are uncomfortable, painful, or confusing and they want clinicians to help them feel better. Emotions, then, are usually what motivate people to seek help. Even in their initial telephone call to schedule an appointment, people will explain, "I feel so bad. I'm thinking about killing myself" or "I worry all the time" or "My husband says I need to stop being so angry" or "My stomach hurts, and the physicians can't find anything wrong with me. Can counseling help?"

Even when people's presenting concerns focus on actual or anticipated events, feelings typically underlie those experiences. For example, the woman who says, "My boss is threatening to fire me if I don't shape up" is probably thinking "I'm terrified that I will lose my job, but I'm also furious at my supervisor." The man who asks, "How can I get my wife off my back about my drinking? I've got it under control" may be feeling angry at his wife and ashamed of his drinking. The teenager who complains, "My parents are from Korea and don't understand what it's like to be a young person in America" may feel caught between his longing for peer acceptance and his love and respect for his parents.

Because emotions typically lead people into treatment, clinicians' recognition and acknowledgment of those feelings can engender hope and optimism in clients, even in the first few minutes of treatment. Consider the following two openings:

Example 1

CLIENT: I called for an appointment because I've been feeling very depressed and discouraged. Nothing seems to be going right.

CLINICIAN: What specifically led you to make an appointment at this time?

Example 2

CLIENT: I called for an appointment because I've been feeling very depressed and discouraged. Nothing seems to be going right.

CLINICIAN: Sounds like you're feeling pretty hopeless. I wonder what specifically led you to make an appointment now?

Even though both clinicians ask the same exploratory question, the second clinician shows empathy and acknowledges the person's feelings. The second clinician's use of the word "hopeless" will probably lead the client to reflect further on his or her feelings and perhaps understand them better. The first clinician, on the other hand, sounds very business-like and, by failing to attend to emotions, may seem uncaring and disinterested.

Recognizing and dealing productively with feelings in treatment can accomplish the following goals:

- Clients feel heard and understood.
- Clinicians build rapport and join with their clients in a collaborative relationship focused on helping the clients.
- Clients who believe that their clinicians hear and understand them are more likely to have confidence in those clinicians and to feel optimistic that treatment can help them. This, in turn, enhances the therapeutic alliance, perhaps the most important ingredient in effective treatment.
- Clinicians who attend to their clients' emotions and sensations are likely to feel more caring toward them; to know, as fully as possible, the pain and unhappiness that the clients are experiencing; and to appreciate them as unique human beings.
- By assessing the nature and intensity of people's feelings, clinicians can formulate specific treatment goals and interventions and can measure progress.
- Many people not only experience painful emotions but also berate themselves for having those feelings. Discovering that their feelings are normal and understandable can be very reassuring.
- Promoting clients' expression and understanding of painful feelings can enable them to change the antecedents, the personal meaning, the nature, and the expression of those feelings, leading to relief of symptoms.

Dimensions of Emotions and Sensations

Emotions are complicated. All emotions have some type of regulatory role to play, according to Damasio (1999), and are "biologically determined processes dependent on innately set brain devices, laid down by a long evolutionary history" (p. 51). The biological function of emotion is twofold. The first is an innate process that ensures survival. The second purpose is regulation of the internal state of the organism. According to Damasio, emotions are not a luxury, but a necessary part of survival.

Damasio (1994, 1999) categorizes emotions as either primary or secondary. Primary emotions are hard-wired in the brain's limbic system and include fear, anger, surprise, happiness, sadness, disgust, and shame. For example, someone who hears what sounds like a gunshot might immediately jump to the floor. The person is experiencing a primary emotion (fear), which causes his amygdala to immediately generate a fight-or-flight response for survival.

Secondary emotions include anger, jealousy, frustration, and embarrassment. Secondary emotions are thought dependent and only come into play after we begin to process cognitively what has happened. As the man in the above example starts to pick himself up off the floor, he begins to feel embarrassment (a secondary emotion) when he realizes the noise he heard was not a gunshot, but the sound of a car backfiring. Secondary emotions are more complex and blend cortical, limbic, and somatic processes. They are sometimes referred to as cognitive or social emotions.

Feelings take many forms. They can be experienced primarily as *emotions,* as *physical sensations,* or, most often, as a combination of the two. Examples of physical sensations include queasiness, headaches, muscle tension, and chills. Physical and emotional feelings often go together. For example, when we feel sad, we sometimes lose our appetite, feel tired and heavy, and have no sexual desire. When we feel happy, we may feel buoyant, relaxed, and alert.

Feelings can be *overt* or *covert* or a combination of the two. Overt feelings are evident to other people through either words or nonverbal clues. For example, a person can express anger by saying, "You make me really mad when you do that," or by scowling, shouting, or making an obscene gesture. Covert feelings are concealed. Sometimes when we attend a social event or go into a situation such as a dissertation defense where we believe others will judge us, we experience anxiety and tension. However, we often hide those feelings so we can make a positive impression. Fear of rejection and disapproval, shame about our feelings, and lack of awareness of our emotions may lead us to conceal or even deny our feelings.

Feelings may be both overt and covert—for example, when we share only a part of our feelings. Before a final exam begins, nearly everyone feels apprehension and anxiety. However, some students conceal the enormity of their feelings so that they do not seem more fearful than most of the others.

Feelings can be *positive, negative,* or *neutral.* Some emotions such as affection, happiness, and amusement usually are positive. Others such as worry, rage, and disappointment generally are negative. Still others such as curiosity and sleepiness may be neutral. Of course, categorization of feelings is often a complex process. Emotions may be experienced differently by different people. For example, Aasif enjoyed feeling rage; it gave him a sense of power and control, and he liked to intimidate others. Reema, on the other hand, viewed anger as a negative emotion; she had been brought up to be self-effacing and was afraid that people would disapprove if she expressed even mild annoyance. Emotions may also be helpful or unhelpful.

The *intensity* of emotions varies greatly depending on the person and the circumstances. Our anger may be mild when someone takes a parking spot that was justifiably ours but intense when we discover that our home has been burglarized. Be sure to consider intensity when assessing people's feelings. Emotions themselves may be appropriate, yet their intensity can cause misunderstandings and relationship difficulties.

People may be *aware* or *unaware* of their emotions and sensations. For example, Rand felt envious of Charleton, his supervisor, but had difficulty recognizing those feelings and admitting them to himself. However, Rand spoke negatively of Charleton to others, avoided working late, and fabricated excuses to miss meetings with his supervisor. Charleton sensed Rand's displeasure and tried to discuss it, but the conversation was not productive. Rand received a satisfactory performance evaluation but was not recommended for a promotion; his lack of understanding of the reasons for this contributed further to his resentment toward Charleton.

Emotions that, like Rand's, are evident to others and guide our behaviors and reactions but are largely out of our awareness are especially challenging in treatment. Such emotions may not emerge or be available for discussion until a strong therapeutic alliance has been established. Clinicians who hurry clients' awareness of their emotions may alienate the clients and inhibit successful treatment.

Appropriateness of feelings is another important dimension, affecting how we are perceived by others and our relationships with them. A wedding, for example, provides a context that can elicit a variety of emotions, both appropriate and inappropriate. The nostalgic tears of the mother of the bride, the pride of her father, the love of the groom, the joy of the bride, the shared happiness of the wedding party, and the pleasure, perhaps coupled with some mild envy, experienced by some of the guests are all classic and appropriate emotions. Inappropriate emotions such as the groom's obvious anger at the cost of the wedding, the noisy grieving of the bride's former suitor, or the rudeness of the servers are particularly intrusive because of the context of the wedding. Contexts, as well as precipitants for emotions, determine the appropriateness and impact of the emotions.

Congruence is another variable to consider. When feelings are expressed congruently, verbal and nonverbal clues to emotions all give the same message. A person expressing words of love will speak softly, maintain good eye contact, and have an open and welcoming posture. However, if that person verbalizes love but has poor eye contact, an angry tone of voice, or a tense and closed posture, conflicting and confusing emotions are communicated. The receiver may not know what to believe, only pay attention to part of the message, misinterpret the message, or discredit the message because of its delivery. People sometimes unknowingly sabotage their efforts to communicate with others by giving mixed and confusing messages. Self-observation and feedback can help people to increase the congruence, clarity, and impact of their emotional messages.

Finally, emotions may *help* or *hurt* people, depending on the variables we have discussed. Expressing emotions can enhance our lives and our relationships, move us toward achievement of our goals, and increase pleasure in our lives. Expressing emotions can also do harm and can contribute to failed relationships, physical symptoms, unsatisfying careers, and unrewarding and unsuccessful lives. When assessing emotions, our own as well as those of our clients, family, friends, and associates, consider the eight dimensions of expression of feelings just discussed:

1. Primarily emotional, physical, or a combination
2. Overt, covert, or a combination
3. Positive, negative, or neutral
4. Level of intensity
5. In or out of awareness
6. Appropriateness for context and stimulus
7. Congruence
8. Helpful or harmful.

Awareness of these dimensions can help us to better understand the nature and impact of feelings and to find ways to modify unhelpful emotions.

Multicultural Factors and Emotions

Clinicians seeking to understand clients' emotions need to keep multicultural factors in mind. Research demonstrates that gender, age, and cultural background all affect the nature and intensity of people's experienced and expressed emotions.

GENDER AND EMOTIONS In a study of sex roles, Jakupcak, Salters, Gratz, and Roemer (2003) found that gender differences in intensity of affect and recognition of others' emotions are consistent with gender stereotypes. Although men and women may experience similar emotional reactions to events, women express emotions more strongly and freely. Women are more attuned to emotions in others, especially the meaning of their facial expressions. Men are less likely than women to express emotions, particularly anger, positive emotions, and sadness. This pattern is particularly prominent in men with traditional views of masculinity. Men's avoidance of strong emotions may well result from socialization in which they learned to stay in control, to always appear strong, or not to express anger, for fear they might become too angry. Of course, considerable variability exists in how men and women express emotions.

Content of emotions also is linked to gender (MacGeorge, 2003). Men are more likely than women to follow an "ethic of justice," emphasizing blame and responsibility in their reactions to themselves and others. Women, on the other hand, maintain an "ethic of care" (Gilligan, 1982) and are more likely than men to seek help for being victimized and mistreated.

Hutson-Comeaux and Kelly (2002) found that people react differently to the same emotions in men and women, depending on whether those emotions are gender-consistent. Strong emotional reactions that conform to gender stereotypes, such as happiness in women and anger in men, are viewed as less sincere than emotions that are counter to type (e.g., happiness in men and anger in women). Clinicians should monitor their own reactions for such instances of gender bias.

AGE AND EMOTIONS Both generational and age differences affect expression of emotion, with research disputing the idea that depression increases with age. Charles, Mather, and Carstensen (2003) concluded, "Currently a growing number of empirical studies have revealed an age-related pattern better characterized by relatively positive emotional experience and improved emotional control" (p. 310). This seems related to the tendency for people to "place increasingly more value on emotionally meaningful goals" (p. 310). Older adults report experiencing less anxiety and depression, more contentment, and shorter periods of negative mood than younger adults do. Older adults also recall relatively more positive information than do younger adults.

Generational differences suggest that younger men and women have patterns of emotional expression that differ from those of their elders. For example, younger men tend to have more androgynous gender roles, probably associated with greater facility in emotional expression.

CULTURE AND EMOTIONS Culture is yet another variable that has an impact on emotional experiences and expression. Mesquita and Walder (2002), for example, observed that "In order to judge an excess or deficit in emotion, one needs to be aware of the 'normal amount' of emotion. . . . Thus cross-cultural assessment of emotional disturbances requires the consideration of standard—i.e., modal and normative—emotion practices" (p. 789). In addition, emotions that are compatible with a cultural model are more likely to be activated, whereas those that are not well accepted in the culture are less likely to be experienced. For example, American culture values happiness and includes an abundance of awards, celebrations, and expressions of praise designed to evoke pleasure. Anger and disapproval are other emotions that are congruent with American culture. On the other hand, in Japanese and other cultures that devalue anger and encourage maintenance of relationships, self-blame is a more common emotion. Knowledge of cultural models and values helps clinicians distinguish between unhealthy emotions and those that may seem dysfunctional in one culture but are compatible with a person's culture of origin.

Summary

This chapter reviewed the place and importance of emotions and sensations in counseling and psychotherapy. It provided a brief overview of the humanistic theories we will be learning about in Part 3: person-centered, Gestalt, existential, and the postmodern approaches of narrative, solution-focused, and feminist therapy. The chapter also provided a list of eight dimensions that can help clinicians understand and analyze feelings.

CHAPTER 8

Carl Rogers and Person-Centered Counseling

"No one since Freud has had more influence on psychotherapy than Carl Rogers. His positive, humanistic approach to counseling and therapy has become extremely popular" (Hergenhahn & Olson, 2007, p. 463). This is largely due to three factors: (1) Outcome research on the core conditions continues to verify that Rogers was correct—empathy, unconditional positive regard, and a sound therapeutic alliance have all been shown to be effective ingredients in positive therapeutic outcomes (although little research has been conducted on congruence, what has been published in the literature appears to be positive); (2) this approach has broad applications and can be integrated easily into other treatment models; and (3) its positive and optimistic nature is appealing.

Perhaps one of Carl Rogers's greatest contributions to the field of psychotherapy was "teaching us to listen with sensitivity and caring" (Cain, 2008, p. 177) and without judgment. Rogers's optimistic view of the person and his belief in the person's innate striving for self-actualization changed the focus of psychotherapy from one of pathology to that of viewing clients as people who come to therapy to help themselves live more fully and function in more satisfying ways. His synthesis of humanism with the scientific method revolutionized psychology, turning it from an art form into a science.

CARL ROGERS

Carl Rogers was born on January 8, 1902, in Oak Park, Illinois, a suburb of Chicago. Carl was the fourth child born of Walter and Julia Rogers and he enjoyed the position of youngest child for more than 4 years before two younger brothers were born in succession. Both of his parents were college educated; his father was a successful civil engineer who managed projects around the country, and his mother was a housewife and devout Christian. Rogers's recollections during these early years were of being socially isolated from children other than family, being teased mercilessly by his older brothers, and developing a closeness with his mother, perhaps in large part due to several illnesses he suffered in childhood. Carl learned to read at the age of 4 and did not start school until he was 6 and a half, beginning in the second grade.

When Carl was 12, his father built a manor house on farmland and moved the family 25 miles west of Chicago to Glen Ellyn. Rogers biographer Howard Kirschenbaum (2009) wrote, "It is widely known that Carl Rogers grew up on a farm, but not so widely known that the farm was approached through brick entrance walls and iron gates and that the farm house was actually a brick manor house with . . . eight bedrooms and five baths, *porte cochere,* and a clay tennis court behind the house . . . and at least two farm houses for the farm superintendent, caretakers, chauffeur, and other employees and their families" (pp. 10–11). Yet the Rogers children were raised simply, with strong Midwestern and fundamentalist Christian values. His family instilled in him the importance of hard work, humility, and a sense of responsibility, values that were reflected in his academic pursuits. He was also schooled in the scientific method, because his father insisted that the farm be run scientifically (Hergenhahn & Olson, 2007).

Rogers went off to college at the University of Wisconsin, majoring in agriculture. In 1922 he was selected as one of 10 students to attend a World Christian Student Federation seminar in China. During the 6-month trip he was exposed to alternative views on religion, philosophy, and cultures that caused him to rethink the traditional fundamentalist Christian beliefs of his family. It was during this trip that the seeds of his later phenomenological perspective of reality were planted. He started to question whether there was just one true religion and started to consider the interconnectivity of all living beings. Later, in his autobiography, he wrote, "from the date of this trip, my goals, values, aims, and philosophy have been my own" (Rogers, 1967, p. 351).

Rogers returned from China to the University of Wisconsin and changed his major to history. After graduation, in 1924, he married his college sweetheart Helen Elliot. The couple moved to

New York City, where he studied for the ministry at the liberal Union Theological Seminary. It was while he was at Union that Rogers took several courses in psychology and began to realize that he could accomplish his ultimate goal "to help people change, grow, develop, live more satisfying and better lives" (Kirschenbaum, 2009, p. 25) without having to do so under the umbrella of religion. Shortly thereafter he transferred to Columbia University, at that time the leading training school for psychologists in the country, where he received a PhD in psychology.

Helen and Carl Rogers were happily married and stayed so for 55 years until Helen's death. While they were living in New York they started a family. Ironically, they raised their son and daughter following the Watsonian behavioral methods popular at the time. Rogers later joked that Helen's mothering instincts probably overcame any ill effects behaviorism may have had on his children. He continued to read voraciously and also became a prolific writer as well, maintaining a daily journal as well as corresponding with family members and friends—a habit that stayed with him across his lifetime. Kirschenbaum (2009) noted that Carl Rogers's need to be understood, "to communicate in writing," paralleled his need to work and to be productive.

Rogers's career reflected a growing involvement with people and the evolution of his personal philosophy and theory of psychotherapy. He moved to Rochester, New York, to take a clinical position in the Child Study Department of the Society for the Prevention of Cruelty to Children. It was here that he began to question the effectiveness of the psychoanalytic approach (what he referred to as counselor-centered therapy) and to consider that it is the client who knows best the direction in which to go. When he was an intern, Rogers had taken several workshops under Alfred Adler, and it was from Adler that he realized he could learn more by observing how the client is relating in the here and now than he could from mining the person's background. In 1940 he took his first academic position at Ohio State University and later moved to the University of Chicago as professor of psychology and director of counseling. During his 12 years at the University of Chicago, Rogers accomplished several milestones. He conducted the first research ever to be done on psychotherapy sessions (Kirschenbaum, 2009), wrote and published *Client-Centered Therapy* (1951), served as the president of the American Psychological Association in 1946, and received the association's first award for scientific achievement in 1956.

In 1957, Rogers took a position at his alma mater, the University of Wisconsin. From there he moved to California where he and Helen would live for the rest of their lives. In 1968, at the age of 66, he and several of his colleagues formed the Center for the Studies of the Person, in La Jolla. He worked with the center until his death in 1987. During his later years, Rogers focused on using person-centered approaches to reduce interracial tensions, resolve intergroup conflicts, and promote world peace and social justice. He led workshops and encounter groups around the world (Kirschenbaum, 2004). In 1987, he was nominated for a Nobel Peace Prize in recognition of his efforts.

Rogers was a strong and influential leader in his profession. According to Cain (1987), Rogers was the embodiment of the theory he developed, "the most attentive, careful and sensitive listener" (p. 284) he had ever known. Rogers's habits of hard work, self-discipline, organization, and concentration continued throughout his life. He enhanced these strengths with his optimism, his sense of self-actualization, and his ability to be open to experience and live in the moment. He was not afraid to express ideas that were new and innovative and was deeply committed to improving the world. His life and his ideas are inseparable.

THE DEVELOPMENT OF PERSON-CENTERED COUNSELING

The evolution of Rogers's theories closely mirrored his personal development, with his ideas growing richer as his insight, personality, and compassion deepened (Kirschenbaum, 2009).

When Carl Rogers published his first major work, *Counseling and Psychotherapy* (1942), the field was dominated by two systems of treatment: psychoanalytic/psychodynamic approaches and behavioral approaches. Rogers criticized both for their lack of scientific method and for their assumption that clinicians know best and should tell clients how they should change. Instead, he proposed what he called *nondirective counseling,* in which the primary role of the clinician is to help people express, clarify, and gain insight into their emotions. According to Rogers, acceptance, reflection, and genuineness are a clinician's primary tools; he avoided elaborate interventions and diagnostic procedures because of their lack of proven validity and the power they gave clinicians over clients. Even theory was minimized in Rogers's early writings; practice and experience were what mattered.

Rogers's second stage of development was marked by the publication of *Client-Centered Therapy* (1951). Although Rogers maintained his emphasis on the importance of people's emotions, the book signaled several important changes in his thinking. He renamed his approach *client-centered therapy*, reflecting his realization that treatment cannot, and probably should not, be completely nondirective. Rogers now saw the clinician's role as more active and important and believed that by communicating accurate empathy, congruence, and acceptance, clinicians create an environment that is conducive to helping people make positive changes. These three core facilitative conditions—empathy, congruence, and acceptance (also known as unconditional positive regard)—became hallmarks of Rogers's work.

In the 1960s, Rogers began his third developmental period, again signaled by the publication of a major work, *On Becoming a Person* (1961). That book introduced Rogers's conception of healthy and fully functioning people: those who are open to experience, appreciate and trust themselves, and are guided by an inner locus of control rather than by an effort to please or impress others. Such people view their lives as a process and value lifelong growth. Rogers's interest in promoting people's healthy development led him to extend his reach beyond the clinical setting. For example, he promoted the idea of student-centered teaching. Encounter groups based on Rogers's ideas became widely used to promote positive development (Rogers, 1970). His work during the 1960s also reflected his interest in research. Rogers pioneered efforts to identify those elements of the client–clinician relationship and the therapeutic process that are most likely to facilitate positive change.

The last two decades of Rogers's life, the 1970s and 1980s, reflected a continued broadening of his ideas and their application. The term *client-centered* was replaced by *person-centered.* Because Rogers's focus was no longer only on the clinical relationship, the new term better represented his concern with all of humanity. His methods were now used not only in treatment of individuals but also in families, business and administration, education, cross-cultural settings, conflict resolution, and, perhaps most important to Rogers, the promotion of world peace.

Throughout his career, Rogers sought to help people feel powerful and in control of their lives while encouraging them to respect the right of others to have their own feelings of power and competence. His person-centered theory evolved out of the belief that people have within themselves "vast resources for self-understanding" for developing their self-concepts and their self-direction, but "these resources can be tapped only if a definable climate of facilitative psychological attitudes can be provided" (Rogers, 1980, p. 49).

IMPORTANT THEORETICAL CONCEPTS

Carl Rogers's theories are informed by his years of experience working with clients. His theory is comprehensive and based on the assumption that people are basically good and have a natural tendency toward growth. For Rogers, understanding, appreciating, and relating to others in positive ways were the ultimate goals. Underlying the theory of person-centered therapy are the important theoretical concepts of all humanistic therapies: human potential, conditions of worth, organismic valuing, the fully functioning person, and a phenomenological perspective. These concepts are discussed next.

Humanism

Rogers's ideas embody the humanistic perspective. He perceived people as strong and capable and trusted their ability to handle their difficulties, grow and develop, and realize their potential. Consistent with this point of view, he believed that the goal of treatment was to affirm and empower people so that they have enough trust and confidence in themselves to make use of their inner resources.

Human Potential and Actualization

An important aspect of the human potential is people's natural inclination toward actualization, expansion, growth, and health. Actualizing is a universal tendency, although each person's self-actualization efforts are unique as they strive to master ongoing challenges within the context of their shifting social worlds (Adler, 2011). Rogers (1951) wrote, "The organism has one basic tendency and striving—to actualize, maintain, and enhance the experiencing organism" (p. 497). An analogy that Rogers (1980) returned to again and again was an outgrowth of his childhood days on the farm and his scientific interest. He spoke of the potatoes his family would store in the basement during the winter months. Even though kept in the cold and dark, away from the nourishing earth and heat of the sun, the potatoes would still sprout roots that would creep across his basement, extending toward the only small windows that received any sunlight. Even the potatoes would inherently move toward the light. Rogers believed that this tendency to self-actualize was a driving force in every living thing.

Just as plants need rich soil, adequate water, and sunlight in order to grow healthy and strong, Rogers believed that people also need the right conditions to enable them to evolve in holistic and unified ways. It is up to the therapist to provide those necessary conditions. (More will be said about the conditions later in this chapter.) Carl Rogers believed that this innate tendency toward self-actualization is a process that occurs across the life span, manifesting itself as movement toward self-awareness and self-realization, autonomy, and self-regulation.

Conditions of Worth

According to person-centered theory, children's self-concepts are shaped through interactions with important people in their lives and the messages they receive from those people (Rogers, 1961). If children experience *conditions of worth*, judgmental and critical messages that they are only worthwhile and lovable if they think, feel, and act in ways that meet the needs of others, their self-images and growth may be impaired (Barton, 1992; Dolliver, 1995). Environments that are overprotective, dominating, or intimidating exert a particularly negative influence on children's development and make it difficult for them to feel free and powerful.

Children in negative environments typically internalize the criticisms they receive, perceiving aspects of themselves as worthy or unworthy. They tend to devalue, shut down, and inhibit what they perceive as the unworthy aspects of themselves. This creates inner conflicts and incongruities and curtails their natural tendency toward growth. According to Rogers, messages of conditional worth restrict authenticity so that people cannot respond with honesty in their emotions, thoughts, or behaviors. They have not learned to value the self, the total organism, and so they become fragmented. Children such as these have a high likelihood of developing into adults who are timid, inhibited, and conformist or angry and defensive.

On the other hand, children who receive unconditional positive regard—the message that they are special and wonderful just because of who they are, not because of their importance to another or the children's specific behaviors or characteristics—are far more likely to become actualizing and fully functioning adults. This does not mean that parents need to be permissive and condone children's harmful behaviors. However, they should correct undesirable behavior in such a way as to affirm both the child's worth and the parents' worth.

Consider the case of Maddy, who is fearful of inoculations and reacts to her parents' efforts to take her to the physician by kicking and hitting them. Parents who apply conditions of worth to their children might say, "I don't like you when you hit me. Stop acting like such a baby over a little shot." Parents who seek to affirm the child but shape the behavior might say, "I can understand that you are scared of the shot and are angry that I am taking you to the doctor, but you hurt my leg when you kicked me. I love you and we can find ways to help you with your feelings, but I need you to stop kicking me."

Although Rogers (1980) acknowledged the harm that an aversive background can do to a person's development, he was ever optimistic: "Individuals have within themselves vast resources for self-understanding and for altering their self-concepts, basic attitudes, and self-directed behavior; these resources can be tapped if a definable climate of facilitative psychological attitudes can be provided" (p. 115). The goals of person-centered treatment are to provide that climate of acceptance, free of conditions of worth; counteract negative messages that people have received; and enable them to have complete freedom to be and to choose for themselves and to realize their potential as fully functioning, self-actualizing people. Self-acceptance, agency, and the ability to rewrite one's own story are important concepts in psychotherapy and are associated with improvements in mental health (Adler, 2011). Rogers's concepts provided the foundation for the development of narrative therapy, which will be discussed in Chapter 11.

Organismic Valuing Process

"The forces released through the catalytic process of therapy are not adequately accounted for by a knowledge of the individual's previous conditionings, but only if we grant the presence of a spontaneous force within the organism which has the capacity of integration and redirection" (Rogers, 1946, p. 419). Rogers called this spontaneous force the *organismic valuing process* (OVP), which is a person's intuitive ability to know what they need in order to feel fulfilled and self-actualized. "The presumption is that people automatically evaluate their experiences and actions to ascertain whether they are actualizing and if they are not, a 'nagging sense that something isn't right' results which can motivate corrective action" (Sheldon, Arndt, & Houser-Marko, 2003, p. 836). Everyone has a "built in, trustworthy, evaluative mechanism" (Cain, 2008, p. 196).

The person's organismic valuing process turns from an internal to external source. "The child has now developed conditions of worth—that is their personal sense of worth is dependent on how others regard them" (McMillan, 2004, p. 7). As the child abandons his own valuing system, he begins to accept the values of others as a way to maintain their positive regard. According to Rogers, this distorts children's healthy development, and derails their development of congruence as well as their self-actualizing tendencies.

The need for love and acceptance is lifelong—first experienced with parents and other caregivers and later with friends, partners, peers, and society in general. When the person's organismic valuing process comes into conflict with his or her need for approval, confusion results (Mearns & Thorne, 1999), and eventually the person develops a self-concept that loses touch with his or her OVP. Certainly everyone experiences conditions of worth at some points in their lives.

When people are not being true to their own internal senses for making value judgments and instead behave in a manner that they think is expected of them or will please other people, they are considered to be incongruent. Relationships cannot grow in this environment because the person is not being honest with him- or herself. Rather, he or she has built up defense mechanisms and created barriers that prevent effective communication. The greater the truth, honesty, and authenticity in a relationship, the more the other person is likely to express the same, and the end result is an increase in intimacy. People who are incongruent often fail to recognize that the true self is being revealed through their behaviors. Everyone behaves incongruently some of the time, but when incongruence is found in most relationships and situations, it is considered to interfere with the organismic valuing process.

Mike and his wife Shay came to therapy to get help working out problems in their 10-year marriage. Shay admits that Mike is a "wonderful father, a good provider, and that he never drinks in front of the children. But as soon as the children go to bed, out comes the alcohol and the nastiness begins." Mike relates that not only does he not think this is a problem, but he feels nothing is wrong in their marriage that couldn't be changed by his wife "just being nice to me." In a separate, individual session Mike reveals that he married Shay when their daughter was 3 years old and that he feels he and his wife have been incompatible from the start. He now feels trapped into staying in the marriage until his children are grown. "As soon as my son graduates high school," he said, "I'm out of here, that is, if I can wait that long. In the meantime, sure I have a drink at night. But what's wrong with that? It's the only pleasure I have in my life."

Mike is living an incongruent life. He feels the need to present himself as a good father, provider, and husband during the day, but his underlying unhappiness is still expressed, albeit indirectly, through his behavior. It is not surprising that Mike doesn't feel understood. He even tries to convince the therapist he's living up to the ideal role of husband and father. And yet, Mike's need to perform the perfect father role during the day, while drinking at night, is confusing to his wife and has created barriers between them. Mike's "image," based on introjected values he probably developed in childhood, has set up conditions of worth, from which he evaluates his experiences, rather than from his own actualizing tendency.

Rogers viewed incongruence, or not being true to yourself, as the cause of anxiety, adjustment problems, and the need to seek to therapy.

The Fully Functioning Person

In describing the fully functioning person, Rogers (1961) wrote, "The person comes to be what he is . . . in awareness as well as in experience, a complete and fully functioning human organism" (pp. 104–105). Such people have authenticity and can respond with congruence and honesty. Rogers's concept of the fully functioning person reflects his idea of emotional health. According to Rogers (1959), the following personality dimensions are characteristic of the fully functioning person:

- Openness to experience
- Living with a sense of meaning and purpose
- Trust and congruence in self
- Unconditional positive self-regard and regard of others
- Internal locus of evaluation
- Being fully aware in the moment
- Living creatively.

Rogers (1961) explained this more completely: "He is free—to become himself or to hide behind a façade; to move forward, or to retrogress; to behave in ways which are destructive of self and others, or in ways which are enhancing; quite literally free to live or die, in both the physiological and psychological meaning of those terms" (p. 192). In order to help other people, Rogers felt that therapists should work toward becoming fully functioning themselves.

Phenomenological Perspective

Because all of the choices we make in our lives stem from our perceptions, we are, in effect, the focus of our universe. Rogers believed that each person exists at the center of a constantly changing world of experience. Even when we believe we are being objective, our subjective perceptions determine the direction of our lives. Thus, person-centered therapy is phenomenological; each person reacts to life events in a way that is consistent with their own reality.

For example, assume that a group of people in an office hears a loud noise. Timi, who delights in social gatherings, believes the noise is a balloon bursting at a nearby party and wishes she were there. Kane attributes the noise to a car backfiring and is reminded that his own car needs repair. Tom, who experienced combat in the military, thinks the noise might be gunfire and feels apprehensive, while Alice is so immersed in her work that she does not even hear the noise. This example illustrates how people can distort, interpret, and organize objective information based on their perceptions of the world, with those perceptions leading to thoughts ("I really should get my car repaired"), behaviors ("I'm going to check out that party"), and emotions ("I feel afraid").

Every moment of the day, we have perceptions that evolve out of our experiences and influence all aspects of our lives. Understanding ourselves, our relationships, and our clients depends on our awareness and acceptance of these subjective perceptions. Only by understanding people's perceptions of reality can we fully appreciate them and the ways in which they direct and organize their lives.

Consistent with his strong emphasis on phenomenology and people's internal frames of reference, Rogers wanted nothing but clients' own experience to inform their treatment (Dolliver, 1995). He believed that no authority, including the clinician's, should take precedence over clients' direct experience. Correspondingly, Rogers drew heavily on his own experience and perceptions, both in his interactions with clients and in the development of his theories. He believed that self-disclosure, used carefully and deliberately, could enhance the therapeutic alliance and advance treatment. More information on the effective use of self-disclosure is provided in the feature on page 157.

TREATMENT USING PERSON-CENTERED COUNSELING

Person-centered counseling is primarily a way of being with clients and providing the therapeutic conditions of congruence, empathy, and unconditional positive regard that will facilitate change. When these conditions are present, "actualizing forces take over, denial and distortions of experience diminish, and the person becomes a more fully functioning human organism" (Fernald, 2000, p. 174).

The Necessary and Sufficient Conditions of the Therapeutic Process

Carl Rogers (1959) identified the following six conditions as "necessary and sufficient conditions for the initiation of constructive personality change" (p. 103):

1. A relationship exists—two people are in psychological contact.
2. The client is in a state of incongruence, which causes him or her to be vulnerable or anxious.
3. The therapist is congruent (genuine or authentic) in the relationship.
4. The therapist experiences unconditional positive regard for the client.
5. The therapist experiences and attempts to express an empathic understanding of the client's internal frame of reference.

6. The therapist's unconditional positive regard, empathic understanding, and congruence must be perceived by the client, at least to some degree.

Of these six conditions, three—congruence, unconditional positive regard, and empathy—form the core conditions used by the therapist to create "a psychological atmosphere in which the client can work. If the counselor can create a relationship permeated by warmth, understanding, safety from any type of attack, no matter how trivial, and basic acceptance of the person as he is, then the client will drop his natural defensiveness and use the situation" (Rogers, 1946, p. 417). Other than the core conditions, techniques or other therapeutic tools are not used in a pure person-centered approach. Rather person-centered counseling is primarily a way of being with the client and providing the therapeutic conditions that will facilitate change. Each of the three core conditions will be discussed in greater depth later in this chapter.

Goals

In the early 1960s, Rogers became interested in bettering his understanding of the process of person-centered counseling. To do this, he spent many hours listening "as naively as possible" to recorded sessions (Rogers, 1961, p. 128). He found that, early in treatment, people were characterized by remoteness, rigidity, and a limited awareness of their inner selves. By the end of treatment, however, people were able to live in and experience the present and trust both themselves and the therapeutic process.

A central goal of person-centered counseling, then, is to facilitate people's trust and their ability to be in the present moment. This enables them to become more honest with themselves and their clinician and to express fully their emotions and thoughts, even those that are painful and viewed as unacceptable by others. Additional treatment goals include promoting self-awareness, empowerment, optimism, responsibility, congruence, and autonomy. Development of these strengths, in turn, helps people build an internal locus of control, become more aware of external reality, make better use of their potential, gain the ability to manage their lives and resolve their concerns, and become more actualized. Rogers's approach does not focus on the resolution of specific presenting problems but on developing fully functioning people with deeper self-understanding who are capable of creating rewarding lives and dealing successfully with life's joys and challenges. Carl Rogers's and the person-centered tradition is a positive and self-directed philosophy of life. It is not surprising then, that it has had a profound influence on the development of positive psychology (Kirschenbaum, 2009). Psychologists Martin Seligman, Michael Csikszentmihalyi and others continue to search for answers to questions such as "What is psychological health?" "How do people develop resilience in the face of what life offers?" and "Why do optimistic people live longer and enjoy better health than those who are pessimistic?" The literature continues to support Rogers's underlying assumptions about the importance of the therapeutic alliance and the power of positive emotions to enhance the person's development of a strengths-based focus in life.

Therapeutic Alliance

Study after study has indicated the importance of the therapeutic alliance in treatment. In a meta-analysis, Horvath and Symonds (1991) concluded that the effects of that alliance were very robust. Glauser and Bozarth (2001) stated, "The variables most related to success in counseling outcome research are the client–counselor relationship and the personal and situational resources of the client . . ." (p. 142). More studies supporting this conclusion are cited in Chapter 1. The person of the clinician and the relationship of the client and the clinician are essential ingredients for change; so essential, that research into what constitutes a successful therapist is expected to be the "next frontier" in research (Miller, Hubble, Duncan, & Wampold, 2010). Not only do clinicians need to establish a positive therapeutic alliance, but they also need to communicate the core therapeutic conditions, which we discuss in this section.

No matter what theoretical orientation a therapist adheres to, they all "share a common debt to Carl Rogers, who made the word 'empathy' almost synonymous with the notion of therapeutic relationship" (Erskine, Moursund, & Trautmann, 1999, p. 2). Study after study has pointed to the importance of the therapeutic alliance in treatment. Rogers believed that if the therapist could only create a nonjudgmental acceptance of client feelings, expressing a sensitive empathy, accompanying a client on the internal search for themselves, trusting in the wisdom of the organism, and helping the client to experience his or her feelings fully, the therapist sets in motion the conditions in which change can occur. Additional emphasis is on promoting self-awareness, congruence, and autonomy. The development of these strengths, in turn, helps people build an internal locus of control, become more integrated and genuine, and gain the ability to manage their lives and resolve their concerns.

Rogers (1942) wrote: "Insight comes spontaneously, providing the clinician does not impose interpretations, praise, criticism, or advice, but concentrates on helping the client clearly to see and accept those feelings which he is able to express." (p. 433). Specifically, Rogers noted, clients become stronger and more independent, begin to take positive steps, and develop a sense of courage which allows them to be more open and honest with the therapist in the counseling session, and eventually in all of their relationships. Eventually they no longer need therapy.

As mentioned earlier, Rogers identified three core conditions—congruence, unconditional positive regard, and empathy—as being necessary to create a climate in which a person can grow, become self-actualizing, and ultimately strive to become a fully functioning person. Rogers believed that providing such a positive climate allowed the client to be free to trust his or her feelings and, ultimately, allowed self-directed change to occur. He believed these conditions were necessary regardless of whether it was a therapy session or a relationship between parent and child, teacher and student, or leader and group. Later we will see how Rogers applied the facilitative conditions to education, encounter groups, and even for the benefit of fostering world peace.

In his 1980 book, *A Way of Being,* Rogers more clearly defined the three facilitative conditions and noted that they apply not only in the therapeutic relationship, but in any situation in which personal growth is the goal.

The first condition is congruence, or genuineness. Rogers wrote: "The more the therapist is himself or herself in the relationship, putting up no professional front or personal facade, the greater is the likelihood that the client will change and grow in a constructive manner," (1980, p. 115). The second condition, according to Rogers is unconditional positive regard, also described as acceptance. When the therapist truly accepts clients as they are, in the moment, with all of their emotions, both positive and negative, without trying to change them, then the client is more likely to feel accepted, empowered, and connectede. "When functioning best, the therapist is so much inside the private world of the other that he or she can clarify not only the meanings of which the client is aware but even those just below the level of awareness . . . listening, of this very special kind, is one of the most potent forces for change that I know" (Rogers, 1980, p. 116).

CLIENT–CLINICIAN RELATIONSHIP Rogers (1967) stated, "Significant positive personality change does not occur except in a relationship" (p. 73). His view of this relationship evolved over many years (Rogers, 1961). In his early writings, he described a distant and impersonal therapeutic relationship, perhaps reflecting his early training. However, in 1955, he wrote, "I launch myself into a relationship. . . . I risk myself. . . . I let myself go into the immediacy of the relationship where it is my total organism which takes over" (Rogers, 1955, p. 269). By the 1960s, he acknowledged that although he initially feared being trapped by a close and loving involvement with his clients, he now found a close client–clinician relationship to be something that added to the lives of both participants (Rogers, 1961). Clinician and client are conceived of as two equal and capable human beings who become collaborators in a shared journey in which both grow and are enriched by the process.

Facilitative Conditions

Consistent with the emphasis Rogers placed on the importance of the clinician in the therapeutic process is his belief that effective clinicians have certain qualities that they communicate to their clients. These qualities help create a positive client–clinician relationship and promote clients' self-awareness and ability to direct their lives in positive ways. The most important of these are congruence, unconditional positive regard, and empathy but other qualities also enhance treatment.

CONGRUENCE Congruence refers to clinicians' ability to be genuine and authentic, well integrated, and aware of themselves and how they are perceived by others. People who are congruent transmit messages that are clear and coherent; their inner and outer selves are consistent.

Rogers believed that the therapist should be genuine, real, and not put up a professional front or façade for the client. The more the therapist could be authentic and open in the therapeutic relationship, the more likely the client would change and grow in a positive manner. When the therapist is transparent, then "what he or she is experiencing is available to awareness, can be lived in the relationship, and can be communicated, if appropriate" (Rogers, 1980, p. 116). Congruence, then, is a way of being, in that particular moment, between the therapist and the client, that brings in sync what is being experienced, what is present in the room, and what is expressed to the client.

In his writings, Rogers makes it clear that congruence relates to what is going on inside of the therapist in the moment. Unlike classical psychoanalysis in which therapist self-disclosure interferes with the transference process and is thus discouraged, the person-centered therapist responds spontaneously; is congruent in thoughts, mannerisms, and communication; and is genuine, sincere, and real. Clinicians' genuineness and consistency promotes clients' trust and openness, establishes a relationship that is free of deception and hidden agendas, and provides a positive role model. For some clients, this sort of relationship is new and can help them see that such relationships are possible in other settings.

But how honest and open should a therapist be? Rogers (1980) shared many examples through his writings, transcripts of therapy sessions, and videotapes: "By this I mean that when my experiencing of this moment is present in my awareness and when what is present in my awareness is present in my communication, then each of these three levels matches or is congruent. At such moments I am integrated or whole, I am completely in one piece" (p. 15).

In person-centered therapy, the careful and deliberate use of self-disclosure can enhance the therapeutic alliance and advance treatment. For example, the therapist uses present-moment awareness (what psychoanalysts refer to as countertransference) to illuminate the therapy. If therapy is not being productive, the therapist finds a way to express that to the client. Rogers (1980) notes that when he trusts this gut feeling, and is able to communicate it in a nonthreatening way to the client, "it is likely to strike some deep note in him and to advance our relationship" (p. 15).

Carl Rogers on Congruence

After his move to La Jolla, California, in the 1960s and his work with encounter groups, Carl Rogers became more comfortable sharing his own feelings and seemed to really resonate the meaning of congruence in a helping relationship. Indeed he strove for genuineness in all relationships. His biographer, Howard Kirschenbaum (2009), relates the story of a time when Carl Rogers walked out of a group therapy session that appeared to be stuck in discussions of trivia. Rogers got up, left the room, and went to bed. The following day when members of the encounter group expressed anger that he had walked out, he explained that while the group kept returning to discussions of trivia, at least he was being congruent by making his behavior match his feelings! Congruence can also relate to the clinician's behavior outside the counseling session. Especially for clients from collectivist cultures or those in which traditional healers and therapists are both part of and separate from society, how the clinician interacts as a community member, a member of society, and exhibits (or does not exhibit) social responsibility can be important attributes in the client's eyes and may enhance, or reduce the effect of the therapeutic alliance (Singh & Tudor, 1997).

Congruence in the treatment process requires sensitivity, openness, and self-awareness on the part of clinicians. To maximize their ability to be genuine and congruent and to participate in clients' experiences, clinicians must be in the present moment, aware of and attuned to their environment and interactions. Particularly important in person-centered counseling are present-moment interchanges between client and clinician.

Clinicians should be aware that clients' subjective interpretation of information may lead to misinterpretation. Clinicians need to be aware of both their verbal and their nonverbal messages, maintain consistency between the two, and address clients' reactions if clinicians inadvertently give confusing or potentially negative messages. Recent research on the client-clinician relationship reinforces Rogers's beliefs and indicates that attention must be paid to the relationship throughout the course of treatment. It is not enough to foster an alliance early on and then assume that all is well. Clinicians must notice and address any ruptures or tears in the relationship, even those that seem minor or inconsequential. Clinicians who are attuned to their clients, develop an intuitive sense of when and how to intervene, what to say, and equally as important, when not to say anything.

The timing of interventions is important to ensure the information is appropriate and likely to be received well.

UNCONDITIONAL POSITIVE REGARD Rogers's writings emphasize the importance of what he called unconditional positive regard: caring about, respecting, liking, and accepting people for who they are without placing any requirements on them to act, feel, or think in certain ways to please their clinicians. Rogers viewed people as inherently worthy, although he recognized that people have both positive and negative impulses and feelings (Kirschenbaum, 2004). Communication of warmth and positive regard is essential in helping people to like themselves, emphasize their positive impulses and emotions, feel powerful enough to successfully cope with their difficulties, and become more fully functioning.

Unconditional positive regard does not mean that clinicians view everything people do or think as wise and appropriate but simply that clinicians see people as doing the best they can at the present time. Person-centered clinicians are consistent in their acceptance of and confidence in the person, although they might express concern about that person's choices. Rather than saying, "You seem to be an angry person," they might say, "You sounded angry when I could not change our appointment time." This perspective is reflected in current child-rearing practices that advocate focusing feedback and evaluation on the behavior, not on the child. Parents are encouraged to comment specifically on the child's behavior, and not on the child herself. Saying, for example, "You did a great job picking up your toys," rather than, "You're such a good girl for cleaning your room."

The first comment focuses specifically on the behavior ("picking up your toys") while the second comment is too general and focuses on the child rather than the behavior.

Communication of acceptance and unconditional positive regard helps people believe that they are worthy and can trust their own feelings and thoughts. It can counter devaluing messages they have received throughout their lives. It allows people to recognize that they can change undesirable behaviors, thoughts, and feelings while still viewing themselves as likable and worthwhile. Knowing that they will be accepted no matter what also enables people to disclose to clinicians aspects of themselves that cause them shame or discomfort. Rogers (1980) believed that the more clinicians prize and value people for who they are, the more likely it is that they will make positive changes.

What Constitutes Appropriate Therapist Self-Disclosure?

Anderson and Anderson (1989) identified three types of therapist self-disclosure: (1) information related to the personal identity and experiences of the therapist, (2) emotional responses of the therapist to the client, and (3) professional experiences and identity of the therapist.

Research has shown that certain amounts and types of self-disclosure by the therapist can have a positive impact on treatment by demystifying the therapy process, normalizing the client's concerns, showing the universality of the human condition, and providing a role model for positive change (Barrett & Berman, 2001). However, inappropriate self-disclosure or too much disclosure on the part of the clinician may cause harm (Kirschenbaum, 2009).

Self-disclosures that are in-the-moment responses to client comments, that are spontaneous and focused on the client, and that are in the service of enhancing the therapy can help to create a more real, intimate, and genuine client–therapist relationship. What constitutes appropriate self-disclosure is complicated, unique to the relationship, and open to therapist judgment about what, at that particular moment in time between those two specific people, would be in the best interest of the client. Certainly an appropriate self-disclosure for one client may be completely inappropriate for another.

Potential drawbacks to therapist self-disclosure include the possibility of evoking negative reactions, client's lack of boundaries, client's fear of intimacy that results from such disclosure, and the therapist being left vulnerable.

What constitutes appropriate and helpful self-disclosure in person-centered therapy is a question that would benefit from additional research, although such research is difficult to undertake due to the very specific nature of each self-disclosure in terms of type, timing, and client–clinician relationship (Sue & Sue, 2008).

EMPATHY Rogers (1980) defined empathy as: "temporarily living in the other's life, moving about in it delicately without making judgments; it means sensing meanings of which he or she is scarcely aware, but not trying to uncover totally unconscious feelings, since this would be too threatening. . . . It means frequently checking with the person as to the accuracy of your sensings" . . . (p. 142).

Rogers viewed sensitive, accurate, and active listening—deeply grasping the subjective world of another person and transmitting understanding of that world to enhance a person's own self-awareness—as the most powerful force for change. To "perceive the internal frame of reference of another person with accuracy and with the emotional components and meanings . . . as if one were the other person, but without losing the 'as if' condition" (Rogers, 1959, p. 210). Therapists must always remain aware that they have not walked in their clients' shoes and, therefore, cannot possibly know *exactly* how the client is feeling in that moment. Thus, empathy is never expressed by saying "I know exactly how you feel," rather empathic expressions maintain the respectful distance of the "as if" condition.

Neither is empathy sympathy. Sympathy can make people feel pitiful and can communicate a distance between the sympathizer and the other person, whereas empathy brings people closer together in a shared experience. Empathy opens the door for further discussion, usually at a deeper level, and is empowering. Sympathy, on the other hand, encourages people to view themselves as wounded victims and limits productive conversation. The following example illustrates the difference:

CLIENT: I can't believe the terrible grade I got on the exam. I hope no one finds out.
SYMPATHY: I'm sorry you did so poorly on the test.
EMPATHY: I can hear the deep sense of shame you feel about your grade.

True empathy is transmitted to the client through genuine reflection of feeling, by closely tracking the client's words and changing felt meaning as it occurs in the moment, and through the continued expression of nonjudgmental and unconditional positive regard. Empathic reflections are based on respect for the other person, awareness of the person's worldview, and always maintaining the "as if" condition. More will be said about empathy in the Skill Development section at the end of this chapter.

Carl Rogers on Empathy

Rogers (1980) recounted that it was a social worker, steeped in Rankian training, who helped him to learn that the most effective approach was "to listen for the feelings, the emotions whose patterns could be discerned through the client's words" (p. 138). Rogers thought it was this social worker who first suggested that the best response of the therapist was "to reflect these feelings back to the client—'reflect' becoming in time a word which made me cringe. But at that time it improved my work as therapist and I was grateful" (p. 138). He later used the term *validation* to refer to the therapist's empathic confirmation of the client's emotions.

OTHER STRATEGIES Many of the systems of psychotherapy and counseling discussed in this book rely heavily on specialized strategies such as word association, dream analysis, and modification of cognitive distortions to further the treatment. Because the heart of person-centered counseling is the therapeutic relationship, clinicians rarely use techniques such as these, nor do they use elaborate diagnostic and assessment tools. They are viewed as unnecessary and as detracting from the client–clinician relationship. All interventions in person-centered treatment should promote the therapeutic relationship and enhance the client's awareness and empowerment. Strategies that promote and deepen communication and that reflect the clinician's caring and interest probably are the most useful interventions in person-centered counseling. These include empathic reflections, paraphrases, and clinician self-disclosure. Research shows that clients experience relational depth when therapists are trustworthy, real, and genuine. When these qualities were absent from the therapeutic process, therapists were described as distant, powerful, and misunderstanding (Knox & Cooper, 2010).

Nondirectiveness

Rogers originally called his work *nondirective therapy* to distinguish it from the prevailing models of the time (mainly psychoanalytic and behavioral) in which the practitioner was viewed as the expert whom the client looked to for advice on what the client should do (Tudor & Worrall, 2006). Nondirective therapy emphasizes the importance of the client taking the lead and being the focus of the treatment process. Although Rogers later changed the name of his approach to *client-centered counseling* and then *person-centered counseling* to highlight the fact that his theory applied to all relationships, the nondirective aspects of this approach still merit attention.

Person-centered therapists do not manipulate change, but neither are they passive recipients of client input. They are busy creating the necessary conditions that are conducive to client growth. Although nondirectivity has been a part of person-centered therapy since the beginning, Rogers affirmed that complete nondirectivity is impossible. Whether through the choice of questions asked or the reflections chosen, the therapist cannot help but insert him- or herself into the therapeutic process. However, all therapists must have a compelling reason that they can elucidate for the interventions they choose to use and when and why they choose to use them. Perhaps a better course than trying to remain exclusively nondirective would be to consider how best to be directive in the service of the therapy.

APPLICATION AND CURRENT USE OF PERSON-CENTERED COUNSELING

"Person-centered therapy has fundamentally shaped the current practice of therapy in general and of experiential therapy in particular" (Pos, Greenberg, & Elliott, 2008, p. 82). Even therapists who engage in Internet therapy or cybercounseling must be cognizant of how therapeutic conditions can be fostered in an online environment. Research is limited, but one study compared outcomes across three different treatment modalities (face-to-face, video therapy, and audio therapy) and found that differences in outcomes were small (Wilcoxon, Remley, Gladding, & Huber, 2007). This is promising, but more research is needed, including gender-specific research since women seem to have a preference for face-to-face counseling (Haberstroh, Duffey, Evans, Gee, & Trepal, 2007).

Several experiential approaches that have grown out of person-centered theory include focusing, developed by Eugene Gendlin, a student of Rogers who later founded the Focusing Institute; emotion-focused therapy (also known as process-experiential therapy), developed by Leslie Greenberg and colleagues (Greenberg & Johnson, 1988; Greenberg, Rice, & Elliott, 1993; Greenberg & Safran, 1987); and narrative therapy, developed by Michael White and David Epston (1990), which helps people to develop a sense of agency and rewrite the stories of their lives. All of these approaches will be discussed in greater detail in the coming chapters.

Person-centered therapy is also at the core of motivational interviewing, which was originally developed by Miller and Rollnick (2002) to promote behavioral change in people who misused drugs. Motivational interviewing has since grown into motivational enhancement therapy, for use with a variety of client problems and populations. Each of these theories is outlined briefly here. Other process-experiential approaches include dialogical Gestalt therapy (Yontef, 1998), Mahrer's (1996/2004) experiential therapy, and foundations of transpersonal psychology.

Emotion-Focused Therapy

The first goal of all process-experiential therapies is to establish the necessary conditions of a good therapeutic relationship as set forth by Carl Rogers (congruence, unconditional positive regard, and empathy). After a safe, genuine, and helpful environment has been created, goals can be worked on that focus on both content and process.

In content-focused goals, the client chooses an issue that is the most pressing or emotionally alive at the moment (e.g., relationship problems, career change, self-validation) to work on. The therapist provides the process goals by selecting interventions that deepen the client's in-the-moment experiencing.

Therapists may ask the client to talk about where the tension is felt in the body, or where the body is tightening when they talk about a stressful event. Or a therapist may focus on a particular feeling, with the intention of helping the client feel empathically understood, while at the same time drawing attention to the "most poignant aspect" (Greenberg & Elliott, 2002, p. 14) of the experience.

The therapist facilitates the client's experiencing of emotion in the here and now and through empathic attunement focuses on the moment-to-moment shifts in client experiencing and processing in an effort to help them differentiate "the edges of their experience" (Pos et al., 2008, p. 89). "The overarching process goal of experiential therapy, therefore, is to help the client deepen experience and symbolize it accurately in awareness" (p. 101).

EFT combines person-centered empathic responding with the directiveness of Gestalt therapy as the therapist guides the client toward certain emotion-processing activities that will result in new insights for the client. Homework, silence, vocal tone, appropriate therapist nonverbal behavior that indicates interest, experiential teaching—all help clients to tease out their underlying feelings. Clients actively participate in the change process. Put simply, EFT involves a three-step process—bonding, emotion evoking, and emotion restructuring (Greenberg & Elliott, 2002). Change occurs through awareness, regulation, reflection, and transformation of emotion taking place in an empathically attuned relationship.

The experiential process may be continued through homework; for example, if the client is working on his relationship with his daughter, he might be asked to notice how he reacts to his daughter during the week. The awareness homework would not be intended to change the client, but to continue to focus attention on those experiences.

With its emphasis on the importance of the relationship, empathic responding, bodily felt experience, and emotion awareness, access, and regulation, emotion-focused therapy provides an exciting new treatment approach with many applications for specific problems (depression, relationships, trauma) and varied populations. Emotion-focused therapy for couples, which integrates process-experiential theory with attachment theory, has been shown to be effective for relationship distress in couples and for those in which one partner has been traumatized (Johnson, 2004). This increasingly popular and effective treatment methodology is discussed in further detail in the chapter on family systems theory (Chapter 18).

Experiential Focusing

Focusing is a stand-alone experiential therapy as well as a powerful intervention developed by Eugene Gendlin. When using focusing, the therapist invites clients to pay attention to the source of feelings in their bodies. Focusing assumes that the felt sense is a source of information relating to current issues and that if a client can tune in to this feeling in the here and now, he or she can access that information (Pos et al., 2008). Felt sense is an experiential process that interweaves existential and Gestalt processes into a holistic approach to psychotherapy.

For example, Sylvia arrives for her session and reports, "I don't know what to talk about. I feel stuck." The focusing therapist invites Sylvia to consider where she feels that in her body. Sylvia responds, "As I sit here, my stomach feels like it's jumping all around." Sylvia is then asked to stay focused on that feeling and to describe what she is experiencing.

In focusing, the therapist directs attention to the experiential elements of the counseling session as they occur in the here and now. Rather than telling a story or looking for insight, the focusing therapist looks at four layers of interaction between the therapist and client: the body, behavior in the moment (e.g., tapping, moving), interpersonal interaction, and symbolizing the experience in words and reflections (Day, 2008). The therapist often uses metaphors to react to the client's feelings. Continuing with our example of Sylvia:

THERAPIST: So, even though you're sitting here quietly on the couch, inside you feel as if a flagman is inside your stomach.

SYLVIA: That's right!

THERAPIST: Can you sense what that's about?

SYLVIA: I have all this energy and so many things to do, and I need to move forward with finding a place to live and separating from my husband, but inside my stomach there's all this turmoil, like this flagman is waving these flags and making me come to a complete halt once again.

THERAPIST: Once again?

SYLVIA: Yes. Like the last time I was ready to leave my husband, and then couldn't do it at the last moment.

THERAPIST: Can you sense what's behind the flagman right now?

SYLVIA: He's warning me about the danger that lies ahead if I proceed with moving out. I feel like I'm going too fast, rushing into this, and maybe my body is telling me to slow down, and make sure I'm making the right decision.

THERAPIST: Your stomach is telling you to proceed with caution.

SYLVIA: That's right.

Gendlin (1996) calls this somatic feeling "the felt sense" (p. 60) or the feeling before emotion. Recognizing this felt sense enables people to access information from a deeper level than their thoughts or emotions. For many clients, this body sense is unclear and vague at first, but with practice, clients learn to focus on the felt sense with an interested, curious attention. Once attention has been focused on a felt sense, and it has been brought into awareness, it moves, changes, or unfolds. Gendlin refers to this as a felt shift in the body.

An experiential way of knowing concentrates on the bodily "felt sense" in the here and now. Attending to this immediacy in the body heightens the internal process for an organic unfolding. Gendlin (1996) believes that "without experiential concreteness" (p. 15) change will not happen. Interpretations are not sufficient to bring about change, rather "an inwardly sensed connection or any other physical response" (p. 11) is a prerequisite for change to occur.

Six steps are involved in the process of focusing: clearing a space, felt sense, handle, resonating, asking, and receiving (Gendlin, 1996). The six-step process is described briefly here:

1. *Clearing a space:* Clients take time to be still, relax, and focus inwardly on their body before asking themselves how their life is going or what the main issue is.
2. *Felt sense:* Clients choose one issue to focus on and experience what the problem feels like; and allow themselves to feel it.
3. *Handle:* The client is asked to choose a word or phrase that comes to mind to describe the felt sense. It might be a word like *heavy* or *tight,* or it might be an image like a big gray blob.
4. *Resonating:* The client is asked to go back and forth between the felt sense and the word, phrase, or image to check how they resonate with each other. The client continues going back and forth until it feels just right.
5. *Asking:* The client is asked questions such as "What is in this sense?" that illuminate the felt sense and move it forward. The client stays with the felt sense until a shift or release is felt.
6. *Receiving:* The client receives whatever comes with a shift in a friendly way.

Focusing brings insight and relief. It can also bring about new behavior. Focusing therapists discuss the "wisdom of the body" in the sense that a deeper, wiser self exists inside the body. By paying attention to a deeper sense of knowing, the body knows what it needs to become. By just being, and focusing interest and curiosity on the felt sense, a shift is made. Focusing provides the conditions in which this change can happen.

Motivational Interviewing

Motivational interviewing is described by its creators as a "client-centered, directive method for enhancing intrinsic motivation to change by exploring and resolving ambivalence" (Miller & Rollnick, 2002, p. 25). Motivational interviewing is deeply rooted in Rogers's person-centered theory, and helps therapists to meet clients where they are, accept their worldview, and enhance their efforts to change (Arkowiz, Westra, Miller, & Rollnick, 2008). Originally created for the treatment of addictions, motivational interviewing has become a standard intervention with many behavioral-related therapies and many health-related concerns (Rollnick, Miller & Butler, 2008).

Similar to person-centered therapy, motivational interviewing avoids diagnosis and direct attempts to persuade the client, and allows the client to control the agenda. The therapist's role is as partner, not an authority figure. Therapists use empathy, reflective listening, and caring concern to help clients explore their attitudes about change. Resistance is not confronted, rather it is reframed as ambivalence to change (Zinbarg & Griffith, 2008).

Therapists who use motivational interviewing produce the conditions in which the client can choose to change; therefore, the therapist's skills in developing a therapeutic alliance using Rogers's core conditions are not only important, but have been found to be directly linked to the amount of client disclosure, cooperation, and emotional expression that occurs in the session (Moyers, Miller, & Hendrickson, 2005). The goal of motivational interviewing is to help the client work through ambivalence through the use of self-talk and an analysis of the advantages and disadvantages of making changes.

Therapists typically use the guiding style of motivational interviewing early on in therapy to help clients identify obstacles to treatment, elicit intentional statements, and set the agenda. The approach is now being used with a variety of clients (e.g., adolescents, people who are incarcerated, couples, and groups) and for a variety of situations in which resistance is a factor (e.g., eating disorders, alcohol abuse and dependence, dually diagnosed disorders). A meta-analysis of 25 years of empirical research found that therapists who use this intervention are more likely to empower reluctant clients to change (Lundahl, Kunz, Brownell, Tollefson, & Burke, 2010). Overall, motivational interviewing is another example of how Rogers's person-centered approach has evolved over the years in the successful treatment of a wide range of diagnostic groups (Arkowiz et al., 2008; Lundahl & Burke, 2009).

Application to Diagnostic Groups

During the past 70 years, empathy, unconditional positive regard, and congruence have been essential common factors of effective psychotherapy, regardless of treatment modality (Duncan, Miller, Wampold, & Hubble, 2010) or population. Astoundingly, one study of outcomes in marital counseling found that the couples' perceptions of the therapeutic alliance at the third session predicted treatment outcome (Quinn, Dotson, & Jordan, 1997). Overall, Hubble and colleagues (2010) found that the alliance accounts for 6% of the variance in treatment outcome. This is roughly six times the effect of treatment modality. Therapist variables accounted for another 7% or 8%.

Wampold (2010) noted, "It appears that for the most prevalent disorders of adults and children, all treatments intended to be therapeutic are equally effective" (p. 60).

A review of 32 outcome studies comparing client-centered or nondirective/supportive therapies to cognitive–behavioral therapy (CBT) found person-centered or nondirective/supportive therapies to be as effective as CBT in the treatment of anxiety, depression, marital and interpersonal problems, personality disorders, trauma, and schizophrenia (Chambless & Hollon, 1998). A more recent study found that process-experiential treatment is as effective as CBT in the treatment of depression (Watson, Gordon, Stermac, Kalogerakos, & Steckley, 2003).

Person-centered therapy has been found to be equally as effective as other approaches (including EMDR and exposure-based behavioral therapies) for the treatment of post-traumatic stress disorder (PTSD) (Benish, Imel, & Wampold, 2008). This is an interesting finding, because exposure-based treatments had long been considered to be the "gold standard" for the treatment of PTSD, and person-centered therapy does not include exposure.

Other research indicates that person-centered counselors and therapy and the necessary conditions are helpful for a variety of populations and presenting problems, including schizophrenia, crisis intervention, and working with people who have been dually diagnosed (Carrick, 2007; Henderson, O'Hara, Barfield, & Rogers, 2007; Seligman & Reichenberg, 2012). Person-centered therapy provides a way of being with clients who may be too disturbed to participate in therapy as a result of psychosis, disability, or mental retardation. Pre-therapy treatment based on person-centered therapy (Rogers, 1951) accommodates the needs of clients who cannot express their feelings by providing content reflections, such as "It's a beautiful day"; face reflections, such as "You look angry"; and body reflections, such as "Your head is down." Such exchanges have been found to facilitate affective content and to provide a map for more meaningful therapy with clients who are severely disturbed (Sommerbeck, 2011). Similarly, the use of feeling charts with children, adolescents, and others who do not have an emotion orientation can be instrumental in providing a baseline language on which therapy can be built.

Spaulding and Nolting (2006) noted in their work with people with schizophrenia that the "unifying role of the therapeutic relationship instills in the client a sense of hope and an expectation that things can and will change for the better" (p. S105). Clearly, person-centered therapy has a significant place in creating a therapeutic alliance in nearly all populations. Bozarth, Zimring, and Tausch (2001) concluded that "Psychotherapy outcome research supports the major tenets of person-centered therapy. The therapeutic relationship and the client's resources are the crux of successful therapy" (p. 214).

Carl Rogers's vision of person-centered therapy was more than just a treatment modality. It "served as a vision of society based on individual freedom and self-determination as well as underpinning a method of psychotherapy" (Anderson, Lunnen, & Ogles, 2010, p. 144). Specifically, his theory has been applied successfully to training programs for pastoral counseling, nursing, and first responders; and across myriad environments from education to business management, human resources, and peace negotiations in many countries of the world (Kirschenbaum, 2009). Empathy is now being taught in some preschools and elementary schools to help children develop social/emotional intelligence and ward off later bullying and aggressive behavior in schools (Gordon, 2005).

Empirical support is also available for process-experiential therapies that have evolved from the Rogerian tradition. A meta-analysis of 64 studies of experiential therapies supports the effectiveness of emotion-focused therapy in general (Elliott, Watson, Goldman, & Greenberg, 2004) and the benefits of EFT for depression specifically (Goldman, Greenberg, & Angus, 2006; Greenberg, 2010). In addition, experiencing as a process has been shown to enhance positive outcomes in psychodynamic therapy and cognitive–behavioral therapy (Hendricks, 2002). Thus, the process of experiencing may be "an important therapy process regardless of the therapeutic orientation" (Pos et al., 2008, p. 109).

Experiential focusing is a stand-alone theory or it can be used as a technique and integrated into other theories such as emotion-focused therapy and Gestalt. It can be used with individuals or in focusing groups. Focusing has been used successfully to help people make difficult decisions such as those related to abortion (Scharwachter, 2008), in recovery from addictions (Barbieri, 2008; Lee & Rovers, 2008), in cases of trauma, and with people who are incarcerated ((Pos et al., 2008). Gendlin (1996) notes the approach is helpful in any situation in which a person feels stuck.

Application to Multicultural Groups

Person-centered multicultural counseling is an effective way to facilitate learning across age, race, ethnicity, and geographic location (Cornelius-White, 2005, 2007). The respectful and accepting nature of person-centered counseling, coupled with its phenomenological perspective, makes it appropriate for people from a wide range of ethnic, cultural, and socioeconomic backgrounds. Person-centered theory emphasizes the importance of valuing and understanding people, of viewing them from their own frame of reference, of building a positive client–clinician relationship, and of attending to the client's world through that person's perspective (Cornelius-White, 2005). People from diverse cultural backgrounds are likely to accept and respond well to person-centered treatment.

People from some cultural groups may be hesitant to self-disclose and, therefore, might be uncomfortable with experiential therapies that focus on the client's internal emotional state (Sue & Sue, 2008). Sue and Sue warn that "certain socioeconomic groups and ethnic minorities do not particularly value insight" (p. 67). Also, humanistic therapies that assume self-actualization as a goal may not be affiliated with the client's frame of reference, but with the ideals and goals of the practitioner. For these clients, moving outside the "ideological milieu of individualism" (Sue & Sue, 2008, p. 68) may be more comfortable.

Although person-centered theory and treatment do reflect American ideals of independence, self-direction, and individuality, many aspects of this approach are also relevant to a diverse and multicultural society. These include:

- The emphasis on people's rights to their own opinions and thoughts
- The importance placed on respect, genuineness, acceptance, and empathy
- The focus on people's own experience and frames of reference
- The emphasis on personal growth and self-actualization
- The interest in relationships and commonalities among people
- The attention to present-moment awareness and the immediacy of the counseling situation.

These perspectives are pertinent to all people, regardless of cultural background.

Some research supports this point. Abdel-Tawab and Roter (2002), for example, studied the communication styles of personnel in family planning clinics in Egypt. They found that a "patient-centered" model of care delivery involving such qualities as reassurance, approval, empathy, concern, and partnership was associated with better client follow-through and satisfaction than a more authoritarian model. The authors of this study observed that, even in a developing culture with a hierarchical perspective, person-centered methods proved their value. Chang and Page (1991) noted the similarity between Rogers's concept of the actualized person and personality traits such as openness to experience, closeness to nature, and independence in thought and action that are valued in Eastern cultures and in Buddhism and Taoism.

Current Use of Person-Centered Counseling

Rogers and person-centered therapy have made an immeasurable contribution to counseling and psychotherapy. As stated earlier, his views of the self and the role of the clinician in therapy revolutionized the counseling process. His version of the therapeutic alliance and a genuine, supportive, accepting, empathic clinician provided an important alternative to the anonymity of the Freudian analysts and the directiveness of the early behaviorists. Rogers humanized clinicians and taught us that the clinician's use of the facilitative conditions in a positive therapeutic alliance is the most important strategy for change.

Person-centered therapy can be easily integrated with other types of therapy. For example, the combination of humanistic and cognitive approaches is the second-most frequent combination of theoretical orientations, and the combination of humanistic and behavioral approaches is fourth (Prochaska & Norcross, 2009). In addition, person-centered principles have been used in career counseling, play therapy for children and elderly adults, couples, family counseling, and group therapy.

Person-centered therapy has application not just for the counseling profession, but in schools, government, and the workplace (Henderson et al., 2007). For example, person-centered educational theory has spawned learner-centered instruction—an application to teaching and learning that prioritizes facilitative relationships and honors the uniqueness of every learner (Cornelius-White, 2007). Rogers's concept of student-centered teaching involves prizing, accepting, trusting, and empathic attitudes of the teachers toward their students (Rogers, 1967). In a meta-analytic review of more than 1,000 articles, Cornelius-White (2007) found that learner-centered teacher–student relationships are effective. Student-centered teaching has spread to the fields of nursing, organizational psychology, interpersonal relationships, and education. Schools have been developed that are based on these principles.

EVALUATION OF PERSON-CENTERED COUNSELING

Rogers's influence in psychology and the human potential movement of the 1970s has had a far-reaching influence on today's therapists. Experiential groups, focusing, Virginia Satir's play therapy for children, psychodrama, emotion-focused therapy, EFT for couples, body-centered focusing developed by Gendlin, and the roots of transpersonal psychology—all are firmly grounded in the humanistic tradition. (See Chapters 19 and 20 for additional information.)

Limitations

Despite its enormous contributions, Rogers's theory has some limitations. Research has shown that depth of experiencing in therapy is related to outcome. Person-centered as well as other experiential therapies that include focusing and emotion processing are correlated positively with successful outcomes in a variety of orientations and populations (Hendricks, 2002). However, some people are not comfortable expressing emotion; some may have cultural backgrounds in which emotions are suppressed and hearing direct empathic responses might make them uncomfortable. Person-centered therapists who are culturally cognizant and adapt their therapeutic style to the client's needs are more likely to be successful.

The nondirective focus of person-centered therapy may also be unfamiliar to some clients, particularly those who view therapists as experts and are looking for someone to solve their problems. Clients might ask, "Aren't you going to tell me what I should do?"

Person-centered therapy demands much of the therapist. Instead of relying on techniques or manualized workbooks, the therapist uses him- or herself. Therapists must be congruent, genuine, self-actualized, present in the moment, focused, nonjudgmental, patient, and, above all, empathic. Without this finely tuned way of being with the client, therapy is unlikely to be as effective. Some therapists might not be comfortable working from a purely person-centered perspective without the use of homework, manuals, and other techniques commonly found in other approaches.

Strengths and Contributions

Carl Rogers was the first person to measure the effectiveness of therapy (Hergenhahn & Olson, 2007). He opened the field of psychotherapy to research investigation. Rogers was the first to record and publish complete transcripts of psychotherapy sessions. Through his extensive writings for both mental health professionals and the general population; demonstrations, tapes, and transcripts of his sessions; research on the process of treatment; and his emphasis on education and the widespread need for person-centered relationships, Rogers gave us an accessible and comprehensible treatment system.

Rogers's ideal of the client–clinician relationship has infiltrated and influenced all theories of counseling and psychotherapy:

- Carl Rogers developed one of the most comprehensive theories of the self ever created.
- He believed in the dignity and worth of each individual and in people's innate movement toward actualization and growth.
- Although his theory first started to evolve in the 1940s and 1950s, it is still appropriate and relevant today—nearly 70 years later.
- Rather than a fixed theory with proscribed techniques, Rogers created a solid foundation on which future theories can build.
- The theory is optimistic, affirming, and has a positive perspective on human nature.
- Psychotherapy outcome research supports the major tenets of person-centered therapy.
- Person-centered therapy can be easily integrated into other treatment approaches. As mentioned earlier, Prochaska and Norcross (2009) found that the majority of person-centered therapists integrate person-centered therapy with other compatible theories, depending on the needs of the client.

Rogers is credited with being the first to introduce the concept of therapist transparency into the treatment process, a concept that Anderson refers to as "being public" (Anderson, 2012, p. 68). The importance of therapist transparency—of being open, honest, genuine, and revealing any biases or limitations—later became core concepts in the development of narrative therapy and feminist therapy. Both will be discussed in greater detail in Chapter 11.

The work of Carl Rogers is well known internationally, and is the primary form of treatment practiced in England (Cooper, Schmid, O'Hara, & Wyatt, 2007; Totton, 2010) and in the emerging democracies of Eastern Europe, and it is popular in Latin America as well (Kirschenbaum, 2004). His writings have been translated into many languages and he is viewed not only as a leader in counseling and psychology but also as a peacemaker.

His ideas formed the basis for Thomas Gordon's *Parent Effectiveness Training* (1970), a classic text that, for the past 50 years, has helped parents raise children with a focus on empathy and attachment.

Parent effectiveness training (PET) has produced evidence-based outcomes for generations of parents. The use of active listening skills, empathic attunement, nonconfrontational discipline, and creative conflict resolution improves the relationship and attachment between parent and child. Parents learn a new way to interact with their child that does not trigger the child's innate instinct to resist (counterwill). In this evidence-based treatment program, the child begins to cooperate because he or she cares about the relationship with the parent. PET training programs exist worldwide and have been proven effective for working with toddlers, children, and adolescents (Cedar & Levant, 1990).

In the final decade of his life, Carl Rogers's contributions to international peace efforts resulted in his nomination for a Nobel Peace Prize. Rogers was a humanitarian and an educator who traveled the world to bring peace and understanding to groups in conflict with each other. From Northern Ireland, the Soviet Union, South Africa, Central America, and other hotspots around the globe, Rogers spread his emotionally honest approach to conflict resolution, which fosters interaction in private settings with a flexible agenda and allows for intense expression of emotion. His paradigm has been credited with helping President Carter create "Track II diplomacy" in the Camp David Accord between Israel and Egypt (Ryback, 2011) and found expression in the philosophy of "deliberative democracy" employed by President Obama (Packer, 2008). "No greater contribution can be made than to save countries from mortal conflict by having them become more humanistic in their political negotiations" (Ryback, 2011, p. 413). The Center for Studies of the Person in La Jolla, California, and the World Association for Person-Centered and Experiential Psychotherapy and Counseling continue to promote and teach Rogers's ideas.

SKILL DEVELOPMENT: EMPATHIC RESPONDING

Empathy and empathic responding on the part of the therapist help to facilitate a compassionate and safe environment in which a person can feel free to explore deeper emotions. All clinicians, regardless of theoretical orientation, use empathic listening when working with clients.

Rather than a technique that therapists use, Rogers (1980) considered empathy to be a process or a way of being with another person. "This kind of sensitive, active listening is exceedingly rare in our lives. We think we listen, but very rarely do we listen with real understanding, true empathy. Yet listening, of this very special kind, is one of the most potent forces for change that I know" (pp. 115–116).

Empathy is effective for a variety of reasons. First, it helps to normalize a person's feelings—by experiencing empathy, people no longer feel that they are isolated or alone in their experiences. Empathy also promotes examination of the client's subjective experience—hearing their feelings spoken back to them invites an exploration of the nuances of those feelings. And finally, empathy helps the client create new meaning. Greenberg (2002) found that the most effective empathic responses focus "on the leading edge of [a] client's experience, on what is most alive or poignant or what is just at the edge of awareness" (p. 77).

And yet empathy alone is not sufficient. Empathy must be experienced, reflected, and accepted by the client in order for it to be meaningful. Empathic responding begins with the therapist who must first understand the client's feelings and accurately express those feelings to the client; then the client must recognize the empathic attunement (Barrett-Leonard, 1981). All three steps in the process are necessary.

Even so, some people have viewed person-centered therapy as deceptively simple and seemingly easy to master, yet when therapists begin to practice empathic listening they often find it is not quite so easy. Carl Rogers began to deplore the term *reflective listening* because of the implication that the therapist simply mirrored back, or parroted, the other person's words. He wrote: "Being empathic is a complex, demanding, and strong—yet also a subtle and gentle—way of being" (Rogers, 1980, p. 143).

The following skill development exercise focuses on validating client's feelings by making accurate empathic responses. Although there are many different ways to rate empathy, we will only focus on three types of responses:

N = Responses in which no empathy is expressed. Either no emotion was implied in the client's statement, or the therapist was completely off track in the reflection.

I = Interchangeable responses in which the therapist captures the essence of what the client said, but nothing more was added. Such responses can be a direct repetition of the client's words, or an accurate rephrasing of the client's words. Interchangeable responses are considered to be empathic and research indicates they are helpful to clients (Greenberg, Elliott, & Lietaer, 1994; Sachse, 1993).

E = Empathic response. This more valuable empathic response is at the outer border of the client's awareness. Sometimes empathic reflections are followed up with a question to clarify the client's internal experience.

Example:

CLIENT: I am so sick of fighting this disease, I just want to give up.

RESPONSE 1: You don't look sick to me. (No empathy.)

RESPONSE 2: You're really tired of it all and just want to stop fighting. (Interchangeable.)

RESPONSE 3: You've been battling this for a long time, and you're wondering what it would be like if you just didn't do it anymore. (Most empathic response.)

Notice how the first response lacks empathy, does not focus on the client, and rather than uniting the client and therapist in shared experiencing actually inserts distance between them. The second response is an accurate and interchangeable response to what the client said. This type of response can help clients to clarify feelings, hear their own words resonate back to them, and give them time to think about their next response. The third response focuses more on the person's felt meaning. It is noticeably more poignant, and more at the leading edge of what the client has implied in the statement "I just want to give up."

Review the following examples and determine which one is the nonempathic response (N), the interchangeable response (I), and the most empathic response (E).

CLIENT: I miss my husband so much since he died, sometimes I want to claw at his grave to dig him up.

RESPONSE 1: You are so desperately sad since he died, that sometimes you feel like you would do almost anything to see him again.

RESPONSE 2: You miss him so much that sometimes you want to dig him up from his grave.

RESPONSE 3: Oh, don't do that!

CLIENT: Since we've gotten married John and I do absolutely everything together. I'm starting to feel stifled.

RESPONSE 1: You and John do everything together, and it's stifling.

RESPONSE 2: You're not thinking about divorce, are you?

RESPONSE 3: You love your husband but you're starting to wonder if it's okay to want to spend time away from each other.

CLIENT: If I fail this final, my parents will kill me!

RESPONSE 1: I'm sure everything will be fine.

RESPONSE 2: You're feeling anxious about this final exam and worry that your parents will be furious if you don't get a good grade.

RESPONSE 3: You believe your parents would be very angry if you fail.

Now, look at the following examples of client statements, and come up with empathic and interchangeable responses of your own.

1. Yesterday marked my first anniversary with AA.
2. I think my wife might be having an affair.
3. I'm so worried. My cat didn't come home last night.
4. After years of infertility, I just found out I'm pregnant!
5. My girlfriend was a half-hour late to the movie—again.
6. My husband always plays with the kids right when it's time for them to go to bed.

Remember to empathize with clients, not sympathize. Empathy is a response that reassures the client that someone is listening and someone understands what he or she is going through.

Empathy normalizes feelings. As discussed earlier in this chapter, sympathy offers condolence and regret, and distances the client from the therapist.

Carl Rogers believed empathy could be learned, although he never explained how to teach it. Later works by others have evaluated empathic attunement in a variety of ways (Greenberg, 2010; Norcross, 2011; Truax & Carkhuff, 2007). Readers should consider obtaining one of the many excellent resources available for improving skill development in therapy (Murphy & Dillon, 2008; Seligman, 2009).

CASE ILLUSTRATION

The following dialogue between Edie and her counselor illustrates many hallmarks of person-centered treatment, including active listening, communicating empathy, valuing the client, modeling genuineness, congruent therapist disclosure, and focusing on the present.

Edie's responses are abbreviated in order to demonstrate the clinician's use of person-centered approaches. Most person-centered clinicians typically talk much less than do their clients. Edie is working on her relationship with her mother and stepfather, Pete, who has been abusive to Edie in the past.

EDIE: I feel so angry at my mother! Ava and I were visiting her and in came Pete. I could smell the liquor across the room. And my mother said nothing. How could she be like that?

CLINICIAN: You're feeling pretty frustrated that she doesn't assert herself.

EDIE: Yes, and to expose Ava to that.

CLINICIAN: You wish she would have done something to protect Ava.

EDIE: But she never does.

CLINICIAN: She never protects her?

EDIE: Nope. She's always been like that. She didn't protect me from my grandfather either.

CLINICIAN: You're remembering what it was like for you when your grandfather abused you. You know, I may be off base here, but I just had a picture of you as a helpless little girl. . . .

EDIE: Yes! Exactly! I feel like a helpless child again (thinking for a moment, then angrily . . .) but I'm *not* helpless! I'm a wife and mother, I've coped with cancer, and gone back to school, and I can figure out how to protect my child.

CLINICIAN: You've overcome a lot in your life, and you can figure out how to deal with this, too.

EDIE: Darn right I can. I could keep Ava from ever going over there or seeing Pete again.

CLINICIAN: Part of you would like to just cut off ties with them completely.

EDIE: Yes. But then Ava wouldn't be able to see my mother, either. That seems so drastic.

CLINICIAN: So, that seems to you like too big a step.

EDIE: Yes, sometimes I do feel like never seeing them again, but that seems very childish. My mother is Pete's victim just as I was. Maybe I could set some limits . . . tell my mother that if Pete is angry or drunk again around me or Ava we'll just have to leave, even if it seems rude.

CLINICIAN: You're thinking that if you set a boundary around Pete's behavior, and let your mother know ahead of time what you are planning to do, that it will protect Ava and your mother will understand.

EDIE: I don't care what Pete thinks of me, but it's very important to me that my mother understands I have to protect Ava from his behavior.

CLINICIAN: As long as your mother understands and Ava is safe, then it will be worth it.

EDIE: Yes, that's right. I'm starting to feel better about this. I think that I really *can* protect Ava, stand up for myself, and still have a close relationship with my mother. Wouldn't that be great?

EXERCISES

Large-Group Exercises

1. Discuss the strengths and limitations of the dialogue in the case illustration. What would you change, if anything, to improve on this segment of a treatment session?
2. Identify, in the case illustration dialogue, examples of the following key elements of person-centered counseling:
   - Active listening
   - Empathy
   - Reflection of feeling
   - Reflection of meaning
   - Valuing and empowering the client
   - Genuineness
   - Focusing on the present
   - Self-disclosure.
3. Create a round-robin dialogue. One person, teacher or student, should stand or sit in front of the class and assume the role of Roberto or another hypothetical client. This client should engage in a dialogue with the class about a time when he or she had very strong emotions. Each student in turn should make one comment or intervention. Interventions should reflect person-centered treatment, with each successive intervention building on the previous one. Following the dialogue, the class should discuss the role-played interview and its strengths and limitations.

Small-Group Exercises

1. Divide into groups of four students. Each dyad should engage in a 10-minute client–clinician role-play, building on previous dialogues that they have had together. Use self-disclosure at least twice and try to communicate empathy often when assuming the role of clinician.
   After each dialogue, the group of four should discuss the dialogue and its strengths and limitations, providing feedback to each clinician on the following:
   - The nature and effectiveness of the self-disclosures
   - Communication of empathy

- Therapeutic alliance
- Strengths of the role-play
- Ways in which the role-play might have been improved.

2. Divide into your groups of four participants. Using the client statements from the Skill Development section of this chapter, take turns creating three brief role-plays that continue each of the three clinician responses. Focus particular attention on what the client says immediately after the therapist responds in a nonempathic, interchangeable, or empathic manner. Consider the following aspects of each client's responses and then discuss the effect of each intervention:

   - Were the therapist's reflections empathic?
   - How did the therapist's response change the direction of the client's focus, if at all?
   - What impact did the therapist's response have on the client?
   - Did the client explore deeper feelings?

Individual Exercises

1. Listening is something we often take for granted, not realizing that it is an art. Plan an hour of time to practice your listening skills. Use reflection of feelings to let the person know you hear and understand the meaning of what he or she is saying. Maintain good eye contact. Monitor your verbal and nonverbal messages to be sure they are congruent and that you are genuine, caring, and accepting. Write about this experience in your journal.
2. The goal of motivational interviewing is to strengthen the client's readiness and commitment to change. Consider a behavior that you would like to change and answer the following questions in your journal.
   - What change do you want to make? (Include positive statements such as "to increase," "to improve," "to begin to.")
   - What are the most important reasons why you want to make this change? List the consequences of both action and inaction.
   - How will you achieve this change? List specific, concrete, and small first steps that you will take. Include when, where, and how these actions will be taken.
   - How can other people help you? List specific ways in which people can help you. How will you solicit this support?
   - How will you know your plan is working? List the benefits that will occur as a result of this change.

   What might interfere with your plan? Anticipate what might go wrong and list situations, obstacles, or setbacks that might occur. List what you could do in each situation to stay with the plan despite any problems that might interfere.
3. Develop and write in your journal an appropriate clinician self-disclosure in response to the following client statements and questions:

   CLIENT A: There must be something really wrong with me. Everybody else seems to love parties, but I hate going into a big room full of strangers.

   CLIENT B: I finally had a great weekend. I woke up early, took a walk, had brunch with a friend, and then went to that great Georgia O'Keeffe exhibit at the museum.

   CLIENT C: I feel embarrassed that my parents found out I had too much to drink last night and had to have someone drive me home. Did anything like that ever happen to you when you were younger?

CLIENT D: My older brother hits me and pushes me whenever we are alone. Yesterday, when he pushed me, I fell down and really hurt myself. I don't know what to do. I'm afraid he'll get into trouble if I tell anyone.

CLIENT E: It feels like once I let people know I'm a lesbian, that changes all their reactions to me and they don't see me as a person anymore. Sometimes I think that happened here too. When I told you my partner was a woman, your expression changed, and I sensed that you disapproved of me.

Summary

Carl Rogers first developed person-centered counseling in the 1940s and 1950s, as a humanistic and phenomenological approach to treatment that values the dignity and worth of all people as well as their potential to resolve their difficulties. The primary source of healing in person-centered treatment is the establishment, by the therapist, of the core conditions of congruence, unconditional positive regard, and empathy. By accepting clients as they are, and providing a safe environment for them to explore their feelings, treatment moves along a path of growth toward actualization of the person's potential, helping him or her to become more fully functioning and self-actualized. This approach, which focuses on the present rather than past problems or future concerns, transformed thinking about counseling and psychotherapy and provided the first comprehensive alternative to Freudian psychoanalysis and the directiveness of the early behaviorists.

Not only did Carl Rogers establish one of the most comprehensive theories of the self, he also revolutionized treatment by opening the field of psychotherapy to research investigation. He was the first to record and publish complete transcripts of psychotherapy sessions. Through his own experience with clients, and his commitment to scientific research and writing, Rogers delineated the most important strategy for change—the establishment of a collaborative therapeutic alliance. Rogers envisioned his theory as just the beginning of a theoretical orientation on which future theorists would build. His expectations are being fulfilled in the present with theories such as Gendlin's focusing and Greenberg and Johnson's emotion-focused therapy, and in the theoretical underpinnings of transpersonal psychology.

Finally, person-centered therapy, particularly the core conditions of empathy, congruence, and unconditional positive regard first identified by Rogers nearly 70 years ago, are now considered to be necessary to creating and maintaining a sound therapeutic alliance regardless of which therapeutic orientation a clinician chooses. Rogers's work is well known internationally. His writings have been translated into many languages and he is viewed not only as a leader in counseling and psychology, but also as a leader in conflict resolution and as a peacemaker.

Recommended Readings

Arkowiz, H., Westra, H. A., Miller, W. R., & Rollnick, S. (Eds.). (2008). *Motivational interviewing in the treatment of psychological problems*. New York, NY: Guilford Press.

Cain, D. J., & Seeman, J. (Eds.) (2001). *Humanistic psychotherapies: Handbook of research and practice*. Washington, DC: American Psychological Association.

Cooper, M., O'Hara, M., Schmid, P. F., & Wyatt, G. (Eds.). (2007). *The handbook of person-centered psychotherapy and counselling*. New York, NY: Palgrave Macmillan.

Cooper, M., Watson, J. C., & Bolldampt, D. (Eds.). (2010). *Person-centered and experiential therapies work: A review of the research on counseling, psychotherapy, and related practices.* Ross-on-Wye, UK: PCCS Books.

Gendlin, E. T. (1996). *Focusing-oriented psychotherapy: A manual of the experiential method.* New York, NY: Guilford Press.

Greenberg, L. (2010). *Emotion-focused therapy.* Washington, DC: American Psychological Association.

Kirschenbaum, H. (2009). *The life and work of Carl Rogers.* Alexandria, VA: American Counseling Association.

Rogers, C. R. (1951). *Client-centered therapy: Its current practice, implications and theory.* Boston, MA: Houghton Mifflin.

Rogers, C. R. (1961). *On becoming a person.* Boston, MA: Houghton Mifflin.

Rogers, C. R. (1980). *A way of being.* Boston, MA: Houghton Mifflin.

Additional Sources of Information

http://www.adpca.org—The Association for the Development of the Person-Centered Approach holds annual meetings and publishes the *Person-Centered Journal.*

http://www.pce-world.org—Website of the World Association for Person-Centered and Experiential Psychotherapy and Counseling hosts an international conference, provides bibliographies, and links to other person-centered approaches.

http://www.ahpweb.org—This website for the Association for Humanistic Psychology promotes the values reflected in Rogers's work. The association publishes the *Journal of Humanistic Psychology.*

http://www.nrogers.com—This website focuses on Carl Rogers and his daughter Natalie, who provides information on her father's life and vision.

http://www.rootsofempathy.org—Roots of Empathy is an evidence-based classroom program created by Mary Gordon to teach children empathy and social/emotional competence.

http://www.iceeft.com—International Centre for Excellence in Emotionally Focused Therapy, directed by Sue Johnson. Provides articles and publications, certification and training, and workshop opportunities for emotion-focused therapy for couples.

http://www.focusing.org—The website for the Focusing Institute includes information about training, workshops, articles, and publications.

CHAPTER 9

Existential Therapy

To focus on life's purpose, freedom, isolation, meaning, and death; to be free of what has been called "the tyranny of the trivial"; to live a life that balances freedom of choice with responsibility toward our fellow citizens of the world; to work toward a purpose and a goal—what could be more meaningful or important than these pursuits? All of us, therapists and clients alike, grapple with these issues at various points in our lives. Existential psychotherapy, one of the most widely used forms of therapy, provides a philosophical approach with which to address these ultimate concerns.

Events of the early years of the 21st century, including terrorist attacks, wars, and growing financial uncertainty, have contributed to a climate of heightened anxiety, fear of death, and a sharpened sense of loneliness and isolation. Once again, people seem to be turning to religion, spirituality, and psychology to help them cope with tragedies, adjust to change, and attempt to find some meaning in their suffering. Existential therapy is well suited to addressing these concerns.

THE DEVELOPMENT OF EXISTENTIAL THOUGHT

In the 1950s, Rollo May wrote a comprehensive introduction on the beginnings of existential psychology, of which the following provides a brief synopsis and introduction to existential concepts that will be expanded on in this chapter. Interested readers are referred to the second edition of May's book *Existential Psychology* (1969a) for an expanded overview of existential psychology and a bibliography of existentialist concepts.

The roots of existential thought can be traced back to the philosophical writings of Aristotle, Socrates, the ancient Greek and Asian thinkers, and others who addressed issues of personal meaning. The philosophical movement that we now call existential philosophy came in two waves. The first wave took place in late 19th-century Europe with the writings of the Danish philosopher known as the father of existentialism, Søren Kierkegaard, and of Friedrich Nietzsche and Edmund Husserl. The second wave occurred in Europe during the 1940s and 1950s. Social, political, and scientific events during those years contributed to the development of this approach. The deaths of tens of millions of people beginning with World War I and ending with World War II led to a pervasive sense of alienation and meaninglessness. Growing industrialization and urbanization of society, as well as scientific advances, added to this dehumanization. Even psychology, dominated at that time by psychoanalysis and behaviorism, seemed to "conceptualize the person as an assemblage of parts often struggling against one another" (Bauman & Waldo, 1998, p. 15). People needed a force that would restore their sense of humanness and also help them cope with their concerns about the meaning of life in the face of devastation, isolation, and death. Existentialism, which both flows from and contributes to humanistic psychology, evolved in response to those needs.

Kierkegaard (1944), who actually coined the term "existentialism," wrote about anxiety and dread as constant companions to the human condition. He described anxiety as the struggle between the living being and nonbeing—the existential crisis of life against death. Anxiety lies in the middle between the two opposing forces. It is this universal truth that every human being must struggle with that is the focus of existential psychology.

Kierkegaard (1941), and later William James, an American psychologist and philosopher, wrote about freewill. Humans are free to make choices in life. Within the constrictions of what life hands us, we have the ability to rise above it, and to make life meaningful. Existential issues are at the core of human existence, and repeatedly come back to challenge us. Jean-Paul Sartre (1956) wrote, "We are our choices," and May (1960) added, "within the limits of our given world" (p. 13). Freedom then, involves transcendence. Acknowledging this freedom of choice results in anxiety, largely as a result of what we give up when we choose.

German philosopher and mathematician Edmund Husserl (1859–1938) was instrumental in the development of phenomenology. Later, his student Martin Heidegger, in his book *Being and Time* (1962), helped turn attention to the universal experience of man's need to make sense of it all, of what it means to exist. He wrote about *dasein* (being-in-the-world). Later, Sartre, who studied under Husserl and Heidegger, wrote *Being and Nothingness* (1956).

What unites these ideas into a movement is the sense that the prevailing worldview—science, religion, and to a certain extent politics—had dehumanized what it meant to be human. By reducing the lived experience of the person into a series of "universal truths" that applied to everyone, modern thought had negated the uniqueness of the individual, and the fact that every person has freewill. Nietzsche in particular spoke out against Hegel's philosophy of absolute idealism in which human beings were merely fulfilling some grand design set in motion by some unknown entity.

"Existence precedes essence" wrote Sartre (1956). The meaning of this statement, according to Paul Tillich (1952), is that human beings are constantly changing, and no system, whether scientific or otherwise, can adequately explain the ability of human beings to transcend experience. Tillich (1952) wrote, "Man has to shape his world and himself according to the productive powers given to him" (p. 124). If we want to know why this is so, or how life is to be structured, we must first have a doctrine that is holistic and includes body, mind, and spirit.

The European existentialists, Friedrich Nietzsche, Paul Tillich, and Martin Buber, also were key to the development of existential thought. In addition, writers, including Albert Camus, Jean-Paul Sartre, and Franz Kafka, helped to shape European existentialism. Swiss psychiatrists Medard Boss and Ludwig Binswanger created *Daseinsanalysis* (Binswanger, 1963, Boss, 1963), one of the first schools of existential psychology. They drew on Heidegger's notion of being-in-the-world and south Asian spiritual traditions (Cooper, 2008) as a way to help clients understand their own internal experiences through psychotherapy. Around 1929, Viennese psychiatrist Viktor Frankl developed logotherapy, a form of existential psychotherapy that helps people discover purpose in their lives. More will be said about these approaches later in this chapter.

When the ship of existential thought landed on American shores in the middle of the last century, it found a welcome home. Existential psychology is not so much a comprehensive theory of treatment as it is an attitude toward psychology. By accepting that man is much more than drives, instincts, or behaviors that can be measured and predicted, the therapist works from an existential perspective.

Freudian psychodynamic therapy had become the main system of psychotherapy in the United States, and while Freud advanced our knowledge about man in his environment (what existentialists refer to as *umwelt*), Freud's theory was more of a structural foundation, rather than an entire theory of man. Existentialists found Freudian theory similar to industrialization and scientific attempts to explain living phenomenon—it provided some information, but missed the mark. It was missing a soul.

Existentialism, therefore, found a partner in the American humanists, including Carl Rogers and other emotion-focused theorists who valued experience, the organismic valuing process, self-actualization, freedom and responsibility, and the importance of the relationship between client and clinician.

Humanists reject scientific and linear explanations about reality and consider the universe to be constantly changing. This state of flux is considered to be the norm. Rather than an aberration or a problem requiring correction, change is viewed as a natural and innate tendency of all things.

If existence precedes essence, as existentialists believed, then any theory that seeks to explain human behavior must first take a phenomenological perspective. In the words of Rollo May (1969a), "There is no such thing as truth or reality for a living human being, except as he participates in it, is conscious of it, has some relationship to it" (p. 14). Thus, human beings cannot be understood in terms of drives or the behavioral models applied to them. It is more complicated than that. The totality of human existence can only be lived and experienced. As we saw, Freud explained man in relation to nature (*umwelt*); what was missing was man in relation to his fellow man (*mitwelt*), and to himself (*eigenwelt*).

The works of Frankl and May were widely read in the United States during the 1950s and 1960s. Several of May's books, including *Love and Will* (1969b) and *The Courage to Create* (1975), became popular and increased general awareness of existential concepts. Attention to the approach seemed to decline after the 1960s, partially as a result of the growing emphasis on accountability in treatment and the corresponding increase in the use of more structured and empirically validated approaches such as cognitive and behavior therapy. Interest in existential therapy has been kept alive by the writings of Yalom, Bugental, Vontress, and others. With the growing recognition that the therapeutic relationship is an empirically supported intervention in and of itself, and that factors common to most theories are responsible for treatment effectiveness, an increasing number of therapists are returning to the philosophical and holistic underpinnings of existentialism.

Of course, the individual does not exist in a vacuum, and events in the world such as the terrorist attacks of September 11, 2001, the wars in Iraq and Afghanistan, school shootings, and a growing dependency on individual technology that tends to isolate rather than connect people have contributed to the creation of a culture in which people are once again searching for meaning, connection, and some type of guiding principle that explains individual existence in the vastness of the universe.

The past 5 years have seen a resurgence in the popularity of existential counseling as evidenced by the publication of existential counseling and psychology textbooks (Barnett & Madison, 2012; Landridge, 2012; van Deurzen & Adams, 2011), writings that incorporate existential and Eastern spiritual traditions into Western psychology (Hoffman, 2009), and integration of an existential perspective into other theoretical approaches, including art and other expressive therapies (Moon, 2009).

Although relatively few clinicians select existential therapy as their primary theoretical orientation, existentialism continues to exert an influence today, particularly on our conception of the clinician's role and the realization that, for many people, counseling and psychotherapy are not just tools for solving problems but ways to give meaning to lives that seem to lack purpose and fulfillment.

EXISTENTIAL PSYCHOTHERAPY TODAY

Just as existential psychology swept the United States in the 1950s, today Eastern traditions of Taoism, Confucianism, and Buddhism are beginning to influence the practice of existential psychology. Both Eastern and Western traditions concern themselves with the essential elements of the human condition: awareness, impermanence, and the phenomenological experience of aloneness, which have prompted the basic questions that human beings have been asking themselves since the beginning of time.

The future of existential psychology will undoubtedly include existential spirituality, awe-based awakening (Schneider, 2004), and the integration of existentialist thinking into the other theoretical orientations. As this trans-theoretical dialogue continues, psychology will find more ways to incorporate the universal concerns with living—both individually and collectively—into the heart of psychotherapy.

Readers interested in learning more about the ongoing dialogue between Western existential psychology and the Eastern wisdom traditions are referred to the work of Nisbitt (2003) and Hoffman, Yang, Kaklauskas, and Chan (2009).

THE PEOPLE WHO DEVELOPED EXISTENTIAL THERAPY

We have mentioned many names associated with the development of existential psychotherapy. Following are brief biographies of the three men—Viktor Frankl, Rollo May, and Irvin Yalom—who are most strongly associated with existential therapy today. Information on other contributors to this approach also is included.

Viktor Frankl

Viktor Frankl was born in 1905 in Vienna, Austria, and received both MD and PhD degrees from the University of Vienna. Before the Second World War, he was a practicing physician. Between 1942 and 1945, however, he was a prisoner in the Nazi concentration camps in Dachau and Auschwitz. His mother and father, his brother, and his first wife and their children all perished in the camps. Of course, these experiences had a profound impact on Frankl's thinking. Although his interest in existential thought began before his imprisonment, his difficult years in the concentration camps led him to conclude that the will to create meaning and purpose is the prime human motivator (Klingberg, 2001). For Frankl, his purpose became surviving his imprisonment so that he could tell others about those experiences and the terrible impact of war and hatred. *Man's Search for Meaning* (Frankl, 1963) is a powerful description of his experiences, his existential struggles, and what he learned from them. In that book, which the Library of Congress has listed as one of the 10 most influential books, Frankl quotes Nietzsche: "He who has a why to live for can bear with almost any how" (p. 121) and "That which does not kill me, makes me stronger" (p. 130). These quotations reflect Frankl's own triumph over tragedy, his ability to make meaningful the terrible losses and experiences he endured.

Frankl calls his treatment approach *logotherapy*—therapy through meaning. Frankl (2000) was convinced that "in the final analysis there is no situation that does not contain within it the seed of meaning . . . this conviction is the basis of logotherapy" (p. 53). Frankl believed that, even under extreme circumstances, people have choices and "ways to find meaning in life—even up to the last moment, the last breath" (p. 64). The tasks of the clinician are to help people:

- Discover and notice where they possess freedom and the potential for meaning
- Actualize those potentials to transform and make meaning of their lives
- Honor meanings realized in the past (Lantz, 2000).

For Frankl, as for most existentialist clinicians, the central ingredient in treatment is the use of the treatment relationship to accomplish these goals.

Frankl's writings as well as his lectures throughout the world certainly made his life a meaningful one. In addition, he married again in the late 1940s and reportedly found personal as well as professional success. Frankl lived until 1997, continuing to write throughout his life about the most important aspects of all our lives, including meaning, love, work, and society (Frankl, 1978, 1987, 1992, 2000).

Rollo May

Rollo May has been credited with bringing existentialism to the United States with the publication of *Existence: A New Dimension in Psychiatry and Psychology* (May, Angel, & Ellenberger, 1958). His writings were instrumental in elucidating the similarities between existential philosophy and psychology. Both were concerned with the same issues and could be used together to promote better understanding.

Rollo May was born in 1909 into a family of six children and spent his childhood in Ohio and Michigan, where he graduated from Michigan State University. He originally trained as a Lutheran minister and later became a psychoanalyst. He studied with Alfred Adler in Vienna and was influenced by Adler and European existential thought. In addition, May's own difficult life, including an unhappy childhood, two unsuccessful marriages, and two years in a sanitarium with tuberculosis, contributed to the development of his ideas.

His work initially focused on the anxiety he believed all people experience as we struggle with the difficulties of growth and change, our aloneness in the world, our apprehensions about death, and the courage required to pursue goals of independence and growth (May, 1950). Also important to him were people's roles in and relationships with their society, reflecting Adler's emphasis on social responsibility. May believed that often people avoid difficult conflicts and confrontations, such as those with culture and destiny (including death), leading us to neglect the potentials for meaning in our lives. Many of May's landmark writings and studies addressed fundamental human experiences such as love, will, intentionality, isolation, loneliness, evil, and the daimonic. He defined healthy will as "action following vision" and noted that apathy (or unhealthy will) often precedes mental distress. He wrote "I, for one, believe this is the chronic, endemic, psychic state of our society in our day" (May, 1969b, p. 218). May's work has influenced many, including Diamond's work on what he refers to as "pervasive postmodern syndrome" (2007, 2009). As May (1990a) stated, "I do not believe there is a special school of therapy to be put in a category of 'existential.' I think existential, rather, refers to an attitude toward human beings and a set of presuppositions about these human beings" (p. 49).

Like Frankl, Rollo May lived a long and productive life, dying in 1994 at the age of 85. In his obituary for Rollo May, Bugental (1996) said of May's contribution, ". . . so much of what he contributed has entered into our general discourse about such conceptual areas as human nature, the major life issues and dimensions that we confront as individuals and as scientists and professionals. . . ." (p. 418).

Irvin Yalom

Born in 1931 in Washington, DC, Irvin Yalom grew up in a small apartment over his parents' grocery store. His escape from the poverty and danger of his inner-city neighborhood was the library, where he developed an enduring love of reading. Yalom was trained as a psychiatrist and completed his residency at Johns Hopkins University. After some years in the army, he became a professor of psychiatry at Stanford University School of Medicine. Yalom and his wife Marilyn, a scholar of women's studies and French literature, have four children and many grandchildren.

Yalom is a prolific writer on both existentialism and group psychotherapy (Yalom & Leszcz, 2005). His ideas have been influenced by both European and American existential thought. His 1980 book *Existential Psychotherapy* contributed greatly to understanding of this approach, particularly in the United States. "There is a basic aloneness to existence that must be faced," he wrote. "In existential therapy the goal is to help clients be authentic and face their limitations and challenges with courage" (Yalom & Leszcz, 2005, p. 102). Yalom's existential clinical approach can be found in his book *The Gift of Therapy* (2009), among others. Yalom also has written books for the general reader, describing his therapy with people coping with existential issues. In *Love's Executioner and Other Tales of Psychotherapy* (1989), Yalom stated, "I have found that four givens are particularly relevant to psychotherapy: the inevitability of death for each of us and for those we love; the freedom to make our lives as we will; our ultimate aloneness; and, finally, the absence of any obvious meaning or sense to life. However grim these givens may seem, they contain the seeds of wisdom and redemption" (pp. 4–5).

In clarifying the nature of existentialism, Yalom (1980) identified the basic difference between Freudian psychoanalysis and Yalom's concept of existentialism. Freud viewed people as struggling with a conflict between the instinctual strivings of the id and the socialized forces of the ego and superego, whereas Yalom saw our conflicts as stemming "from the dilemma of a meaning-seeking creature who is thrown into a universe that has no meaning" (p. 9). "It's not easy to live every moment wholly aware of death. It's like trying to stare the sun in the face: you can stand only so much of it. Because we cannot live frozen in fear, we generate methods to soften death's terror. We project ourselves into the future through our children; we grow rich, famous, ever larger; we develop compulsive protective rituals; or we embrace an impregnable belief in an ultimate rescuer" (Yalom, 2008, p. 5). Yalom and other existential therapists believe that confronting the fear of death will allow us to live life in a richer, fuller, more compassionate, and meaningful way. Irvin Yalom continues to lecture and write about his ideas as well as his practice of psychotherapy.

Two Other American Existential Therapists: Bugental and Vontress

Because of their groundbreaking and prolific writing, Rollo May and Irvin Yalom have become the best known American existential therapists. However, James Bugental and Clemmont Vontress are two other important existential therapists in the United States.

Since the 1970s, Bugental sought to clarify the implementation of existential therapy (Miars, 2002). He provided information on the therapeutic alliance, the values inherent in existential therapy, and the skills and stance reflective of existentially oriented clinicians. Important in Bugental's theory is the self-in-world construct system, defined as "the conception each of us holds about who and what we are and how our world operates" (Miars, 2002, p. 219). Bugental likened this construct to a spacesuit that helps people navigate through their lives. Existential therapy can help people examine their self-in-world constructs and configure them in more life-enabling ways.

Clemmont Vontress is an African American man who is a leading advocate of the existential approach to counseling and a pioneer in the cross-cultural counseling movement. He was born more than 80 years ago in a racially segregated south. His father was a sharecropper, and his great grandfather was killed by the Ku Klux Klan. The young Vontress left home to attend college, and after a stint in the military and some time spent working as a schoolteacher, finished his master's degree and received a PhD degree in counseling from the University of Indiana. He is professor emeritus at George Washington University, co-author of *Cross-Cultural Counseling: A Casebook* (1999), and the subject of a biography by Moodley and Walcott (2010). He has written more than 100 articles, chapters, and monographs on existential counseling, historical hostility, cultural difference, issues related to men and masculinity, particularly black men in the United States, and traditional healing (Vontress, 1996, Vontress & Epp, 1997). According to Moodley and Walcott, Vontress is "one of the most significant figures in the culture and counseling movement" (p. 4), which he helped to create in the 1960s.

Throughout his 40 years of putting culture into counseling, Vontress has been influential in the United States, Canada, the United Kingdom, Africa, and the Caribbean. He was the first recipient of the Lifetime Achievement Award for Cross-Cultural and Diversity Counseling and Psychotherapy presented by the Ontario Institute for Studies in Education at the University of Toronto. His work has been important in promoting awareness of the dynamics of existentialism and cross-cultural counseling. Moodley and Walcott (2010) document the history of the movement and its evolution toward the current model of diversity counseling in which the "racial, cultural, and ethnic identification of the client is contextualized within the particular socio-political experiences" (p. 8). This will be addressed further later in this chapter.

IMPORTANT THEORETICAL CONCEPTS

The theory underlying existential therapy focuses not on the treatment process but on exploring the universal issues that people face and ways for people to address them that are life enhancing and actualizing. Through their understanding of these issues, clinicians can connect with people on a deep and personal level and help them change their lives so that they have more meaning and fulfillment.

Ultimate Concerns of the Human Condition

For the existentialists, life has no inherent meaning and is replete with challenges. Unless people meet these challenges with awareness, openness, and courage, their emotional development can become blocked or delayed. Existentialist theory suggests that the following four ultimate concerns of the human condition are typically at the root of emotional difficulties:

- ***Inevitability of death.*** From childhood, we realize that our death is inevitable, as are the deaths of our loved ones. No matter how gifted we are, no matter how special our lives are, death is the outcome for everyone. The fear of our ultimate nonbeing can cast a pall over people's lives and make them seem pointless.
- ***Isolation.*** Although we may surround ourselves with colleagues, friends, and family, we are ultimately alone. No one can truly understand us or sense our thoughts and feelings as we do. No one can rescue us from the inevitability of death and other losses we will experience in our lives. Some people seek to fuse with and become dependent on others in an effort to counteract their sense of alienation and loneliness, but those efforts inevitably fail because they detract even further from people's sense of themselves and the purpose of their lives. In fact, loneliness can be most acute when we are with others and are aware of our lack of a true connection with them.
- ***Meaninglessness.*** Life seems inherently meaningless. The only certainties in our lives are birth and death. Beyond that, life seems to be a random process. The lack of meaning in life can lead to hopelessness, discouragement, and a sense of emptiness. All human beings at one point or another ask themselves, "What *is* the meaning of life?" Viktor Frankl (2000) believed "it is not we who should ask for the meaning of life, since it is we who are being asked. It is we ourselves who must answer the questions that life asks of us, and to these questions we can respond only by being responsible for our existence" (p. 56). Early on, Frankl determined there were:

> . . . three groups of values, or possible ways to find meaning in life—even up to the last moment, the last breath. These three possibilities are: (1) a deed we do, a work we create; (2) an experience, a human encounter, a love; and (3) when confronted with an unchangeable fate (such as an incurable disease), a change of attitude toward that fate. In such cases we still can wrest meaning from life by giving testimony to the most human of all human capacities: the ability to turn suffering into a human triumph. (Frankl, 2000, p. 64)

Just as Viktor Frankl found meaning in his efforts to survive the concentration camp so that he could share his ideas with the world, each person is unique and must discover his or her own meaning.

- ***Freedom and responsibility.*** Modern society presents people with an overwhelming and constantly increasing array of choices: choices of lifestyles, choices of experiences, choices of acquisitions, and others. We have both the freedom and the responsibility to make choices that create a worthwhile existence for ourselves in the limited time we have on earth. That is a daunting prospect for most of us!

Existential and Neurotic Anxiety

Everyone experiences the four ultimate concerns of the human condition and, according to existentialist theory, that creates feelings of anxiety in everyone. However, the theory distinguishes between existential (normal) anxiety and neurotic anxiety. Existential anxiety is viewed as an inevitable part of the human condition. It is deeper than anxiety about one's career or health. Rather, it is "a deep feeling of unease that arises from our awareness of the givens: our existence is finite, we are mortal, and there is no purpose but the ones we create for ourselves" (Bauman & Waldo, 1998, p. 19). Existential anxiety is a positive sign rather than a pathological state; it indicates that people recognize the need to accept responsibility for their lives and are engaged in efforts to create a worthwhile and meaningful existence. Such people are living *authentic* lives in which they are aware of their self-in-world construct, strive to make wise choices, and take responsibility for their decisions.

Existential guilt and neurotic anxiety result when we lack awareness of our physical world, our relationships, and our psychological world; fail to take responsibility for making our lives meaningful and worthwhile; and realize that we have not become what we might have. It reflects our awareness that we have not fully realized ourselves as human beings and have allowed our lives to be controlled by chance and circumstance. We may not understand or be able to articulate the reasons for our feelings of guilt but, for many, an underlying sense of deep guilt and regret pervades our lives.

Depression often is the result of efforts to defend against existential guilt and anxiety and avoid the task of making our lives meaningful. Yalom (1980) found, for example, that among people nearing death, depression was greatest in those who had not created meaningful lives, whereas those who felt satisfied with the lives they had created for themselves were more able to accept death.

Human Development and the Development of Emotional Difficulties

Existential therapists do not dispute the importance of early development and the child–parent relationship. However, they link those to existential concerns. Frankl, for example, believed that so-called neurotic difficulties often stem from an upbringing in which parents were punitive and deprived children of freedom (Barton, 1992).

Similarly, existential therapists think of the unconscious in ways that reflect the tenets of existentialism. They concentrate on the unconscious conflict between people's wish to escape the givens of the human condition and lose themselves in lethargy and denial and their wish to achieve fulfillment despite the challenges and responsibilities that achievement entails. For the existentialists, emotional difficulties stem from failure to deal successfully with the inevitabilities of the human condition and to transcend them by creating a meaningful and authentic life for oneself.

Existential therapists pay attention to development throughout the life span and do not limit their focus to early childhood. They view life as a process of creating our own histories, with each choice and phase shaping and contributing to the next. Existence is never static; people are always becoming something new, striving to move toward their possibilities, and making their lives worthwhile.

Dasein

Existentialists speak of *dasein*—translated from the German as being present, being-in-the-world. According to Bauman and Waldo (1998), "The term dasein acknowledges that human beings exist, have consciousness, and are responsible for their own existence" (p. 16).

Unlike other living things, human beings have consciousness. They are aware of their existence and participation in the world around them, and they are aware of this awareness! Binswanger (1963) defined ways of being that describe the phenomenological experience:

> ***Umwelt***—the natural world around us. On a broad scale, this refers to the earth, biology, and the laws of nature. On a more personal level, *umwelt* can be our personal space, living arrangements, or work environment. We interact with and are affected by our physical surroundings.
>
> ***Mitwelt***—refers to being-in-the-world with other people, to relationships, interactions, and concepts we introject about society, race, gender, and religion. *Mitwelt* is subjective, based on personal experience.
>
> ***Eigenwelt***—is our own subjective world. It is our world of thoughts, feelings, and desires; the interrelationship of mind, body, and spirit. It is our beliefs about ourselves—awareness, identity, personal meaning, and our perceptions of ourselves. Binswanger explains *eigenwelt* as our perceptions of ourselves along such dimensions as interests, values, intelligence, motivation, and character. These self-perceptions impact how we live in the world and interact with other people.
>
> ***Uberwelt***—the fourth dimension of being-in-the-world was not developed by Binswanger, but added later by van Deurzen. *Uberwelt* refers to the spiritual or metaphysical dimension. *Uberwelt* is "the domain of experience where people create meaning for themselves and make sense" of the world (van Deurzen, 2002, p. 86).

These four ways of being-in-the-world are subjective, personal, and necessary to a complete understanding of the self and its experiences and perceptions of the world.

It is an interactive process. We are always of the world, but at the same time creating our world. We interact in the world, and the world impacts on us. Things are always in a state of flux. Unlike other living things, we are also aware of the temporary nature of our lives. We are able to contemplate our not being-in-the-world (van Deurzen, 2010).

According to May and colleagues (1958), "Man (or Dasein) is the particular being who has to be aware of himself, be responsible for himself, if he is to become himself. He also is that particular being who knows that at some future moment he will not be: he is the being who is always in dialectical relation with non-being death" (p. 42).

The concept of *dasein* is complex and elusive, but reflects people's ability to simultaneously live in the present, be conscious, and take responsibility for making their lives meaningful, while realizing fully that death will inevitably end their efforts. It reflects a dynamic process of potential and becoming rather than a fixed state.

Concept of Mental Health

Vontress defined mental health as "being in balance and harmony with one's inner-self; with one's friends, family and colleagues; with one's physical environment; and with one's spirituality" (Epp, 1998, p. 9). In other words, mental health exists when all four aspects of *dasein* (*umwelt, mitwelt, eigenwelt*, and *uberwelt*) are in harmony. Existential therapists emphasize the importance of experiencing the unity of self and world. People who are not simply passive victims of circumstances but become the architects of their own lives provide good examples of emotional health. Rollo May (1996) quotes existential philosopher Paul Tillich as having said, "Man becomes truly human only at the moment of decision" (p. 145). Whatever difficulties we encounter in our lives, we always have choices. According to May (1990b), "No matter how great the forces victimizing the human being, man has the capacity to know that he is being victimized and thus to influence in some way how he will relate to his fate" (p. 270).

Potentials of the Human Condition

The inevitable concerns of the human condition, discussed previously, seem to present a bleak picture of life. However, existential therapy is an optimistic and hopeful approach that seeks to integrate the somatic (physical), psychic (psychological), and noetic (spiritual) dimensions of man (Xu, 2010). Existential therapy believes that the human spirit has a healthy core. and what has been called "existential courage" (Moodley, 2010, p. 6). It takes courage to live and to transcend psychological and environmental constraints. Existential therapy recognizes people's many strengths including those discussed next.

AWARENESS People have the capacity for awareness of both themselves and the world. The greater our awareness, the more possibilities that are open to us and the more successfully we can address our fears and anxieties. Although awareness will not always bring us pleasure or peace, it allows us to recognize the limitations and challenges of our lives and make wise choices that can make our lives worthwhile.

Years ago, people often were not told when they had a terminal illness because of the belief that they were better off not knowing about their condition. However, that decision deprived them of the capacity to make meaningful choices about how they would live out their lives and encouraged inauthenticity and deceptive relationships. Now people are almost always told the truth about their medical conditions so they can make choices such as whether to take medication that may hasten their deaths but relieve their pain.

AUTHENTICITY Authenticity has been described as "living the kind of life that is freely chosen and not dictated by the values of others. In such a life, one's own feelings, values, and interpretations act as a guide for conduct" (Hergenhahn, 2009, p. 603). In *The Search for Authenticity* (1965), Bugental described three essential features of authenticity:

1. People are aware of themselves and their relationships with the world.
2. They make choices, knowing that decisions are the inevitable consequences of responsibility.
3. They take responsibility for their choices, recognizing that awareness is imperfect, and sometimes leads to unanticipated results.

Taking responsibility for making choices based on awareness reflects authenticity and allows people to live more fully in the present and be themselves in their relationships. People whose decisions are based on denial, the wishes of others, or dependence are not truly living in the present; they may be driven by past losses or acting out of a hope for future gains. In addition, they are wearing a "mask of inauthenticity" (Frank, 2007, p. 181) that prevents others from really knowing who they are. Boss (1963) explained that emotions and guilt often influence choice and our way of being with others in the world. Each choice we make involves loss of many other alternatives. This ultimately shapes our lives and who we are in the process of becoming.

FREEDOM AND RESPONSIBILITY Freedom can be viewed as consisting of four aspects: awareness, choice, action, and change. Once people accept that they have freedom, no matter what their circumstances are, they have the responsibility:

- To be aware of their past history, their current options, and their future potential
- To make choices that give meaning to their lives
- To exercise courage and thought in taking action toward life-enhancing change.

Once we see that we have choice, we can no longer view our decisions and behaviors as purposeless and accidental, make excuses for ourselves, and shift blame for our unhappiness to others. We must assume responsibility and recognize that ultimately we alone are in charge of our lives. The enormity of that realization can be frightening but also can be empowering, if only we can use our freedom in positive and growthful ways. The choices available to us may not be limitless, but we must recognize that even declining to make a decision, is, in effect, making a decision.

ACTUALIZATION Actualization is an important concept for existential therapists, as it is for person-centered clinicians. Abraham Maslow (1954, 1968) probably best described the nature of actualization. He advanced the idea that each person has an essential nature, part of which is universal and part of which is unique to that individual. Maslow (1954) believed "that full healthy and normal and desirable development consists in actualizing this nature, in fulfilling these potentialities, and in developing into maturity along the lines that this . . . essential nature dictates, growing from within rather than being shaped from without" (p. 340). The will toward actualization is an innate and natural process that leads people toward realization of their potential and toward growth and fulfillment.

Actualization can be blocked by many factors, including a cultural or family background that inhibits creativity, a repressive environment, and overwhelming fear and guilt. People who fail to move toward actualization typically experience confusion, agony, shame, defeat, anxiety, and a perception of life as meaningless (Vontress, 2008a; Yalom, 1980).

MAKING MEANING Existential therapists believe that life has the potential to be meaningful if people use their capacities to bring purpose and worth into their lives. According to May (1969b), our will to love and to live gives us meaning. Our awareness, our recognition that we have freedom, our authenticity, and our will toward actualization all enable us to know and confront disturbing aspects of ourselves and our world, such as the inevitability of death and our ultimate aloneness, and to transcend them by creating meaning in our lives.

Meaning is the purpose and logic of our lives and often is reflected in choices people make. Dreams, visions, and fantasies also provide clues to meaning. Some people have social goals, such as Carl Rogers's efforts to increase world peace; others have competitive goals, such as breaking a world record, or creative goals, such as writing a novel. But most people find meaning in daily activities such as raising healthy children, planting gardens, helping others, and establishing a rewarding business.

Because life itself is a process, we are in a constant state of emerging and evolving, becoming more fully ourselves, and making meaning of each day as well as of the entirety of our lives. According to the existentialists, it is this journey that makes us human.

TREATMENT USING EXISTENTIAL THERAPY

Existential therapy is a process in which two people, client and clinician, embark on a journey to help the client cope more effectively with the inevitable conditions of life and make better use of the potentials of humankind. This approach makes minimal use of techniques but relies heavily on the clinician to effect change.

Goals

The fundamental goal of existential therapy is to help people find value, meaning, and purpose in their lives. Treatment does not specifically seek to ameliorate symptoms. In other words, "The purpose of psychotherapy is not to 'cure' the clients in the conventional sense, but to help them become aware of what they are doing and to get them out of the victim role" (May, 1981, p. 210).

To reach this goal, existential therapists help people confront their deepest fears and anxieties about the inevitable challenges of life including death, isolation, and meaninglessness. Reviewing and reflecting on clients' histories can facilitate this process, especially if it helps them identify barriers that impede their movement toward an authentic and personally meaningful life. In addition, treatment helps people become aware of the freedom they do have, recognize their options, and make choices that help them become more actualized and able to lead a life that reflects their values and priorities.

Therapeutic Alliance: An I–Thou Relationship

Martin Buber (1970) believed that relationships can reflect several possible levels:

1. I-to-I relationships, in which other people are almost irrelevant ("I am all that matters")
2. I-to-it relationships, in which people are viewed as objects in transient interactions
3. It-to-it relationships, in which people have little sense of self
4. We-to-we relationships, involving a lack of individuality and primarily characterizing children's relationships
5. Us-to-them relationships, in which others are viewed as either chosen or rejected, special or lacking, in or out of favor; us (those in good favor) are all that matters
6. I-to-you relationships, involving two people who view each other as separate individuals
7. I-to-thou relationships, in which people have the deepest respect for each other as well as a great sense of relatedness.

I-to-thou relationships are the most profound and meaningful kind. Therapists who can create this type of relationship with their clients are truly sharing a journey with them and empowering their clients through the strong and honoring connection between client and therapist (Bugental, 1978). Therefore, existential therapists expand on Rogers's concepts of empathy and positive regard and focus even more on the therapeutic relationship as an expression of intimacy, openness, and real human exchange.

As the primary vehicle for facilitating change, clinicians who practice existential therapy have considerable responsibility. Their own values are very much a part of the treatment process and clinician self-disclosure is important. Therapists advocate freedom and authenticity (Hergenhahn & Olson, 2007), encourage people to confront their fears, and promote their efforts to make meaningful choices. In keeping with their emphasis on personal freedom, existential clinicians do not hold back their views. They express their values and beliefs, give advice, use humor, and make suggestions and interpretations but always allow clients the freedom to determine how they will use this input. As Bugental (1987) put it, "The therapeutic alliance is the powerful joining of forces which energizes and supports the long, difficult, and frequently painful work of life-changing psychotherapy" (p. 49).

Existential therapists are companions and coexplorers with their clients. Available and empathic, these clinicians experience clients' pain without losing their sense of themselves. To understand their clients' deepest thoughts and feelings about issues such as death, isolation, and guilt, existential therapists need to be with their clients as fully as possible and to listen with both eyes and ears. According to Yalom (1980), clinicians should "implicitly and explicitly, wonder about the patient's belief systems, inquire deeply into the loving of another, ask about long-range hopes and goals, and explore creative interests and pursuits" (p. 471). They communicate respect, support, encouragement, and concern and are genuine, open, and caring. They have no expectations for outcome, no mandates for client behavior, but simply join people in their quest to use their freedom to craft a meaningful and rewarding life. Their focus is on process, rather than on content.

Maintaining relationships of this magnitude and intensity can be very demanding of clinicians. Being an existential counselor requires openness to perpetual learning and the ability to maintain an intense level of involvement with a client through some of their most difficult experiences. Therapists who have not come to terms with their own fears about death and dying may be more likely to avoid or "selectively inattend" to such material presented by their clients (Yalom, 1998, p. 202). Retaining authenticity as a counselor can also be challenging. Existential counselors remain true to their own beliefs while also recognizing and appreciating individual differences. Richert (2010) reminds us that the therapeutic relationship that develops between the client and therapist is always, by necessity, co-constructed. That is, the bond that is created between the therapist and client is reflective of the depth to which each person is willing to go to understand and to be understood.

The Process of Treatment

Because existential therapy is not problem or crisis focused and involves the establishment of a deep relationship between client and clinician, it is almost never time limited or rushed. Typically, treatment has no clear stages or transitions.

However, the process generally begins by developing clinicians' understanding of their clients and clients' awareness of themselves and their world. Clients are encouraged to describe their values, beliefs, and assumptions; their histories and backgrounds; and the choices they have made, as well as the choices they believe they cannot make. Clinicians listen closely so they can comprehend the clients' views of the world and gradually help them express their deepest fears and take greater responsibility for their lives.

The middle phase of treatment enables people to use the information they have shared to find purpose, meaning, and value. Therapist interventions encourage client authenticity during this process.

Treatment moves toward a close when people can implement their awareness of themselves and move forward to establish more meaningful lives. They have learned that they cannot eliminate anxiety completely but have found ways to live full lives despite anxiety about the inevitabilities of the human condition. In addition, they are progressing along a path that seems natural and right for them and is helping them become actualized.

An important and challenging aspect of concluding treatment is the client's separation from the clinician. This can be a reminder of the inescapable endings in life and is often difficult for both client and clinician. However, if both can be present in the moment, authentic, and aware of their reactions to the end of treatment, that process itself can foster growth, helping people face and cope effectively with their fears.

Specific Intervention Strategies

The primary interventions in existential therapy—use of the person of the clinician and the client–clinician relationship—have already been discussed. Existential therapists do not use techniques, but they do focus on important aspects related to being-in-the-world. The approach also uses some other interventions.

SYMBOLIC GROWTH EXPERIENCE Both Frankl (1963) and Maslow (1968) described the learning and growth that came from intense experiences. Maslow referred to these as peak experiences but some of them might also be viewed as cathartic experiences. Willard Frick, building on the ideas of Frankl and Maslow, described a model, the Symbolic Growth Experience (SGE), to explain the relationship between experience and the discovery of meaning. Frick (1987) defined the SGE as "the conscious recognition and interpretation of the symbolic dimensions of an immediate experience leading to heightened awareness, discovery of meaning, and personal worth" (p. 36). The exploration of an SGE has four steps:

1. People are educated about the concept of the SGE.
2. They select a salient past experience and explore its importance and symbolism in their lives.
3. They are helped to understand the meaning embedded in the experience.
4. They have a clearer sense of that meaning and are able to repeat their use of these strategies to grasp the significance of other experiences.

SGE is explored in more detail in the case illustration later in this chapter.

FRANKL'S LOGOTHERAPY AND PARADOXICAL INTENTION Viktor Frankl (1978) termed his version of existential therapy *logotherapy*—"therapy through meaning" (p. 19). He believed that even well-functioning people sometimes perceive life as meaningless and experience a sense of emptiness. He referred to this as "the unheard cry for meaning" (p. 20). Through treatment, he helped people recognize the depth of their need for meaning, reassured them that all people can create meaning in their lives, and supported them in their efforts to find purpose and meaning.

Frankl described a cycle in which fears evoke symptoms that in turn increase the fears. For example, a person who fears heights avoids them; because of the avoidance, anticipatory anxiety develops, the heights become increasingly frightening in the person's mind, and the avoidance as well as the fears increase. As Frankl (1978) put it, "The fear of fear increases fear" (p. 116).

To break this pattern, he recommended a technique called *paradoxical intention* in which clinicians encourage clients to do or wish for the very thing they fear most. For example, a woman was afraid to leave her house lest she faint. Frankl instructed her to go outside and try her best to faint. Not surprisingly, she was unable to faint. His intervention succeeded in both reducing her fear and strengthening her courage by changing the meaning of her fear. She could now accept her fear, as well as the slight possibility that she might faint. As Yalom (1980) stated, "When we take ourselves out of the lie and become distant spectators, things cease to matter" (p. 478).

Yalom (1980) believed that this principle extended to people's search for meaning: "I believe that the search for meaning is similarly paradoxical: the more we rationally seek it, the less we find it; the questions that one can pose about meaning will always outlast the answers" (p. 482). Finding meaning is a lifelong process of facing our fears, developing awareness, and making choices. Paradoxical intention is one technique that has been found to be effective, based on several meta-analytical reviews. In one meta-analytic review of 19 outcome studies, logotherapy was found to be effective (Fabry, 2010). A separate meta-analytic review of 15 studies on logotherapy found that paradoxical interventions are more effective than nonparadoxical interventions (Hill, 1987).

DEREFLECTION Dereflection is a type of paradoxical intervention that is based on "two essential qualities of human existence, namely man's capacities of self-transcendence and self-detachment" (Frankl, 1969, p. 99). Unlike hyperreflection, in which a person becomes self-absorbed in their thoughts, dereflection takes the focus away from the person and helps them concentrate less on themselves and more on other people or goals they find meaningful. Dereflection is intended to reduce compulsive self-observation and redirect clients' attention in a more positive manner, helping them discover meaning in situations in the present moment, rather than becoming trapped in obsessive worry (Graber, 2003).

Dereflection was originally formulated to treat couples with sexual dysfunction. By focusing away from one's own performance anxiety and instead pleasuring one's partner, the end result is less anxiety and less attention being paid to oneself (Schulenberg, Schnetzer, Winters, & Hutzell, 2010).

Dereflection can also be useful in group therapy. Rather than focusing on problems, the group's attention is turned to the present moment. Group members are not allowed to complain about fate, feeling victimized, or other negative emotions, but rather must focus on what are worthwhile, attainable goals. Dereflection is a positive, meaningful, and useful tool.

ADDRESSING THE FOUR DIMENSIONS OF THE HUMAN CONDITION Earlier in this chapter the four dimensions of the human condition that typically underlie emotional difficulties were presented: death, isolation, meaninglessness, and freedom. Theorists have suggested responses to concerns about these four conditions, such as the following (Bauman & Waldo, 1998):

- Faith in our own existence in the present can ameliorate fears of death.
- Love is the authentic response to isolation.
- Drawing on our inner creativity, to find ways to realize our potential, can counteract the inherent meaninglessness of life.
- Responsibility and commitment, making choices and staying with them, help us cope with our overabundance of freedom.

Addressing the four dimensions of the human condition can be effective in working cross-culturally. In an interview with Roy Moodley (2010), Vontress said, "Counselors must concern themselves with the human condition in general before addressing the specifics of the client's culture because people are more alike than they are dissimilar" (p. 12). Therapists who are attuned to universal issues of love, meaning, fear of death, and freedom are more likely to be successful.

APPLICATION AND CURRENT USE OF EXISTENTIAL THERAPY

Existential therapy is a useful approach for many types of problems and people. The following describes its application, as reflected in theory and research.

Application to Diagnostic Groups

Because of its lack of specific interventions, its focus on philosophical issues rather than on concrete problems, and its emphasis on the client–clinician relationship and thoughtful and open dialogue, existential therapy seems most appropriate for people with long-standing, pervasive anxiety (generalized anxiety disorder) or depression (dysthymic disorder) and those who are coping with life and death matters such as grief and loss, diagnosis of a terminal illness, or transitioning between phases of life (entering adulthood, parenting, retirement). People with other anxiety disorders such as post-traumatic stress disorder, agoraphobia, and panic disorder also may respond well to the existential clinician's efforts to help them explore and understand the meaning of their fears so that they can develop an acceptance of what is happening in their lives. Looking at how they have made choices and the meaning of their lives so far might enable people to live their lives more deliberately, create more meaning for themselves, and be more authentic and connected in their relationships.

Application to Multicultural Groups

Existential therapy is based on a universal worldview and is by its very nature adaptive to culturally diverse groups (Vontress, 2008a). Existential therapy is suitable for people from all cultural backgrounds. Vontress, whose work has been described as connecting "the existentialism of Europe and the spirituality of Africa" (Moodley, 2010, p. 10), reminds us that philosophers from Asia and other non-Western areas have addressed issues of the meaning of life for many more years than have Western philosophers. For more than 40 years, Vontress has been integrating existential therapy with cross-cultural counseling. Moodley and Walcott (2010) credit Vontress for his culture-centered focus. He has been "instrumental in bringing to consciousness the critical value of infusing culture, race, and ethnicity into counseling theory and practice" (p. 8).

Bojuwoye and Sodi (2010) highlight that not all Western psychological models have been found effective when applied to the needs of non-Westerners because of the heavy reliance on natural science, while ignoring the role of social conditions, power relations, and societal institutional arrangements in shaping a person's conceptualization of illness and associated help-seeking behaviors. Western traditional healing models tend to segment people into physical, psychological, social, and spiritual parts in order to treat each separately. Alternatively, non-Western healing models are holistic and treat the "whole" person, employing interventions targeted at all symptoms and causes of ill health in order to ensure well-being, harmony, or ideal human functioning.

Opportunities to integrate traditional healing into psychotherapy are challenging, however, because they are comprehensive and concerned with illness prevention as well as cure. Medication and nonmedication therapies, such as acupuncture, thermal therapy, yoga, and other mind–body therapies, can become part of an integrated psychological practice, where counselors and traditional healers work together.

For example, in some African cultures talk therapy is frowned upon because it is considered a taboo to talk about family problems to strangers. Similarly, in some South East Asian countries, people do not talk about personal feelings and needs with those outside of the family because of mistrust of strangers (Bojuwoye & Sodi, 2010). In East Asian cultures, individuals often seek out family members, shamans, or religious leaders for advice, not therapists (Chae & Foley, 2010). A holistic existential perspective that addresses mind, body, spirit, and cultural considerations seems to provide a broader focus for the helping professions.

Application to Other Groups

Studies have looked at the impact of existential therapy on specific client groups, for example, family survivors of homicide (Miller, 2009), those in palliative care facing end-of-life issues (Burnett, 2009), and in the treatment of anorexia (Fox & Leung, 2009). Although the scope and sample size of these studies are insufficient to firmly establish the approach's effectiveness, research does suggest a broad application for existential therapy (Burnett, 2009), especially when considered in the context of the common factors discussed in Chapter 1 that are effective across all theoretical boundaries.

Logotherapy addresses the spiritual core at the center of every human being. It provides a strengths-based approach to help those who are aging to gain a sense of meaning and self-acceptance at the end of life. Coming to terms with death, and integrating this knowledge into life, can help people to transcend suffering and fear. Xu (2010) writes "the hidden story of successful aging is about positive attitudes towards life and death, about the spiritual and existential quest, and about personal growth in wisdom and spirituality" (p. 184). Logotherapy can help people to find that sense of meaning and has been associated with positive outcomes including better physical and mental well-being; improved self-esteem, self-acceptance, and happiness; and improved health in elderly adults (Krause, 2004; Melton & Schulenberg, 2008).

An existential approach has been found helpful with individuals, couples, and groups. Lantz and Gregoire (2000) presented two studies on couples therapy that reflect the beneficial impact of an existential approach. They wrote, "The therapist pays close attention to the importance of the treatment encounter, to freedom and responsibility, to opportunities for growth to be found in tragedy and crisis, and to the central human desire to notice, actualize, and honor the meanings and meaning potentials in marital and family life" (p. 317).

Existential issues are common to many therapy groups addressing both psychological and somatic illness. Topics such as alcohol abuse, midlife adjustment, and serious mental illness regularly touch on issues of an existential nature. For example, women with breast cancer who participated in existential group therapy were able to share their concerns about their cancer treatment and discuss their fears about death and dying. At the end of 10 sessions, the women reported being more optimistic and positive (Breitbart & Heller, 2003; Yalom, 2009). Goldner-Vukov and colleagues (2007) found existential group therapy to be helpful for people with bipolar disorder, and studies are under way to look at the effectiveness of deeper spiritual, religious, and existential treatment to address addictions to alcohol and other substances (Mercadante, 2010; Mills, 2002).

Existential therapy can be particularly useful in group therapy, counteracting participants' sense of meaninglessness and isolation with the opportunity to connect with others with similar problems. In a group of older adults facing death, the group leader was able to build on this experience to encourage group members to find meaning by giving back and helping others outside of the group (Garrow & Walker, 2001).

These studies reflect the type of person and situation for whom existential therapy seems best suited:

- People coping with life-threatening and chronic illnesses
- Those whose lives have challenging limitations, such as people who are incarcerated, people with disabilities, and people living in poverty
- Those who have suffered important losses, such as bereavement, disappointments in relationships, and failure to achieve their goals
- People who have had traumatic experiences
- People with long-standing mild-to-moderate anxiety or depression
- People at a crossroads in their lives who are looking for direction, such as those who are recently divorced, approaching midlife, retired, or graduated from college.

It quickly becomes apparent that every human being at some point in their lives can benefit from existential therapy. Anyone experiencing what Diamond (2009) has referred to as "pervasive postmodern symptoms" such as excessive anxiety, apathy, alienation, nihilism, avoidance, shame, addiction, despair, or purposelessness, as well as those who are seeking meaning in life, truth, self-actualization and transcendence, can benefit from an existential approach to psychotherapy. In other words, existential therapy seems relevant to all types of people, in all age groups. It can even be useful in working with children and adolescents.

Current Use of Existential Treatment

Existential therapy's themes of meaningfulness, authenticity, freedom, and responsibility continue to have great relevance and broad application. The more our lives seem to be out of our control, the more we hear about terrorism, school violence, and bullying; and the more we are troubled by our own overcommitted lifestyles, the more many of us search for meaning and purpose in what we do and struggle to maintain a sense of freedom and authenticity.

Of course, end-of-life issues and living with chronic or terminal illnesses require a more holistic approach to treatment than what standard treatment modalities offer. Existential therapy provides a comprehensive and integrative method for exploring these complicated and yet universal issues.

Existentialist therapy is also inherently conducive to the current focus on time-limited approaches to treatment. Both a short-term existential integrative therapy (Bugental, 2008) and a modular approach that can be administered in 12 to 15 sessions have been developed. Working within a time-sensitive framework offers clients a focus, but also provides flexibility and allows additional support and more sessions to be added, if necessary, based on the client's needs (Strasser & Strasser, 1997).

In recent years, spirituality has emerged as an acceptable and important topic in counseling and psychotherapy. This emphasis on spirituality is consistent with an existential viewpoint. Although existentialism does not advocate any specific religious beliefs, it reminds us of the importance of having a sense of meaning that transcends our immediate and finite lives. Whether that meaning comes from traditional religion, the spirituality of nature, watching a child grow, or another source, it can help people cope with the challenges of the 21st century. One can find many similarities between existential therapy and Buddhist mindfulness practice. Both focus on acceptance of the finality of life, transcendence of self, and staying grounded in the here and now. These concepts are essential to self-acceptance and finding contentment in life (Claessens, 2009; Xu, 2010).

Addressing existential and spiritual needs can be an important part of a holistic approach to counseling. Particularly with an aging population, an existential approach, either alone or in combination with other approaches such as logotherapy and narrative therapy (Xu, 2010), can be quite effective. Existential therapy integrates well with other approaches, including positive psychology (Thompson, 2011; Wong, 2010), narrative therapy (Richert, 2010), and brief therapy (Mobley, 2005). More will be said about integrative theories in Chapter 19.

The majority of the literature on the effectiveness of existential therapy relies on in-depth case studies (Bugental, 1990; May, 1983; Yalom, 1980). Existentialist therapy also falls under the larger umbrella of experiential-humanistic psychotherapies, for which there is growing empirical support (Cain & Seeman, 2001; Schneider, 2008).

EVALUATION OF EXISTENTIAL THERAPY

Like all approaches to counseling and psychotherapy, existential therapy has both strengths and limitations. As with many types of therapy, additional research is necessary to empirically validate existential therapy. However, some interventions, particularly interventions using paradoxical intention, have been found to be effective.

Limitations

Existential therapy relies heavily on developing a strong client–clinician relationship and on verbal communication. It is an individualized approach in which the clinician offers little structure or direction. This approach takes a stance that responsibility, choice, and self-determination are desirable but does not offer specific steps and has few strategies for intervention. Treatment may be a leisurely and lengthy process. Because of these limitations, many people may be skeptical of its value, reluctant or unable to engage in the thinking and self-exploration that it requires, and find its underlying philosophy unacceptable. Of course, clinicians need to respect those feelings and select carefully the people for whom existential therapy is recommended.

In addition, this approach does not seek to directly ameliorate symptoms and its practitioners acknowledge that symptoms may or may not abate after existential treatment. People struggling with prominent symptoms such as drug or alcohol dependence or mania probably are not good candidates for this approach.

Strengths and Contributions

The existential approach to treatment does have many strengths. Its greatest contribution is probably not as a separate approach to psychotherapy and counseling but as a philosophy of human development that can be infused into other treatment systems. This idea was advanced by May and Yalom (1995), who stated that their primary objective was the integration of the theory's goals and concepts into all approaches to psychotherapy. They wanted all clinicians to become aware of the importance of choice, meaning, actualization, and the therapeutic alliance. May and Yalom believed that this process was already well under way. Certainly, few would argue with the premise that counseling should promote people's overall wellness, help them live fully and authentically, and encourage them to take responsibility for their lives, make more positive and deliberate choices, and create meaning for themselves (Bauman & Waldo, 1998).

Existential therapy has made many important contributions to the fields of counseling and psychotherapy. Like person-centered counseling, it emphasizes the importance of a collaborative, respectful, and authentic client–clinician relationship. Current research has given ample support to the connection between the treatment alliance and the outcome of treatment.

Existential therapy has broadened the reaches of psychotherapy beyond pathology and symptoms and legitimized inclusion in the treatment process of deep and philosophical issues such as existential anxiety, isolation, fear of death, actualization, freedom, and the meaning of life. It is a holistic and growth-promoting approach that de-emphasizes pathology and has relevance to everyone.

Eisenberg (1989), for example, used Frankl's logotherapy along with other humanistic and emotionally oriented interventions such as Rogers's facilitative conditions, meditation, and relaxation to treat people in an Israeli prison. Participants were helped to increase their awareness, find meaning and alternatives in all situations, and use their guilt as a catalyst for positive change. They were encouraged to make a conscious choice to "straighten themselves out" (p. 90) and to be more open and authentic. A theme of treatment was the existential message: "Place one thing above everything else: To master life under all circumstances. This foremost self-transcending endeavor immunizes against despair. By forgetting yourself, by transcending yourself, you become truly human" (p. 90). The treatment approach yielded positive results and still is used in this setting.

Although it was developed more than 75 years ago, existential therapy is compatible with current trends in counseling and psychotherapy. It takes a broad perspective on the meaning of spirituality and affirms its importance in our lives. It is phenomenological and emphasizes the importance of meaning making. While espousing an emphasis on people's commonalities, existential therapy also attends to the importance of each person's experience within his or her cultural context. It acknowledges the importance of people's thoughts and values flexibility and creativity in thinking. Existential treatment also encourages balance in our lives, another important contemporary value.

Although existential therapy de-emphasizes techniques, Frankl's paradoxical intention has been found to be helpful in treating anorexia nervosa, agoraphobia, anxiety, urinary retention, and insomnia. A series of studies during the past 5 years on the empirical efficacy of logotherapy have found paradoxical intent to be helpful with populations as diverse as at-risk urban adolescents (White, Wagener, & Furrow, 2010) and nurses working in palliative care settings (Vachon, Fillion, Achille, Duval, & Leung, 2011). Family therapists and cognitive–behavioral counselors, in particular, use this intervention in their work and find it to be a powerful tool for change, although one that must be used carefully.

Inventories and assessment scales developed by existential thinkers provide other potentially useful tools. Some of these are:

- Reker's (1994) Life Attitude Profile for assessing meaning and purpose in life
- The Sources of Meaning Profile, also developed by Reker, measuring how meaningful people find aspects of their lives
- Purpose in Life Test (Bauman & Waldo, 1998), which measures level of existential meaning and future time perspective.

Inventories such as these can promote discussion and awareness, helping people give meaning to their lives. Cross-cultural validation of selected logotherapy tests, including the Purpose in Life Test, have been undertaken in Nigeria, Iran, and other countries and have been found to be valid among graduate students cross-culturally (Asagba, Alarape, & Chowen, 2009).

Existential therapy is a hopeful, optimistic, and timely approach, differentiated from other theories by "the overarching philosophical attitude toward human existence" (Vontress, 2008a, p. 162). Existential therapists focus holistically on the person's *dasein* (being-in-the-world), on the environments that influence their personal journey, and on the universal themes of life, death, love, and responsibility—constructs that people live with every day. "Existential therapists try to connect with others across cultural, national, racial, and other boundaries on a spiritual level" (p. 169).

SKILL DEVELOPMENT: VALUES CLARIFICATION

Understanding people's values is relevant to existential therapy as well as to other treatment approaches. Our values are an important aspect of our identities and affect the choices we make. Our success in leading lives that are consistent with our values is strongly connected to the meaningfulness of our lives and our sense of fulfillment. Values can be expressed, manifested in our daily activities, and assessed via inventories. Ideally, people's expressed, manifest, and inventoried values all will be congruent. However, sometimes discrepancies emerge, particularly between expressed and manifest values. This can lead people to feel unfulfilled and unmotivated.

Wanda, for example, reported that she valued close interpersonal relationships, spending time in nature, and demonstrating her creativity. However, her manifest values were different. She worked long hours as a bank manager and made a high salary but had little time for friends and leisure activities. In addition, she lived in a small apartment in an urban setting. Her place of residence did not allow her to grow a garden, make space for her painting, or have much contact with the beauty of nature. Not surprisingly, Wanda reported that she was unhappy with her life and felt unmotivated at work.

Seeing the discrepancy between her expressed and manifest values prompted her to take a more honest look at her values. She realized that the security and income of her job were important values to her but that she was neglecting the interpersonal and creative values that also mattered. She was able to transfer to a bank in a more rural area and purchased a small house. These changes allowed her more time and opportunity for hiking, painting, and gardening. Although Wanda did take a cut in pay, she was able to maintain an adequate and stable income and decided that the loss in income was more than offset by her ability to realize some of her other values.

Expressed Values

Looking at values from several perspectives can provide useful information. The usual place to start is with people's expressed values. This might involve asking questions such as the following:

- What do you view as the most important and meaningful parts of your life?
- What accomplishments have you had that make you particularly proud?
- If you had only 1 year to live, how would you want to use your time?
- What do you view as your three most important values?
- If you were to write a brief biography of yourself for publication in a national magazine, what information would you include?

Of course, these questions can be modified and adapted to ensure that they are well received by a particular client.

Manifest Values

Manifest values are reflected in how people lead their lives, including their personal and professional activities, the distribution of their time, their lifestyles, their objective accomplishments, and neglected areas of their lives. Questions such as the following can elicit manifest values:

- Describe a typical day (or week or month) in your life.
- If someone who did not know you read a biography of your life, what would that person view as your greatest accomplishments? Your greatest disappointments?
- Assume that you have 16 waking hours each day. Tell me the number of hours you typically spend in each of the following roles and what you usually do in that role:
  - Spouse/partner/friend
  - Parent
  - Career person
  - Self-care (e.g., exercise, meditation, walking in nature)
  - Life manager (e.g., shopping, cleaning, paying bills)
  - Other roles.
- If you could redistribute your time among these roles, what changes would you make?
- How have your activities and the ways in which you spend your time changed during the past 5 to 10 years?
- When you awaken in the morning, what parts of your life do you look forward to and engage in as much as possible and what parts do you avoid whenever you can?
- What do you enjoy doing when you are on vacation?

Inventoried Values

Many inventories, both standardized and nonstandardized, are available to assess values. Sometimes paper-and-pencil or computerized inventories elicit more objective responses than do discussion questions such as those just listed. The following is a simple written assessment of values that can provide another perspective on what is important to a person. Either of the two sets of instructions can be used with the accompanying list of values, depending on which seems more likely to engage a person's interest and cooperation. Discussion of the person's responses should follow completion of the inventory to clarify the information provided.

> ***Instructions 1:*** Review the following list of values. Place a check mark by all of the values that are important to you. Then review the values that you have checked and list, in priority order, the three that are most important to you.

Instructions 2: Assume that you have $1,000 to spend at an auction of values. Review the following list and decide how you would allocate your money. Allocating too little to any one value may mean you will lose the auction for that value, but allocating too much to a value limits how much you can allocate to other values.

List of Values	
Achievement	Learning and Knowledge
Beauty	Love and Romance
Career Success	Nature/Outdoor Activities
Child Rearing	Order
Creativity	Possessions and Wealth
Fame	Power
Friendship	Prestige and Admiration
Health and Fitness	Security
Helping Others	Spirituality
Independence	Variety and Excitement

CASE ILLUSTRATION

The following dialogue illustrates use of a Symbolic Growth Experience (SGE) with Edie. As you learned earlier in this chapter, processing an SGE entails four steps:

1. People are educated about the concept of the SGE.
2. They select an important past experience and explore its importance and symbolism in their lives.
3. They are helped to understand the meaning in the experience.
4. They develop a clearer sense of meaning and can repeat their use of these strategies to understand the significance of other experiences.

Assume that Edie has already been educated about the concept of the SGE. As you read the following dialogue, observe how exploration of the significance of past experiences helps her develop a greater sense of meaningfulness in her life as well as an understanding of some of her emotions and choices. Also note the existential clinician's role.

CLINICIAN: Edie, I see great sadness on your face today.

EDIE: Yes, the weekend was tough. I told you that Roberto and I were planning to attend my twentieth high school reunion. I bought a new dress, got my hair styled, picked out pictures of Ava to show off. I thought it would be wonderful, but it was horrible.

CLINICIAN: How did something you were so looking forward to bring you so much pain?

EDIE: You remember my telling you that when I was ten years old, I was diagnosed with cancer. No one thought I would survive, except maybe my father. I had chemotherapy and lost all my hair. And I took steroids to help with the nausea and that made me gain weight. There I was, disgusting-looking, maybe dying . . . and I was supposed to go to school, if I could drag myself there. The other children would make fun of me, laugh at me, call me baldy. I know they didn't understand, but it was so awful.

CLINICIAN: That must have been such a difficult time for you, not only coping with cancer but also with the teasing. How is the reunion connected with that?

EDIE: I guess I wanted to show everyone that I had survived, that I was attractive now and had a family. But when I got to the reunion, all those feelings I had when I was ten came back to me.

CLINICIAN: So in your mind, the reunion was to be a life-affirming experience, but somehow it was just the opposite. What sense do you make of that?

EDIE: I don't know.

CLINICIAN: Edie, you have talked quite a bit about the impact cancer had on your life and your concern that it might recur despite the doctors' reassurances. Perhaps that strong fear of death has never left you and the reminder of the reunion intensified that fear.

EDIE: That's true. You know, when I hit the tenth anniversary of my cancer diagnosis, the doctors said I was cured, but I never really believed it.

CLINICIAN: And you're still living as though death is imminent.

EDIE: Yes, I am. I felt like a fake at the reunion. How could I present myself as a woman who had survived when I knew inside that I was really dying?

CLINICIAN: Most of us have anxiety about death, but for you, of course, it is particularly strong. How do you think this fear affects your life now?

EDIE: I worry a lot about dying before Ava is grown. She needs me so much, and I don't want to abandon her. I try to do all I can for her while I still have time, but I never feel like I do enough. Roberto can't understand. He says I pamper her and I should stop, but she's my only child. I couldn't get pregnant again because of the cancer. It's a miracle I got pregnant with Ava. She's like a gift from God.

CLINICIAN: I hear you saying so many important things. Ava's birth and your role as a mother have given meaning to your life, and you want to make the most of that. But I also hear a sense of urgency, a fear that time might run out for you before Ava is grown and that terrifies you.

EDIE: Yes, I still feel like it's just a matter of time before the cancer catches up with me again. Why can't Roberto understand that?

CLINICIAN: You feel very alone. I think one of the hardest things about being human is that no matter how much other people care about us, they can't really know what it is like to feel the way we feel. That can be very lonely.

EDIE: That's true. I know Roberto loves me and Ava, but he never does seem to really understand me. Maybe I've been too hard on him and expected too much.

CLINICIAN: What could you choose to do differently?

EDIE: Instead of blowing up at him, I could remind myself that he hasn't been through what I have, that there's no way he could really understand, and that's all right. I have a better awareness of myself now that I understand why I treat Ava the way I do.

CLINICIAN: How does that fit with the importance in your life of being a good mother?

EDIE: I love Ava and do all I can for her. Roberto says it's not good for her, though—that she needs more independence and confidence in herself.

CLINICIAN: I know your anxiety pushes you to do everything possible for Ava and to be a different parent to her than your parents were to you. Could it be that your anxiety makes it hard for you to see any value in what Roberto is saying?

EDIE: You mean that I'm scared something bad will happen to Ava if I don't keep a close watch on her? Yes, I guess I can be overprotective . . . and I know that's not really good mothering. I want her to feel confident and good about herself, not the way I felt when I was growing up.

At this point, Edie has developed a clearer idea of the meaning, for her, of both her experience with cancer and the recent reunion. She is more aware of the impact that her fear of death and her sense of aloneness have on her. She has gained some clarification about the primary purpose of her life—to stay alive so that she can continue to be a good parent to Ava—and has begun to increase her awareness of both her own behavior and the possible validity of Roberto's words. She is now in a better position to make choices that will help her to move toward the meaning she has created in her life, to feel more actualized, and to improve her relationships with both Ava and Roberto.

EXERCISES

Large-Group Exercises

1. Conduct a values auction in class based on the list in the Skill Development section. Notice the items for which you bid, how much you wager to win values of importance to you, and how you feel when you win or lose values on which you have bid. Did any of your wagers or reactions surprise you? What have you learned from this exercise about your values?
2. Are clinicians who focus primarily on profound issues of the human condition doing people a great service, or are they doing them a disservice by de-emphasizing the immediate problems and symptoms that led people to seek treatment? Create a debate in the classroom, with a group of people taking each side of this question.
3. Engage in a round-robin counseling dialogue, with one person assuming the role of either Roberto or another hypothetical client and the class assuming the role of the clinician. Focus on helping the client increase the sense of meaning in his or her life.

Small-Group Exercises

1. Divide into your groups of four students. Each dyad should have an opportunity to assume clinician and client roles for a dialogue of approximately 15 minutes in length. The client in each dialogue should present an experience in his or her life that was probably a Symbolic Growth Experience (SGE). The clinician should help the client explore the importance of that experience and the connection it has to the meaning the client has created in his or her life. Take particular note of themes and connections in the information presented by the client.

   Feedback about the dialogue should focus on the following:

   - Ability to incorporate existential issues into the dialogue
   - Clarification of the meaning of the SGE
   - Use of empathy

- Use of questions
- Therapeutic alliance.

2. Vontress writes about universal culture—truths in life (such as love, death, guilt, responsibility) that affect everyone regardless of race, gender, culture, religion, or sexual orientation. Take 3 or 4 minutes to silently contemplate the following: Think of some examples of the beliefs you hold or issues that you struggle with that could be considered universal. In contrast, what values reflect the larger society, culture, or family environment in which you live? Spend 15 minutes in your small group sharing your answers. When finished, each group should make a list of universal truths to share with the class.

Individual Exercises

1. Viktor Frankl said, "When we are no longer able to change a situation, we are challenged to change ourselves." Ponder this for a moment. Has there ever been a time when something occurred in your life that you could not change? How did you react? What did you do? Write about this in your journal. Over time, how did you adjust to the situation?
2. Imagine that you are home alone reading a book, when you hear an explosion outside. Within minutes you are told by the fire department that you must evacuate the building immediately because of the risk of fire. Knowing that time is precious, and that your home might be destroyed, what items do you choose to take with you? What do you leave behind? Journal about the experience.

Summary

Existential therapy grew out of a European society devastated by two great wars. It seeks to help people deal with the deep and powerful issues that affect everyone. Both a philosophy and a psychological system of treatment, the approach addresses deep dimensions of the human condition such as the inevitability of death and loss, loneliness and alienation, meaninglessness, and guilt. Clinicians and their relationships with their clients are the primary instruments of change; establishment of a genuine, caring, supportive, and authentic client–clinician relationship is essential in this treatment model. Existential therapy enables people to become more actualized, aware, and connected to others, which can help them make wise and responsible choices and create meaning in their lives.

Recommended Readings

Bugental, J. F. T. (1987). *The art of the psychotherapist.* New York, NY: Norton.

Bugental, J. F. T. (1990). *Intimate journeys.* San Francisco, CA: Jossey-Bass.

Frankl, V. (1963). *Man's search for meaning.* Boston, MA: Beacon.

Hoffman, L., Yang, M., Kaklauskas, F., & Chan, A. (Eds.). (2009). *Existential psychology East–West.* Colorado Springs, CO: University of the Rockies Press.

Klingberg, H. (2001). *When life calls out to us: The love and lifework of Viktor and Elly Frankl.* New York, NY: Doubleday.

May, R. (1969). *Love and will.* New York, NY: Norton.

Moodley, R., & Walcott, R. (Eds.). (2010). *Counseling across and beyond cultures: Exploring the work of Clemmont E. Vontress in clinical practice.* Toronto, Canada: University of Toronto Press.

Van Deurzen, E., & Adams, M. (2011). *Skills in existential counseling and psychotherapy.* Thousand Oaks, CA: Sage.

Yalom, I. D. (2008). *Staring at the sun: Overcoming the terror of death.* San Francisco, CA: Jossey-Bass.

Yalom, I. D. (2009). *The gift of therapy: An open letter to a new generation of therapists.* New York, NY: Harper Collins.

Additional Sources of Information

http://www.existentialanalysis.co.uk—This is the website for the Society for Existential Analysis, a London-based membership organization that provides training, holds conferences, and publishes the *Journal of the Society for Existential Analysis.*

http://www.yalom.com—Irvin Yalom's website includes lectures, articles, Yalom's biography, and a complete bibliography of the writings of this existential therapist and author.

http://www.viktorfrankl.org—The website of the Viktor Frankl Institute in Vienna.

http://ehinstitute.org—The Existential-Humanistic Institute in San Francisco offers training, articles, and links to those interested in existential and humanistic therapy.

http://www.existentialpsychology.org—The International Society for Existential Psychology and Psychotherapy is a membership organization based in Toronto, and publisher of the *International Journal of Existential Psychology and Psychotherapy.*

CHAPTER 10

Gestalt Therapy

What distinguishes Gestalt therapy from other humanistic approaches is its emphasis on the *Gestalt,* which Laura Perls (1992) defined as "a structured entity that is more than and different from its parts. It is the foreground figure that stands out from its ground, it 'exists'" (p. 52). According to Gestalt therapists, people experience psychological difficulties because they have become cut off from important parts of themselves such as their emotions, bodies, or contacts with others. The purpose of Gestalt therapy is to help people become aware of these neglected and disowned parts and restore wholeness, integration, and balance.

Gestalt therapy was developed primarily by Fritz Perls, with contributions from his wife Laura Perls. Erving and Miriam Polster also contributed important enhancements to Gestalt therapy. Widely used during the 1960s and 1970s, it has evolved and matured into a widely used treatment methodology and has influenced other approaches to treatment.

THE PEOPLE WHO DEVELOPED GESTALT THERAPY

Frederick Perls, known as Fritz Perls, was born in 1893, the middle child and only son of a middle-class Jewish family living in Berlin, Germany. Although Perls was not always a motivated student, he succeeded in receiving an MD degree with a specialization in psychiatry (Perls, 1969b). Interested in becoming a practicing psychoanalyst, Perls moved to Vienna, home of Sigmund Freud, where he met many of the leaders in his field. Perls studied with Karen Horney and was psychoanalyzed by both Horney and Wilhelm Reich. Reich's emphasis on the use of facial, bodily, and linguistic cues to promote understanding and personal growth had a powerful influence on Perls and on the concepts and strategies of Gestalt therapy (Wulf, 1998).

Perls also was strongly influenced by several other experiences. During World War I, he served as a medical corpsman, a powerful personal experience. After the war, he worked with neurologist Kurt Goldstein at the Frankfurt Neurological Institute, a treatment facility for people with brain injuries. Both experiences led Perls to reflect on the workings of the human mind, on Gestalt psychology, and on better ways to help people (Simkin, 1975; Wheeler, 1991). Even early in his career as a psychoanalyst, he was becoming disenchanted with psychoanalysis as well as with behaviorism.

The versatile and extroverted Perls also worked as an actor in the 1920s. He later reported that his experiences in the theater gave him an understanding of and appreciation for nonverbal communication, an essential aspect of Gestalt therapy. In 1930, Fritz Perls married Laura Posner, a concert pianist and dancer (Serlin, 1992). Whereas Fritz Perls emphasized independence and confrontation, Laura Perls advocated support and connections. She studied existentialism with Martin Buber and Paul Tillich and drew on this background as she became involved in developing Gestalt therapy.

When Hitler came into power, the couple left Europe, relocating first in Holland and then in South Africa, where Fritz Perls served as a captain in the South African Medical Corps. During his years in South Africa, he outlined his theory of personality integration, which later became Gestalt therapy (Simkin, 1975). In 1946, the couple immigrated to the United States, where Fritz Perls published *Gestalt Therapy: Excitement and Growth in the Human Personality* (Perls, Hefferline, & Goodman, 1951). In 1952, he established the Gestalt Institute of America.

The most important impetus for the growth of Gestalt therapy was Fritz Perls's work between 1962 and 1969 at the Esalen Institute in Big Sur, California. He became best known there for his use of the "hot seat" in his workshops and soon was regarded as an innovative and charismatic advocate of the human potential movement.

Perls's personality enhanced the popularity and success of Gestalt therapy. An outspoken free spirit, unafraid to challenge and reject established traditions and procedures, both Perls and his work were in tune with the 1960s, when many people sought more fulfillment in their lives and new ways to live. As he stated, "The meaning of life is that it is to be lived; and it is not to be traded and conceptualized and squeezed into a pattern of systems. We realize that manipulation and control are not the ultimate job of life" (Perls, 1969a, p. 3).

Fritz Perls died in 1970, when the popularity of Gestalt therapy was at its peak. Many clinicians abandoned traditional systems of treatment in favor of this exciting approach, while others incorporated elements of Gestalt therapy into already-established treatment approaches. After her husband's death, Laura Perls continued their work on Gestalt therapy until her death in 1990.

Others continue to develop and refine Gestalt therapy. Particularly important were Erving and Miriam Polster. Both served for many years as codirectors of the Gestalt Training Center in San Diego, expanded on Perls's ideas, and emphasized the importance of theory to increase the credibility of this treatment system (Polster & Polster, 1973). Others, including Yontef (1993, 2012), Evans and Gilbert (2005), and Lichtenberg (2012), have contributed to the maturation of Gestalt therapy during the past 60 years (Finlay & Evans, 2009).

THE DEVELOPMENT OF GESTALT THERAPY

Like many other treatment approaches, Gestalt therapy has its roots in Europe. A group of Gestalt psychologists in Berlin, including Max Wertheimer, Kurt Koffka, and Wolfgang Köhler, laid the groundwork for Gestalt therapy with their studies of perception and integration of parts into perceptual wholes. These theorists believed that understanding knowledge in "units of wholes, Gestalten" is more useful to the expansion of knowledge than dissecting the parts (Wulf, 1998, p. 86). In other words, they believed that the whole is greater than the sum of the parts. They also viewed people as having a natural tendency toward closure and equilibrium, which leads to thinking in terms of wholes rather than parts. For a comprehensive discussion of the history of Gestalt, see Hergenhahn (2009).

Although Gestalt psychologists provided the name and a basic premise for Gestalt therapy, Perls drew on many sources of knowledge in developing his treatment system, including Kurt Lewin's field theory, existentialism, and Eastern thought (Sapriel, 2012). The ideas of Sigmund Freud, Karen Horney, Wilhelm Reich, and Otto Rank also helped to shape Gestalt therapy.

In addition, Jacob Moreno's psychodrama, along with Perls's own experiences as an actor, are reflected in the development of Gestalt therapy. Psychodrama encourages people to work out personal difficulties by creating dramatizations of problematic situations such as a family fight. With the help of a therapist, members of the audience assume family and other roles and give the protagonist an opportunity to relive and change painful experiences. Feedback from observers both enhances the impact of the process and affords observers vicarious benefits. Perls's techniques, including the empty chair, role-plays, group feedback, and perhaps even the hot seat, were influenced by Moreno's ideas, as was Perls's emphasis on spontaneity, creativity, and enactment (Wulf, 1998).

During Perls's lifetime, the highly charged techniques associated with his approach received attention because of their use at Esalen, their powerful impact, and their application to encounter groups, widely used during the 1960s and early 1970s. Since then, Gestalt therapy has become less sensational and more solid. Practitioners of mindfulness meditation will recognize concepts of Buddhist thought woven throughout Gestalt theory. Fritz and Laura Perls first became familiar with Zen Buddhism through their friend Paul Weisz who was a doctor and a serious student of Zen (Clarkson & Mackewn, 1993). Weisz trained in Gestalt theory with Fritz Perls and introduced him to Eastern ideas, which Perls wholeheartedly incorporated into his work. Buddhist theories such as the paradoxical notion of change, the polarity of life, and present moment awareness are core concepts of Gestalt. Clinging and aversion, Buddhist concepts that are considered hindrances to mindfulness meditation, correspond with Gestalt concepts, as do self-acceptance and maintaining a nonjudgmental approach to life, free of "shoulds" and "oughts" (Kim, 2011). Perls believed his exercises offered a Zen-like experience for Westerners. He later studied Zen Buddhism in Kyoto, Japan. He was also influenced by Alan Watts, philosopher and author of *The Wisdom of Insecurity,* 1951; and *The Way of Zen,* 1957.

IMPORTANT THEORETICAL CONCEPTS

Although Perls often used distinctive terminology, his theoretical concepts are in many ways consistent with person-centered and existential approaches. However, Perls and his associates did add their own ideas, which distinguish Gestalt therapy from other treatment systems. In addition, the strategies used in Gestalt therapy represent a considerable departure from existential and person-centered treatment approaches, which make minimal use of specific intervention strategies.

View of Humankind

Like other humanists, Perls had an optimistic and empowering view of people and placed great importance on self-actualization: "Every individual, every plant, every animal has only one inborn goal—to actualize itself as it is" (Perls, 1969a, p. 33). He believed that people were basically good and had the capacity to cope with their lives successfully, although he recognized that they sometimes needed help. According to Perls, healthy people engaged productively in the tasks of survival and maintenance and intuitively moved toward self-preservation and growth. Gestalt therapy helps people develop awareness, inner strength, and self-sufficiency. These qualities enable them to recognize that the resources they need for positive growth and change are within themselves rather than in a partner, title, career, or clinician.

Wholeness, Integration, and Balance

As its name implies, Gestalt therapy is a holistic approach that emphasizes the importance of integration and balance in people's lives. People cannot be separated from their environment nor can they be divided into parts (such as body and mind) (Murdock, 2009). Perls (1969a) said of the human organism, "We *have* not a liver or a heart. We *are* liver and heart and brain and yet, even this is wrong—we are *not* a summation of parts but a *coordination* of the whole. We do not have a body, we *are* a body, we *are* somebody" (p. 6).

To some extent, this polarization and denial of parts of the self stem from a drive toward homeostasis. People have difficulty dealing with ambiguity or disequilibrium and prefer stability and cohesiveness. This may lead them to stay "stuck" in an unsatisfying marriage because they fear the alternative, or to exclude from awareness the parts of themselves that seem incongruent or cause discomfort, in a misguided effort to force equilibrium.

INTEGRATING POLARITIES People's need for homeostasis also can lead them to view themselves and their world in terms of *polarities* or extremes. The world may seem easier to understand if we categorize people as either good or bad. However, these polarities generally reflect internal or interpersonal conflicts. To truly achieve wholeness, people must become aware of and integrate their polarities, especially the polarities of the mind and the body. Unless we accomplish that, the neglected or rejected side of the polarity is likely to build barriers against our efforts toward growth. For example, people who believe they must always be independent may deny the part of themselves that craves connection and intimacy, whereas people who believe that their intellect is their greatest gift may cut themselves off from their emotions and sensations.

FIELD THEORY: INTEGRATING FIGURE AND GROUND Although people strive for homeostasis, our lives and our world are always in flux, always changing. People constantly experience disequilibrium and then naturally try to restore balance. We are hungry, so we eat. We are tired, so we nap. We shift priorities based on the nature and importance of the rising needs to be met.

Perls incorporated Lewin's field theory, which was popular in physics, into the concept of the *figure/ground* to clarify this constant flux. The metaphor of driving a car illustrates how we must live our lives in the here and now, using our best judgment and knowledge to react to the constantly changing needs on the road. We cannot possibly control every experience on the road, nor can we get in a car with a predetermined goal of driving 70 miles an hour until we reach our destination. Rather, certain elements come into the foreground, depending on the environment. The figures that emerge require different levels of focus and attention. The self is the fluid part of this environmental field, and the one that is always shifting and changing. This shift in the figure/ground is a process that attends to the immediate needs of the organism. Not to change results in stagnation and the sense of being "stuck."

This process—shifting back and forth between figure and foreground—is the crux of psychotherapy. According to Perls, the basis of the Gestalt approach is the paradoxical situation that the organism has a two-part existence: both the awareness of what is happening in the present moment, and the relationship that this is in contrast with. Foreground implies background and vice versa. According to Perls, recognizing these splits and activating both is the goal of psychotherapy. Through awareness, boundaries become fluid, disappear, and then reappear. Similar to our car analogy, something is always receding into the background or moving into the foreground.

The therapist can use his or her perspective as part of the field as a tool in therapy. Through the use of Gestalt techniques such as the empty chair and the two-chair technique, the therapist helps the client become aware of the background–foreground, to recognize the duality, and to conclude that things are not "either/or," but "both/and." This both/and way of thinking results in a paradigm shift for the client that reduces judgmentalness, increases compassion, and eventually brings about change (Neff, Kirkpatrick, & Rude, 2007).

More significant figure/ground shifts lead to sudden and often important changes in our understanding of events and experiences. For example, after dating for 10 months, Kristen arrived about 45 minutes late to pick up her boyfriend Luke for a party at his supervisor's house. Before she could explain that an accident had caused her delay, Luke became enraged and hit Kristen in the face. He had become angry with her before and had come close to hitting her, but Kristen had overlooked those signs of Luke's violent behavior; she had grown up in an environment in which anger and shouting were acceptable and even desirable expressions of feeling. However, when Luke actually hit her, she saw those early warning signs in a new light, integrating figure and ground. She recognized that Luke presented a danger to her and that they did not have a healthy relationship.

EGO BOUNDARY Just as the figure/ground relationship changes, so does the ego boundary. Perls (1969a) described the *ego boundary* as "the organism's definition in relation to its environment . . . this relationship is experienced both by what is inside the skin and what is outside the skin, but it is not a fixed thing" (p. 7). The two polarities of the fluid ego boundary are identification and alienation. Identification, as with our parents, our bodies, and our jobs, brings those aspects of our lives into our ego boundaries, whereas alienation, for example, from other people or parts of ourselves, leads us to put those aspects outside our ego boundaries. According to Perls, "So the whole idea of good and bad, right and wrong, is always a matter of boundary, of which side of the fence I am on" (p. 9).

Gestalt therapy, like the other approaches discussed in Part 3, is *phenomenological:* It recognizes that people's perceptions of a situation can vary widely; that even within a person, perceptions can change; and that our perceptions greatly influence our thoughts, emotions, and behaviors. Perls first introduced field theory in his seminal work (Perls et al., 1951) and was consistent with scientific writings at the time, including Einstein's theory of relativity (O'Neill, 2012; Perls & Philippson, 2012). Current use of the unified field perspective in Gestalt therapy considers the self as an interactive part of the larger environmental field. The person exists in a larger field, and cannot be understood outside of that context (Perls et al., 1951).

HOMEOSTASIS VERSUS FLUX Perls used a great many terms, including figure/ground, ego boundary, and polarities, to refer to the constant state of flux that people experience. These constructs all pose threats to our homeostasis. Clearly, people cannot achieve a state of fixed homeostasis and then freeze the action. Our lives are always changing. However, through awareness of and identification with all aspects of ourselves, we can deal successfully with flux and still have a sense of integration and wholeness. Homeostasis can be explained by the organism's need "to complete all unfinished situations in the sequence of the survival importance" (Perls & Philippson, 2012, p. 169).

Awareness

For Gestalt therapists, awareness is an essential element of emotional health: "Awareness per se—by and of itself—can be curative. Because with full awareness you become aware of this organismic self-regulation, you can let the organism take over without interfering, without interrupting; we can rely on the wisdom of the organism" (Perls, 1969a, p. 17). Awareness is both a hallmark of the healthy person and a goal of treatment.

Several possible causes have been identified for people's limited awareness. Preoccupation is one of the foremost. We may be so caught up with our pasts, our fantasies, our perceived flaws or strengths, that we lose sight of the whole picture and become unaware. Another reason for lack of awareness is low self-esteem: "The less confident we are in ourselves, the less we are in touch with ourselves and the world, the more we want to control" (Perls, 1969a, p. 21). Low self-esteem makes it difficult for people to trust themselves, to allow their natural health and strength to propel them toward growth and self-actualization. Rather, people with low self-esteem typically set out to control themselves and others in an effort to realize an idealized self-image rather than to truly become actualized. The result is often exactly the opposite of what is intended.

Awareness is facilitated in Gestalt therapy by the use of experiments, a here-and-now focus, and process statements. Because it is not enough for clients to merely talk about their feelings—talking leads to intellectualization—Gestalt therapists do not practice reflective listening. Rather, they focus on their clients' nonverbal language—the way they sit, their tone of voice, or a tapping finger. By attending to these and other body movements, the therapist requires clients to go deeper, to reexperience their emotions in the here-and-now environment of the therapy session, and to understand the physical as well as verbal meaning of what they are projecting.

ENVIRONMENTAL CONTACT TO PROMOTE GROWTH People engage in many efforts to achieve awareness, and contact with the environment is one of the most important. Contact is made through seven functions: looking, listening, touching, talking, moving, smelling, and tasting (Polster & Polster, 1973, pp. 129–138). Contact is necessary for growth; when we make contact with other people or aspects of our world, we must react and change. The experience of contact teaches us about ourselves and our environment and helps us to feel a part of our world, while defining more clearly who we are. People who avoid closeness with others and live isolated and circumscribed lives may believe that they are protecting themselves, but, in reality, they are preventing their growth and actualization.

Perls (1969a) identified five levels or stages of contact and growth:

1. ***The phony layer.*** People play games, assume roles, react in stereotyped and inauthentic ways, and are insincere.
2. ***The phobic layer.*** People avoid pain, hide their real selves to prevent rejection, act out of fear, and feel vulnerable and helpless.
3. ***The impasse layer.*** Having passed through the first two layers, people feel confused, stuck, and powerless; they seek help from others.
4. ***The implosive layer.*** People become aware that they have limited themselves and begin to experiment with change, to deal with unfinished business, to lower defenses, and to move toward greater integration. People connect with their possibilities and give up old layers. This implosion turns into an explosion in the fifth layer.
5. ***The explosive layer.*** People experience reintegration and wholeness, become their authentic selves, gain access to great energy, feel and express emotions, and become more actualized.

Treatment often involves helping people progress through the layers, peeling away each one like the skin of an onion to expose the next healthier layer of the adult personality. In this way, people truly become their authentic, actualized selves, capable of full contact with the environment, other people, and themselves.

HERE AND NOW Another way to increase awareness is to live in and be conscious of the present moment rather than remaining tied to the past or trying to control the future. According to Perls (1969a), "Nothing exists except the here and now. . . . The past is no more. The future is not yet. . . . You should live in the here and now" (p. 44). When we are centered in the present, we are more likely to be congruent—to have our minds, our bodies, and our emotions integrated. When we are not fully in the present, we may be fragmented. Our emotions may be stuck in past hurts and our thoughts may wander to future anticipations while we talk with people in the present. When we are not centered in the present, we give confusing messages to others, have a poorly integrated sense of ourselves, and have difficulty making contact because we are not fully present.

Gestalt therapy takes place in the here and now. The therapist reacts in a genuine, empathic, and transparent way to the client's material. This transparency may include disclosures from the therapist, but any disclosure must be made in the best interest of the client. Finlay and Evans (2009) caution that the use of the here and now is not a technique to be selected for use with the client, but a way of being that reflects the I–thou relationship found in all humanistic therapies (Buber, 1970; Yontef, 1993). More will be said about the I–thou relationship in the discussion of the therapeutic alliance.

RESPONSIBILITY Like the other humanistic theorists, Gestalt therapists place importance on accepting responsibility for our own lives rather than giving that power away or blaming and resenting others for our disappointments. Gestalt therapists believe that people must make their own choices rather than allowing others to choose for them.

Perls's focus, in keeping with the climate of the 1960s, was on the individual; but contemporary Gestalt therapists have modified the concept of responsibility. Now it refers not only to taking care of ourselves but also to recognizing that from birth we rely on the presence of interdependent relationships. To maintain a healthy balance between interconnectedness and independence, we must have awareness and self-acceptance, which lies at the core of the healthy person.

The Nature of Growth Disorders

Although Perls sometimes used the term *neuroses* to describe emotional problems, he believed that these difficulties should more accurately be referred to as "growth disorders" (Perls, 1969a, p. 30).

This term is used in connection with people who deny or reject aspects of themselves and their environment, are not living in the present, are not making fulfilling contact with others, lack awareness, and are not becoming actualized. Rather than changing or growing, they have become stuck. Change is an inevitable part of life, and those who do not change stagnate.

Avoidance and resistance, what Perls referred to as creative adjustment, keep people trapped in this unhealthy state. They avoid dealing with uncomfortable feelings, remain unaware, and circumscribe their lives to minimize flux or change. They make extensive use of ego defenses such as projection of disowned aspects of themselves onto others, distraction, failure to set boundaries between themselves and others, and introjections and withdrawal from their surroundings. Wholeness, integrity, freedom of choice, and actualization are sacrificed to the illusion of safety and homeostasis. Such people do not allow themselves to be aware of, anticipate, and cope successfully and flexibly with the changes in their lives. Rather, they persist in unsuccessful defensive maneuvers to avoid change. Paradoxically, as Perls observed, even stagnation indicates that movement has occurred and there is hope. Ironically, it can result in greater turmoil and discomfort than those who are aware of and use their own powerful resources to manage their lives.

People who are not developing in healthy ways often have a great deal of unfinished business. According to Perls (1969a), "Our life is basically practically nothing but an infinite number of unfinished situations—incomplete Gestalts. No sooner have we finished one situation than another comes up" (p. 15). Healthy people may be disconcerted by the constant unfinished business in their lives but learn to use their resources to deal with it effectively. People who do not adapt to life's changes develop growth disorders. This malfunction or breakdown in the process of living is not a medical problem, but rather "one possibility of existence" (Levine, 2012, p. 9). Because they are alienated from many aspects of their environments and themselves, they cannot deal effectively with the demands of their lives, so they accumulate more and more unfinished business. Their energy is sapped by their unproductive efforts to cope, leaving them depleted of the resources they need to live their lives successfully. People who are overwhelmed by unfinished business typically feel stuck or blocked and may experience physical symptoms. Their current issues tend to mirror unresolved past issues and are never finished because they are not addressed in the here and now. Gestalt therapists serve as facilitators of growth and self-regulation, not as change agents. One of the major goals of Gestalt therapy is to help people become aware of their backlog of unfinished business and bring it to closure—finish it so that they are able to live more fully in the present.

TREATMENT USING GESTALT THERAPY

Unlike person-centered counseling and existential therapy, Gestalt therapy includes a rich array of strategies that facilitate treatment. These strategies have been developed to further what Perls et al. (1951) identified as the four major emphases in Gestalt work:

1. To pay attention to experience and become aware of and concentrate on the actual present situation
2. To maintain and promote the integrity and interrelationships of social, cultural, historical, physical, emotional, and other important factors
3. To experiment
4. To encourage creativity.

Goals

Many of the treatment objectives of Gestalt therapy are similar to those of person-centered and existential therapy. However, others are unique to this approach. The most important goals of Gestalt therapy are:

- Promoting attention, clarity, and *awareness*
- Helping people live in the *here and now*
- Improving people's sense of *wholeness, integration,* and *balance.*

Additional goals of significance in this treatment system include:

- Enabling people to bring *closure* to their unfinished business
- Increasing people's appreciation of and *access to their own considerable resources*
- Promoting responsibility, appropriate choices, and *self-sufficiency*
- Promoting self-esteem, self-acceptance, and *actualization*
- Facilitating people's efforts to have *meaningful contact* with all aspects of themselves, other people, and their environment
- Developing the skills people need to *manage their lives successfully* without harming others.

According to Perls (1969a), "The difference between Gestalt therapy and most other types of psychotherapy is essentially that we do *not* analyze. We *integrate*" (p. 70). The ultimate aim of Gestalt therapy is to promote the natural growth of the human organism and enable people to live aware and actualized lives—not just to solve problems or promote adaptation but also to help clients feel more fulfilled and whole.

How People Change

Gestalt clinicians believe that awareness is the primary vehicle of change. If people can gain awareness of their unfinished business (the areas in which they are blocked and alienated) and their own strengths and resources, they can grow and become more actualized. Particularly important is awareness gained through the body since, according to Gestalt theory, most people overemphasize intellectual awareness and ignore messages from the body and the senses.

Therapeutic Alliance

Like the existential therapists discussed in the previous chapter, Gestalt therapists seek to create an I–thou relationship in contrast to the I–it relationship, which is the type of everyday relationship that moves us forward throughout the day but does not involve deep meaning. The I–thou relationship is a willingness to truly know the other person as he or she is, as well as the willingness to be transparent and to be fully known. Although I–it ways of relating are not to be shunned (because they make up the bulk of our communications), Crocker (2005) noted that they miss the depth of our humanity. She writes: "Being constantly open to the revelation of Thou, whenever and from wherever it comes—even while busy in the workings of I–it—and being willing to reveal oneself as Thou to an other's I when the opportunity presents itself—that is being faithful to oneself as a person. For Buber, the unique individuality of the Other is revealed and received, and from this mutual process rises true community and thus the fulfillment of life" (p. 72).

Gestalt clinicians strive to be genuine and aware of their own feelings, experiences, and perceptions. They build relationships with clients in which both client and clinician are free from judgment, narcissism, or expectations; are respectful and accepting of the other; are open; and are fully present in the here and now (Buber, 1970; Finlay & Evans, 2009). They do not urge or persuade people to change or tell people how they should be. Rather, they establish a climate that promotes trust, awareness, and a willingness to experiment with new ways of thinking, feeling, and acting. Clinicians and clients enter into a partnership in which both are committed to and active in the treatment process. However, clients take responsibility for their own development and decide for themselves how they will use the information that emerges in their sessions.

This bringing into awareness is often referred to as the paradoxical principle of change. "Change occurs when one becomes what he is, not when he tries to become what he is not" (Beisser, 1970, p. 77). It is only through ownership and integration of previously disavowed aspects of the self that change becomes possible. When a clinician observes that a client's attention is wandering, that conflicts are emerging, or that a person seems fragmented or out of contact, the clinician calls attention to these phenomena in the "here and now" of the session. The clinician makes this observation without interpretation or judgment, but simply to provide information that is likely to refocus attention, create awareness of blocks, and help people maintain contact with their present activities and experiences. Instead of trying to figure out their clients, Gestalt therapists focus on listening and helping clients find their own way.

Experience in the here and now is the process used to increase awareness. Awareness occurs in the present experiential moment, so even though the client may be addressing a past experience, the focus in therapy is on the "present moment where the past is embedded and therefore alive and obvious" (Melnick & Nevis, 2005, p. 105). It is only through this web of relational interconnections that we know ourselves (Finlay & Evans, 2009).

Experiments

One task of Gestalt therapists is suggesting experiments or learning experiences for their clients. These are individually tailored to each client in order to accomplish a purpose relevant to that person, usually to promote awareness and bring problems and unfinished business into the present where they can be resolved. These experiments should not be threatening or negative; instead, they should be positive and growth promoting. Presentation of suggested experiments should always be respectful, inviting, and carefully timed. Although confrontation may be used to encourage involvement, clients are never demeaned and can always choose whether or not to involve themselves in the experiments.

Experiments might take the form of enactments, role-plays, homework, or activities for clients to accomplish between sessions (Polster & Polster, 1973). For example, a Gestalt therapist suggested to a withdrawn and guarded woman who wanted to have closer relationships with people that she tell a friend something about herself that would surprise and please the friend. Spending time thinking about what she would tell the friend promoted the woman's self-awareness, and the eventual sharing increased the closeness between the woman and her friend.

Use of Language

Language plays an important part in Gestalt therapy. By choosing their words carefully, clinicians create an environment that encourages change.

EMPHASIS ON STATEMENTS Although questions are part of Gestalt therapy, clinicians typically prefer statements. They are more likely to say, "I am experiencing a loss of contact between us," than "Where has your attention gone?" The immediacy and direct person-to-person contact of a statement promotes a collaborative client–clinician relationship. Questions, on the other hand, are reminiscent of a teacher–student relationship in which the power differential may undermine the process. Talking *with* someone rather than *at* someone is critical in building a connection.

"WHAT" AND "HOW" QUESTIONS When Gestalt therapists do ask questions, they usually begin them with "what," "how," or sometimes "where," but rarely with "why." Questions such as "What are you experiencing when you stamp your foot?" and "How does it feel when you stamp your foot?" are more likely to keep the client in the present moment and promote integration than are questions such as "Why are you stamping your foot?" "Why" questions typically lead to a focus on past experiences, as well as blocks and manifestations of resistance.

"I" STATEMENTS Gestalt therapists encourage people to own and focus on their own feelings and experiences rather than talk about other people (they) or events (it). Statements beginning with "I" such as "I feel angry" and "In the dream, I am lost" encourage ownership and responsibility as well as integration. Statements such as "My mother made me angry" and "My dream was about being lost" take the focus off the client and the present moment and promote fragmentation and externalizing of responsibility.

THE PRESENT TENSE Even when clients talk about past events, Gestalt clinicians encourage them to focus on their present experience of the events—to bring events into the room and into the moment. For example, rather than focusing on a client's perceptions of how his father abandoned him when he was a child, the therapist might suggest that the client describe how that early abandonment affects his feelings and behaviors in the therapy session. This fosters awareness as well as a true connection with the clients' experience of the events.

ENCOURAGING RESPONSIBILITY Gestalt therapists encourage people to take responsibility for themselves, their words, their emotions, their thoughts, and their behaviors in order to facilitate integration. Language can help further that goal. For example, the clinician might suggest that people temporarily begin all their sentences with the phrase "I take responsibility for . . ." to help them recognize and accept their feelings. They might also apply to themselves statements they have made about others to facilitate awareness of their projections. The woman who says, "My sister only thinks of herself," might be asked to say, "I think only of myself," and then talk about what feelings this brings up for her.

Another way to encourage people to take responsibility for themselves is for clinicians to help them make the implicit explicit. For example, a woman assured her husband that she would be happy to accompany him to church as he requested. However, each Sunday she told him that she had work to do so she could not go to church. Her therapist encouraged her to make her feelings explicit by stating, "I really don't want to go to church with you; I feel uncomfortable and out of place there because it is not the religion I was brought up to believe."

Dreams

Dreams occupy an important place in Gestalt therapy. Perls viewed dreams as the royal road to integration rather than the royal road to the unconscious, as Freud had viewed them. Perls believed that the parts of a dream represent projections or aspects of the dreamer. Awareness comes from assuming the various roles or parts of the dream and enacting the dream as though it is happening in the present.

For example, a man had a dream about a rabbit, which was being chased across a field by a fox, escaping into a burrow. Freud, of course, would focus on the unconscious meaning of the conflict between the fox and the rabbit and the possibly sexual significance of the burrow. Perls, on the other hand, would encourage the man to assume the roles of each of the salient parts of the dream. One at a time, the client would enact the roles of the frightened rabbit, the menacing fox, the open field, and the protective burrow, speaking the thoughts and feelings that arose for him in each role. For example, he might say, "I am that rabbit, running scared, afraid that I will be swallowed up. I am always running for cover, safe just in the nick of time, but knowing that I might not make it the next time."

This approach to understanding dreams puts the client in charge of the process. It also allows people to take responsibility for their dreams, see their dreams as part of themselves, increase integration, and become aware of thoughts and emotions reflected in the dream that they might otherwise disown. Many concise examples of dreamwork can be found in Perls's book *Gestalt Therapy Verbatim* (1969a).

Fantasy

Fantasies, like dreams, can help people become more self-aware. Clinicians might use guided imagery to take people on a journey into their imaginations. Clients might be encouraged to imagine themselves walking through a beautiful meadow with a ramshackle house, looking around to see who is with them, and deciding what to do in that situation. Clinicians might make the fantasy more productive by asking questions to promote exploration and suggesting actions the person might take in the fantasy.

As with dreams, Gestalt therapists assume that the parts of the fantasy represent projections or aspects of the person. When the fantasy is completed, clinicians encourage people to process the experience by becoming the parts of the fantasy, speaking as though they are each part. This technique, as with the exploration of dreams, often helps people become more aware of and in contact with their feelings and more able to express their emotions.

Fantasies also can be used to bring closure to unfinished business. For example, a woman who had undergone surgery was left with some angry feelings about her surgeon and the need to have her surgery redone. When she called to express her feelings to the physician, he failed to return her telephone calls. To help her reach closure, her clinician led her on a guided fantasy in which she expressed her feelings to the physician and affirmed her ability to take care of herself and have the unsatisfactory surgery corrected.

Role-Play Using Empty Chair Methods

Role-play, in various forms, is an essential tool of Gestalt therapists. Although Perls was influenced by Moreno's psychodrama, Gestalt therapy rarely uses other people to play roles, in part because that might encourage fragmentation. Rather, an empty chair is more often used to represent a role.

THE TWO-CHAIR METHOD FOR ADDRESSING AN INNER CONFLICT This common type of role-play is intended to help people become aware of and resolve inner conflicts, develop clarity, and gain insight into all aspects of a problem (Strumpfel & Goldman, 2002). It can also help people become aware of their self-judgments, how they respond to their self-judgments, and help them to develop compassion for themselves (Barnard & Curry, 2012). Two chairs are used, representing two parts of the person that are in conflict, perhaps the intellect and the body or love and anger. Resolving conflicts involving anger, accompanied by emotions such as shame, grief, and sadness, seems especially therapeutic. The client spends time sitting in each chair and talking from the perspective represented by that chair.

Underlying this exercise is the Gestalt concept of the top dog and the underdog. Perls believed that "we constantly harass ourselves with . . . the top dog/underdog game where part of ourselves attempts to lecture, urge, and threaten the other part into 'good behavior'" (Fagan & Shepherd, 1970, p. 4). The top dog, a sort of superego or conscience, makes judgments and tells the underdog how it should feel, think, or act. The underdog tends to be meek and apologetic but does not really try to change. Although the top dog may seem more powerful, the underdog really has control by refusing to change or cooperate despite feelings of guilt. In addition to having both a top dog and underdog within them, people may cast another person into the role of top dog while they assume the role of the guilty but ineffectual underdog. Some clients seek such a relationship with their clinicians, creating a hierarchical and nonproductive relationship.

When the two-chair method is used to address an inner conflict or split, the dialogue generally begins with the top dog or dominant part of the person expressing strong criticism of the other part, which is likely to become defensive and vulnerable. As the dialogue continues, the clinician encourages the critic to become even harsher while prompting the underdog to express its pain and sadness. Recollections, misunderstandings, and previously unspoken and unacknowledged feelings may surface at this point. This, in turn, creates what Perls has described as an "ah-ha" experience: the shock of recognition in which people gain new emotional awareness and understanding. The goal of this exercise is to avoid an impasse and enable the two parts to achieve resolution; the critic becomes more tolerant and accepting, while the underdog gains self-confidence and a direct means of self-expression. People become more able to own and integrate both parts of themselves.

The polarity of the top dog versus the underdog is one of the most well known of the Gestalt polarities. As the name suggests, the top dog polarity is our underlying need to be right, to be in charge, and to appear to be "one up" on other people; at the opposite pole, the underdog is the inclination to be the victim, to act lazy, stupid, or passive, in order to avoid the responsibility of being the top dog. Although each of us swings between these two polarities, the healthy person finds balance, whereas the unhealthy person clings to one of the polar extremes in an effort to avoid emotional pain. This is true with all of the polarities, whether it is connection/separation, strength/vulnerability, or others (Prochaska & Norcross, 2009). If people stay in the either/or mode of the polarities and fail to accept that they are also the opposite of what they pretend to be, they will not experience the entirety of life, the full Gestalt. The full Gestalt takes a both/and approach to life.

THE EMPTY CHAIR METHOD FOR ADDRESSING UNFINISHED BUSINESS According to Strumpfel and Goldman (2002), ". . . significant unmet needs represent unclosed gestalts that have not fully receded from awareness" (p. 196). The empty chair dialogue is a way of addressing and resolving in the imagination those unclosed gestalts. The empty chair might represent another person, a troubling and confusing part of a person's dream or fantasy, or a physical symptom the client is experiencing such as a headache.

Clients visualize in the empty chair a person (or symptom or part of a dream) with whom they have important unfinished business. They then express their thoughts and feelings to that person, in an effort to complete a process that had been interrupted. The goal of this experience is a resolution in which clients develop greater understanding and acceptance of the other person or issue, as well as growth in their own self-confidence.

Sujata, a woman who was born in India, had unfinished business with her father. Constantly trying to earn his approval, she proudly called him with each professional and academic achievement. His usual response was to ignore her information or ask when she was going to produce another grandchild for him. When she finally earned her doctorate after many years of hard work and received the same reply from her father, she became discouraged and devalued her accomplishments. Through an empty chair dialogue with her father, she came to understand the influence of his cultural background and the messages he had received from his parents. This led her to become more tolerant and accepting of his values while maintaining pride in her own accomplishments.

The Body as a Vehicle of Communication

Gestalt therapy seeks to give people a sense of wholeness, enabling them to access and be aware of their thoughts, emotions, and physical sensations. Many people have fairly good awareness of their thoughts and emotions. However, they ignore or cut themselves off from their bodily sensations. Consequently, Gestalt therapists pay particular attention to the messages of the body.

The following strategies are especially useful in focusing attention on the body:

- ***Identification:*** Clinicians remain alert to bodily messages. If they notice that a part of a person's body is in a reactive state, such as fingers tapping on a table or a leg strenuously swinging, they call attention to the movements and ask about their message. A clinician might say, "I notice that your leg began swinging when we started to talk about your relationship with your sister. What is your leg saying?" or "Become your leg and give your leg a voice. What is your leg feeling?"
- ***Locating emotions in the body:*** Another strategy is helping people locate their emotions in the body so that they can more fully experience their feelings. A clinician might say, "You have told me that you feel rage toward your sister. Show me where you are experiencing this rage." Once the client locates the rage, perhaps in her stomach, the clinician can explore the client's physical sensations, enabling her to more fully connect with and express her feelings.
- ***Repetition and exaggeration:*** When they observe body movements or symptoms, clinicians often encourage clients to repeat and exaggerate them. For example, a clinician might say, "I notice you are tapping your foot. I would like you to exaggerate the tapping, do it as hard as you can, and then talk about what feelings come up." The techniques of exaggeration or repetition also can be applied to a tone of voice or a meaningful phrase that the person uses. This intervention focuses attention on where energy is located and can succeed in releasing blocked awareness and energy.

THE USE OF GESTALT THERAPY IN GROUPS

Initially, Gestalt therapy usually took the form of individual therapy practiced in a group. Today, individual therapy is the primary mode of treatment, but use of this approach in a group setting offers many benefits. Gestalt therapy groups focus on both interpersonal dynamics and the dynamics of the group system. Feedback and support from both the clinician and the group members can accelerate the process of awareness and empowerment. Members also can learn vicariously from each other. The use of Gestalt therapy in a group setting has led to the development of several useful techniques.

The Hot Seat

Fritz Perls's work in Big Sur at the Esalen Institute emphasized the use of the hot seat in a group setting. This powerful technique brought him considerable attention, and it was widely adopted by encounter groups during the 1960s and 1970s. The hot seat is a chair, placed in the middle of the group, usually with a box of tissues nearby since sitting in the hot seat often evokes strong emotions. Group members volunteer, one at a time, to spend 5 to 10 minutes in the hot seat, becoming the center of the group's attention. When people are in the hot seat, they are encouraged to express and stay with their feelings. Feedback from the group on their body language and verbal messages promotes their awareness of themselves and their feelings.

Making the Rounds

When making the rounds, people in the hot seat speak to each member of the group, perhaps identifying something they want from that person or something in him or her that reminds them of themselves. Alternatively, group members might take turns giving people in the hot seat feedback, perhaps on their strengths, in an effort to empower them. Like many of the other experiments used in Gestalt therapy, this is a powerful technique that is likely to have an enduring impact on people.

As in all Gestalt therapy, figure/ground dynamics, field theory, and intersubjectivity are considered in Gestalt group therapy (Gaffney, 2012). Gestalt group work can also be applied to clinical supervision (Gaffney, 2008).

TRANSACTIONAL ANALYSIS

Developed by Eric Berne, transactional analysis (TA) has its roots in psychoanalysis but today is often integrated with Gestalt therapy and psychodrama. TA de-emphasizes the unconscious and instead focuses on responsibility, emotional health, and social relationships (Totton, 2010). However, Berne, who originally trained as a psychoanalyst, also stressed the importance of early childhood development and of parental messages. Like Alfred Adler, Berne believed that people form life scripts in childhood that guide their lives. Berne sought to reduce the complexity and increase the relevance of psychoanalytic concepts. His book *Transactional Analysis in Psychotherapy* (1961) was soon followed by *Games People Play* (1964), a bestseller that led to widespread interest in TA. Berne died in 1970, having published eight books and 64 articles.

Theoretical Concepts and Development of Transactional Analysis

Although not as popular as it once was, TA continues to be used, either alone or in combination with Gestalt or other treatment systems. The following information is provided for readers who want to learn more about this approach.

HUMAN DEVELOPMENT AND EGO STATES Berne suggested that people evolve through developmental stages. Although Freud's and Erikson's influences are evident, Berne put his own stamp on the stages through his concept of the three ego states: child, adult, and parent.

- The *child ego state* contains early experiences, emotions, intuitions, inquisitiveness, and the capacity for both joy and shame. The child ego state may talk in superlatives, focus on the self, and manifest such nonverbal behaviors as tears, whining, giggling, and squirming.
- The *adult ego state* is like a computer; it is objective and rational, emphasizes logic over emotion, processes information, integrates messages from the other ego states, and solves problems. This ego state is straightforward, gives opinions, and asks questions. It cannot erase material in the parent or child ego states, but it can integrate or minimize the input from those states.
- The *parent ego state* has two parts: the nurturing parent, which provides support, affirmation, and caring but can be overprotective; and the critical parent, which makes judgments, disapproves and criticizes, and sets standards. The critical parent grows out of the rules, reprimands, praise, and rewards that children receive from parents, teachers, and other authority figures and reflects their conceptions of right and wrong (Harris, 1967). The parent ego state tends to use words such as *always, never,* and *should* and focuses on *you* ("You need to clean your room" or "You aren't doing a good job"). Nonverbal signs include pointing, sighing, and a raised voice. The parent ego state may provide clear guidelines or give mixed messages.

Ideally, the three major ego states (child, adult, and parent) are in balance in the personality. However, if a person relies too heavily on one or two of the ego states, or if one ego state contaminates or intrudes on another, the person is likely to develop difficulties, especially in relationships. For example, the person who has too little adult is likely to be illogical, whereas the person with too much adult will probably be uninteresting. Similarly, the person with too little free child is likely to be constricted and rigid, whereas the person with too much free child may be irresponsible. A structural analysis can assess ego state balance.

TRANSACTIONS Transactions are the basic units of behavior. They involve an exchange of verbal or nonverbal messages between two people. TA describes three types of transactions characterized by the source of the transaction, its target, and the replying ego state:

1. ***Complementary transaction.*** The target and the replying ego states are the same, and the reply is directed to the source ego state. Complementary transactions are likely to lead to interactions and relationships that are clear, open, and rewarding. People say what they mean and can understand what other people are saying. Any disagreements are evident and can be addressed.

   Example A (Figure 10.1)
   Parent (source ego state) to child (target ego state): Please pick up your toys.
   Child (replying ego state) to parent (target of reply): All right, I will.

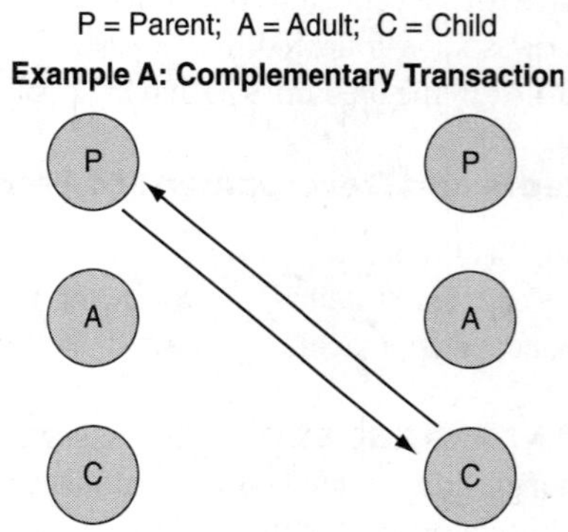

FIGURE 10.1 Complementary Transaction.

2. ***Crossed transaction.*** The target ego state and the replying ego state differ. In crossed transactions, the responses people receive usually are different from what they anticipated, and they may feel ignored and misunderstood.

   Example B (Figure 10.2)
   Adult to adult (target ego state): It's cold out. Do you want to get your coat?
   Child (replying ego state) to parent: Don't tell me what to do!

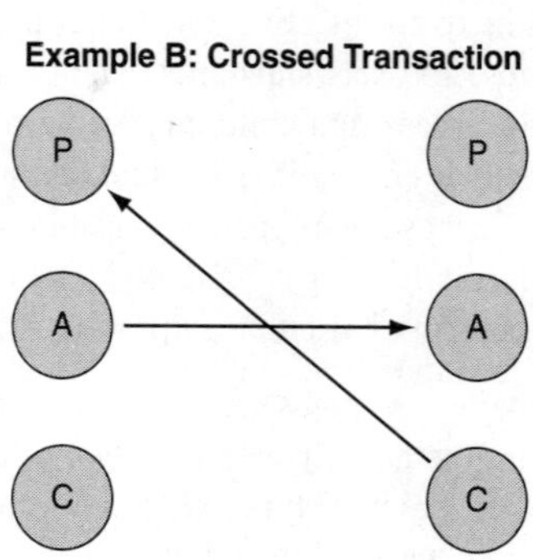

FIGURE 10.2 Crossed Transaction.

Example C (Figure 10.3)

Parent to child (target ego state): Your desk is a mess. Aren't you ever going to clear off that junk pile?

Adult (replying ego state) to adult: You know, I realized the other day that my desk really has become a mess. I'm planning to clear it off as soon as I finish this project.

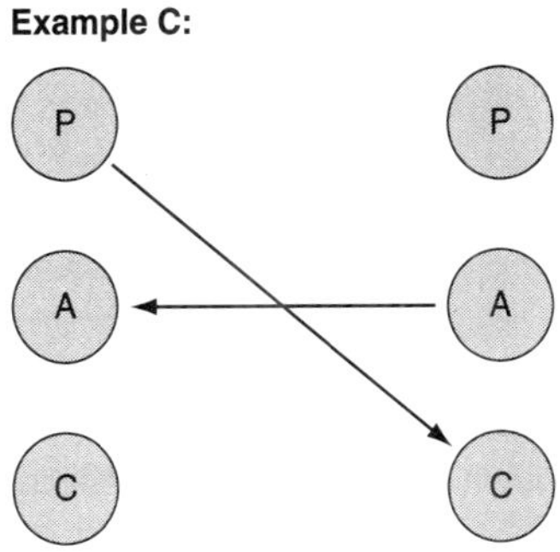

FIGURE 10.3 Example C.

3. ***Ulterior transactions.*** These transactions take place on two levels of communication simultaneously: an overt or social level and a covert or psychological level. They involve more than one ego state as a source or target of a communication. Ulterior transactions are the most problematic: The overt communication is incongruent with the covert communication, and neither person really knows what is in the mind of the other. A continuing pattern of ulterior transactions is likely to lead to a dysfunctional relationship or one that is terminated.

Example D (Person 1 to Person 2, after Person 2 arrives home late; Figure 10.4)

Adult to adult (overt message): Is it after 11 P.M. already? I don't know where the time went tonight.

Parent to child (covert message): I want you to know I noticed that you came in after your curfew. Don't expect an extended curfew this weekend!

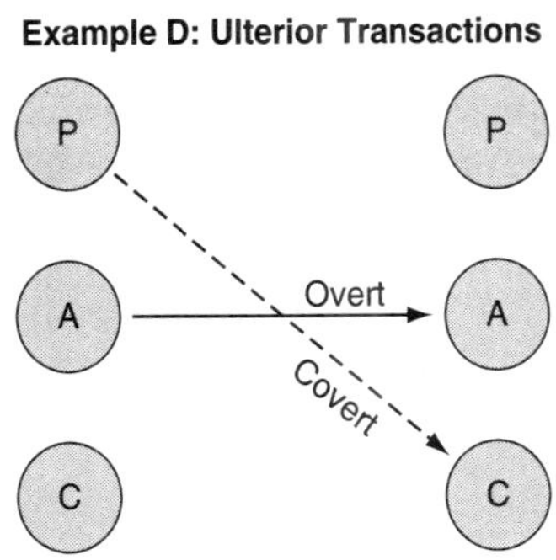

FIGURE 10.4 Ulterior Transaction.

Example E (Person 2 to Person 1; Figure 10.5)

Adult to adult (overt message): Yes, it is after 11. Excuse me; I need to read my e-mail.

Child to parent (covert message): There she goes again, ready to give me a hard time because I came in a few minutes late. I'll go into my room so she won't bother me.

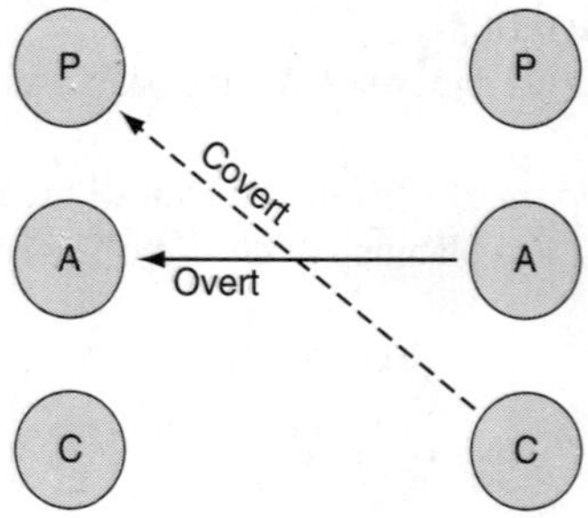

FIGURE 10.5 Example E

The overt transactions in these last examples appear to be complementary transactions from adult to adult. However, the covert transactions are actually from parent to child and from child back to parent, as the thoughts behind the words reflect.

STROKES AND INJUNCTIONS Children's emotional and ego state development is largely determined by the messages and responses they receive from their caregivers. Berne identified two types of messages. *Strokes* are positive messages and are best when they are unconditional, whereas *injunctions* (negative strokes) express disapproval and dislike and include criticisms and prohibitions. Positive and negative strokes may be verbal (such as words of praise or criticism) or nonverbal (such as a hug, a slap, or a lack of eye contact). According to Berne (1961), strokes are the basic motivation for human interaction; and even negative strokes are preferred to no strokes—that is, being ignored and discounted.

BASIC LIFE POSITIONS According to Harris (1967), people develop basic life positions that reflect the value they perceive in themselves and others. These positions can be identified by the age of 5 (Harris & Brockbank, 2011) and are revealed in people's thoughts, feelings, and behaviors. Harris (1967) described four possible life positions:

1. ***I'm not OK; you're OK.*** This position is appropriate for young children who perceive themselves as weak and helpless and seek strokes from others who appear powerful and in control. However, if this position persists, it can cause difficulties. In this position, people typically feel guilty, depressed, powerless, and inferior to others, although they long for acceptance and appreciation. They may have a constricted free child or a rigid adapted child, always following the rules in hope of acceptance. On the other hand, they may act out, viewing themselves as unworthy of positive strokes and preferring negative strokes to none.
2. ***I'm OK; you're not OK.*** This position also might characterize people who received few positive strokes. However, they survived through self-stroking. They grow up believing that they must rely totally on themselves. They treat others in angry and punitive ways and have a sense of entitlement and grandiosity. They blame others for their difficulties and have little empathy or caring for others. They may engage in criminal behavior or abuse of others.
3. ***I'm not OK; you're not OK.*** This is the most negative of the four positions. As children, people in this position typically were deprived of strokes. Consequently, they become hopeless and even suicidal, seeing no value in themselves or others.
4. ***I'm OK; you're OK.*** In this position, people feel good about themselves and others. While they need strokes, they can be caring and reciprocate those strokes. Harris viewed this as the healthiest of the four positions. These people focus on win–win situations and have a good balance among their ego states.

SCRIPTS According to TA, people develop scripts that guide them through life. These scripts are shaped primarily by the internalized strokes and injunctions that they received as children and reflect their life positions. Scripts lead people to envision their lives a certain way. If life scripts are based on outdated or erroneous information, faulty life scripts such as psychosis, substance abuse, or suicide can result (Totton, 2010). TA believes these faulty life scripts were created by people and can, therefore, be changed.

Treatment Using Transactional Analysis

The goal of TA is not insight into the unconscious but autonomy. According to Berne (1964), this is comprised of awareness, spontaneity, and intimacy. In addition, TA helps people move into an "I'm OK; you're OK" position, achieve balance among their ego states, and make healthy use of their time.

In TA, clinicians assume a flexible role, adapting to the needs of the clients, while always conducting sessions from the adult ego state (Harris & Brockbank, 2011). Collaboration between clients and clinicians is important. Both participate actively and share responsibility for the treatment. Clinicians provide education on the language and concepts of TA and guide the therapeutic process. Clients are expected to be open, responsible for themselves, and willing to take risks to make positive changes. Clinicians are alert to the possibility that the ways in which clients communicate with them may reflect childhood patterns. Carefully used reparenting is sometimes part of TA; clinicians take on a reparative role, providing strokes to compensate for a lack of strokes in the client's childhood.

Contracts are an important component in TA (Muller & Tudor, 2002). They clarify the nature of the treatment process and affirm the roles and responsibilities of clinicians and clients. TA was one of the first approaches to use such an agreement to establish a collaborative and effective client–clinician relationship.

According to Harris (1967), people are prompted to change when they are hurting or bored or discover that they can change. The goal is to obtain a clear picture of the following in each client:

- The balance of the ego states forming the personality
- The nature of the person's transactions with others
- Their games and rackets (dysfunctional, manipulative roles and interactions)
- The person's basic position (e.g., "I'm not OK; you're OK")
- The person's life script.

By analyzing and understanding this information, people become more aware of their patterns and why those patterns developed. This, in turn, frees people to modify patterns and choose healthier ways of relating to others. It enables them to form a more positive picture of themselves and of the people in their lives: "I'm OK; you're OK."

Application of Transactional Analysis

Although it is lacking in an overall theory, as a tool, TA can be easily combined with other experiential therapies. Totton (2010) noted that "TA is inventive, imaginative, observant, eloquent, and fun" (p. 15) and is easily applied and relevant to the problems people bring to treatment. The combination of TA and Gestalt therapy is particularly effective, with TA emphasizing the cognitive and analytical aspects of the person and Gestalt drawing in the affective parts. Transactional analysis has also been integrated with brief psychoanalytic therapy (Mothersole, 2002) and short-term cognitive therapy (Hargaden & Sills, 2002).

TA's combination of systemic and intrapsychic thinking helps couples to differentiate and has been found to be helpful in working with both high-conflict and conflict-avoidant couples. The games people play and transactional lingo is so easy to comprehend that it is also being used to help children and adolescents develop a new way of looking at problems, and for improving the parent–child relationship (Tudor, 2008; Zadeh, Jenkins, & Pepler, 2010).

Harris and Brockbank (2011) promote the use of TA in supervision to help supervisees recognize their own ego states, both in their interactions with clients and in supervision. Ideally, the supervisor relates to supervisees adult to adult, providing feedback in a straightforward and supportive manner. More information on supervision, training programs, family and couples work, and integrating TA with other forms of treatment is available from the International Transactional Analysis Association (http://www.itaaworld.org).

APPLICATION AND CURRENT USE OF GESTALT THERAPY

Current trends in Gestalt therapy integrate relational themes, emotion focus, and attachment theory and the use of experiments in a relational therapy. Clients explore topics of identity, trauma, childhood abuse, and other developmental bruises that may have shaped their early years (Finlay & Evans, 2009). Gestalt therapists focus on the relationship and use much more caring confrontations than was the norm in the 1970s. They help clients to understand the subjective interconnectedness of everything, while also helping them to take responsibility for their own feelings and actions. Topics such as male identity, women's aggression, and ruptures in the therapeutic alliance may all be fodder for discussion in the here and now of the therapy session. For example, the therapist and client might discuss the client's feelings of shame and guilt that resulted from her parent's overly strict socialization process, how that shame is erupting in her current relationship with her husband, what triggers it, and how it impacts the therapy session.

Several meta-analytical analyses of Gestalt effectiveness studies found evidence supporting the use of Gestalt therapy in the treatment of affective disorders, personality disorders, and substance use disorders (Strumpfel, 2006; Strumpfel & Martin, 2004). In addition, research suggests that the positive treatment results from Gestalt therapy are enduring.

Application to Diagnostic Groups

Case studies in the literature show Gestalt therapy being adapted for treatment of a wide range of problems that impact emotion regulation including sexual trauma, narcissistic self-hatred, shame, and aggression (Bloom & Brownell, 2011). Clinicians who work with children and adolescents will find Gestalt play therapy, as developed by Virginia Oaklander (1994, 1997), to be a highly experiential, existential "here-and-now" philosophy for work with children (Blom, 2006). As mentioned earlier, Gestalt family therapy combines a systemic perspective with field theory and provides an integrative and holistic model for couples counseling (O'Neill, 2012).

Gestalt therapy may be helpful to people with eating disorders including anorexia nervosa and bulimia nervosa (Angermann,1998), people with substance use disorders (Clemmens, 2005), and for people who channel emotional concerns into their bodies. Such people might be diagnosed with somatoform disorders (often called psychosomatic illnesses) in which they report physical complaints that have no medical basis. Several relatively large-scale research studies have been conducted using Gestalt therapy with clients such as these. Results show reductions in both physical and psychosocial symptoms (Strumpfel & Goldman, 2002).

Application to Multicultural Groups

Because Gestalt therapy views the individual holistically, it is by definition an inclusive approach. People cannot be understood in isolation, but only within the broader perspective of their historical and social backgrounds. Thus Gestalt innately attends to "cultural difference, historical background, and social perspectives" (Mackewn, 1997, p. 51).

When working with people from a variety of cultures, therapists must be careful to select culturally appropriate interventions that respect non–Western European communication styles. Traditional Asian or Native American clients may view direct and confrontational forms of therapy such as Gestalt to be lacking in respect and sensitivity (Duran, 2006). Similarly clients from cultures that value restraint of strong emotions, unassertiveness, or filial piety, as do many Asian cultures, are likely to feel uncomfortable or intimidated if the counselor uses role-plays, behavioral rehearsal, or the Gestalt empty chair technique (Sue & Sue, 2008). Rather than taking a universal perspective or a one-size-fits-all approach, Sue and Sue recommend therapists show respect for the client's cultural background and adapt their techniques, interventions, energy level, and tone of voice to match the client's. Recognizing when Gestalt techniques such as the empty chair or the hot seat should not be used is equally as important as knowing when to use them.

For example, when working with Asian American clients, using the empty chair technique can be appropriate if the client is struggling to have a conversation with parents about moving out of the family home to be independent and suppressing one's own desires and wishes as an expression of respect and sensitivity to elderly authoritative figures. In comparison, the empty chair technique may not be suitable for the same client with a higher level of psychological distress when exploring and confronting feelings from a traumatic incident such as a history of childhood sexual trauma, causing a strong emotional reaction that is unproductive and harmful.

Gestalt therapy seems particularly appropriate for treatment with people who have disabilities. It could promote their responsibility for themselves, their self-awareness, and the integration of their mind and body (Livneh & Sherwood, 1991).

Gestalt therapy is likely to help people who are dealing with issues of grief and of death and dying because of its emphasis on living life to its fullest in the present. For example, this approach has been used to treat homosexual men diagnosed with HIV/AIDS who were experiencing symptoms of depression (Mulder et al., 1994).

Enns (1987) suggested integrating Gestalt and feminist therapy (discussed in Chapter 11), believing that the Gestalt approach could empower women, promote their self-awareness and establishment of healthy interpersonal boundaries, and facilitate the expression of denied or suppressed emotions. Gestalt therapy also seems likely to help men who are dealing with gender issues, feelings of powerlessness, and impaired awareness of themselves and their emotions.

Application to Other Groups

Gestalt therapy has been used with low-achieving adolescents and high school students (Strumpfel & Goldman, 2002); to help middle school students deal with the suicide of a classmate (Alexander & Harman, 1988); and to help pregnant women prepare for the birth of their children. Gestalt therapy's present orientation, as well as its use of powerful exercises, can quickly bring all aspects of an issue into awareness and encourage closure as well as growth. Used skillfully, and adapted to the needs of a particular client or group, the range of this approach is almost unlimited.

Current Use of Gestalt Therapy

Bowman (2012) speaks of the growth of Gestalt therapy during the past 20 years as nothing short of a Renaissance. He attributes this resurgence in Gestalt popularity to the fact that Gestalt therapists have become even more aware of the importance of the client–clinician relationship and strive to establish a true I–thou collaborative relationship rather than adopting the charismatic and powerful role modeled by Fritz Perls. At the same time, they have de-emphasized pathology and reduced reliance on techniques.

Gestalt therapy is flexible enough to be easily integrated with a broad range of other treatment systems. The empty chair and two-chair dialogues of Gestalt therapy as well as other strategies also have been integrated into new process-experiential therapies discussed earlier in Chapter 8. The Gestalt approach to dreamwork, as well as the use of role-plays, continues to play a prominent part in treatment.

Gestalt therapy is actively evolving through the work of many practitioners and at more than 60 Gestalt therapy institutes around the world (Wagner-Moore, 2004). Although Fritz Perls was the embodiment of Gestalt therapy during his lifetime, his ideas have attracted many followers and live on.

EVALUATION OF GESTALT THERAPY

Like other treatment approaches, Gestalt therapy has both strengths and limitations. Because of its powerful nature, clinicians need to be particularly aware of its limitations and appropriate use.

Limitations

Gestalt techniques are not for everybody. They can be powerful motivators for change, or have limited applicability, especially with people who have severe cognitive disorders or impulse control disorders—acting out, delinquency, and explosive disorders—or with people who have sociopathic or psychotic symptoms (Saltzman, 1989). Gestalt techniques may even cause harm if not used carefully (Wagner-Moore, 2004). Other criticisms of the therapy include that it focuses too much on felt bodily sensations and not enough on cognitions, and that getting in touch with internal polarities to relieve emotional problems sounds too much like blaming the victim. Due to its emphasis on self-regulation, people who come from collectivist cultural backgrounds and those who are uncomfortable putting themselves first may have difficulty with the "I-ness" instead of "we-ness" of Gestalt therapy (Prochaska & Norcross, 2009, p. 197).

Polster and Polster (1993) addressed other possible shortcomings, expressing concern about the risk of oversimplification as well as of neglecting important past concerns in the service of promoting immediacy. They also speculated that some clinicians might be more concerned with replicating the charismatic style of Fritz Perls than finding their own way to use this approach and really understanding its underlying theory and philosophy. Gestalt therapy also runs the risk of overemphasizing emotions and ignoring cognitions, which most clinicians now view as important determinants of emotions and vehicles for modifying feelings.

In addition, Gestalt therapy tends to evoke strong emotional reactions. In one group therapy session, a woman in the hot seat became so anxious that she lost control of her bladder, which led her to experience shame and social withdrawal. Thus, just as this approach has the power to do good, it also has the power to do harm. Its strategies are appealing and may seem deceptively simple, but in reality they require a skilled and experienced clinician who can determine their appropriate use, guide people through the treatment process, and protect them. This is more likely to happen if clinicians do not take on the powerful role embodied by Fritz Perls but, instead, temper that role with support, education, exploration of cognitions, and recognition of the importance of culture and background (Stoehr, 2009). In addition, combining Gestalt strategies with those from other approaches, including process-experiential and cognitive–behavioral therapy, reduces the risk of overemphasizing emotions and creates a more supportive treatment environment.

Strengths and Contributions

Despite these limitations, Gestalt therapy has many strengths. Studies on the impact of the empty chair and two-chair experiences have been particularly positive. In one study, when compared to empathic responses, the two-chair technique resulted in greater depth of experience and greater awareness than the empathic techniques (Greenberg, Elliott, & Lietaer, 1994; Strumpfel, 2006). The two-chair technique has also been empirically validated for reducing marital conflict, indecision, conflict splits, and other interpersonal difficulties (Strumpfel & Martin, 2004; Wagner-Moore, 2004). When research compares Gestalt therapy to cognitive–behavioral therapy, the two have comparable positive outcomes. In two large studies of Gestalt therapy, 73% of the clients showed "a strong to mid-range improvement in the symptoms and problems that led them to seek therapy; only 5% suffered a worsening in their symptoms. . . . Ninety percent of all clients reported that they had learned strategies in Gestalt therapy with which to successfully combat any reappearing symptoms" (Strumpfel & Goldman, 2002, p. 204). One comparison of cognitive, Gestalt, and supportive, self-directed psychologies for depression found that all treatments were effective, and that Gestalt therapy tends to work best with clients who have low resistance, are overly socialized, and are internalizing (Beutler, Consoli, & Lane, 2005).

The flexibility of Gestalt therapy is one of its strengths, making it naturally integrative. It has been successfully combined with other treatment approaches including transactional analysis, cognitive–behavioral therapy, person-centered therapy, mindfulness meditation, and brief therapy. A manualized approach to Gestalt therapy has been developed and is used for research as well as practice.

Gestalt therapy is a philosophy of life, growth, and change and also provides specific ways to help people realize that growth. It respects the individual and adapts treatment to the needs of each person. Its emphasis on process and the client–clinician relationship is consistent with current understandings of how counseling and psychotherapy effect change. Gestalt therapy is a compassionate approach that can empower people and enable them to have more joy and fulfillment in their lives.

Gestalt therapy has made many contributions to counseling and psychotherapy. The concepts of field theory, of immediacy and wholeness, and the importance of mind–body integration are particularly important and have been assimilated into other theoretical systems (Woldt & Toman, 2005). Similarly, many innovative strategies, including the empty chair, the emphasis on nonverbal messages, Perls's approach to processing dreams, and "I" statements, have achieved wide acceptance. Chair work has been so well accepted that many forget its Gestalt origins. The Gestalt approach to dreamwork has become an often-used and powerful alternative to psychoanalytic dream interpretation. In addition, the work of Gestalt therapists, along with that of the person-centered and existential theorists, established the importance of phenomenological, experiential, and humanistic approaches to treatment as well as the realization that the therapeutic alliance is probably the most important element in successful therapy.

Levin and Levine (2012) sum it up nicely: "The Gestalt philosophy of being can stimulate, inspire and encourage a different view of human nature—a more human vision of and for the future" (p. 1). This Gestalt philosophy transcends cultural boundaries and understands the contextualization of human experience (Polster, 2012). As we move from cultural, political, and religious absolutes to increasing relativity, it is remarkable that Perls's initial theories were right all along. They mesh nicely with what we now know about the world, and set the stage for our discussion of three post-modern constructivist theories—narrative, solution focused, and feminist—which we will consider in the next chapter.

SKILL DEVELOPMENT: GESTALT CHAIRWORK

Gestalt therapy employs various experiential exercises to help clients reexperience (rather than retell) emotionally charged incidents in the here and now of the therapy session. The most effective experiments are those that arise spontaneously in the therapy session as a result of the client's needs in that given moment. Chair work is one of the most effective and frequently used experiments or techniques in Gestalt therapy (Paivio & Greenberg, 1995), developed by Fritz Perls to help people overcome blockages in awareness and work through unfinished business. Rather than intellectualizing or talking about their problems, in Gestalt therapy the client is asked to reexperience the feelings in the here and now of the therapy session.

Clients easily learn the steps in this exercise, and are supported in their emotions and encouraged by their clinicians. Two-chair work includes the following steps (Houston, 2003):

1. Ask the client if he or she wants to participate in chair work.
2. Repeat the names of the two polarities that will be the focus of the work.
3. Ask which polarity is more present in the chair where the client is seated.
4. Encourage the client to make statements from the vantage point of one polarity to the other chair.
5. When the client is ready, suggest that the client move to the second chair and assume that polarity.
6. Remind the client of the statements made from the other seat. Ask for feelings and a response.
7. Continue to suggest that the client move back and forth between the two seats, as appropriate.
8. If the dialogue seems stuck, ask the client what he or she needs from the other polarity. Consider whether there is movement toward change.
9. If not, consider that for the moment, the client has decided to retain the same feelings.
10. If change does occur, continue the two-chair dialogue until the client has integrated the new insight and feelings.

Example

A 37-year-old woman has come to therapy because she is having difficulty accepting responsibility for her failed marriage. She has been experiencing some anger, and in this session begins to recognize that she might have some unfinished business left over from childhood.

CLIENT: I think I'm angry at my mother. It's silly because my mother died before my marriage fell apart, so what could I be mad at her for?

CLINICIAN: Would you like to explore that using the empty chair?

CLIENT: Sure, I guess so.

CLINICIAN: So, you will be exploring the anger that you never expressed to your mother before she died. Which position feels more real for you where you are seated?

CLIENT: Me. Me and my anger.

CLINICIAN: Okay. Now, imagine that your mother is sitting in the other chair. What would you like to tell her?

CLIENT: Mom, I am so mad at you for the way you always coddled Mark [her older brother]. You always yelled at me. I always got in trouble. Even when he did something wrong, you punished *me* for his bad behavior. It was so unfair.

CLINICIAN: Okay. Stay with that feeling. . . .

CLIENT: (raising her voice) I just can't get past how unfair it was. Now that he's an adult he has this sense of entitlement. He doesn't work, and Dad has to support him. It just really makes me mad. You did both of us a disservice. It's not fair. Now that my husband is gone, I need support, too. And where are you? Where is any help for me?

CLINICIAN: Would you like to change chairs and respond from your mother's perspective? Your daughter is very angry at you.

CLIENT (CHANGES CHAIRS):
I know. Honey, I'm sorry you're hurt and upset, but your brother was always so needy. It took him longer to do things, and you know how socially inept he was. I don't believe that I ever punished you for your brother's bad behavior. . . .

CLINICIAN: Switch chairs. Do you have a response to your mother?

CLIENT: I sure do! Of course you knew! You made me hold his hand and walk around the yard smiling as if we were best friends! I was so embarrassed when the neighbors saw us. What were you thinking?

CLINICIAN: Can you keep going with that?

CLIENT: (CHANGES CHAIRS; THINKS FOR A MOMENT FROM HER MOTHER'S PERSPECTIVE THEN RESPONDS THOUGHTFULLY):
Maybe I hoped you would be a good influence on him; you were always so friendly and active. You were the cheerleader, the good student, the good daughter. I never had any problems with you. I hoped you would somehow influence your brother in a positive way.

CLIENT (CHANGES BACK TO HER OWN CHAIR):
Oh, I never thought of that before. I never looked at it from my mother's perspective.

CLINICIAN: Stay in the role.

CLIENT (BEGINS TO CRY SOFTLY):
I never realized how difficult it was for you, Mom. You had to raise us and Dad was always working, then it seems as soon as I went to college you got sick, and I never had a chance to know you as an adult. We never had time to have these conversations.

CLINICIAN (GENTLY):
It sounds like you're feeling very sad.

CLIENT: It never occurred to me that my mother was frustrated, too.

CLINICIAN: What's it like for you to see your mother's frustration?

CLIENT: It's like she's human. She had her issues, too, and as a mother I think she tried to do the best that she could. I just wish she hadn't died so young. I would really like to talk to her.

This example illustrates how use of the two-chair technique can quickly stir up emotionally laden content. Therapists should remember to use caution when employing this technique and to avoid using the two-chair technique with populations in which it is contraindicated.

CASE ILLUSTRATION

The following dialogue illustrates the use of the two-chair technique with Roberto to address a split within him. This is one of the most powerful and widely used of the Gestalt strategies.

CLINICIAN: Roberto, you have talked about feeling like there is a split within you between your tough side and your caring side and how hard it is for you to express that caring side. I have set up two chairs here, one to represent your tough side and one to represent your caring side. I would like you to role-play each side of you while sitting in the chair that represents that side.

ROBERTO: All right. I'll start out with the tough side. That's the easy one. I was the biggest bully on the block.

CLINICIAN: Would you talk in the present?

ROBERTO: Okay. I am the biggest bully on the block. No one messes with me. I have quite a reputation. My father is proud that I can take care of myself. I protect the younger kids.

CLINICIAN: Now change seats.

ROBERTO: Well, here I am, in the caring seat. I'm not sure what to say. I do care deeply about my family, Edie and Ava. I make sure they are safe, that we have enough money, that Ava goes to a good school. But they say that's not enough. I feel invisible. No one seems to see me and all that I do.

CLINICIAN: What do you look like?

ROBERTO: I am small and weak.

CLINICIAN: Continue to be the caring side and talk to the tough side in the empty chair.

ROBERTO: I feel overshadowed by you. I try to let people know I'm here, but you're all they notice. I feel powerless and helpless.

CLINICIAN: Now change chairs and have the tough side talk to the caring side.

ROBERTO: I know you're there, but I want to keep you hidden. What will it do to my reputation if people see you? They won't think I'm the tough guy anymore. You're not worth much to me.

CLINICIAN: Change chairs and continue the conversation.

ROBERTO: Yes, I know your tough reputation is important to you. But I'm important too. Without me, you don't get along very well with people. Edie gets mad at you, and Ava goes off and cries. You need me even if you don't know it. I don't want to be as big as you, but maybe you could let me grow a little bigger.

CLINICIAN: How could the caring side grow?

ROBERTO: It . . . I could exercise. That's how the tough side got so big. Practice. If I could just keep the tough guy from sitting on me every time I try to show my face. . . .

CLINICIAN: Can you tell him that?

ROBERTO: Yeah. Hey, tough guy, how about giving me a little space? I won't take over your turf. You don't have to be afraid of me ruining your reputation. I have respect for you. You worked hard to get where you are. Can you give a little guy a chance?

CLINICIAN: Change chairs again and respond.

ROBERTO: Yeah, I guess I could do that. As long as we agree that I run the show, I'm in charge . . . at least for now.

Roberto has a top dog and an underdog as well as a split within himself. His tough side has served him well, and he identifies strongly with that aspect of his personality; but he has nearly cut himself off from his caring side. This dialogue increased his awareness of these two sides of himself and the negative impact the neglect of his caring side has on his life. Although Roberto is still apprehensive about revealing his caring side, he has moved toward integrating the two sides and allowing them to coexist. He also has begun to recognize that he does not need to choose between the two.

EXERCISES

Large-Group Exercises

1. You now have had the opportunity to learn about three approaches to counseling and psychotherapy that emphasize the importance of emotions and sensations. Discuss and list the similarities and differences among person-centered counseling, existential therapy, and Gestalt therapy. Then discuss which approach is more appealing to you and the benefits each has to offer clients.
2. Review the illustration of the use of the two-chair experience with Roberto. Using this dialogue as a starting point, discuss how a Gestalt therapist would continue to work with him. What blocks and impasses do you see in Roberto? From what you know about him, can you identify other splits that he might be struggling with in addition to the tough/caring one? What unfinished business do you think Roberto has? What do you imagine Roberto would look like if his body expressed his emotions? How would he sit? What would his eye contact be like? Would he have characteristic gestures? Plan experiments you might suggest to Roberto to promote his awareness and integration.
3. Look around you, at your clothes, your books and other possessions, and the contents of the room. Pick an object with which you identify. Write down the object as well as a few "I" statements, speaking from the point of view of the object, such as "I am a chalkboard. I am blank and impressionable. I have little character but am here to reflect the ideas of others." Have volunteers share their objects and accompanying statements.

Small-Group Exercises

1. Each dyad should engage in an exercise using the two-chair or empty chair technique. The person in the client role should identify an internal or external conflict that can be represented by two chairs. With the help of the person in the clinician role, the client should engage in a 10-minute dialogue between the two people or aspects that represent the conflict. Be sure to bring closure to the experience.

Feedback following the exercise should focus on:

- The effectiveness of the exercise
- The use of questions and other interventions that reflect Gestalt therapy
- How Gestalt therapy might help the client deal with the split or conflict that has been presented
- The nonverbal messages of both client and clinician
- The therapeutic alliance
- The strengths of the role-play
- Ways in which the dialogue might have been improved.

Individual Exercises

The individual exercises in this chapter are especially challenging. If you want to engage in these exercises but have difficulty doing so, you might seek help from your professor, a counselor, or someone else you trust.

1. Observe your own body language, your eye contact, the way you sit, the way you use your hands, and any other body movements you display. What messages do they seem to give? What can you learn about yourself from your body language? Did you notice any incongruities between your verbal and your nonverbal messages? Think about whether your body language reflects any internal splits or disowned parts of yourself. Write about this in your journal.
2. Conduct an experiment with yourself using the top dog/underdog technique. Sit quietly in a room with two empty chairs and think for a moment about a situation in the past week in which you struggled with yourself. Perhaps you procrastinated on a homework assignment, or were rude to your friend. Voice the dialogue of the top dog as he justifies his actions. Now, move to the second chair and respond from the underdog position. Pay attention to how you talk to your "two selves." Notice any judgments in how you talk to yourself. Instead of being judgmental, try to compassionately defend yourself. Write down in your journal what you noticed, how it felt to be superior and "right" on the one hand, and what it felt like to be judged. What price do you pay for listening to the judgmental self? Write some ideas about how you can be less critical and more compassionate in your self talk. What did you learn about yourself from this exercise?
3. Think about a criticism you recently made of someone else. Turn the statement around so that you apply it to yourself. For example, instead of saying, "My friend is an irresponsible person," say "I am an irresponsible person." Think about whether the new statement has any truth to it. Write about this in your journal.

Summary

Fritz Perls, along with his wife Laura Perls, developed Gestalt therapy in the 1950s. This is a humanistic and phenomenological approach that pays particular attention to emotions and sensations. The concept of Gestalt implies that patterns and wholes are important to people. Gestalt therapists believe that we all have a natural drive toward integration, homeostasis, and self-actualization. However, people sometimes deny or become alienated from parts of themselves or their world. This can lead to fragmentation, an overload of unfinished business, and what Perls termed growth stagnation.

Gestalt therapy is an active approach that emphasizes the importance of a trusting, collaborative, I–thou relationship between client and clinician. The security of that relationship enables people to engage in growth-promoting experiments developed by the clinician to meet the needs of each client. Techniques such as dreamwork, the hot seat, the empty chair, the two-chair technique, the fantasy trip, the use of "I" statements, a focus on "what" and "how," and attention to nonverbal communication all help people achieve the goals of Gestalt therapy, which include awareness, integration, and actualization.

Recommended Readings

Berne, E. (1961). *Transactional analysis in psychotherapy.* New York, NY: Grove.

Berne, E. (1964). *Games people play.* New York, NY: Grove.

Buber, M. (1970). *I and thou.* New York, NY: Scribner.

Harris, T. A. (1967). *I'm OK—You're OK.* New York, NY: Avon.

James, M. (1996). *Born to win: Transactional analysis with Gestalt experiments.* Reading, MA: Addison Wesley.

Levine, T. B. (2012). *Gestalt therapy: Advances in theory and practice.* New York, NY: Routledge.

Oaklander, V. (2007). *Hidden treasure: A map to the child's inner self.* London, UK: Karnac Books.

Perls, F. (1969a). *Gestalt therapy verbatim.* Lafayette, CA: Real Person.

Perls, F. (1969b). *In and out of the garbage pail.* Lafayette, CA: Real Person.

Philippson, P. (2009). *The emergent self: An existential-Gestalt approach.* London, UK: Karnac Books Ltd.

Polster, E., & Polster, M. (1993). Fritz Perls: Legacy and invitation. *Gestalt Journal, 16*(2), 23–25.

Woldt, A. L., & Toman, S. M. (Eds.). (2005). *Gestalt therapy: History, theory, and practice.* Thousand Oaks, CA: Sage.

Additional Sources of Information

http://www.aagt.org—Website of the Association for the Advancement of Gestalt Therapy.

http://www.gestalt.org—The Gestalt Therapy page. Includes a bookstore, a news board, and online access to the *Gestalt Journal*, the *Gestalt Review*, and the *International Gestalt Journal.*

http://www.gestalttherapy.net—The Gestalt Therapy Network maintains both a directory of Gestalt practitioners and a continuously updated bibliography of Gestalt resources. A news board, forum, and discussion groups are accessible to people interested in this approach to treatment.

http://www.newyorkgestalt.org—This website for the New York Institute for Gestalt Therapy offers suggested readings, a message board, articles, and training opportunities.

http://www.gestalttherapy.org—Website for the Pacific Gestalt Institute.

http://www.itaaworld.org—This website for the International Transactional Analysis Association provides information on events, products, training, certification, and members of the association. It is home to the online journal—*TAJ*—which has been published since 1970.

CHAPTER 11

Emerging Approaches Emphasizing Emotions and Sensations

As in all dynamic fields, new theories and strategies of counseling and psychotherapy continually emerge, while established approaches undergo expansion and revision. This chapter, which concludes Part 3, introduces three approaches that emphasize emotions and sensations and that take a postmodern, constructivist approach to psychotherapy: narrative therapy, solution-focused brief therapy, and feminist therapy. All three have much to offer when used either on their own or when integrated with other treatment approaches.

The three approaches reviewed in this chapter are consistent with humanistic theories that focus on emotions. They share experiential, relational, and existential constructs with the other theories we have learned about in Part 3. They also share the following attributes; they are:

- Holistic
- Sensitive to issues of diversity, multiculturalism, individual differences, and people's multiple roles and perspectives
- Supportive of a clinician role that is more facilitator than expert
- Appreciative that therapy is a bidirectional process and that both client and clinician are affected and changed by psychotherapy.

More information on the hallmarks of each of the three approaches covered in this chapter is provided in the discussion of each treatment system. First, however, we consider a brief overview of postmodern, constructivist philosophy.

CONSTRUCTIVIST THEORY: THE HEART OF POSTMODERN PSYCHOLOGY

A worldwide paradigm shift is changing the way in which we view reality. This new way of thinking permeates the sciences, the arts, and all aspects of life. In effect, the very foundations of objective knowledge, so central to the institutions of science and education, are eroding. The increasing awareness of the validity of multiple perspectives makes it futile to look for one objective reality. Concepts of truth, honesty, and authenticity are subjective, based on the individual and his or her perception of the world. Instead of one fixed, agreed-on reality, reality is co-created, constructed by the individual based on what he or she perceives and experiences. "Constructivism" is the term used to describe this philosophy.

This new way of thinking is reminiscent of the classic tale of the blind men encountering an elephant. Each touched a different part of the elephant and so described the elephant in a different way. Their perceptions of the elephant were colored not only by their direct and limited contact with the elephant, but by their own life experiences and interactions, which gave them the language and comparisons they used to understand what the elephant was like.

According to Mahoney (1988), "Constructivist theories recognize that psychological realities are inherently private, even when they are shared collectively, and that the forum of psychological changes lies in the domain of those dynamic processes referred to as the self" (p. 9). He further stated, "Psychological construction refers to a family of theories that share the assertion that human knowledge and experience entail the (pro)active participation of the individual" (p. 2).

Five Basic Themes of Constructivism

Mahoney (2003, p. 4) identified five basic themes that further clarify the nature of constructivism:

1. ***Active agency.*** People are active participants in shaping their lives. Through choices, actions, and the focus of our attention, we continuously influence our experiences.

2. ***Order.*** People seek order and organization and to make meaning of their experiences. Too much order can lead to emotional overcontrol, whereas too little order can lead to loss of balance and direction.
3. ***Self and identity.*** According to Mahoney (2003), "Relationships with self are critical to life quality. These include self-concept, body image, self-esteem, and capacities for self-reflection and self-comfort" (p. 33). When our sense of self becomes inflexible or fragmented, we are likely to experience both intrapersonal and interpersonal difficulties.
4. ***Social-symbolic processes.*** Order, meaning, and identity stem largely from social interactions and symbolic processes (e.g., language, images, stories).
5. ***Dynamic dialectical development.*** People experience constant cycles of experience that can lead to organization or disorganization. We seek balance and may resist change in healthy and self-protecting ways. At the same time, some disorganization is necessary for reorganization.

While agreeing that reality can never really be known, there are three important distinctions in constructivist thinking: radical constructivism, social constructivism, and critical constructivism. Each of these schools of thought differs in the nature of the relationship between the person and the world.

Radical constructivists believe that reality is different for everyone and is limited by the biological structure of the brain and its abilities. Therefore it is impossible to know if reality exists outside the boundaries of our mind.

Social constructivists believe that reality is created through social constructs such as language, culture, and the society in which a person is born and raised. Therefore there is not one objective reality, but rather multiple ways of viewing the world based on these and other variables. Viewed in this way, the development of a cohesive sense of self is impossible. As Gergen (1991) relates in his book *The Saturated Self,* the person is overwhelmed with multiple culturally defined selves interacting with the multiple selves of others.

Critical constructivists are similar to the social constructivists, but also believe that "both individual and social processes contribute to the creation of reality" (Neimeyer & Raskin, 2001). Meanings are enacted between the person and the world and although we can't know it directly, the universe is real (Kelly, 1955).

Many approaches to therapy have emerged from the postmodern, constructivist perspective. Narrative therapy and the writings of White and Epston (1990), Anderson (2001), Gergen (1985), and others are an outgrowth of social constructivism, as is positive psychology and other strengths-based practices including solution-focused brief therapy. Feminist therapy and multiculturalism have their roots here as well. All of these theories are phenomenological and experiential and focus on people's perceptions of themselves and their worlds. These approaches adopt the postmodern assumption that there is no such thing as universal, objective knowledge and that our perceptions reflect the language, values, and beliefs of our particular community or social system. These theories are holistic and seek to understand people fully and from many perspectives. They also assume that the creation and experience of meaning are central to human life (Mahoney, 2003).

In all constructivist theories the therapeutic alliance is collaborative and nonauthoritarian. Client and clinician co-create a connection in which they differ only in terms of roles and training. Clinicians do not direct the process or seek to persuade, analyze, or instruct. Rather, they use empathy, encouragement, affirmation, reflection, elaboration, and metaphor to advance the treatment. They provide clients a safe place, focus on clients' strengths and abilities, and are caring and compassionate. Clinicians help people "construct more coherent and comprehensive self-theories or, as coauthors, assist clients in the identification and revision of central themes in their personal narratives," but it is the clients who are the primary change agents (Neimeyer, 1993, p. 230).

Constructivism views people in positive and optimistic terms, seeing them as "pro-active, goal-directed, and purposive organisms" (Neimeyer, 1993, p. 223). People operate according to the knowledge they possess, reflecting their construction of their experiences and actions. Knowledge evolves and changes with new experiences and perceptions. A central goal of constructivist treatment is helping people develop possibilities and recognize that experiences have alternative meanings and interpretations. People's knowledge can then be assessed and either changed or validated, leading to knowledge that allows more satisfying ways of being.

Treatment initially begins with a focus on current problems and distress, then shifts to an exploration of patterns or recurrent difficulties, and finally moves to an understanding of underlying processes or constructions that perpetuate patterns. This can enable people to develop more rewarding ways of being and coping.

Constructivist approaches situate the self in the social context (Neimeyer, 1993) and suggest that people can best be understood and helped if attention is paid to that context. Constructivist clinicians pay considerably more attention to background than do other treatment approaches discussed in Part 3 of this book and believe that early attachment plays an important part in shaping who we are. They also attend to thoughts, actions, and emotions to help people achieve a sense of integration (Mahoney, 1988). In his work as a psychologist and professor in the Midwest, George Kelly (1905–1967) developed the idea of the "personal construct." Basically the idea is that people create roles or ideas about themselves and then check them out, much like a scientist tests a hypothesis (Fransella & Neimeyer, 2005). Kelly's early work on self constructs laid the foundation for the later development of narrative, solution-focused, and feminist therapies.

Narrative therapy is *postmodern* because it is constructivist in nature, emphasizing the belief that our personal realities and self-images are not absolute but are created and maintained by our societies and historical contexts. "There is no stable, fixed, knowable or essential self or identity, as self and identity can emerge only within linguistic, cultural, and relational practices" (Brown & Augusta-Scott, 2007, p. xv).

Although constructivist therapy is not associated with a specific group of techniques, some strategies are emphasized in this approach. Language is an important focus in constructivism; people make meaning through language. As Lynch (1997) stated, language not only labels human experience; it forms it. Deconstructing or loosening constructs is another frequently used strategy, as are co-creating new constructs, promoting empowerment, exploring themes and metaphors, expanding people's behavioral options, externalizing, and helping people create support or referent groups (Richert, 2010). Strategies that integrate mind, body, and spirit such as breathing exercises, meditation, and relaxation also are important tools used in constructivist therapy (Mahoney, 2003).

Constructivist therapy has captured the attention of many clinicians because of its compatibility with postmodern clinical thought. It appreciates the importance of the individual in society, diversity, and the client–clinician collaboration. It is holistic, integrative, and flexible. It is respectful and optimistic, viewing people's efforts to cope as sources of knowledge that can promote positive change.

The *Journal of Constructivist Psychology* promotes and disseminates the rapidly expanding research on this treatment approach. According to Mahoney (2003), constructivist themes run through all areas of contemporary society including education, government, science, and human resources. The expressions of constructivism in psychology will continue to grow in importance and influence globally, impacting spirituality, ethics, and discourse on world peace. Now we look more deeply at three postmodern constructivist approaches: narrative, solution-focused, and feminist therapy.

NARRATIVE THERAPY

According to narrative therapy, people are interpretive beings who make meaning of themselves and their world through the language of stories that have become part of themselves, as well as their understanding of those stories. Narrative theorists believe that through exploration, deconstruction, and revision of problematic stories, people can shift their perceptions and create alternative scripts, leading to greater empowerment and the ability to more successfully manage their lives.

Narrative therapy takes the phenomenological emphasis of humanistic treatment systems one step further; not only do narrative therapists believe that people's perceptions determine their realities, but they believe that loosening and changing people's perceptions are the best routes to facilitating their positive development. Rather than looking at clients as having pathological disorders, narrative therapists often consider people who consult them to be "under the influence of problem-saturated stories" (Malinen, Cooper, & Thomas, 2011, p. 13). With narrative tools such as mapping, scaffolding of conversations, externalization, and others that will be discussed later, narrative therapists collaborate with clients to deconstruct their stories and then create new ones to essentially reauthor their lives. This is the essence of narrative therapy.

The Development of Narrative Therapy

Narrative therapy had its roots in Australia in the work of Michael White and David Epston (1990). However, clinicians and researchers worldwide have shown interest in its application and study. Important influences on narrative therapy include the ideas of Gregory Bateson, George Kelly, and French philosopher Michel Foucault.

But it was the collaborative efforts of White and Epston that led to the development of narrative therapy. Until his death of a heart attack in 2008, White lived in Adelaide, Australia, where he was codirector of the Dulwich Centre. Other important influences on White's philosophy and thinking included family systems theory, cybernetics, and Vygotsky's social development theory.

In his eulogy of his colleague and friend, Epston, a New Zealand therapist and coauthor of the seminal work on narrative therapy *Narrative Means to Therapeutic Ends* (1990), noted that Michael White "caught the wave of post-modernism earlier than anyone else in the field of psychology" (Epston, 2008, p. 6) and was able to combine his interest in philosophy, particularly the post-structuralist philosophy of French philosopher Michel Foucault, with his desire to help people, especially those who had become disenfranchised or marginalized by society. Bateson suggested that, in order to detect and acquire new information, people must engage in a process of comparison in which they distinguish between one body of information and another (Monk, 1997). Building on this concept, White discovered that by drawing people's attention to subtle changes in their lives, he could foster new insights, promote empowerment, and help people develop better ways to resolve difficulties.

French philosopher Michael Foucault's writing on the interrelationship of knowledge and power led White to address the damaging effects of encouraging people to adjust and comply with stereotyped standards of behavior that could undermine their efforts to lead a life of their own design (Monk, 1997; White & Epston, 1989). White believed that only through knowledge could people truly be the authors of their own lives.

In several important ways, narrative therapy represents a departure from conventional counseling and psychotherapy. White has been described as a "therapeutic anthropologist" (Lee, 1997, p. 5), and referred to himself as a consultant. He did not seek to heal or fix people but to learn about them, understand them, and provide a different and helpful perspective.

Lee (1997) summarized the narrative approach to treatment as addressing "the human dilemma of existence in a postmodern world by focusing on the linguistic and discursive ways that people construct their lives. It assumes that humans are interpretive beings in the phenomenological sense, active in the interpretation of everyday life and in the attribution of meaning through stories or self-narratives" (pp. 5–6). In other words, narrative therapists believe that people's lives are created and interpreted through stories: the ones they hear, the ones they create in their own minds, and the ones they tell and retell. There are no essential truths; realities are constructed and maintained through language, social interactions, and story (Mascher, 2002).

Consider the following example. Suki, a young woman from an Asian background, sought counseling because of her difficulty trusting others, her inability to form close relationships, and what she termed her "self-hatred" that led her to cut herself repeatedly. Suki's mother had told her the following story many times since Suki was a young child: "When I became pregnant with you, I was living with your father. He was a terrible man. He beat me, he stayed with other women, and he took all the money I had. I wanted so badly to leave him. When I found out I was pregnant, I was devastated. I thought I would never be able to escape. So I went to a wise woman in the village and asked her to help me abort you. I did everything she told me, but it didn't work. I went back to her, and she told me other things to do. I did everything again, but it still didn't work. Then I decided that this baby was meant to be. I packed up everything I could carry and ran away. I found my way to the home of my aunt, who took me in and helped me until you were born."

Hearing this story again and again led Suki to adopt a negative view of herself and her world. She perceived herself as unwanted by both her father and her mother. She saw herself as a burden to her mother and viewed men as abusive and untrustworthy. She believed that she could only survive if she avoided closeness and intimacy with others; at the same time, she viewed herself as unworthy of survival and thought that everyone would have been happier if the abortion had been successful. Her self-injurious behavior and her inability to trust reflected views of herself and the world that grew out of the story her mother had told her. Although Suki's mother later married an American man who brought Suki and her mother to the United States and was a loving father to Suki, the story continued to have an impact. Stories give messages and can become the road maps of our lives. Narrative therapy helped Suki to deconstruct those stories, consider alternatives, choose a preferred path, and improve her life.

NATURE OF THE STORIES People have a large repertoire of stories that they carry with them. All stories are accepted as legitimate and important in narrative therapy. However, stories tend to fall into several categories. Many people have a single dominant story that shapes who they are, as did Suki. A dominant story typically acts as a sort of tyrant that censors and changes a person's other stories and can send those stories into oblivion. What White (1986) called *specifications of personhood*—the information in the stories that tells people how to behave as individuals or family members—act as restraints and keep people stuck in and limited by their dominant stories.

Lost, untold, or marginalized stories also need to be told and may serve people better than their dominant stories, particularly if the lost stories portray a life in which problems are either solved or absent. Suki's stepfather told her stories about how she used to make up poems when she was a child and how much he enjoyed reading her poems. However, as long as her single dominant story was in control, Suki paid little attention to her stepfather's stories, which reflected appreciation for her intelligence and creativity. Accessing those untold stories and others helped Suki value herself and use her intelligence and creativity to relate more successfully to others.

People are constantly trying to make sense of life's events. It is the narratives they tell themselves that determine self-identity. Richert (2010) identifies three types of stories that result in unhappiness or dysfunction:

1. Some narratives are too constricting but have become accepted by the dominant culture. Therefore, people who do not have all options available to them become labeled or otherwise

constrained, which leads to personal frustration and dissatisfaction. Narratives around themes of gender or psychological illness are frequently impacted by such conventions.

2. When a person's story is fragmented or disorganized, distress can occur. When this happens, the person's reality becomes fragmented and difficult to cope with, leading to stress, anxiety, depression, and ultimately, an inability to conduct goal-oriented behavior.
3. If disrupted, a personal narrative can also result in psychological distress. Disruptions occur when a person is no longer able to participate in the construction of his or her life lives, or if they fail to recognize or take up the process of storytelling. Richert (2010) makes an important distinction between the distress that occurs from these "disorders of construction" as opposed to the previous two which result in "construction of disorders" (p.18).

In all cases, narrative therapists believe the solution is to help people open up new pathways and possibilities for living so they can find greater satisfaction in life. The work begins by eliciting stories.

Therapeutic Alliance

In narrative therapy, the clinician is a consultant in a partnership. Clients are the experts on themselves and their stories, whereas the clinician is the expert on narrative therapy. The two are coauthors and collaborators, sharing the responsibility for shaping the treatment process. According to Brown (2007) "both bring knowledge and agency to the conversation" (p. 4).

Malinen and other narrative therapists have referred to themselves as "collaborationists" to describe the live interactions and encounters that a therapist has with clients that reflect working with clients to create a shift in consciousness rather than solving problems. "In the sea of collaboration," he wrote, "there are many waves" (Malinen et al., 2011, p. 12).

Narrative therapists place great emphasis on being respectful and encouraging of clients' strengths and resources. Although clinicians do share their own perceptions and stories, including those about the clients, they assume a tentative stance, never prescribing or judging. Concepts such as resistance, denial, and mental pathology, which may give the clinician the upper hand, are not a part of narrative therapy. In fact, resistance is viewed as the client's effort to make the pace of treatment more comfortable for them.

Narrative clinicians encourage and facilitate rather than change people. They are inquiring rather than knowing, asking questions about the content and context of stories, as well as their meaning to the person. They are active in suggesting exercises, offering new viewpoints, and soliciting feedback (Richert, 2003). They help their clients appreciate themselves and enable them to play an important part in their treatment. Clinicians use careful listening, empathy, summarization, and paraphrasing to give people ownership over their right to create themselves and to listen to themselves in new ways that engender courage, hope, and resourcefulness.

Typical of the treatment approaches discussed in this chapter, narrative clinicians remain aware of the part they play in clients' development and often discuss this with them. Narrative therapists are "participatory witnesses" who engage in "interactive mirroring," which they openly acknowledge to the client reflects themselves as well as the client. Narrative therapists are active, asking questions designed to help people deconstruct old stories and identify new possibilities that can lead to fresh outcomes (Richert, 2010). This collaborative process between client and clinician is called co-construction or co-authoring of stories, and is an essential part of the therapeutic process. Brown (2007) writes: "Narrative therapy emphasizes the resurrection of the suppressed voice" (p. 77) and brings into the open knowledge that has been disqualified. Clinician and client work together to share meanings and identify expectations inherent in the culture, gender, race, or other relevant frameworks, to put them in context and therefore decrease their power or effect on the client.

Similarly, every effort is made to "elevate" the client and decrease the therapist's position of power. In narrative therapy, clients are encouraged to ask questions about the reasoning behind the therapist's questions, and therapist self-disclosure is considered helpful because it reduces the power differential in the relationship (Richert, 2010).

Strategies

ELICITING STORIES Most people produce stories spontaneously and typically enjoy telling stories. However, those stories that support the dominant theme are usually closest to the surface and most accessible. Narrative therapists have strategies to encourage people to tell a wider variety of stories (Carr, 1998):

- They may ask people to tell alternative stories about a single event or emotion.
- They may suggest that people create a story about themselves and their lives as if they were another person or ask them to assume a different perspective.
- They may suggest that people extend their stories into the future.
- They may ask about neglected aspects of the stories.
- They may ask people to tell stories in which they are more powerful than their problems.

DECONSTRUCTION OF STORIES Before stories can be changed, they must be taken apart, analyzed, and understood. Narrative therapists use several strategies to accomplish this, with their goals being to identify themes and metaphors that are prominent in the stories, enable people to recognize the influence the stories have had on them, and help people see that they did not totally create their stories themselves.

Bruner (2002) speaks of landscapes of consciousness and landscapes of action. *Landscapes of consciousness* are the backdrops of values, feelings, motives, beliefs, and attitudes that recur in a person's stories. *Landscapes of action* are the sequences of behaviors related to events in people's lives that similarly pervade and recur in a person's stories. Questions help people identify, reflect on, determine the meaning of, and perhaps change these landscapes. In Suki's stories, the landscapes of consciousness generally reflected hopelessness, sorrow, and pain. People in her stories usually experienced rejection and loss. In the landscape of action, Suki usually was withdrawn and ineffectual.

Mapping is another approach that can help people reflect on their stories. Clients' presenting problems are identified and linked to their stories, illustrating how their problems emerge and are handled in the stories. Similarly, people are encouraged to look at how their positive interpersonal experiences mesh with and potentially change their dominant stories and landscapes.

White spoke of the difficulty inherent in making changes. He noted that clients need to build scaffolding that bridges the gap between familiar actions and new possibilities. Narrative therapists do not view such agency as coming from within or being independent, but as a series of small steps that integrate support, assistance, learning, and an understanding of the influences that shape important new values. Based on Vygotsky's (1986) model, White (2007) developed a "scaffolding conversations map" (p. 275) that therapists can employ to guide therapeutic conversations and help clients successfully bridge this gap. This technique is discussed further in the Skill Development section at the end of this chapter.

Externalizing is the process of separating people from their problems. Therapists use externalizing language to reinforce that the problem is having an effect on the person rather than the problem being intrinsic to the person or existing within him or her (Payne, 2006). For example, a clinician might say "Anger has power over you" or "Anxiety robbed you of your peace" to help clients separate their identities from the problems. Externalization is facilitated by helping people identify the threads connecting many stories and the assumptions the stories suggest about the self and the world. Once externalization occurs, access points for changing the story can be identified. Careful and deliberate use of language by the clinician facilitates externalization and can empower clients.

This process of externalization seems to conflict with the emphasis of Gestalt therapists on helping people own and take responsibility for their difficulties. However, narrative therapists believe that externalizing and objectifying problems reduces feelings of failure and guilt, decreases unproductive discussions about fault and blame, provides people with new perspectives on their difficulties, reduces blocks to action and change, and opens the way for people to reclaim their lives from their problems (White, 1988–1989). Instead of believing they are the problem, people can mobilize their resources to combat the problem, which is now separate from who they are. They can establish new views of their problems and themselves, seeing themselves as competent and powerful people who have some problems that need attention rather than people who are problem ridden and flawed.

REVISIONING AND REAUTHORING Once stories have been told and deconstruction has begun, the stories can be modified or revisioned. Only the clients have the right to make and accept changes to their stories, although clinicians often suggest alternative viewpoints and elicit stories of power and resourcefulness.

Revisioning entails both changing the story and changing people's visions of their lives. The two are inseparable; as people come to see more clearly the rules and meanings that govern the old stories, their vision changes, a new interpretation of their lives emerges, and the stories can be revisioned. As revisioning proceeds, it provides opportunities for further deconstruction, which in turn allows for more story revisioning. Gradually, alternative stories that offer exceptions to the dominant story emerge, and other perspectives become available for incorporation into the stories. White (1989) referred to this as the *insurrection of subjugated knowledge.*

Reauthoring now can take place. Possibilities for thoughts, actions, and emotions are expanded as therapists and clients share new descriptions of old stories (Gottlieb & Gottlieb, 1996). People have come to understand their meaning constructions and can move toward a more productive version of their self-narratives in terms of their feelings about themselves and their relationships with others (Lee, 1997).

Through revisioning and reauthoring, people are empowered to develop alternative and preferred self-narratives extending into the future, in which the self is viewed as more powerful than the problem (Carr, 1998; White, 1995). People are now ready to solidify their gains and share them with others.

THERAPEUTIC DOCUMENTS Therapeutic documents are materials, usually prepared by the clinician in collaboration with the client, that reinforce and provide evidence of accomplishments. Both client and clinician decide on the form for the documents, how they should be prepared, when and how they should be consulted, and with whom they should be shared (Crocket, 2008). The documents may take the form of literary productions such as personal letters, lists, reports, certificates and awards, news releases, personal declarations, letters of reference, or manifestos that articulate people's problems, contradict the dominant plots of their lives, and suggest ways for them to deal with these problems (White & Epston, 1990). An exchange of letters between client and clinician is another form of documentation; these may be used to promote clients' reflection and to put their ideas and alternatives into a concrete form that can be kept as a resource. Writing about the effectiveness of such therapeutic documents, Crocket said: "David Epston reported that his informal research with clients suggested that a letter was worth '4.5 sessions of good therapy'" (p. 506).

IMPORTANCE OF THE SOCIAL NETWORK Narrative therapists believe that stories have a cultural and interpersonal basis and that their meanings are generated in social interactions (Richert, 2003). Consequently, they maintain awareness of people's social and cultural contexts and incorporate them into treatment in several ways. Stories may be passed from one person to another, shaped along the way, and given to people as a legacy from their families. Clients are encouraged to recognize the family origins of some of their stories and to find people in their social and family networks who have similar experiences and problems. Drawing on those relationships and learning about ways in which other people have addressed similar problems can provide support, resources, and education about problem solving.

Because of the importance of people's social systems in creating and forming their stories, narrative therapists also use social systems to promote and solidify people's revisioned stories. Clients may be encouraged to tell their new stories to significant members of their social system who are chosen to hear and witness the new self-narrative (Carr, 1998). This public declaration helps solidify changes and puts others on notice to expect people to reauthor their lives.

Clinicians practicing narrative therapy also encourage people to share their learning with others. In what has been called the *bringing-it-back process,* people prepare a written account of their new knowledge and behaviors to share with future clients who have similar difficulties. The authors of the written accounts are then invited to share in person the narratives of how they solved their problems (Carr, 1998). These innovative procedures not only help new clients but also solidify and reinforce the gains of those who already have made progress through treatment.

Current Status

Until recently, there was not much research available on the effectiveness of narrative therapy, but in the past decade there have been a large number of investigations into the construct of narrative identity, spanning almost every theoretical orientation in psychology including personality and life-span development, cultural and clinical psychology, existential and end-of-life issues, and cognitive therapy (Adler, 2012). In addition, a longitudinal study of narrative identity development and mental health seems to suggest that increased agency brought about by creating new stories may lead to symptom relief and improved mental health among people who are exposed to narrative therapy. Clearly, more research is necessary to adequately draw this connection, but the results are exciting in terms of identifying robust trends. Still to be determined is the temporal sequences of change. In other words, "which comes first, feeling better, or telling a new story?" (Adler, 2012, p. 368).

A recent empirical study found narrative therapy to be as effective as interpersonal therapy or cognitive–behavioral therapy (CBT) in the treatment of depression (Vromans & Schweitzer, 2011). Separate research (Ridge & Ziebland, 2006) considered the strategies people use to recover from depression. What they found was that people in recovery from depression had developed a set of "narrative tools" that they used in a self-agentic sort of way. These tools included yoga, talk therapy, and medication, among others. During the course of the study, the authors found that in the very process of explaining the tools they used in recovery, the study participants were creating a recovery story that reinforced their recovery. In addition, Ridge and Ziebland found that the therapists who were collaborative and served as "recovery allies" as opposed to "experts" were the most helpful. The collaborative therapist "helps the person select the narratives and the recovery tools that feel most true to them" (Lewis, 2011, p. 493).

A description of the use of narrative therapy with people who misuse alcohol makes clear its distinctive characteristics (Winslade & Smith, 1997). Rather than accept the stance of Alcoholics Anonymous that encourages people to internalize their problem ("I am an alcoholic"), clinicians help them to externalize the problem, give it a name ("Al"), and then divorce him. In this way, people separate themselves from a close identification with alcohol and are in a better position to combat its influence. In addition, rather than assuming the role of expert and teaching people skills to change their behaviors, clinicians help clients discover and use the knowledge they already have about ways to deal with the problems alcohol has brought into their lives. In his work with adolescent substance users, Sanders (2007) shifted away from this "deficient identity (alcoholic, addict), and toward re-authored identities" (p. 66). Rather than pathologizing clients, they are empowered to develop agency through the reauthoring of their stories. Sanders believes it is through the acceptance that comes from being heard as they attest to their stories that young adults begin to reflect on their choices, develop hope for the future, and start to create "alternative threads of identity" (p. 69).

Narrative therapy seems particularly helpful for the treatment of people who have been victimized and disenfranchised by others, such as women, elderly adults, and those from some ethnic and cultural groups. Drauker (1998), discussing the use of narrative therapy with abused women, wrote: "A therapy that challenges sociopolitical conditions that contribute to violence, highlights women's personal insurrections against these conditions, and supports the reauthoring of their life stories should be considered as a potentially useful approach for women who have been victimized throughout their lives" (p. 168). Similarly, when used with older people, narrative therapy can be positive and life affirming, transforming stories that are based on loss and worthlessness into those that reflect a rich and full life. Narrative therapy also can provide a respectful way to understand people from diverse cultural backgrounds, giving them the opportunity to tell the stories of their lives and revise those stories in ways that give them greater power and control and also are consistent with the values and beliefs of their cultures.

Because the approach does not focus on diagnosis of pathology and is deeply respectful of people's ownership of their own lives, it can be useful with a broad range of clients and concerns. White (2011) used narrative therapy in his work with couples who were experiencing conflict, survivors of suicide, women with eating disorders, and men who were perpetrators of violence. Narrative therapy has also been used successfully to help people cope with trauma (Brown & Augusta-Scott, 2007); to treat delinquency, bullying, and other conduct problems in children; to help people cope with grief and loss (Baddeley & Singer, 2010); and to help people diagnosed with schizophrenia (Gruber & Kring, 2008; White, 2011).

Incorporating people's stories and their revisions into treatment seems to be a useful strategy, so narrative techniques are frequently integrated into other treatment approaches. In psychiatry, for example, doctors are discovering the value of using a narrative approach in medicine to create empathic and meaningful connections with clients (Lewis, 2011). Although narrative therapy clearly has value for a broad range of people, clinicians still must take care when applying this approach. It may be unsuitable for people who cannot engage in a coherent conversation because of their poor contact with reality, for those who seek a quick solution to a specific problem or are in crisis, and for those who anticipate little benefit from treatment. In short, like all approaches to counseling and psychotherapy, narrative therapy has limitations but does offer a new perspective on the treatment process as well as considerable promise. Now we turn to another constructivist-inspired theory—solution-focused brief therapy.

SOLUTION-FOCUSED BRIEF THERAPY

Solution-focused brief therapy has become a popular and well-known treatment system in recent years. This approach seeks solutions, rather than focusing on underlying problems. Treatment is usually brief, although progress is measured by results, not by number of sessions.

The Development of Solution-Focused Brief Therapy

The people most frequently associated with the development of solution-focused brief therapy (SFBT) are Steve de Shazer and Insoo Kim Berg. De Shazer was born in Milwaukee, Wisconsin, and in the 1970s and early 1980s worked with Milton Ericksen and others at the Mental Research Institute in Palo Alto, California (Presbury, Echterling, & McKee, 2008). Their vision of treatment is reflected in the following statement: "We try to base our conceptions and our interventions on direct observation in the treatment situation of *what* is going on in systems of human interaction, *how* they continue to function in such ways, and *how* they may be altered most effectively" (Weakland, Fisch, Watzlawick, & Bodin, 1974, p. 150). Initially, treatment was generally limited to 10 sessions. Typical interventions encouraged people to reverse or alter what they were doing, not just do more of the same (de Shazer & Dolan, 2007).

Insoo Kim Berg was born in Korea and came to the United States in 1957. After obtaining a graduate degree in social work, she moved to Palo Alto to train at the Mental Research Center, where she first met Steve de Shazer. They married and in 1978 cofounded the nonprofit Brief Family Center in Milwaukee, Wisconsin. In the 1980s and 1990s, de Shazer (1985, 1988) and Berg (De Jong & Berg, 2012) developed what they called *solution-focused brief therapy*. De Shazer probably is best known for his use of the miracle question (discussed later in this chapter). De Shazer died in 2006 and Berg died in 2007. She had written 10 books and 35 papers. However, their contributions to brief therapy go far beyond that. Their legacy continues to evolve and gain in importance, especially in light of considerable pressure from managed care, schools and agencies, clients, and clinicians themselves to be accountable and demonstrate results.

De Shazer, Berg, and their colleagues used a decision tree to determine which interventions to use with a client. They generally began treatment with a standard task such as suggesting that clients observe and describe what was happening in their lives that they wanted to continue to happen. If clients completed such a straightforward task, treatment continued in a fairly traditional way. However, if people failed to complete suggested tasks, indirect treatment strategies were tried, such as the use of metaphors or paradoxical interventions. De Shazer, Berg, and their colleagues were known for creative use of clues or suggested tasks to help people find solutions to their problems. They also sometimes used a reflecting team that observed treatment sessions and interrupted with suggestions or ideas.

Brief treatment, building on natural, spontaneous, and ongoing changes in people, can be very powerful. Effective interventions can begin in the first moment of contact with a client. Change can happen quickly, usually in less than six sessions (Winbolt, 2011). Many SFBT therapists begin the first session by asking what changes have occurred since the person first made the appointment.

Important Theoretical Concepts

Solution-focused brief therapy lacks many of the features associated with a well-developed treatment approach. Its literature does not offer a detailed understanding of human development, nor does it address at length the impact of past experiences on present difficulties. Neither does it elaborate on mental disorders it can treat successfully.

These omissions might be interpreted to mean that SFBT is an emerging approach rather than a full-fledged treatment system. However, these omissions are consistent with the nature of the approach, which pays little attention to the origins of people's difficulties and touches lightly, if at all, on their histories. Adopting an idea suggested by Albert Einstein, this treatment system maintains that a problem cannot be solved at the same level it was created. Therefore, SFBT focuses on the present and the future rather than on the past and emphasizes even small glimmers of health and positive change rather than past pathology (de Shazer, 1985). It is included in this book because of its widespread use, its impact on counseling and psychology, and its internal coherence and consistency, even though it lacks some elements that might be viewed as essential in a fully developed treatment system.

UNDERLYING ASSUMPTIONS Solution-focused therapists assume that people's complaints involve behavior that stems from their view of the world. These behaviors are maintained when people do more of the same in the belief that there is only one right and logical thing to do.

Clinicians believe they usually need only limited information about a complaint to resolve it and do not seek to discover the cause or purpose of a complaint. SFBT spends little time helping people figure out why they have been unable to resolve their problems and carefully avoids giving people the message that they have been deficient in their efforts to help themselves. Instead, it assumes that people are doing the best they can at any given time. The thrust of treatment is to increase people's hope and optimism by creating expectancy for change, no matter how small. In this way, people become more aware of what is working rather than what is not. As they become cognizant of the possibilities for positive change, their empowerment and motivation increase correspondingly, creating a beneficial circle; positive change fuels people's belief that change can happen, which enhances their motivation and efforts to change, which in turn leads to more positive changes.

Solution-focused therapists believe that change is constant, that things cannot *not* change. Often, all that is needed to help people is to enable them to notice and build on positive changes that are already happening. To do that, therapists help co-construct solutions to problems, foster independence rather than dependence, and strive to make themselves unnecessary as soon as possible (Winbolt, 2011).

SFBT assumes that exceptions to the problem (i.e., times when the problem is absent) give clues to effective solutions. Identifying these exceptions and building on the ingredients that created them provide further impetus to change. Finally, clinicians practicing SFBT believe that solutions may not directly relate to the problems. Rather, clinicians often suggest "skeleton keys" that help people transform a variety of problems into solutions.

STAGES IN TREATMENT SFBT typically proceeds according to seven stages (de Shazer, 1985):

1. *Identifying a solvable complaint* is an essential first step in treatment. Not only does it facilitate development of goals and interventions, but it promotes change. Client and clinician collaborate to create images of the complaints that place their solutions in the client's hands. For example, "making my spouse stop his abuse" probably is out of the client's hands and is not a readily solvable complaint. However, "remaining strong and taking care of myself when my spouse is abusive" are within the client's control.

Clinicians phrase questions so that they communicate optimism and expectancy for change and empower and encourage. People's difficulties are viewed as normal and able to be changed. Clinicians might ask, "What led you to make an appointment *now?*" rather than "What problems are bothering you?" or they might ask, "What do you want to change?" rather than "How can I help you?"

Clinicians use empathy, summarization, paraphrasing, open questions, and other active listening skills to understand the client's situation in clear and specific terms. They might ask, "How do you express your anxiety?" "What would help me to really understand this situation?" and "How does this create a problem for you?"

In SFBT, presenting complaints are not viewed as symptoms or evidence of pathology. Rather, they are seen as a function of unsuccessful interactions with others or the mishandling of everyday experiences. People often believe that what they are doing is the only right way and, hence, keep doing more of the same, even though they are unsuccessful. As a result, "the solution becomes the problem" (Weakland et al., 1974, p. 31). People may fail to take necessary action, take action when none is indicated, or take action in the wrong way. SFBT assumes that if people's actions and interactions change, their complaints can be alleviated.

Like other behaviorally oriented clinicians, solution-focused therapists often use scaling questions to establish a baseline and facilitate identification of possibilities and progress. The clinician might ask, "Let's say one stands for how bad you felt when you first came to see me with this concern and ten stands for how your life will be when you don't need to see me anymore. On a scale between one and ten, where would you put yourself today?" (Berg & Miller, 1992, p. 362). This scale also can be used to assess specific areas of focus, including symptoms and relationships.

2. *Establishing goals* continues the treatment process. Clinicians collaborate with clients to determine goals that are specific, observable, measurable, and concrete. Goals typically take one of three forms: *changing the doing* of the problematic situation; *changing the viewing* of the situation or the frame of reference; and *accessing resources,* solutions, and strengths (O'Hanlon & Weiner-Davis, 1989). Again, questions presuppose success: "What will be the first sign of change?" "How will you know when this treatment has been helpful to you?" "How will I be able to tell?" Detailed discussion of positive change is encouraged to obtain a clear view of what solutions look like to the client.

One of the most useful ways for solution-focused clinicians to establish treatment goals is to use the *miracle question* (de Shazer, 1991): "Suppose that one night there is a miracle and while you were sleeping the problem that brought you to therapy is solved. How would you know? What would be different? What will you notice different the next morning that will tell you that there has been a miracle? What will your spouse notice?" (p. 113). This question enables people to imagine that their problems are solved, instills hope, and facilitates discussion of how to make the miracle a reality. People's responses to the miracle question usually provide clinicians with potential solutions to clients' concerns.

Delivery of the miracle question is important to its success. Clinicians typically speak slowly, using an almost hypnotic tone of voice, when presenting this question. This engages clients and evokes openness and responsiveness. The miracle question can be adapted to be compatible with the client's concept of the divine. Berg and Miller (1992), for example, suggest that the miracle might be presented as a magic pill, divine intervention, a silver bullet, or a magic wand, depending on the client's beliefs.

Solution-focused therapists accept and use whatever clients present. For example, when asked the miracle question, one woman replied, "The first thing I will notice is that my husband has brushed his teeth before returning to bed for some romance." She had tried to tell her husband that his morning breath bothered her, but increasing nagging yielded no results. After determining that the woman and her husband were playful, the clinician suggested that the woman hide a toothbrush and toothpaste under her pillow and whip it out to brush her husband's teeth the next morning. She felt empowered by having something to do other than complain, and tried this suggestion. This conveyed her message to her husband and also introduced humor into their interaction.

3. When *designing an intervention,* clinicians draw on both their understanding of their clients and their creative use of treatment strategies to encourage change, no matter how small. Typical questions during this stage include "What changes have already occurred?" "What worked in the past when you dealt with similar situations?" "How did you make that happen?" and "What would you need to do to have that happen again?"

4. *Strategic tasks* then promote change. These are generally written down so that clients can understand and agree to them. Tasks are carefully planned to maximize client cooperation and success. People are praised for their efforts and successes and for the strengths they draw on in completing tasks.

Careful assessment of the client is essential in determining an appropriate task. De Shazer (1988) identified three types of tasks, each linked to the level of client motivation:

- If people are *visitors or window shoppers* who have not presented clear complaints or expectations of change, clinicians should only give compliments. Suggesting tasks prematurely is likely to lead to failure that can jeopardize the treatment process.
- If people are *complainants* who have concerns and expect change, but generally in others rather than in themselves, clinicians should suggest observation tasks. This helps people become more aware of themselves and their situations and more able to describe their wants. The clinician might suggest, "Between now and our next appointment, I would like you to notice things that are happening in your life that you want to continue." Observation tasks require little client effort or motivation and, once suggested, usually are done almost automatically.
- Finally, if clients are customers who want to take steps to find solutions to their concerns, clinicians can suggest action tasks with the expectation that they will be completed. Tasks should both empower clients and effect a change in their complaints. For example, Neva had many fears, including learning to drive a car and initiating conversations. Her counselor suggested she ask at least two people to tell her how they learned to drive. Neva found that people enjoyed talking about this topic. She not only gained useful information on driving but initiated several conversations.

5. *Positive new behaviors and changes are identified and emphasized* when clients return after they have been given a task. Questions focus on change, progress, and possibilities and might include "How did you make that happen?" "Who noticed the changes?" and "How did things go differently when you did that?" The problem is viewed as "it" or "that" and as external to the client; this helps people view their concerns as amenable to change, not as an integral part of themselves.

Particularly during this stage of treatment, solution-focused clinicians serve as a sort of cheering squad for their clients. They provide compliments and highlight areas of strength and competence.

6. *Stabilization* is essential in helping people consolidate their gains and gradually shift their perspectives in more effective and hopeful directions. During this stage, clinicians might actually restrain progress and predict some backsliding. This gives people time to adjust to their changes, promotes further success, and prevents them from becoming discouraged if change does not happen as rapidly as they would like.

7. Finally, *termination* of treatment occurs, often initiated by the clients who have now accomplished their goals. Because SFBT focuses on presenting complaints rather than resolution of childhood issues or significant personality change, it recognizes that people may return for additional treatment, and clients are reminded of that option. At the same time, SFBT is not just seeking to help people resolve immediate concerns. Through the process of developing confidence, feeling heard and praised rather than blamed, and finding their strengths and resources, people treated via SFBT can become more self-reliant and capable of resolving future difficulties on their own.

TIMING Most therapy or counseling relationships are relatively brief, whether or not that is planned and regardless of treatment approach. SFBT capitalizes on this pattern, and both clinician and client are aware from the outset that treatment is likely to be short. Because SFBT emphasizes present-oriented efficient treatment that seeks solutions to specific concerns, treatment usually requires fewer than 10 sessions with an average treatment length of between 3 and 5 sessions (Prochaska & Norcross, 2009). However, duration is not determined by an artificial conception of how long therapy is supposed to be; rather, treatment is as long as it needs to be to help people meet their goals and resolve their complaints. Clinicians do not hesitate to extend treatment as long as positive change and forward movement are evident.

Solution-focused therapists tend to be flexible in scheduling appointments. Breaks within sessions allow clinicians the opportunity to develop clues, sometimes in consultation with a reflecting team. Clinicians might plan treatment intervals of one or more months to give clients time to implement suggested strategies and allow changes to evolve. Clinicians also use extended follow-up if people need continued reinforcement. Adapting treatment to the individual is essential.

FINDING SOLUTIONS Finding solutions or clues to resolve complaints is an essential component of SFBT. Clinicians put considerable thought into identifying strategies that are likely to succeed and avoiding those that are discouraging or likely to fail. The following guidelines can help clinicians work with clients to find effective and empowering solutions:

- View clients as experts on their complaints as well as on what solutions will work.
- Assume they have the strengths and resources they need to change.
- Focus on natural and spontaneous changes that are already in progress.
- Expand and build on positive exceptions.
- Interrupt and change repetitive and nonproductive sequences of behavior.
- Provide a rationale to explain how tasks can be helpful, to increase clients' motivation to perform the tasks. If people are skeptical, tasks might be presented as an experiment that they can stop at any point.
- Make interventions congruent with people's worldviews (de Shazer, 1982).
- Learn from past solutions when formulating future solutions. For example, if people respond to direct suggestions, keep providing them; but if they do the opposite of what is suggested, create paradoxical interventions in which doing the opposite is desirable.
- Embed compliments in suggestions to promote optimism and encourage follow-through on tasks.
- Encourage new behaviors rather than simply cessation of old and ineffective ones.
- Create an expectancy for change and a context in which people can think and behave differently.
- Make solutions practical and specific.

Treatment Using Solution-Focused Brief Therapy

Although the process of solution-focused therapy is important, the outcome determines whether treatment has been successful. SFBT helps people use the strengths and resources they already possess to effect positive change in their lives.

THERAPEUTIC ALLIANCE The client–clinician relationship is an important element in solution-focused brief therapy. Like the approaches discussed earlier in this chapter, SFBT therapists develop a collaborative therapeutic alliance and maximize client involvement to empower people and enhance their commitment to change (Presbury et al., 2008). Although clinicians have primary responsibility for creating and suggesting solutions and presenting them in ways that promote action, they view the relationship as a reciprocal process in which clients can help the clinician as the clinician helps the client in the treatment process.

Clinicians *create an environment that is conducive to change*. Tone of voice, metaphorical stories, and suggestions embedded in discussions promote such a state. This enables people to become more open to new possibilities and interpretations, more creative, more amenable to changing the ways they have always behaved, and more able to assess neglected or overlooked alternatives.

SFBT clinicians use a wide variety of interventions. Active listening, empathy, open questions, explanation, reassurance, and suggestion all are important, while interpretation and confrontation are rarely used. Clinicians engage actively with their clients, communicating acceptance, promoting cooperation, serving as role models, telling metaphorical stories, and suggesting actions to effect change. Because they recognize the importance of people's social systems, clinicians may use resources in the environment and involve clients' significant others in the therapeutic process to further the goals of treatment. Osborn (1999) suggested the following helpful guidelines for clinicians: "Listen, do not label; investigate, do not interrogate; level, do not lecture; cooperate, do not convince; clarify, do not confront; solicit solutions, do not prescribe them; consult, do not cure; commend, do not condemn; explore, do not explain; be directive, not dictatorial" (p. 176). Clinicians maintain a positive, respectful, and health-oriented focus and assume that every session is important, that change is inevitable, and that problems will have a solution.

STRATEGIES As we have seen, solution-focused brief therapy uses a broad range of strategies. Some are particular to SFBT and some integrate cognitive and behavioral techniques into the process. We have already discussed the miracle question, the use of scaling to measure change, and the use of suggested solutions. The following are other interventions often used in SFBT (de Shazer & Dolan, 2007).

Identifying exceptions to people's problematic patterns can lead to solutions to their complaints. Although people commonly come into treatment with a desire to vent and process their difficulties, solution-focused therapists believe that a negative focus stabilizes the system and makes change difficult. They believe that a positive focus is far more likely to lead to beneficial transformations. As a result, solution-focused clinicians encourage people to examine times when their difficulties were absent, as sources of information about ways to effect desired change.

For example, Fredda, in her first job as a teacher, sought help with anxiety that she experienced nearly every morning before beginning to teach. Rather than focusing on her unpleasant feelings, the clinician asked whether she could remember a morning when she did not experience anxiety. Fredda described one morning when she got to school early, organized her materials for the day, and then had tea with another teacher who gave Fredda some good ideas about managing a difficult student. This exception suggested several routes to alleviating Fredda's symptoms: arriving early, being well prepared, relaxing before class, and seeking advice from more experienced teachers. By building these behaviors into her routine, Fredda gained control over her anxiety and also began to form friendships at work.

If clients cannot readily recall exceptions to their difficulties, clinicians can take an active role in promoting exceptions. They might suggest a strategic change in behavior. They might predict an exception if one seems likely to occur. They also might encourage clients to search for exceptions, a strategy that is likely to be fruitful if exceptions seem to go unnoticed. Questions such as "What is different about the times when the difficulty does not happen?" "When is the problem less severe?" "How does your day go differently without the problem?" "How is that different from the way you handled the situation the last time it occurred?" "How did you resolve this concern before?" and "What would you need to do to have that happen again?" focus attention on exceptions.

Solution talk is an important tool in SFBT. Clinicians choose their words carefully so that they increase clients' hope and optimism, their sense of control, and their openness to possibilities and change. The focus is on solutions, not problems. Some examples of how language can be used to enhance treatment follow:

Solution Talk

- Emphasize *open questions.*
- Use *presuppositional language* that assumes that problems are temporary and that positive change will occur. For example, clinicians speak of *when,* not *if,* the problem is solved: "When this problem is solved, what will you be doing?"
- *Normalize people's problems* to provide reassurance and reduce feelings of inadequacy. A clinician might say to a parent, coping with a child's drug use, "Your son seems to be engaging in some risky behaviors and it makes sense that you are worried."
- *Focus on coping behavior* via questions such as "What has kept you from harming yourself?" and "How do you manage to keep going?"
- *Reinforce and notice strengths and successes.* Congratulate and compliment people for their improvements and efforts; avoid emphasizing problems and failures.
- *Create hypothetical solutions* such as "If you weren't feeling afraid, what might you be feeling and doing instead?" This expands possibilities and encourages change.
- *Concentrate on describing and changing behaviors* rather than thoughts or emotions.
- *Use rituals, metaphors, stories, and symbols* to convey indirect messages that can promote change. For example, Mary envisioned a formidable brick wall standing between her and the sort of life she wanted. Her counselor suggested that she remove one brick, leaving it up to Mary to determine how she would complete this task. She responded by changing several behavioral patterns and reported that she had made a hole in the wall big enough for her to crawl through.
- Make frequent use of words such as *change, different, possibility, what,* and *how* that suggest change.
- Use *inclusive language* such as "and" that allows potentially incompatible outcomes to coexist. Rather than saying, "You might feel like you can't do it, but you can do it," the clinician might say, "You might feel like you can't do it, *and* you can do it."
- *Use reframing and relabeling* to offer different perspectives. For example, an event might be viewed as an opportunity for learning rather than a disappointment, and a person might be depicted as "taking the time to sort out options" rather than "stuck" or "paralyzed by fear."
- *Match clients' vocabulary or style of talking* to promote a collaborative therapeutic alliance. Then change the language to encourage change in clients' perspectives.

Make Suggestions

- Recognize that *indirectness and implied suggestions* are sometimes more powerful than direct suggestions and advice.
- *Solution prescriptions,* a common form of suggestion in SFBT, are tasks designed to help people discover ways to resolve their concerns. These may be designed to fit a particular person or situation or may be a standard prescription in the clinician's repertoire. Commonly used prescriptions include "Do one thing different," "Continue doing something that has been successful," and "Notice times when the problem is slightly less of a problem and what you did to bring that about" (Sklare, 2000, p. 442).

Application and Current Status of Solution-Focused Brief Therapy

The scope of solution-focused therapy has expanded beyond treating people with mild or moderately severe problems to successfully treating people in crisis, those who have been given court mandates requiring therapy, people with addictions, and children in protective services settings (Tarragona, 2008).

APPLICATION TO DIAGNOSTIC GROUPS Some of the concepts and strategies associated with SFBT—notably attention to motivation, emphasis on small successes, and efforts to find exceptions—are likely to enhance treatment for people with personality disorders, somatoform disorders, impulse control disorders, and substance use disorders. Shilts (2010) suggested using the scaling question to determine readiness for treatment for clients seen in school, mental health, and substance abuse treatment programs. Scaling can also provide a means of assessment if used in the initial session with clients who are beginning treatment with antidepressants (Thomas, 2010b).

Solution-focused brief therapy can be helpful in work with adolescents who have ADHD (Nelson, 2010), and to help counteract bullying in public schools (Young, 2010). An alternative to the miracle question can be used at the end of treatment to help clients recognize progress and solidify gains. Nelson (2010) suggests asking the client, "If I run into you six months from now and you tell me all of the changes you have made, what will you tell me?"

APPLICATION TO MULTICULTURAL GROUPS Solution-focused therapy "is an incredibly culturally respectful approach to working with clients of diverse backgrounds because it discourages diagnoses and focuses on the client's personal frame of reference" (Erford, Eaves, Bryant, & Young, 2010). Because each client is seen as "the expert on his or her own life," SFBT inherently values the cultural backgrounds and resources of all clients. De Jong and Berg (2012) see much in SFBT to give this approach multicultural relevance including its flexibility and its emphasis on health, resources, strengths, client dignity, collaboration, empowerment, and self-determination. In addition, SFBT's respect for people's views of the world, its recognition of the importance of people's connections with their environment and with others, and this treatment approach's brief and nonintrusive nature all seem to make it suitable for use with a broad range of people. Solution-focused therapists recognize the importance of client motivation, and efforts to promote clients' involvement in treatment make SFBT useful with people who are hesitant or leery about treatment.

APPLICATION TO OTHER GROUPS Solution-focused therapy seems useful with children and adolescents as well as with adults, although it might need to be modified for treatment of children. Because it is an active approach that provides positive talk and solutions, it is well suited for people with eating disorders, substance use disorders, and other impulse control and behavioral problems (Erford et al., 2010). Increasingly, SFBT is being used in crisis situations, to reduce suicidal risk, and to help those who have been the victims of domestic violence or trauma. SFBT's focus on resilience and coping skills seems particularly helpful to people seeking to move past a traumatic situation and rebuild a future.

Corcoran and Stephenson (2000) found that treatment via solution-focused therapy yielded significant improvement when used with children presenting behavior problems in their schools. Positive changes were reflected in the Conners' Parent Rating Scales assessing conduct, learning, and psychosomatic problems, as well as impulsivity and hyperactivity.

SFBT can also be effective in a broad range of settings, including work environments, employee assistance programs, schools and colleges, and corrections and medical settings. Bezanson (2004) recommends the use of solution-focused therapy in employment counseling, and Berg and

Szabo (2005) integrated SFBT into a model for brief coaching. Metcalf's (1998) writings are especially helpful for clinicians who want to use this approach with groups in both school and mental health settings.

CURRENT STATUS Because SFBT encourages thoughtful use of interventions and homework tasks, it lends itself well to integration with other treatment approaches, particularly those that take a phenomenological perspective and focus on behavior change. For example, Fernando (2007) combined an existentialist approach with SFBT in his work in Sri Lanka with survivors of the devastating tsunami that occurred in 2004. SFBT has also been easily integrated with cognitive behavioral, rational emotive behavior therapy, Adlerian, and reality therapies (Carlson & Sperry, 2000).

SFBT has been noted for achieving positive effects in less time than long-term therapy. The approach came out of a social constructivist, family systems perspective and can be useful for couples, individuals, children, and adolescents as well. SFBT works with all types of problems from PTSD and substance abuse to mediation (Bannink, 2007). It is generally well received by clients, is encouraging and empowering, and offers new ways of thinking about helping people. It addresses immediate problems while enabling people to make better use of their strengths and resources in addressing future difficulties.

Evaluation of Solution-Focused Brief Therapy

Although most of the literature on solution-focused treatment consists of case studies and descriptions of treatment strategies, additional empirical research is expected to enhance the reputation of this powerful approach.

LIMITATIONS Solution-focused brief therapy has limitations, which many of its practitioners seem to realize. Unless clients and clinicians carefully co-create problem definitions, the approach can cause clinicians to focus prematurely on a presenting problem and thereby miss an issue of greater importance. Solution-focused treatment is not usually appropriate as the primary or only treatment for severe or urgent emotional difficulties or when clients do not have the skill or internal resources to cope with their problems. In addition, its implementation appears easier than it is. In reality, this approach requires well-trained clinicians who are skilled and experienced in assessment, goal setting, treatment planning, and effective use of a range of creative and powerful interventions.

Another drawback to SFBT is the misconception among some clinicians and clients, as well as some managed care organizations, that brief treatment is all that is ever needed to treat clients successfully. This is, of course, a dangerous overgeneralization, with the result that people may fail to receive the intensive treatment they need. Clinicians should exercise caution when using SFBT to be sure that this approach is adequate to meet their clients' needs.

SFBT has provided clinicians with powerful new interventions. Its use of the miracle question, its emphasis on exceptions and possibilities, its use of presuppositional and other solution-focused language, and its emphasis on small behavioral changes are innovative concepts that are changing the way many clinicians think about and provide treatment. The miracle question, in particular, has gained widespread acceptance as a useful tool to facilitate information gathering and goal setting.

FEMINIST THERAPY

Historically, feminist therapy had its beginnings in three waves of feminism (Bruns & Trimble, 2001). The first wave was in the late 1800s with the suffrage movement seeking voting rights for women. The second wave, based on Betty Freidan's women's liberation movement of the 1950s and built on in the 1970s by Gloria Steinem and others, gained prominence with women's struggle for equal rights. Women started to have a voice and to be encouraged to move into leadership positions. These two waves were of greatest relevance to upper middle class educated white women. The third wave of feminist thought coming into prominence today is egalitarian and inclusive. Reflective of social constructivism, it is not concerned with trying to develop one reality or truth, but rather embraces concepts of meaning and connection.

Postmodern feminist therapy is directed toward both women and men, and toward people of all sexual orientations, races, classes, age groups, cultures, and abilities. It is designed to combat limiting and harmful influences and to empower all people so they can fight oppression while developing full and rewarding lives. Despite its misleading name, feminist therapy is a gender-sensitive approach that strives to help both men and women change themselves and their societies and act together to make a difference. As you read this section, keep in mind this current and broad goal of feminist therapy.

The Development of Feminist Theories

Unlike most of the other theories in this book, feminist therapy has no single unified theory nor are specific people credited as founders (Enns, 2004; Indelicato & Springer, 2007). Rather, feminist therapy has been shaped by several important tenets:

1. The personal is political.
2. The experiences and perceptions of all people must be heard and valued, whether they belong to powerful or marginalized groups. Attention must be paid to understanding and addressing the impact of power and gender, race, socioeconomic status, ethnicity, ability, sexual orientation, culture, and religion in social interactions and situations.
3. Egalitarian relationships are prized, both inside and outside of therapy, therefore the therapeutic process is demystified.
4. Women's experiences are valued and understood in the context of multiple roles and relationships. Women's "ways of being" are not only valued, but intuition, instinct, and the concept of a collective sisterhood are cherished. Women are not considered to be an aberration from a male "norm," but are unique in and of themselves.
5. Feminist therapy is positive and strengths based. Mental health is reframed from a resources perspective rather than considered to be pathological. Instead of looking at dysfunction as resulting from disease, it is reframed from a sociological or survival perspective.
6. Feminist therapy involves a commitment to social change. Feminist therapists are not only concerned about interpersonal issues, but are concerned with economic, social, political, and educational issues, and often advocate for their clients in these areas as well.
7. Group membership (e.g., gender, race, age) has a pervasive impact on our lives, affecting perceptions, emotions, conflicts, styles of relating, and more.

Feminist therapy has been strongly influenced by humanistic and phenomenological approaches as well as by cognitive therapy and existentialism. Like constructivism, it postulates that people's internal and external worlds, the subjective and objective, are interconnected and that both must be part of the therapeutic process. Feminist therapy is an intentionally culturally competent model with its emphasis on "making central issues of oppression, identity, and power, and its reliance on a culturally informed knowledge base" (Brown, 2010, p. 102).

FEMINIST THERAPY AND WOMEN Many of the emotional, cognitive, and behavioral difficulties experienced by girls and women can be directly linked to societal messages. For example, the increase in eating disorders in females has been caused, at least in part, by messages equating beauty with thinness. Depression and anxiety, much more common in women than in men, probably have both biological and societal roots, with women experiencing these symptoms in response to feelings of powerlessness, loneliness, and role confusion. Recent research on the psychology of women has led to new areas that were previously overlooked in therapy: domestic violence, the long-term impact of childhood sexual abuse, adolescent depression, and an examination of traditionally female values such as altruism and affiliation (Day, 2008; Nolen-Hoeksema & Hilt, 2009).

Feminist therapy recognizes that many women come from cultures that foster and value interdependence, community, and collectivism (Enns, 2004). For example, in Japanese society "relationships within the inner circle of family and relatives are characterized by oneness between persons, unconditional love, affirmation, and indulgence" (Enns, 2004, p. 238). In many cultures, including Asian, Hispanic, and African American cultures, responsibility extends beyond the individual to include collective responsibility for the extended family. The importance of this interdependence to many women of color underscores the need for feminist therapies that incorporate and build on these values.

FEMINIST THERAPY AND MEN Clients of feminist therapy may be men or women just as feminist therapists may be women or men. Many problems that are experienced by men are particularly well suited to a feminist treatment approach. Gender role strain, difficulty expressing emotions, deconstructing internal scripts, and issues of anger and rage are just a few examples. Therapy is considered feminist as long as the treatment approach supports feminist models and outcomes, is used in the service of empowerment and egalitarianism, addresses issues of bias and power, and contributes to a greater understanding of the impact of social factors and patriarchy on well-being and distress (Brown, 2010).

Research and writing suggest that men, like women, often develop difficulties as a result of conformity or nonconformity to traditional gender roles. Societal expectations surrounding fathering, communication and connection with their mates, and the expression of emotion can all lead to "discrepancy strain" if men perceive themselves as not conforming to traditional masculine norms (Levant & Wimer, 2009; Levant, Wimer, Williams, Smalley, & Noronha, 2009). Others may feel conflicted and confined by their efforts to conform to masculine norms and suppress any feminine elements in themselves (dysfunction strain). A third type of gender role strain is trauma strain, which can result when young boys are forced to conform to uncomfortable gender roles. Gender role strain is associated with higher levels of anger, aggression, anxiety, health-risk behavior, depression, and distress and with lower levels of self-esteem. (Of course, many men have flexible conceptions of the masculine role and do not experience gender role strain.)

Another perspective on the impact of gender role constriction was advanced by Mahalik, Good, and Englar-Carlson (2003) who suggested that many men adhere to masculine scripts such as strong-and-silent, player, winner, and homophobe. These scripts can act as barriers, curtail men's options, and prevent them from seeking help.

Anger is another issue that is often seen in therapy with men, especially when it is expressed inappropriately through substance abuse or violence. The egalitarian focus at the core of feminist therapy helps therapists to develop strategies for working with this population, including those men who abuse their power or are vocally or physically violent. Anger management groups for men and consciousness-raising groups for men who batter women are examples. Such programs are often run by therapists of either gender who practice from a feminist framework. Ganley (1988), Levant (1996, 2001), and Nutt and Brooks (2008) describe their experiences as male feminist therapists in their work with other men.

Feminist therapy can help both men and women address issues of gender role strain, lack of empowerment, and consciousness raising. Treatment would promote understanding of societal messages and their impact, flexibility in thinking, self-awareness and self-acceptance, gender role analysis, distress tolerance, and relaxation (Enns, 2004).

Therapeutic Alliance

Descriptions of feminist therapists resemble those of constructivist therapists in general. Clinicians are respectful, empathic, empowering, collaborative, and encouraging. They are authentic, enthusiastic, and open to new perceptions and experiences. Clinicians are resources and support systems rather than experts. They work collaboratively with clients to establish goals and decide on pacing. They discredit traditional ideas of resistance, transference, and countertransference and, instead, view those processes as reflective of meanings and information that need attention. Countertransference, termed a "symbolic relationship" by feminist therapists, can be a particularly fruitful source of information (Brown, 2001).

Feminist therapists work to create an egalitarian relationship with their clients. Therapy often begins with a discussion of the relationship. Feminist therapists seek to deconstruct barriers to equality and to increase awareness of power structures and differentials in society as a whole and within the therapeutic relationship in particular. To do this, the therapist increases self-disclosure, openly recognizes and discusses the power differential, actively works to empower clients, and encourages clients to establish power within relationships outside of therapy. Treatment goals, strategies, and interventions are openly discussed between the client and clinician and determined collaboratively.

Relational Power

Feminist therapy also discusses the construct of *relational power*. One of the hallmarks of feminist therapy is the focus on relationships and connections. Both the creation of the relational-cultural model at the Stone Center and Carol Gilligan's research on the importance of relationships and care in human development and in the development of morality (1977, 1996) have been instrumental in the development of a feminist theory of personality.

Gilligan's (1977) work on the morality of care in girls found that issues of responsibility and concern for other people is at the heart of women's sense of self. Connectedness and interdependence, concepts that had not been a part of most theories of human development, appear to be at the core of women's identity development. Specifically, the ability to create and maintain relationships provides girls with positive psychological strength and resilience. "Relationship brings the oxygen of experience into the psyche" (Gilligan, 1996, p. 258).

Gilligan's (1982) work with Kohlberg (1981), who created the stage model of moral development, showed that moral judgments are not always made based on linear or rational judgments. Especially in girls and women, moral decisions can be based on an ethic of care and an honoring of relationships. As a result, theories have emerged that value the relational and cooperative dimensions of women's experiencing (Enns, 2004).

More than 35 years ago, Jean Baker Miller and others at the Stone Center in Wellesley, Massachusetts, developed the self-in-relation theory. Now known as relational-cultural therapy, RCT is a separate school of feminist thought that, according to Laura Brown (2010), developed "in parallel with separate streams of feminist therapy" (p. 7). It was originally developed to explain women's psychological experiences but has since been found to be appropriate for all human interactions, especially those involving a power or privilege differential. The literature shows RCT to be useful in reducing racism, sexism, depression, eating disorders, substance misuse, and trauma (Hartling & Ly, 2000). RCT can be used with individuals, with couples of any type including

Relational-Cultural Theory: The Stone Center Approach

In 1976, feminist and psychoanalyst Jean Baker Miller outlined an exciting new theory in her book *Toward a New Psychology of Women*. Miller wrote about the centrality of relationships to women's lives and hypothesized that for women psychological well-being occurs in the course of mutually empathic relationships. Instead of viewing self-sufficiency or personal growth as the goal, this theory views the establishment of relationships, and the movement toward connection, as being of primary importance to women's psychological health and fulfillment. This concept is referred to as "the self-in-relation" (Surrey, 1991, p. 51).

In 1981 Miller was appointed director of the Stone Center at Wellesley College, with the mission to explore psychological development and ultimately reduce psychological problems.

For nearly 35 years, Miller and her colleagues at the Stone Center—Judith Jordan, Irene Stiver, and Janet Surrey—brought together scholars, researchers, and other professionals in workshops and seminars. The center's researchers have published more than 100 working papers that have become the core foundation of relational-cultural theory. These core concepts include the proposition that all people yearn for connection and when healthy connections occur, people grow as a result. Miller (1976) believed connection occurs through mutual empathy and empowerment. It is only then that people can grow, take control of their lives, and change. Miller delineated the following five characteristics of a growth-fostering relationship:

1. Increased vitality (Miller referred to this as "zest")
2. Empowerment (an increased ability to take action)
3. Improved clarity of self and relationship
4. Enhanced self-worth
5. A desire for additional relationships.

In addition to connection, relational-cultural therapy believes that disconnection is an inevitable part of any relationship. Disconnections can result from empathic failures, violations of the relationship, and injuries. If the injured person is able to confront the situation, express her feelings, and have those feelings responded to empathically by the other, the rupture may be repaired and the relationship strengthened. This ability to effect change and feel empowered within the relationship is referred to as *relational competence* (Jordan, 1999). However, if the injured person is not able to communicate her feelings, or if the feelings are denied or ignored, she will begin to withdraw parts of herself from the relationship in order to maintain the relationship. This causes the injured person to act inauthentically and ultimately diminishes the relationship. Miller and Stiver (1997) refer to this as the *central relationship paradox*. The person uses survival strategies to disconnect, while adapting to the relationship that is available to him or her. Robb (2006) describes this paradox as "keeping your true feelings out" (p. 307) of the relationship in an attempt to save the relationship. This cycle eventually leads to less satisfaction in relationships by reducing the five good things Miller identified (zest, empowerment, clarity, warmth, and growth), and results in the person's natural tendency toward connection becoming a signal of danger. The person learns to dread the vulnerability required to be fully connected in relationships.

mother/daughter couples, and with the family system. It can be implemented in a time-limited framework as well as with intermittent or spaced therapy (Jordan, Handel, Alvarez, & Cook-Nobles, 2004). RCT therapy stresses continuity of the relationship, even when therapy is not taking place.

In session, RCT therapists are likely to discuss different forms of unearned advantage (classism, sexism, racism, homophobia) and how the experiences of dominance and privilege suppress authenticity and mutuality in relationships (Hartling & Ly, 2000). This, then, becomes the goal of the relational-cultural therapist's work: to identify the sociocultural and interpersonal dynamics that serve to isolate and marginalize people, to create a meaningful therapeutic connection with the client that will eventually lead to change and growth, and, ultimately, to achieve the healing that results from connection.

The following case example illustrates relational power. See the boxed feature for a more complete history of RCT and the Stone Center.

EXAMPLE CASE ILLUSTRATING RELATIONAL POWER Angela, a married African American woman in her early 40s with two young children, sought counseling shortly after she was diagnosed with early-stage cancer. She deliberately sought help from a clinician about her own age who had cancer 8 years earlier. Her clinician, Lesley, was married, had one child, and was Caucasian. Angela's presenting concerns included dealing with her fear of not living long enough to see her children grow up and of wanting to clarify her priorities so that she could live a more fulfilling life.

Although Angela's concerns shaped the treatment, counseling involved considerable sharing between the two women and each learned from the other. Early in treatment, they discussed their common experiences (cancer, marriage, motherhood, age, education) as well as their differences (race) and the probable impact these would have on Angela's treatment. At Angela's suggestion, and with the counselor's encouragement, Angela provided considerable information on role expectations for African American women, the importance her mother and sisters had for her, the value she placed on her professional job, and the challenges she had encountered in finding a suitable partner, leading her to defer marriage until her mid-30s. Both women shared thoughts and feelings on the challenges of combining a family and a professional career, as well as on how race made that challenge somewhat different for each of them.

Angela realized that she had been devoting most of her attention to her well-established career and now wanted to reduce her work hours so she could spend more time with her children. Her increased acceptance of traditional female roles and her ability to reduce her unwarranted fear of living in poverty like her mother helped her make this change with comfort. She regained the powerfulness and hopefulness she had lost as a result of her medical diagnosis and coped effectively with changes in her body image resulting from her cancer treatment. She initiated an exercise program and formed a support group of other African American women dealing with cancer; these activities reflected her sense of empowerment and further enhanced her powerfulness.

As a participant in this process, Lesley learned a great deal about the special role of the African American woman and also gained insight into her own rejection of some traditional female attitudes and behaviors, stemming from her need to carve out a different path for herself than that of her mother. In addition, Lesley saw more clearly the influence on her of growing up as a white middle-class woman, a condition of privilege. Although these insights were shared only briefly with Angela, Lesley did make clear that she, too, had learned and grown through the mutuality in the treatment process.

Strategies

Interventions frequently used in feminist therapy include analysis of gender roles and power, empowerment, and integrated analysis of oppression. Relabeling and reframing are helpful ways to look at coping skills that have outgrown their usefulness. Group work is often included for psychoeducation, support, and raising consciousness:

1. ***Consciousness-raising.*** By increasing awareness of oppression of women and other marginalized groups, consciousness-raising helps people to clarify the changes they want to make.
2. ***Gender role analysis.*** The goal of gender role analysis is to examine the effect of cultural expectations on the client. The media's portrayal of thinness as the norm for women, or the idea that men should be aggressive and competitive while women are nurturing and empathic,

are just two examples of gender role expectations. This intervention is a threefold process. First, societal messages about behavior must be recognized and identified. Second, people reflect on the pros and cons of such messages. The third part involves planned challenges to such beliefs either with the system or individually. The impact on both helps clients to see how societal roles and experiences reinforce gender-based bias.

3. ***Relabeling and reframing.*** Symptoms and problems are reframed from the framework of being a woman in American society. For example, a woman who just gave birth to a newborn baby 6 weeks ago is now experiencing panic attacks every time she thinks about returning to work. Reframing the situation would consider the larger cultural perspective and view the problem as resulting from living in a society in which economic needs force a mother to return to work when she is not ready. Looking at it from this perspective reduces the person's negative beliefs ("What is wrong with me? Everyone else can do this, why am I so emotional?") and puts it in a broader political perspective ("What is wrong with a society in which a mother has to make a choice between taking care of her child or paying the rent?"). This results in anger rather than self-blame.
4. ***Assertiveness training.*** Assertive behavior requires a person to be honest about their own needs without violating the rights of others. Feminist therapists empower clients to be assertive by expanding the client's range of options. Through role-plays of potentially difficult interpersonal situations, clients can learn how to speak assertively without being aggressive. When clients are too passive and do not speak up for themselves, they may experience anxiety. It they speak up too assertively, they may fear sounding angry. Role-playing empathic assertiveness—in which the client first puts herself in the other's shoes before responding—can help clients get the language right and defuse potentially difficult interpersonal relationships. Empathic assertiveness is illustrated in the following example:

   "I'm sure you didn't realize you were leaving a message on my home phone. In the future, I would prefer you use my cell phone number to remind me of appointments."

   The Case Illustration at the end of this chapter provides a role-play on assertiveness with Edie and Roberto's 10-year-old daughter Ava.
5. ***Therapy-demystifying strategies.*** Just as feminist therapists seek to reduce the power differential with their clients, they also want them to feel comfortable and equal in therapy and not feel that they are participating in some mysterious process. Therapists do a number of things to make therapy more egalitarian, including having their clients call them by their first names, providing information, and a generous use of self-disclosure. One therapist, for example provides her clients with a 10-page handout before the first session, which provides information about the session (length, frequency, fee), and also explains her therapeutic style and what the client can expect out of therapy. In the first session, client and therapist collaborate on the goals for therapy, and both sign a treatment plan. Most feminist therapists provide information, when appropriate to the session, on, for example, decision-making skills, mindfulness techniques to help clients stay in the moment, or assertiveness skills. Feminist therapists are also more lenient than other types of therapists in what they disclose to clients, frequently using examples from their own lives if it will help the client. For example, a disclosure from the therapist that she also "took the five-year plan to finish college" can normalize the client's situation and provide a successful role model. This can empower a young person who is struggling with her perceived "failure" at needing an extra year to complete her degree. Such disclosures are always made for the client's benefit, and not to help the therapist.

Feminist therapy emphasizes the here and now, the importance of self-actualization, and both individual and group empowerment. It promotes people's efforts to construct language, stories, and symbols drawn from their own experiences that strengthen and expand possibilities. It stresses the importance of relationships that respect diversity and that are nonhierarchical. Gender, race, and other contexts are explicitly discussed. Inclusiveness and plurality rather than discrimination are advocated. Narratives are elicited and viewed from individual and cultural perspectives. Interventions include analysis of gender roles, messages, and power differentials in social interactions, and encouragement of clients to use and develop their self-awareness, strengths, and resources.

Existential, Gestalt, psychoanalytic, family systems, and cognitive–behavioral therapy are some of the treatment systems that are commonly integrated with feminist therapy. Several models used to treat complex trauma integrate feminist concepts at their core (Brown, 2008, 2010). Feminist family therapy goes beyond traditional family therapy to explore gender role biases and the impact of socialization and culture on the family system (Nystul, 2006). Psychoeducation, particularly assertiveness training and role-plays, is used to empower women, improve self-esteem, and help them to overcome stereotypical gender roles.

Feminist therapy often eschews traditional diagnosis in favor of a more sociocultural approach to problems. By recognizing and discussing the fact that women are more likely than men to be diagnosed and treated for depression and anxiety (Seligman & Reichenberg, 2012), as well as other "relation-related" illnesses (e.g., dependent personality disorder, histrionic personality disorder), feminist therapists are more likely to look at underlying societal expectations and biases that contribute to women perceiving themselves as powerless, dependent, and unfulfilled. Feminist therapists then work to change the context, rather than label a client with a particular diagnosis.

Current Status

Feminist therapy provides an important perspective for counseling and psychotherapy. It emphasizes human potential and people's ability and right to make choices that enable them to live their lives in rewarding ways. It is integrative and reflects "an ultimate feminist perspective; that mind and body and spirit must be addressed together in order to make therapy effective" (Brown, 2001, p. 1011). It can, and usually is, combined with other approaches including humanistic, narrative, and brief psychodynamic therapy. Working with faulty cognitions, mindfulness and relaxation techniques, and other experiential techniques such as focusing can also be helpful. Feminist therapy can be particularly helpful to couples who are struggling with gender role conflicts and confused and unmet expectations. It emphasizes the importance of context and of social change, encouraging clinicians to focus their efforts at both individual and societal levels.

Much of the literature on feminist therapy emphasizes the multicultural relevance of this approach. Funderburk and Fukuyama (2001), for example, described the convergence of feminism, multiculturalism, and spirituality—three forces that emphasize "consciousness, context, and connection in order to heighten awareness regarding suffering, liberation and enlightenment" (p. 6). All three "encourage the examination of socially, culturally, and cognitively constructed worldviews and beliefs" (p. 8) and "are interested in liberating the individual and transforming oppression and suffering in society and accomplish this, in part, by deconstructing 'social realities'" (p. 8).

The literature reflects the application of this approach to multicultural groups including GLBT and questioning clients, African American and Chicana/Latina women, and adolescent girls. In recognition of the increasingly diverse and complex roles of women in society, the American Psychological Association (2007) adopted a set of guidelines for consideration in therapeutic practice with women and girls. The APA guidelines for working with women have been adapted for working with women with disabilities, an area that Banks (2010) believes has been left out of the literature. "Traditional feminist psychology has seldom considered the influence and impact of disability on women's lives. Ableism continues to be a covert, but still detectable and powerful, force in feminist psychology"

(p. 432). Banks notes that women with disabilities are more likely than men to be dependent on other people for personal assistance and at higher risk of abuse. Therapists of all treatment modalities are reminded that cultural competence includes being competent to work with people with disabilities.

Limitations of a feminist approach include the lack of one theory that drives the movement; each therapist tends to pull from his or her own experiences in combination with the specific client's needs. Because it is a relatively new approach and initially focused on treating women, empirical research on its effectiveness is limited, although feminist therapy is considered effective because of its use of "the empirically supported common factors" (Brown, 2010, p. 102).

Several studies show promise for the use of feminist therapy with specific populations, such as those who have experienced domestic violence or other trauma, and in the treatment of self-inflicted violence (SIV). A feminist approach to narrative therapy has also been shown to be helpful in treating people with anorexia (Olson, 2001) and those coping with chronic and life-threatening illnesses. More research is needed on specific concepts such as mutuality, therapist self-disclosure, and values as they relate to women.

Like all constructivist therapies, feminist therapy has made important inroads into 21st-century thought. Originally developed to focus on women, feminist therapy has expanded during the past 40 years to center on an analysis of gender, power, and social location. As increasing emphasis is placed on culturally competent counseling, the scope of people for whom feminist therapy can be helpful has broadened (Brown, 2010). Counseling that takes into account societal biases and privileges seems to provide a practical, egalitarian method in which to further advance our knowledge of human development and improve and protect relational connectivity.

Now we turn to the skill development of mapping, a narrative technique that is highly adaptable to usage in all of the constructivist approaches.

SKILL DEVELOPMENT: MAPPING

An earlier section of this chapter presented Michael White and David Epston's theory of narrative therapy. A narrative approach assumes that people live their lives based on the stories they tell themselves and the stories they are told. This constructivist approach believes that these stories shape our reality. By deconstructing the stories, narrative practitioners help people to see the parts of their stories that they have overlooked in their focus on problem-laden narratives. In this overlooked material may be stories of resilience, hope, and courage—certain lived experiences that are more desirable than others. Unpacking the influence of the problem on the person's life and helping the person to recognize the restrictive cultural assumptions that might lie beneath are the goals of narrative mapping. After a client's problems have been externalized and the effects of the stories have been mapped and deconstructed, the person is ready to create new alternative narratives that empower him or her to move forward with life.

White (2007) delineates four categories of inquiry to help the therapist:

1. Developing an experience-near position of the problem
2. Mapping the influence of the problem in the person's life
3. Evaluating the problem's effects
4. Justifying the problem.

Each category of inquiry includes a certain line of questioning by the therapist to help clients tell their stories.

Developing an experience-near position of the problem. In the first stage of mapping, the therapist seeks clarification of the presenting problem as it is experienced from the client's unique perspective. Especially with children, clients may believe that they are the problem and become resigned to the fact that nothing can be done. Through therapist questioning about the problem, a distinctive shape of the problem emerges. The person is able to talk about the problem in a very real, experience-near, manner.

Mapping the influence of the problem in the person's life. After the problem has been externalized, outlined, given a name, or discussed as an object onto itself rather than viewed as part of the person, it becomes less personalized and easier to discuss. For example, Antika came for counseling to help her overcome her shyness at school. She was embarrassed to sit with others at lunchtime and was ashamed to discuss her problem with anyone. After a few sessions she labeled her problem as a big caped man that spreads his shadow over her whenever she is around people. As it became visible and developed its own outline, the problem became less personal and Antika was able to recognize the control this shadowman had on her life and to take action in a more positive direction.

By asking questions that probe the size (length, breadth, and depth) of the problem, the therapist begins to get a picture of the extent of the problem's influence on every aspect of the person's life including home, school, work, relationships, motivation, dreams, aspirations, and even the future. Talking to Antika about times when the shadowman came around, where she was at the time, how far the shadow extended, how long it lasted, and its impact on her relationships with classmates and family helped her to see the problem as separate from herself and provided hope that it could be changed. Questions for Antika might include any of the following:

- What has the shadowman persuaded you to think about yourself?
- What has it convinced others to say about you?
- How does it convince them of these things?
- What decisions does the shadowman make for you?
- Are there any benefits of having the shadowman around sometimes?
- What are its intentions for your future?

Mapping the influence of the person in the life of the problem is another line of questioning that begins to pave a road to recovery. By looking for unique outcomes or times when the problem hasn't been a problem, the therapist uncovers powerful messages that can be used to form an alternative narrative. Not surprisingly, Antika said the shadowman only came into her home when strangers were present such as when her father invited colleagues home for dinner. During those times she was able to overcome her shyness because she told herself her father would protect her. This lead to a discussion of exceptions such as:

- Have there been other times when you've overcome or ignored the shadowman?
- How did you feel when this happened?
- How might you stand up to it in the future?
- By ignoring the hold that this shadowman has over you, do you think you are becoming less vulnerable? Stronger?
- What will the future be like without this dominating your life?
- How is this future different from the one that the shadowman would have planned for you?

Evaluating the problem's effects. Once the therapist has a handle on the extent of the problem for the person, it is helpful to question the larger effect it has on their lives. Beginning with a summary, or what White (2007) refers to as "editorials" (p. 45), the therapist makes a brief statement about the problem and its attendant consequences. With Antika the summary went like this:

THERAPIST: Antika, I understand that apart from the shadowman, people tend to treat you differently as a result. Students stay away from you, no one calls you to go to the movies, and you said you spend a lot of time alone.

ANTIKA: Yes, that's right.

THERAPIST: What is that like for you?

ANTIKA: Lonely. I don't like it.

THERAPIST: You don't like it. What other words might you use to explain this?

ANTIKA: Sad. I hate being alone. I feel left out of everything and my parents think I'm a loser.

THERAPIST: And you don't want to be a loser?

ANTIKA: No! I want to be like everyone else!

Justifying the problem. In the fourth stage of mapping, White (2007) recommends asking why questions such as these: Why is this situation not okay with you? Why do you want this to stop? Why do you feel the way you do? Such questions are not asked in a judgmental way, or in a manner that elicits defensiveness, but more out of curiosity in an effort to discover the values and assumptions that underlie a person's narrative. "Why" questions can be a lead-in to reauthoring conversations and revelations about what the client had intended life to be like, replacing problem definitions with aspirations and goals for the future. With Antika, the question of why she wanted the shadowman to go away elicited a wealth of information about her goals for the future. She reported that she wanted friends, relationships, and one day to have a career. "Don't I deserve to be happy?" she asked. "I want to overcome this; to get this shadowman behind me and just be like everyone else."

Externalizing conversations and mapping are powerful interventions used by narrative therapists to help people rewrite their stories. Mapping can also be documented through the use of a chart (White, 2007).

CASE ILLUSTRATION

Following is an example of a feminist therapist working with Ava Diaz who is now in the fifth grade and is having some difficulty making friends at school. Notice how the therapist uses self-disclosure to equalize the power imbalance in the relationship. She also uses the countertransference and stays in the here and now of the therapy session to help Ava develop appropriately assertive behavior.

CLINICIAN: Ava, your mother tells me you've been having some problems at school. What's going on?

AVA: (Looks down at the floor.) Nothing. I guess I'm just shy.

CLINICIAN: I was shy when I was your age.

AVA: Really? You were?

CLINICIAN: Sure. I always sat in the back of my classes, and at lunchtime I pretty much stayed to myself. I thought no one liked me, but when I look back at my behavior I can see that it was the way I was acting that made them think I wasn't really interested in being friends with them.

AVA: What did you do?

CLINICIAN: I acted tough so they wouldn't see that I was really hurting inside.

AVA: I do that sometimes, too. The other day in the lunchroom I really wanted to sit with a bunch of people from my English class. When I walked past their table, one of them said "Hey." I said "Hey" back, but I didn't know what else to say. So I ended up sitting alone. They were all having fun together, and I just felt left out.

CLINICIAN: Ava, I've noticed that you have a hard time making eye contact with me when you talk. Is that part of your feeling shy?

AVA: (softly, without looking up) Yes.

CLINICIAN: Sometimes if you don't look at the people you are talking to, it tells them that you aren't feeling very confident about yourself. Could that be how you're feeling?

AVA: I don't feel very confident.

CLINICIAN: Okay. Why don't we role-play a scenario in the cafeteria. I'll play you, and you play the part of one of the girls you'd like to sit with. What's her name?

AVA: Caylin.

CLINICIAN: (Stands up and walks towards Ava, carrying a book as if it were a lunch tray. Smiles and looks her directly in the eyes, and says:)
Hey, Caylin. Boy, that English test was hard, wasn't it? Do you mind if I sit with you?

AVA: Ah, sure. Go ahead.

CLINICIAN: How do you think you did on the test?

AVA: Fine.

CLINICIAN: (Sitting down next to Ava.) Now you try it.
(Ava repeats the role-play; being herself this time.)

CLINICIAN: Great! How did that feel to you?

AVA: It was easy!

CLINICIAN: Ava, you know everyone deserves to be treated with respect. And you have the same rights as anyone else to sit with your classmates at the lunch table. Another thing you can do is to make "I" statements.

AVA: What's an I-statement?

CLINICIAN: That's when you start a sentence with the word "I" to ask for what you want. Like "Hi Caylin. I'd like to sit with you at lunch."
Or in class, you might tell your teacher: "I don't think I did my best work on that paper. Is there anything I can do to make up the grade?"
Or sometimes if people are trying to get you to do bad things, you could say "I don't want to do that."
Do you think you could try making an I-statement tomorrow at school?

AVA: (Looks the therapist in the eye and smiles.)"I think so."

CLINICIAN: Now there's an I-statement!
(The clinician and Ava both laugh.)

Feminist therapists make use of material in the here and now of the therapy session to help clients work on their problems. In this short vignette, the clinician helped Ava to recognize how she is seen by others, and provided suggestions to help her overcome her awkwardness in social situations and be appropriately assertive. By sharing her own experience making friends, the therapist normalizes Ava's feelings. Finally, she gave her suggestions for how to be more assertive and through the use of role-play, helped Ava to verbalize her feelings.

EXERCISES

Large-Group Exercises

1. Generally counselors and therapists are entreated not to ask "why" questions. Such questions can be regarded as judgmental, can spur people to be cautious and consider their answers carefully, or can lead to intellectualizations and defensiveness. Even so, Michael White (2007) took up the cause of the why question and reported that in his experience "why questions play a profoundly significant role in helping people to give voice to . . . their purposes, aspirations, goals, quests, and commitments, and their understanding about what they value in life, their knowledge about life and life skills, and their prized learnings and realizations" (p. 49). Consider the impact of why questions in the counseling process. Certainly there are times when asking "why" could lead to defensiveness and justification of a person's actions, and other times when it could help explore underlying meanings and values. Discuss as a group the situations in which you might use why questions, how you would frame it, and what responses might result. Discuss also some of the negative ramifications of asking why. Are there particular circumstances (or types of clients) in which you might not use this particular intervention?
2. As a class, conduct a solution-focused round-robin with one person role-playing Edie or a different person. Each person in the class should select one of the interventions listed in the solution talk section. Choose your words carefully to be as hopeful and solution oriented as possible. After the round-robin, discuss the effectiveness of your interventions.

Small-Group Exercises

1. Form into your groups of two dyads. Each dyad should take a turn conducting a four-part mapping exercise similar to the example outlined in the Skill Development section. Spend 15 minutes each. Make sure you externalize the problem; ask questions about the effect of the problem on the person's life; look for exceptions; and plant seeds of hope that the client can move toward a solution. After each role-play, group members should provide feedback. How were the why questions responded to?
2. Form into your small groups. Each person should draw a large circle on a piece of paper. Now divide the circle into eight pieces, as if you were cutting a pie. Finally, draw a circle equidistant between the outer ring and center of the circle.

Label the Outer Circle with the following:

1. Person of color
2. Female or transgendered person
3. Child, elderly adult
4. Physical, cognitive, or emotional disability
5. Lesbian, gay, bisexual
6. Working class or below
7. Catholic, other Christian, atheist, Jewish, Muslim, Hindu, Shaman, Taoist, other
8. Refugee, illegal immigrant, or temporary resident

Label the Inner Circle with the following:

1. European American
2. Male
3. Young or middle adult
4. Temporarily able-bodied
5. Heterosexual
6. Upper or middle class
7. Protestant
8. Citizen

Now look at the words in the inner and outer circles, and choose the words that best describe you. If any of your selections are located in the inner circle, turn your paper over and write any privileges that you enjoy as a result of belonging to this group. Now take 15 minutes to share your results with your group. Were you aware of privileges you enjoy that others do not? Why are some of the privileges hidden or not noticeable? Is anyone in your group completely in the outer group? Completely in the inner group? How might one's social location affect their worldview?

Individual Exercises

1. Consider the influence of societal gender role expectations over the course of your lifetime. Think back to your childhood. What messages did your parents send you that reinforced traditional gender distinctions? Were you encouraged or discouraged from participation in play activities, household chores, manner of dress because that was or was not what girls (or boys) were expected to do? What about adolescence? What did you learn about how to act around boys (or girls)? Who gave you these messages? Did you feel that there were specific rules about same-gender friendships, career choices, or personal appearance that you were expected to follow? What about now? Do you see any difference in gender in any of your college course selections or majors? Where do you get messages about femininity or masculinity? Have your ideas remained the same? If not, how have they changed? Write about this in your journal.
2. Externalization is an important technique in narrative therapy. By placing the problem outside of themselves, people can be empowered to do something about it. Think about a problem you have had over the years. Imagine what it looks like. What color is it? Give it a name. Write a short autobiography from your problem's perspective.
3. Identify a problem or concern you are currently experiencing. Then find at least one exception to the problem or a time when you handled a similar problem successfully. Plan a small change based on this information. Write about this in your journal.

Summary

This chapter provided information on three postmodern constructivist approaches to counseling and psychotherapy: narrative therapy, solution-focused brief therapy, and feminist therapy. All of these approaches are holistic, attending to background as well as emotions, thoughts, and actions. They view people in a social context and believe that each person has a subjective psychological reality that has grown out of his or her life experiences. They also emphasize the reciprocal relationships we have with our world.

- Narrative therapy suggests that people's conceptions of themselves and their lives come from the stories they have made a part of themselves. By helping people to explore, understand, and modify their stories, clinicians can enable them to revision and reauthor their lives.
- De Shazer and Dolan (2007) summarized the main tenets of solution-focused therapy: "If it isn't broke, don't fix it. If it works, do more of it. If it's not working, do something different. Small steps can lead to big changes. The solution is not necessarily directly related to the problem. The language for solution development is different from that needed to describe a problem. No problems happen all the time; there are always exceptions that can be utilized. The future is both created and negotiable" (pp. 2–3).
- Feminist therapy seeks to help both men and women overcome rigid gender and other roles. This approach encourages people to appreciate the special attributes of their gender while expanding their options and promoting empowerment and egalitarian relationships.

All three approaches emphasize emotions and sensations, and all offer new and emerging ways for clinicians to treat their clients more effectively.

Recommended Readings

Constructivist

Journal of Constructivist Psychology—all issues.

Narrative

White, M. (2007). *Maps of narrative practice*. New York, NY: Norton and Company.

White, M. (2011). *Narrative practice: Continuing the conversation*. New York, NY: Norton.

Solution-Focused Brief Psychotherapy

De Jong, P., & Berg, I. K. (2008). *Interviewing for solutions* (3rd ed.). Pacific Grove, CA: Brooks/Cole.

de Shazer, S. (1988). *Clues: Investigating solutions in brief therapy*. New York, NY: Norton.

de Shazer, S. (1991). *Putting difference to work*. New York, NY: Norton.

de Shazer, S., & Dolan, Y. (2007). *More than miracles: The state of the art of solution-focused brief therapy*. Binghamton, NY: Haworth Press.

Feminist Therapy

Ballou, M., Hill, M., & West, C. (Eds.). (2008). *Feminist therapy theory and practice: A contemporary perspective*. New York, NY: Springer.

Enns, C. Z. (2004). *Feminist theories and feminist psychotherapies: Origins, themes, and diversity* (2nd ed.). Binghamton, NY: Haworth Press.

Gilligan, C. (2008). *Exit-voice dilemmas in adolescent development*. New York, NY: Analytic Press.

Jordan, J. V. (2010). *Relational-cultural therapy*. Washington, DC: American Psychological Association.

Robb, C. (2006). *This changes everything: The relational revolution in psychology*. New York, NY: Picador.

Additional Sources of Information

http://www.Dulwichcentre.com.au—Website for the Dulwich Centre in New Zealand. Site provides information on narrative therapy, interviews with leaders in that treatment approach, a bibliography, plus an archive of Michael White's articles.

http://www.narrativepractice.com—Website of the Institute of Narrative Training in the United Kingdom.

http://www.narrativetherapycentre.com—Website of the Narrative Therapy Centre of Toronto.

http://www.narrativeapproaches.com—Website includes workshops, papers, and links to additional resources on narrative therapy.

http://www.feminist-therapy-institute.org—Website of the Feminist Therapy Institute, a membership organization that holds conferences and provides information for people interested in feminist therapy.

http://www.wellesley.edu/JBMTI—The Jean Baker Miller Training Institute located at the Wellesley Centers for Women at Wellesley College. The institute focuses on relational-cultural theory and offers workshops, training, and publications.

http://constructingworlds.googlepages.com—Website of the Society for Constructivism in the Human Sciences. It provides information about leaders and publications in constructivism. Includes a discussion forum, listserve, and journal for those interested in constructivist theory, research, and practice.

http://www.sfbta.org—This website is home to the Solution Focused Brief Therapy Association begun in 2002 by Steve de Shazer, Insoo Kim Berg, and colleagues. The website provides information on the history of SFBT, conferences and training, access to articles, videos, tapes, and other resources including biographies and memorials to de Shazer and Berg.

http://www.brieftherapy.org.uk—Based in England, this website offers research articles, training, and conferences for SFBT therapists.

CHAPTER 12

Overview of Thought-Focused Treatment Systems

Thoughts, like emotions and sensations, are our constant companions. We wake up thinking about our plans for the day, fall asleep reviewing the day's experiences, and have myriad thoughts in between. The term *stream of consciousness* has been applied to the constant flow of thoughts we all have.

Part 4 of this book focuses on approaches to counseling and psychotherapy that view thoughts and cognitions as the primary avenue to change—the third of the four elements in the BETA (background, emotions, thoughts, actions) model. Cognitive therapists believe that thoughts lead to emotions and behaviors and that, through awareness and modification of their thoughts, people can change their feelings and actions.

DEVELOPMENT OF THOUGHT-FOCUSED TREATMENT SYSTEMS

Cognitive therapy emerged in the 1960s, largely as a result of the work of two very different and distinctive individuals—Albert Ellis and Aaron Beck. Ellis, a native of New York City with a PhD from Columbia University, trained as a psychoanalyst. Beck, a Yale-educated physician trained in psychoanalysis, worked at the University of Pennsylvania. Although they did not know each other at that point, both became disillusioned with psychoanalysis, the leading theoretical orientation at that time. Ellis preferred to be more directive in helping people with their problems, so he developed rational emotive therapy, later changed to rational emotive behavior therapy (REBT). REBT uses persuasion, teaching, and evidence gathering to help people dispute and modify their irrational beliefs and learn to accept themselves.

Meanwhile, in Pennsylvania, Beck was conducting research on the efficacy of psychoanalysis for depression and became disillusioned with the results. Beck had come to the conclusion that it was the way people think, the thoughts they tell themselves, and the manner in which they react, that is the most important element in their therapeutic recovery. He developed a theory of his own which he called cognitive therapy. Like Ellis, who was influenced by the writings of Epictetus, Beck also traced his theories back to the Stoic philosophers (Beck, Rush, Shaw, & Emery, 1979).

Even though their work evolved separately and independently from each other and resulted in two very different types of treatment, Ellis's and Beck's approaches are both considered to be cognitive therapies. This type of therapy seeks to help people overcome difficulties by identifying and changing dysfunctional thinking, behavior, and emotions. To do this, clients are taught skills to help them identify distorted thinking, modify beliefs, relate to others in different ways, and ultimately to change their behavior.

Beck and Ellis did exchange letters and ideas over the years. In his autobiography, *All Out!* (2009), Ellis included correspondence he exchanged with Aaron Beck during a 10-year time period. The letters highlight the fond relationship the pair had developed as well as the philosophical differences between REBT and cognitive therapy.

USE OF COGNITIONS IN COUNSELING AND PSYCHOTHERAPY

Either alone or in combination with other theoretical approaches, cognitive treatment systems are powerful and flexible approaches with broad application. Focusing treatment on thoughts has many strengths and benefits.

Beck and others have extensively researched cognitive approaches to treatment, and the effectiveness of these approaches is well established. Here are a few reasons why:

1. Thoughts are readily accessible. When we attend to our thoughts about a subject, we typically have little difficulty becoming cognizant of them and articulating them.
2. Asking people about their thoughts is usually less threatening than asking them about their feelings.
3. Cognitions are amenable to change and analysis. Thoughts can be written down, their validity and helpfulness can be assessed, and, if appropriate, they can be disputed and modified.

   For example, assume Pablo is at home reading a book when the doorbell rings. He thinks, "I bet that is my brother wanting to borrow some money." He feels unhappy and apprehensive. The reality of his thought can easily be tested; all he needs to do is answer the door. If it is not his brother, Pablo's thought will change, leading to a shift in his emotions. However, focusing directly on Pablo's emotions and trying to change his apprehensions probably will be a more complex process; for some people emotions feel amorphous, difficult to identify, and even harder to explain and analyze.

4. Changing thoughts can be relatively rapid. Experiencing positive gains early in treatment increases people's motivation and optimism, which can accelerate the course of treatment.
5. Learning to identify, dispute, and change thoughts can be empowering. Those skills can give people a greater sense of control over their lives and provide highly effective strategies for addressing problems.

TREATMENT USING COGNITIVE APPROACHES

REBT and Beck's cognitive therapy have much in common in terms of their theories of human development, concepts of effecting change, and strategies used. Both treatment systems are phenomenological models, as are person-centered counseling, existential therapy, Gestalt therapy, and other approaches discussed in earlier chapters. However, cognitive therapies focus on the meaning that people give to experiences through the way they *think* about them instead of how they *feel* about them. Although cognitive therapies recognize that background, emotions, and behavior are important and worthy of attention in treatment, they view thoughts as the primary determinant of both emotions and behaviors, as well as of mental disorders and psychological health.

Cognitive therapists believe that the basic material of treatment is a person's transient automatic thoughts and their deeply ingrained and fundamental assumptions and schemas. Once these have been identified, clinicians draw on a variety of interventions to help people test and modify their cognitions. Replacing dysfunctional cognitions with thoughts that are more accurate, helpful, and healthy enables people to cope more successfully with their immediate difficulties and leads to more rewarding lives.

Goals

The goal of cognitive therapy is to teach people how to recognize, identify, and respond to dysfunctional thoughts. To do this, cognitive therapists employ a variety of techniques. Cognitive therapists use inventories, assessments, suggested tasks or homework, and other techniques and strategies to advance treatment goals. Because cognitive therapy is based on research and clients' practical experience of what works best to fit their needs at that particular time, the approach is constantly evolving. Many techniques are borrowed from behavior therapy and integrated into cognitive therapy to provide more of a hybrid of behavior management and action. We will learn more about the integration of cognitive therapy with behavior therapy and with newer acceptance- and mindfulness-based approaches in Part 5 of this book.

Therapeutic Alliance

Even though cognitive therapists are directive in their approach, they still must focus on the common factors of a collaborative therapeutic relationship; a supportive and healing environment characterized by respect, genuineness, and unconditional positive regard; a holistic understanding of clients and their backgrounds; a sense of direction or goals; a shared understanding about the nature of the problems to be addressed in treatment; and the use of a valid treatment approach to address the client's symptoms. When working with Middle Eastern clients, for example, Constantino and Wilson (2007) recommend a two-way negotiation of therapy in which the therapist initiates an open exploration of a client's ideas about what she believes will alleviate her distress. Through the negotiation process, differences between the therapist's and the client's beliefs about change are brought into the open and expectations can be discussed.

Application of Cognitive Therapies

Beck, who was trained in psychoanalysis, created a methodology that is easily replicated and lends itself to clinical trials. He developed a model of therapy that worked for depression and anxiety and was also testable. Research continues to support the use of cognitive therapy with all of the anxiety disorders (Clark & Beck, 2011), mood disorders, personality disorders, and schizophrenia (Clark, Hollifield, Leahy, & Beck, 2009). Not only are cognitive therapy and REBT effective treatments, but they have also been found to be cost effective (Sava, Yates, Lupu, Szentagotai, & David, 2009).

Cognitive treatment approaches also lend themselves to the use of manuals. Treatment manuals can provide guidance for therapists and tend to be specific to a disorder. They are generally research based and provide a process, techniques, and other guidance for therapists to be able to replicate evidence-based practices.

Application to Multicultural Clients

Treatment systems that emphasize thoughts are likely to be comfortable for and make sense to a wide range of people. Particularly important, a focus on thoughts can make the counseling process more acceptable to people who are not used to sharing their emotions, including some men, many older people, and some people from Asian and other cultural backgrounds who may view expression of emotions to a stranger as inappropriate, weak, or in conflict with their upbringing and self-images.

Experiments and Homework

Both REBT and Beck's cognitive therapy rely on experiments or homework assignments to help clients recognize underlying thoughts and to reinforce efforts made during therapy sessions. Ellis, for example, often prescribed what he called "shame-attacking exercises" to help clients overcome their shame when others disapproved of their actions. Asking silly questions in a classroom or talking in a movie theater are homework assignments he designed to overcome feelings of shame or disappointment by other's disapproval. Clients would be told to repeat the exercise until they no longer felt anxiety or fear of other's disapproval. We turn now to the planning and processing of homework, which is an integral part of all cognitive–behavioral treatment approaches.

PLANNING AND PROCESSING HOMEWORK

The mere mention of homework can bring up negative images for both clinicians and clients—memories of deadlines, failures, and blame for poor performance. However, homework, or what Aaron Beck called task assignments, also can be an asset to treatment; homework can help people feel empowered, encourage them to take credit for their gains, and accelerate treatment. According to Judith Beck (2011), some researchers have shown that "therapy patients who carry out homework assignments progress better in therapy than those who do not" (p. 294). The guidelines that follow can help make homework a positive experience for both clients and clinicians.

Terminology

For some people, the words *homework* and *assignment* have negative connotations. Those words also imply that the clinician/teacher is telling the client/student to complete a requirement. This can create a hierarchy rather than a collaboration, which is undesirable in cognitive therapy. Finding more acceptable language can help. Terms such as *tasks, between-session projects,* and *experiments* may be more acceptable. Clinicians should use language that will elicit a positive response from clients.

Determining the Assignment

Collaboration. Clients and clinicians should collaborate in determining assignments. Although initially suggestions may come primarily from clinicians, clients should have the opportunity to shape the tasks in ways that make them meaningful. They also should have the right to accept or reject any assignments. As clients progress and become familiar with cognitive therapy, clinicians can encourage them to suggest tasks they find meaningful.

Relating assignments to sessions. Clinicians should clarify for clients the rationale behind each assignment. The assignments should continue progress or address issues that arose during the current session. For example, a woman who expressed thoughts of self-blame related to the abuse she and her younger sister received from their mother was urged to draft a letter to her mother, expressing her thoughts and feelings about the abuse of her sister. The woman could think more clearly about the abuse of her sister than about her own abuse. The letter-writing assignment helped her become more aware of those thoughts so she could eventually believe similar thoughts about her own abuse. This letter was not actually mailed but served as a learning experience.

Making assignments specific. Assignments should be specific so that people know exactly when and how to complete them. This reduces resistance and barriers to the assignment. Rather than suggesting that a client "have more contact with friends," the assignment might involve "having telephone conversations of at least 5 minutes with two friends on Wednesday evening and inviting at least one of them to lunch."

Ease of accomplishment. Assignments should be fairly easy to accomplish. This, too, reduces resistance and makes it more likely that people will complete the tasks. In addition, success in accomplishing tasks can help them feel empowered and optimistic about their treatment. Graded task assignments are assignments that gradually increase in difficulty. They are particularly useful in helping people build on past successes and confront increasing challenges. Again, clinicians should plan carefully when making tasks more difficult, always seeking success. Assigning tasks that are too hard for clients or that bring up strong negative feelings is likely to undermine treatment and increase clients' self-doubts.

Practicing tasks in the session. Clinicians can increase the likelihood of clients' completing suggested tasks by starting or practicing a task in the session before asking people to complete tasks on their own. For example, a man who wanted to stop thinking negative thoughts about his failure to graduate from college with honors was encouraged to deliberately think the negative thoughts in the session and then practice thought-stopping followed by an affirmation to curtail his negative ruminating. Coaching and encouraging him through this process in the session increased his motivation to use these skills outside of the session.

Addressing possible barriers. Clinicians should address possible barriers to accomplishment of assignments, as well as potential negative outcomes, to prevent them from interfering with treatment. Elinor, a woman who had been adopted as an infant, had successfully modified cognitions about her unlovableness. Her newfound confidence led her to decide to contact her biological mother. She and her counselor spent time talking about the possible responses of her biological mother to prepare Elinor to handle any outcome. In addition, the clinician helped Elinor focus on the personal achievements that enabled her to take this step, rather than the outcome of her interactions with her mother, to determine whether this experience was a success or a failure. Role-plays and cognitive rehearsal are useful strategies for helping prepare people for challenging tasks.

Minimizing excuses. Clinicians also should plan assignments so that they minimize the likelihood of excuses. For example, "If I go out to dinner with my mother and if she orders a glass of wine, I will tell her my thoughts about her excessive use of alcohol" is a weak assignment. It has too many ifs and possible pitfalls. Create assignments that depend on the client rather than on other people or external circumstances.

Addressing clients' reactions. Clinicians should address clients' reactions to the concept of homework assignments. Some people have a strong need for perfection, may fear failure or judgment, or may be very eager to please the clinician. Clinicians should explore clients' feelings about completing task assignments, making sure that people understand the reason for the homework and know that the clinician will not judge them. Keeping clients' reactions to homework in mind when suggesting or processing tasks should increase the likelihood that they will enhance treatment.

Offering options. For people who are beginning treatment or who may be apprehensive about completing assignments, offering options can be helpful. For example, identifying three tasks but encouraging a client to complete only two of them gives the person some control as well as the message that this is not school where all assignments must be done.

Writing down assignments. Task assignments should be written down, by either the client or the clinician, in a place where the client can easily locate them. Some clinicians have space on the back of their appointment cards for assignments, some give clients a form at the end of each session that lists their suggested tasks, and others have clients bring a notebook or date book to each session to record their homework for the week. Clinicians also should note the homework in their own records so that they can follow up appropriately in the next session.

Processing Homework

Clinicians should be sure to discuss and process homework in the session following the one in which it was suggested. Most clients invest considerable effort in completing their tasks and want to share their accomplishments with their clinicians. Processing homework is likely to improve clients' self-esteem and cooperation with the completion of future tasks, and also helps identify and reinforce the learning that has come from the task.

Of course, clients will not always complete homework, and their experiences with assignments may not always be rewarding. Even under these circumstances, homework can be viewed as a learning experience so that something positive always emerges from that process. For example, in an effort to develop her social skills and relationships, Mary joined a cooking class. Unfortunately, traffic problems delayed her arrival at the class. When she got there and saw that the class was already in progress, she became anxious and left the class. Although this disappointed her, she could take credit for making an effort to attend the class and learned that she needed to plan her next social experience more carefully to maximize her comfort level. The experience also gave Mary an opportunity to identify an automatic thought, "I am a failure at whatever I undertake," and replace it with "I was wise to know that coming into the class late was too much for me. I can learn from this and be more successful next time."

Homework can be a rewarding and reinforcing experience for clients and provide an opportunity for clinicians to use their creativity and understanding of clients to craft meaningful, interesting, and growth-promoting tasks. One clinician who made regular use of homework reported that many of her clients kept a file of their assignments over the course of treatment and viewed them as a reflection of how much they had accomplished.

Summary

This chapter reviewed the importance of thoughts in understanding and counseling people. It introduced cognitive and rational emotive behavior therapy, two types of therapy developed by Aaron Beck and Albert Ellis that help people assess and, if indicated, modify thoughts, as well as their accompanying emotions and actions. The last section in this chapter focused on planning and processing homework, a valuable tool for all types of cognitive interventions. What you have learned in this chapter provides a foundation on which to develop your understanding of cognitive approaches to treatment as presented in the remaining chapters of Part 4.

CHAPTER 13

Albert Ellis and Rational Emotive Behavior Therapy

Rational emotive behavior therapy (REBT) emphasizes thoughts. REBT initially was developed by Albert Ellis in the 1950s. Ellis continued to be the primary advocate and spokesperson for this approach until his death in 2007 at the age of 93. In his obituary, the *New York Times* (Kaufman, 2007) referred to Ellis as irreverent and charismatic, and he has been called the Lenny Bruce of psychology. Indeed, his creativity, humor, and crackly personality made him a dynamic speaker and trainer. Ellis was voted by his peers as the second most influential psychologist (after Carl Rogers).

The REBT approach to treatment assumes that people's cognitions are the primary source of their difficulties. Although rational emotive behavior therapists believe that thoughts, emotions, and behaviors are interrelated (Ellis & MacLaren, 2005), they view helping people think more rationally as the most effective route to improving all three areas of functioning.

Cognitive therapy and REBT have much in common in terms of their theories of human development, concepts of effecting change, and strategies used. Both treatment approaches are structured and active, while emphasizing the human element in treatment. However, the two approaches also have differences. REBT has its own approach to disputing and modifying distorted cognitions. Persuasion and teaching, along with gathering evidence, are important strategies for rational emotive behavior therapists.

ALBERT ELLIS

Albert Ellis, the originator of REBT, was born in 1913 in Pittsburgh. He moved to New York as a young child and lived there for most of his life. Ellis's family of origin included an independent mother, a father who cared about the family but was often absent, and a younger brother and sister (Bernard, 2011). Ellis was apparently the family favorite. He got along well with the others in his family, although in many ways he had a difficult childhood. At an early age, he perceived his family as "pretty crazy" and stated that he basically raised himself from the age of 7 (Ellis, 2009). In addition, Ellis, was sickly as a child and was often hospitalized, usually for nephritis. Ellis noticed that he frequently worked himself into a miserable state, and it was then that he decided not to be miserable about his circumstances and maintained strong positive thoughts about his competence and worth (Ellis, 1997, 2009). Thus, at an early age he learned that the way people think can enable them to overcome adversity.

In the 1940s, Ellis received MA and PhD degrees in clinical psychology from Columbia University and began practicing as a marriage, family, and sex therapist. Seeking to help people achieve profound change, he obtained training as a psychoanalyst with an emphasis on the work of Karen Horney (Ellis & Dryden, 2007). However, his dissatisfaction with the inefficiency of psychoanalysis as well as his readings in Greek and Asian philosophy led him to develop a way to treat people that focused on their thoughts.

Ellis began practicing what he initially called rational therapy in 1955, founded the still-active Institute for Rational Emotive Therapy (now the Albert Ellis Institute) in 1959 to offer both treatment and training in this approach, and published the first of his many works on REBT in 1962. A prolific writer, Ellis authored more than 800 academic papers and 80 books and monographs. His final book, titled simply *Rational Emotive Behavior Therapy*, was published posthumously (Ellis & Ellis, 2011). He received many awards, including the Distinguished Professional Psychologist Award in 1974 and the Distinguished Professional Contributions Award in 1985, both from the American Psychological Association.

Ellis was open about his personal life and often used himself as a role model in his work. A classic story he told about himself was that, as a young man, he was apprehensive about asking women for dates. To overcome his fears, he forced himself to approach 100 women and invite them out. Although all refused, this experience of forcing himself to do repeatedly what he feared most enabled him to overcome his anxieties. Ellis's shame-attacking exercises (discussed later in this chapter) recall this experience.

THE DEVELOPMENT OF RATIONAL EMOTIVE BEHAVIOR THERAPY

Now more than 50 years old, rational emotive behavior therapy has evolved considerably, although its basic premise—that emotions and behavior can best be modified by changing thinking—has not changed. Early influences on REBT include the writing of the philosopher Epictetus, Buddhist and Taoist philosophy, and writings on happiness, secular humanism, and behaviorism. Alfred Adler's emphasis on the social system, the importance of goals and purpose, and use of live demonstrations also are apparent in REBT. In addition, Karen Horney's concepts, especially about the power of "shoulds" in our lives, are evident in REBT.

Ellis changed the name of his theory twice. In 1961, rational therapy became rational *emotive* therapy (RET), reflecting the attention this approach paid to feelings. This modification may, at least in part, have been a response to the popularity of Carl Rogers's ideas, which emphasized the importance of emotions. RET became rational emotive *behavior* therapy in 1993, reflecting its increased emphasis on behavior, especially as a vehicle for reinforcing and implementing changes in thinking (Ellis, 1995). As practiced today, REBT emphasizes thoughts, but views emotions, behaviors, and thoughts as intertwined and inseparable. To maximize success, treatment must attend to all three.

Since its initial development, the theories, structure, and strategies of REBT have become less absolute and more compatible with postmodern treatment approaches, including narrative therapy, constructivist therapy, and existential therapy. Ellis's emphasis on people's perceptions of the world have led some to view him as constructivist in his outlook (Ellis & MacLaren, 2005). Interventions used in REBT have become more varied and eclectic. In addition, REBT now pays greater attention to understanding the background and viewpoints of each client and is more accepting of people's religious and other beliefs, as long as they are not rigid and harmful. Rational emotive behavior therapy was the first cognitive therapy to be developed (Ellis, 1957).

IMPORTANT THEORETICAL CONCEPTS

As with all cognitive therapies, REBT focuses on helping people identify, evaluate, and modify dysfunctional cognitions. However, rational emotive behavior therapists differ from cognitive therapists following Beck's approach (which will be discussed in the next chapter) in terms of the strategies they use and their conception of healthy development.

Human Development and Emotional Health

According to REBT, dimensions of psychological health include the following (Ellis & Dryden, 2007, pp. 18–19):

- Awareness, acceptance, and appreciation of oneself and others
- Social interest; recognition that contributing to the world enhances our own happiness
- Self-direction and personally meaningful goals
- Involvement in long-range, absorbing creative pursuits; commitment to something outside oneself
- Long-range hedonism; the ability to enjoy the present as well as the discipline to defer immediate gratification and seek pleasure in the future
- Acceptance of uncertainty and ambiguity
- Flexibility, ability to adapt to change
- High frustration tolerance so we are not devastated by disappointments
- Ability to think in a clear, logical, scientific, and rational way
- Willingness to take sensible risks, experiment, and be reasonably adventurous
- Recognition that we cannot always be totally happy and that life will not always go exactly as we hope
- Acceptance of responsibility for our own emotional difficulties.

SELF-ACCEPTANCE Self-acceptance is an important concept in REBT. This approach suggests that emotional difficulties often are found in people with conditional self-acceptance; they value themselves because of their accomplishments rather than because of their basic worth as a person. When they experience failures or disappointments, they tend to rate themselves harshly and their self-esteem plummets as a result (Bernard, Froh, DiGiuseppe, Joyce, & Dryden, 2010). According to Ellis, people should have a realistic sense of their strengths and weaknesses and take pride in their achievements. At the same time, they will feel happier and more stable if they accept, value, and believe in themselves even when they are disappointed in their behaviors or experiences. REBT teaches people to assess their thoughts and behaviors, not themselves.

ORIGINS OF EMOTIONAL DISTURBANCE REBT suggests that, because irrational thinking is so widespread, people must have a strong biological tendency to think dysfunctionally and believe that life should go their way. However, people do vary in their propensity to think irrationally. REBT recognizes that childhood difficulties and traumas may contribute to a person's tendency to think and act in unhealthy ways. Emotional disturbance, then, results from a combination of an innate predisposition toward irrational thinking and life experiences.

Despite its recognition of the impact of biological, social, and other forces on human development, REBT maintains an optimistic view of human nature. It emphasizes will and choice and perceives people as having inborn drives toward actualization and happiness (Ellis & MacLaren, 2005). REBT perceives people as able to exercise choice, to see that their thoughts are responsible for disturbing them, and to actively and continually work toward positive change and fulfillment (Ellis & MacLaren, 2005).

Secular Humanism

With its focus on the perceptions and responsibility of the individual, REBT is rooted in secular humanism. According to Ellis (1992), "Secular humanism is relativist, skeptical, and nondogmatic and emphasizes the best and most practical aspects of the scientific method together with human choice and meaningfulness" (p. 349). Secular humanists view people as unique individuals who usually value and choose to live in interdependent social groups. They see people as neither good nor bad but simply human; only people's acts are evaluated. People who adopt a philosophy of secular humanism typically are concerned with social systems and advocate peace, fairness, and democracy. They seek possibilities and alternatives rather than absolute truths. Overall, REBT encourages people to develop a rational philosophy of life.

Thoughts as the Route to Change

According to REBT, change only occurs when people recognize and accept that they are largely responsible for creating their own emotional problems (Ellis, 1988). Regardless of when and how the problems began, REBT maintains that emotional problems stem primarily from irrational beliefs. As Shakespeare wrote, "Things are neither good nor bad but thinking makes them so" (DiGiuseppe, 1996, p. 6). Rational emotive behavior therapists have found that, through hard work and practice, people can change their absolute and irrational beliefs and correspondingly alleviate their emotional difficulties.

FOCUS ON PRESENT THOUGHTS REBT focuses on present thoughts rather than past events. Although clinicians recognize the significance of the past, they discourage lengthy, in-depth exploration of people's backgrounds and the origins of their thoughts. Instead, they believe that a present-oriented focus is more meaningful to people, more likely to enhance rapport, and in keeping with the idea that people's current thoughts and behaviors maintain their self-defeating thoughts, whatever the origins of those thoughts.

Believing that irrational thoughts underlie all psychological problems, clinicians use forceful and creative strategies to help people identify and dispute their irrational beliefs; REBT asserts that positive results are obtained when people gain awareness of their irrational beliefs and take effective action to change them (Dryden & Branch, 2008). Like other cognitive therapists, clinicians practicing REBT provide people the skills they need to become their own therapists—to enable them to use the methods of REBT throughout their lives to identify and change their self-destructive thoughts.

REBT'S VIEW OF INSIGHT Helping people gain insight into the origins of their problems and emotional disturbances is not an essential part of REBT. Not only is insight viewed as insufficient for change, but it is seen as potentially harmful, leading to self-blame and immobilization. However, gaining insight into the principles of REBT is important. Ellis (1988) described three levels of insight, which he views as necessary for people to make positive changes:

1. The insight to see that we choose to upset ourselves
2. The insight to see that we acquired our irrational beliefs and to see how we continue to maintain them
3. The insight to see that we need to work hard to change.

REBT'S VIEW OF EMOTIONS Clinicians using REBT do not spend a great deal of time exploring the background behind emotions nor do they seek to change them directly. However, clinicians recognize that if people can become aware of their emotions and their impact, this can facilitate their efforts to identify and change their irrational beliefs.

Ellis (1986) distinguished between inappropriate/self-destructive emotions and appropriate/nondefeating emotions. *Self-destructive emotions* are enduring, immobilizing, and nonproductive; reflect overreactions to stimuli; and lead to negative self-images and actions. Dryden (2011) identified eight emotional problems: guilt, shame, jealousy, hurt, anxiety, depression, envy, and unhealthy anger. On the other hand, *appropriate emotions* are transient, manageable, in proportion to the stimulus, and enhancing of self-acceptance. They include both positive emotions such as joy, satisfaction, and peacefulness and negative emotions such as annoyance, regret, and sadness. Of course, we all have negative reactions when we experience losses and disappointments. However, our thoughts about those disappointments determine whether we develop emotions that are inappropriate and self-destructive or appropriate and nondefeating.

REBT'S VIEW OF BEHAVIOR Like emotions, behaviors are a secondary focus of treatment. They provide a measure of progress, are used to modify and reinforce thoughts, and are a prime target of homework assignments. Although REBT views behaviors, emotions, and thoughts as having a reciprocal relationship, thoughts are the primary route to change. Changing thoughts and the accompanying self-statements leads to changes in both actions and emotion.

Irrational Beliefs

Irrational beliefs usually are characterized by at least one of the following themes: awfulizing, self-deprecation including global evaluations of human worth and self-criticism, and frustration intolerance (Ellis, 2001).

REBT identifies thoughts as either rational beliefs or irrational beliefs. Rational beliefs are logical, pragmatic, and based in reality. They are flexible and not extreme (Dryden, DiGiuseppe, & Neenan, 2010). Irrational beliefs often include words such as *should, ought,* and *must* and may include immediate demands about the self, others, and the world (Ellis, 1984, p. x; 2003, pp. 236–237):

1. I must act perfectly and be achieving and lovable at all times. If I do not, I am incompetent and worthless. (This belief usually leads to feelings of anxiety, depression, and low self-esteem.)
2. Other people must always treat me kindly and fairly or I can't stand it and they are terrible, evil people who should be punished for mistreating me. (This belief typically leads to rage and vindictiveness.)
3. Life must go the way I want it to go and must never be too difficult or frustrating. Otherwise, life is terrible and I cannot bear it. (This belief often results in inaction, low frustration tolerance, self-pity, anger, and depression.)

Irrational beliefs are typically absolutes about oneself, other people, or one's circumstances. They tend to be evaluative and judgmental, viewing life in extremes. They are illogical, inconsistent with reality, and prevent people from attaining their goals (Dryden et al., 2010).

Common types of irrational beliefs identified by clinicians practicing REBT (Ellis & Dryden, 2007) are similar to Beck's cognitive distortions, which will be described in the next chapter. Examples of irrational beliefs include thoughts such as these:

VINCE: I must have a date for New Year's Eve by tomorrow, or I will be the laughing stock of my fraternity.

MARTIN: My supervisor should praise me and is a jerk for not seeing how hard I work.

NATASHA: I ought to spend every evening with my family. I am a terrible mother if I don't do that.

Here are rational versions of the same beliefs:

VINCE: I would like to have a date for New Year's Eve so that I can join my friends in that celebration.

MARTIN: I believe that my supervisor is not really familiar with my work and so is not giving me the praise I would like.

NATASHA: My family and I enjoy spending time together and I believe that is helpful to my children, but I can take some time for myself and still be a good mother.

The preceding irrational beliefs are extreme statements that promote negative emotions and difficulties in relationships. They do not facilitate problem solving or constructive action because they view success or failure in extreme terms, are demanding and inflexible, and blame people rather than assess a situation clearly. The rational beliefs, on the other hand, reflect preferences, hopes, and wishes. They do not judge, but instead look at possibilities. Problem solving and constructive action are facilitated because, without extremist thinking, many options and solutions are available. Vince can take steps to find a last-minute date but still may be able to celebrate the holiday with his friends even if he doesn't have a date. Martin can plan to acquaint his supervisor with the quality of his work. Natasha can build in more time with her family while not demanding perfection from herself. Ellis (1995) defined a rational belief as a "cognition that is effective or self-helping" as well as "empirically or logically valid" (p. 85).

THE FORMAT OF SESSIONS

Sessions in REBT tend to follow a relatively predictable pattern. A typical session includes the following 10 steps (Walen, DiGiuseppe, & Dryden, 1992, p. 65):

1. Review old business from the previous session.
2. Check up on mood, behavior, thoughts, symptoms, and medication.
3. Elicit new business, especially any major life changes.
4. Follow up on homework.
5. Establish the agenda for the sessions.
6. Do the work according to the *ABC* format (discussed later in this chapter).
7. Summarize the work that has been done.
8. Assign new homework.
9. Obtain feedback on the session.
10. Close the session.

Inclusion of additional steps at the beginning and end of the treatment process is invaluable in maximizing the success of REBT. Clinicians typically begin by explaining the theory of REBT and familiarizing clients with its procedures and with what is expected from them as clients. Although clinicians who practice REBT are less likely to use a formal assessment process incorporating many inventories than are other cognitive therapists, they, too, engage in assessment during the first few sessions of treatment, exploring clients' history and background, thoughts, emotions, behaviors, and symptoms. Once that has been accomplished, focus shifts to helping clients recognize that they largely create their own disturbance, understand that psychological difficulties typically stem from irrational beliefs, and see that they can change their beliefs and alleviate their difficulties.

Homework assignments are an important part of the treatment process and help to reinforce lessons learned. Even if the client has not completed the previous week's homework, the lesson should be reviewed (Neenan & Dryden, 2011).

By the end of treatment, clients should have learned to evaluate and dispute their own beliefs using a variety of strategies, and be prepared to continue that process throughout their lives. Follow-up sessions facilitate people's efforts to continue REBT on their own. Relapse prevention is especially important for people who have made significant philosophical changes and may need help in continuing to maintain those changes.

Although REBT is often a relatively brief process, clinicians generally do not predetermine the number of sessions. Rather, treatment lasts as long as necessary to help people accomplish their goals. Efficiency rather than brevity is valued.

TREATMENT USING RATIONAL EMOTIVE BEHAVIOR THERAPY

Clinicians who practice REBT foster the therapeutic alliance and use a wide range of strategies, particularly the *ABC* approach to modifying irrational beliefs. Many of these are described here.

Goals

REBT is a goal-oriented treatment system that focuses on outcomes such as changes in beliefs and reduction in symptoms. It de-emphasizes processes such as exploration of early development and insight into the impact of the past on the present. Although REBT helps people to become more aware of their thoughts, emotions, and behaviors, this approach is primarily concerned with helping people to learn cognitive skills that promote rational thinking and lead to greater happiness and self-acceptance (Ellis & Ellis, 2011).

Therapeutic Alliance

Clients and clinicians have a collaborative relationship in REBT. Clients assume some responsibility for planning and implementing their treatment, just as they are encouraged to take considerable responsibility for their difficulties. Clinicians teach clients about rational and irrational thinking; help people identify, dispute, and modify their irrational beliefs; and facilitate their efforts to develop a more rational philosophy of life. Although problem solving is part of treatment, REBT clinicians go beyond problem solving and help people to establish more balanced, logical, and rewarding lives.

Rational emotive behavior therapists are highly involved in the treatment process, often using their influence on clients to effect change. Ellis had a directive, sometimes brusque, therapeutic style. He was genuine and authentic, and recognized that flexibility is important (Dryden & Branch, 2008). Clinicians in REBT do not hesitate to use persuasion, praise, exaggeration, instruction, humorous songs, and anecdotes from their own lives to help people think more rationally and make positive changes. According to Ellis (1992), clinicians should not be blank screens; they should be highly active, genuine, and directive, revealing their own thoughts and experiences, but always maintaining a professional relationship with clients. Of course, Ellis recognized that the degree to which a clinician is active and directive is a personal choice (Dryden & Ellis, 2001).

Ellis and Dryden (2007, p. 29) suggest that clinicians practicing REBT be:

- Structured but flexible
- Intellectually, cognitively, and philosophically inclined
- Active and directive in their style
- Comfortable using behavioral instruction and teaching
- Untroubled by fear of failure and willing to take thoughtful risks
- Emotionally healthy, accepting of themselves and others as fallible
- Practical and scientific rather than mystical and magical
- Comfortable with a variety of interventions.

Clinicians practicing REBT assume many roles. They are teachers, coaches, role models, confidence builders, cheerleaders, and motivators. They strive to communicate acceptance and caring to their clients, helping them to overcome problems and lead happier lives.

REBT follows the beliefs first set forth by Carl Rogers of unconditional positive regard, congruence, and authenticity being necessary conditions for change to occur. Ellis referred to it as unconditional other acceptance (UOA), unconditional self-acceptance (USA), and unconditional other acceptance-multicultural (Ellis, 2007). REBT clinicians do not judge their clients, but they may disapprove of their behaviors. Ellis often told clients he disliked some of their behaviors and would not want to befriend them in social situations—certainly a powerful message.

Ellis cautioned against clinicians becoming gurus and creating a situation in which clients change to please the clinician rather than themselves. In REBT, self-acceptance is paramount.

Most clinicians practicing REBT do not seem to emulate Ellis, rather, they have many different yet effective styles. As we have seen in the chapter on Carl Rogers, rapport and empathy are essential to building a therapeutic alliance. These traits are also compatible with an active and directive treatment stance like REBT. Creating a positive therapeutic alliance and being able to adapt

REBT to the needs of each client are essential to effective treatment. Using the client's words, and incorporating language that is meaningful to the client can help to improve rapport (Dryden, 2011).

Identifying, Assessing, Disputing, and Modifying Irrational Beliefs

REBT uses a structured format for identifying, assessing, disputing, and modifying beliefs—a plan represented by the letters *ABCDE* (Ellis & Ellis, 2011). The REBT Self-Help Form or the Attitudes and Beliefs Inventory (Lega & Ellis, 2001) is sometimes used to help people identify their beliefs. To illustrate the *ABCDE* model, we consider Martin's beliefs about his supervisor (presented earlier in this chapter).

A, the first step, is identification and description of the *activating event.* This is the external and objective source of discomfort, the experience that initiates the process of irrational thinking and precipitates the negative thoughts, emotions, and behaviors.

> ***Martin A:*** "My supervisor gave me an average rating on my evaluation."

B is the person's *belief* about the activating event, evaluating that stimulus as positive, negative, or neutral. The belief may be rational or irrational. REBT holds that people may not have a choice about experiences or activating events but do have a choice about their beliefs related to those activating events.

> ***Martin B:*** "My supervisor should praise me more and is a jerk for not seeing how hard I work. It is awful that I work so hard and am not valued as I ought to be."

C stands for the *consequences* of the belief. Of course, the activating event itself can produce negative consequences; but according to REBT, beliefs mediate between events and consequences, with beliefs being a major determinant of most consequences. By assessing the nature and consequences of a belief, clinicians can determine whether the belief is irrational and harmful to the client or rational and either neutral or helpful. If the belief is irrational, consequences are likely to be unhealthy and harmful and might include inappropriate and self-destructive emotions (e.g., rage, anxiety, depression) and inappropriate and self-destructive behaviors (e.g., excessive use of alcohol, blaming self and others, withdrawal). Rational beliefs usually lead to healthier and more constructive consequences such as appropriate emotions (e.g., disappointment, annoyance) and appropriate behaviors (e.g., taking effective steps to change the situation or distracting oneself with exercise or a creative pursuit).

Initial consequences of a belief can lead to subsequent reinforcing consequences that themselves become activating events. For example, if Martin expressed his anger toward his supervisor in loud and attacking ways and the supervisor reacted with further disapproval, Martin's irrational beliefs and negative emotions probably would be reinforced.

> ***Martin C:*** Martin experienced anger, shame, and anxiety about the possibility of losing his job. His behaviors included berating his supervisor.

D, dispute (also referred to as debate), is the next step in the process. Exploration of beliefs and their consequences determines whether they are rational or irrational. In general, clinicians begin by focusing on irrational beliefs about immediate situations and then move to more generalized and abstract irrational beliefs.

Later in the chapter, we will talk more about the many strategies available to help people contest their irrational beliefs. Some are similar to strategies that will be discussed in Chapter 14. However, in REBT, clinicians rely more on persuasion, teaching, and techniques that elicit strong emotions than do other cognitive therapists, who rely more on logic.

> ***Martin D:*** Strategies to dispute irrational beliefs include cognitive, behavioral, and emotional approaches to change. For Martin, all three are relevant. Cognitive approaches might involve examining the logic of his belief, including the adequacy of the supervisor's information on Martin's performance and whether receiving an average evaluation was truly awful or simply undesirable. Ellis would probably have used emotional methods, pointing out Martin's awfulizing, his tendency to catastrophize, and his perfectionistic need to have his life be exactly as he wishes. Ellis might have encouraged Martin to feel appropriate and nondestructive emotions such as annoyance and disappointment, which contribute to rational thinking, rather than shame and anger, which are self-destructive and inappropriate emotions. Martin might also benefit from behavioral strategies, such as meeting with his supervisor, providing her additional information about his work, and planning an outing or creative project to help him focus on rewarding aspects of his life.

E, the last step, stands for *new rational effect or beliefs,* describing the desired outcome of the disputation. The outcome of REBT is likely to include both effective rational beliefs and an effective new philosophy. Out of this philosophy flow new feelings and behaviors and greater, long-lasting happiness (Bernard et al., 2010).

> ***Martin E:*** After disputing his beliefs, Martin developed more rational beliefs such as: "Although I am disappointed that my evaluation was average, it is not the end of the world. I will take steps to familiarize my supervisor with my work and obtain a more positive evaluation next time."

Although the *ABCDE* process may seem simple and straightforward, changing irrational beliefs to rational ones is a challenging and complex process. It requires effort and practice on the part of the client, as well as well-chosen and skillfully used interventions on the part of the clinician. The process can be complicated by the tendency of many people to have second-order disturbances: to feel bad about feeling bad. This creates several layers of irrational beliefs that need attention. In addition, people sometimes prefer their familiar discomfort to the risk of the unknown discomfort of change (Ellis & Dryden, 2007). They also may value the sympathy, attention, and other secondary gains they receive as a result of their problems.

Approaches to Disputing Irrational Beliefs

Even if people can intellectually grasp the *ABCDE* model and the message that our beliefs, rather than activating events, are the primary source of our disturbance, people often have difficulty modifying their thoughts. Ellis (2003) explained this by saying ". . . they tend to *keep* holding these irrational beliefs and upsetting themselves by them, not because they held them in the past but because they are still actively, though unconsciously, reaffirming them and acting as if they are still valid" (p. 241). "Work and practice" (p. 242) are the ways to address these entrenched beliefs. Using a combination of cognitive, emotive, and behavioral interventions in a forceful and persistent way, REBT clinicians actively work with clients to identify their irrational beliefs, dispute them, and replace absolutist and irrational beliefs with flexible preferences.

Beal, Kopec, and DiGiuseppe (1996) described four *strategies of disputation:*

1. *Logical disputes* identify magical thinking and leaps in logic. Example: "Just because your sister seemed quiet and distracted when she visited you on her birthday, it doesn't logically follow that she is rejecting a close relationship with you."
2. *Empirical disputes* focus on an accumulation of evidence. Example: "You told me that after her visit, your sister called to tell you what a good time she had and suggested you visit her

soon. You also told me that your sister is a quiet person. When we examine this evidence, there is little reason to believe that your sister is withdrawing from you. In fact, the evidence suggests just the opposite."

3. *Functional disputing strategies* focus on the practical consequences of people's beliefs, looking at whether their beliefs get them what they want. Example: "Believing that your sister is withdrawing leads you to withdraw from her and brings up memories of past wrongs you believe she has done to you. This belief isn't helping you rebuild your relationship with your sister, as you want to do."
4. *Rational alternative beliefs* offer a viable alternative belief. Example: "I know your sister is going through a difficult divorce. I wonder if another possible explanation for her quietness could be that she felt sad because she wasn't with her husband on her birthday."

Beal et al. (1996) also describe *four disputing styles:*

1. A *didactic style* is explanatory, educational, and efficient but involves giving information rather than using dialogue. Example: "Marnie, I think you may be jumping to unwarranted conclusions about the significance of your sister's behavior. Keep in mind that she is still recovering from her divorce and that may be affecting her mood."
2. A *Socratic style* involves using questions to promote client reasoning. This is the most common REBT technique. Example: "What do you make of your sister's call and invitation to visit? Do those behaviors suggest she is withdrawing from your relationship?"
3. A *metaphorical style* uses analogies, especially from the client's own experience, to dispute beliefs. Example: "Your reaction to your sister's visit reminds me of the time you believed your supervisor was dissatisfied with your work because she did not offer you a ride to a conference. Then later you learned that she had to leave the meeting early because of a medical appointment and so could not give you a ride. I think that was the same month you received a top evaluation from your supervisor."
4. A *humorous style* disputes the belief in a lighthearted way. Clinicians should be sure never to make fun of people, only of their thoughts and behaviors. Example: "So let's see. . . . It sounds like you are equating the number of words a person speaks to you with how much they like you. How about for the next day you count how many words each person you encounter says to you. Then we can determine which one likes you best."

The four strategies of disputation and four disputing styles can be combined to form 16 different ways in which clinicians can approach the process of disputing beliefs. This great variety of strategies allows clinicians to adapt their approaches to disputing beliefs to the needs of a particular client as well as to the clinician's own personality.

Other Intervention Strategies

Rational emotive imagery (REI) is used to reinforce positive change after people have learned to identify irrational beliefs. Ellis believed that experiential techniques that are active, directive, and vigorous lead to more rapid change. As mentioned earlier, strategies commonly used by clinicians practicing REBT are cognitive, behavioral, or affective. Cognitive techniques are almost always combined with behavioral or emotive ones (Ellis, 1996; Ellis & Dryden, 2007). Following are some strategies that help solidify behavioral change:

Cognitive Strategies

- Detecting, evaluating, disputing, and modifying irrational cognitions
- Writing to express and explore thoughts and feelings

- Teaching the difference between rational and irrational beliefs
- Confronting irrational beliefs
- Identifying disadvantages of particular thoughts, actions, and feelings
- Socratic questioning
- Reducing thinking to absurdity
- Identifying and changing self-talk
- Reframing a situation by changing labels and language
- Listing ways to cope with the worst that might happen
- Rating experiences on a continuum to counteract awfulizing
- Generating alternatives
- Distracting oneself
- Using visualization and imagery
- Rating degree of conviction in beliefs and then rerating after change
- Formulating, writing down, and repeating rational coping statements
- Promoting a focus on happiness
- Exercising high frustration tolerance.

Behavioral Strategies

- Using relaxation strategies
- Engaging in shame-attacking exercises (potentially embarrassing experiences such as singing loudly on a bus to insulate oneself against feelings of shame)
- Creating challenging situations and then coping with them
- Role-playing
- Taping sessions for later review
- Reversing roles; clinician takes on client's irrational beliefs, and client talks clinician out of those beliefs
- Using two chairs to represent a rational and an irrational belief, person enacts a dialogue between the two beliefs, moving from one chair to another
- Acting as if a person is someone else; stepping out of character
- Reading self-help books and listening to tapes intended to effect change
- Training in skills such as assertiveness and effective communication
- Planning pleasurable activities and involvement in an absorbing interest or long-range pursuit.

Affective Strategies

- Imagining the worst that might happen
- Providing emotionally powerful stories, metaphors, and parables
- Using emotionally charged language
- Persuading
- Eliciting inappropriate emotions via imagery and then practicing changing them
- Using humor
- Encouraging willpower and determination to change
- Promoting unconditional clinician- and self-acceptance.

Strategies such as these may be incorporated into homework or used within sessions. As in cognitive therapy, use of task assignments is viewed as an essential part of treatment and is planned collaboratively. This promotes client responsibility, builds optimism, and facilitates progress.

APPLICATION OF RATIONAL EMOTIVE BEHAVIOR THERAPY

REBT is a well-established and widely used approach to treatment. It is appropriate for a broad range of people, problems, and settings, although not everyone is a suitable candidate.

Application to Groups, Families, and Psychoeducation

REBT is a flexible approach. It is appropriate for use in individual, group, and family counseling. Because it emphasizes teaching and is a fairly straightforward approach that can be readily learned and applied, REBT has been widely used for psychoeducation with client groups, as well as for "large groups, classroom courses, workshops and seminars, intensives, and other mass applications" (Dryden & Ellis, 2001, p. 339). Many video and audiotapes, pamphlets, self-help books, and other resources are available to facilitate instruction on REBT.

REBT is also appropriate for use with couples and families. Rational emotive behavior couples therapy focuses on common irrational beliefs about relationships such as "My partner should know intuitively what I want" and "Romantic love will always endure." Treatment goals include modifying cognitions, resolving disturbances, and increasing relationship satisfaction.

REBT is particularly useful in helping family members realize they have little power to change others but need to take responsibility for themselves. It is recommended for people dealing with a severely disturbed family member; treatment encourages the family to accept that person as a fallible human being and enables them to increase happiness in the family.

REBT also is well suited for group counseling, offering participants an opportunity to observe and try out behaviors and to share feedback and reactions. Group members are encouraged to take responsibility for helping each other as well as themselves. Ellis and Dryden (2007) recommend a group of 8 to 10 participants, meeting weekly for $2\frac{1}{4}$ hours for at least 6 months. However, groups as large as 20 or 30 people also can be successful. People who are reasonably well functioning can begin treatment in a group setting, whereas 5 to 15 sessions of individual REBT are recommended first for people who are shy or have other significant interpersonal difficulties. REBT also is used for time-limited groups focusing on the development of communication and other specific skills.

Application to Diagnostic Groups

REBT is appropriate for treatment of many mild to moderately severe mental disorders, including depressive disorders, anxiety disorders, and adjustment disorders. In addition, symptoms that often respond well to REBT include anger and aggression, obsessiveness, sexual difficulties, unassertiveness, and low frustration tolerance. The literature suggests that REBT also can be effective with problems of drug and alcohol abuse. SMART Recovery, the self-help group for people with substance use problems, is another outgrowth of this theory. An alternative to Alcoholics Anonymous (AA) and other 12-step programs, SMART Recovery diverges from AA in its belief that people are not always in the process of recovering but can actually recover from drug and alcohol problems. In addition, unlike AA, which emphasizes the importance of a higher power, SMART Recovery focuses on personal responsibility for effecting change.

Despite its broad application, REBT, with its forceful and directive nature and its emphasis on client responsibility, should be avoided or used with extreme care in treatment of people with some mental disorders. REBT does not seem appropriate for people with psychotic disorders, dangerous impulse control disorders, or other severe mental disorders or for people who are highly suicidal or very fragile. In addition, REBT should be used with great caution, if at all, for people who have had traumatic childhood experiences (Ellis & Dryden, 2007). Misapplication of REBT may lead inexperienced clinicians to ask those who have survived traumas whether their experiences were "really so awful" or whether they "really can't stand the feelings and flashbacks." Questions such as these may retraumatize or otherwise harm such clients. People who are unwilling to complete homework, manifest narcissistic or histrionic symptoms or rebellious behavior, have severe intellectual limitations, or have a very low tolerance for frustration also do not seem to be good candidates for REBT. However, careful integration of some of the concepts and strategies of REBT with those of other treatment approaches may extend the application of REBT to some of the severe mental disorders.

Application to Multicultural Groups

Ellis notes that REBT practitioners are almost "intrinsically multicultural." Through the use of unconditional other acceptance-multicultural (UOA-M) they accept people from other cultures "as they exist" (Ellis, 2001, p. 196).

Sue and Sue (2008) note that therapy that is active, directive, and short term is compatible with many cultural expectations. People who are highly motivated, fairly resilient, pragmatic, logical, and tough minded are most likely to enjoy this energetic and interactive approach and appreciate the characteristic directness and humor of the REBT clinician. However, just as clinicians vary in their comfort with the active and directive stance of REBT, so do clients vary in their reactions.

Clinicians should exercise care in using REBT with people from non-Western backgrounds, especially those whose cultures stress interdependence, privacy, and respect; those who may not have the background needed to appreciate the humor and linguistic subtleties of REBT; and those whose strong or mystical spiritual beliefs may conflict with REBT's pragmatic stance. Nielsen and Ellis (1994) cautioned clinicians not to attack beliefs that are strongly anchored in people's ethnic, religious, and cultural backgrounds unless they are clearly self-defeating.

Ellis (2002) points out that therapists are not a very diverse group themselves. Most are politically liberal, and may be prejudiced against conservative points of view. Therapists, like other people, need to guard against being narrow-minded and intolerant. By practicing unconditional acceptance of others (UAO), they can provide good role models (Ellis, 2002).

REBT also has application for work with people of all age groups (Banks & Zionts, 2009; DiGiuseppe & Bernard, 2006; Vernon, 2009). REBT has an extensive history of use by child therapists, many of whom use the ABCDE technique for disputing irrational beliefs (Esposito, 2009). Frustration Tolerance Training for Children uses rational emotive behavior therapy to help children accept that life will not always go their way. By learning "to live with unpleasant feelings without magnifying them" (Knaus, 2005, p. 145), children learn to delay gratification, improve acceptance of things as they are, and self-regulate their emotions. As a result, the child's frustration tolerance improves as does performance in school, in social situations, and overall behavior. Banks and Zionts (2009) found REBT useful for adolescents who have behavior problems at school, and in their book *Optimal Aging,* Ellis and Velten (1998) help people moving into their later years dispel the myths of aging. By confronting head-on their fears about getting old and facing the unknown of physical, emotional, and cognitive decline, Ellis and Velten use logic to dispute faulty beliefs and help people overcome any regrets they might have about their lives, set realistic goals and objectives, and face the final years of life with renewed interest and vitality. Manuals are available for using REBT preventively with adolescents in school settings and for teaching their parents how to incorporate the principles of REBT into their interactions with their children (Ellis, 2003; Vernon, 2006a, 2006b). Stories, fables, plays, films, and other resources have been developed to teach the elements of REBT in simplified ways. These resources probably also can be used with people who have mild impairment in intelligence.

EVALUATION OF REBT

Like other cognitive approaches to treatment, REBT has many strengths and has proven its value through empirical and theoretical research. Of course, it also has limitations.

Limitations

As with many of the theories considered in this book, more empirical research on the effectiveness of REBT is needed. The use of REBT with specific diagnostic groups and with people from diverse cultural, religious, and ethnic backgrounds needs more study. Ziegler (1999) and others have emphasized the need for REBT to have "a more comprehensive and detailed theory of personality at its base" (p. 19). REBT sometimes pays too little attention to clients' histories and moves too rapidly toward promoting change; clinicians should be sure to allow adequate time to assess and understand people before moving forward. Vernon (2009) notes that humor must be used judiciously by the therapist. Also, he warns that irrational beliefs cannot simply be recognized or expressed. Insight is not enough. Rather, the client must do the work necessary to change the irrational beliefs.

Strengths and Contributions

REBT has many strengths. An efficient and positive approach, it can lead to a rapid reduction in symptoms as well as philosophical change. It teaches and empowers people to help themselves after treatment has ended. Its theory is relatively straightforward and clear. Because it draws on a broad range of interventions, REBT can be adapted to a wide variety of people and problems and used for prevention and psychoeducation as well as treatment.

REBT is compatible with and can be integrated into many other treatment approaches, although it seems most easily combined with existential and humanistic approaches. The importance that clinicians practicing REBT place on the intrinsic value of each individual is similar to Rogers's unconditional positive regard. The importance they attribute to each person's finding a personally meaningful and rewarding direction is consistent with existential therapy. A phenomenological approach, REBT maintains that people's views of reality are the source of their disturbance; this is compatible with narrative therapy and constructivism. Of course, as we will see in the next chapter, great overlap exists between Beck's cognitive therapy and Ellis's REBT.

Many inventories have grown out of REBT, including the Attitudes and Beliefs Inventory and the Jones Irrational Beliefs Test. Most help identify irrational beliefs. According to Dryden and Ellis (2001), "The tests have been shown to distinguish reliably between various kinds of disturbed individuals and control groups" (p. 337).

Although much of the writing on REBT is theoretical and clinical, many empirical studies of its impact have been conducted. DiGiuseppe (1996) reported that more than 240 studies of REBT were conducted before 1995, and many have been conducted since. (Of course, many more studies have been conducted on cognitive therapy, which has much in common with REBT.) Although REBT cannot be viewed as superior to other cognitive and behavioral approaches to treatment, it has clearly demonstrated its effectiveness.

REBT also lends itself to the use of technology by using mobile mind maps to enhance the counseling process (Warren, 2012). REBT's most important contribution, however, is probably raising awareness of the importance of thinking in people's lives and the need to attend to and change cognitions in treatment. Information on the differences between rational and irrational thinking, the *ABCDE* model, and the many interventions associated with REBT have shaped psychotherapy and counseling, and contributed to the development of Beck's cognitive therapy, which is discussed in the next chapter.

SKILL DEVELOPMENT: RATIONAL EMOTIVE IMAGERY

The technique of rational emotive imagery (REI) helps people practice changing their unhealthy and inappropriate negative emotions into healthy and appropriate ones. Clinicians teach clients the steps in this exercise during a session in which they can learn and practice REI. Then clinicians encourage clients to spend at least 10 minutes a day practicing REI on their own.

REI includes the following steps (Thompson, 2003):

1. ***Visualize an unpleasant activating event.*** "Picture yourself or fantasize, as vividly and intensely as you can, the details of some unpleasant activating experience (*A*) that has happened to you or will likely occur in the future" (Thompson, , p. 115).

   Example
   "I met a man over the Internet; Gary was his name. We exchanged e-mails and IMs for a week and then decided to meet. We agreed that, no matter what, we would have a pleasant time—just have dinner together and get better acquainted. I was very apprehensive. I hadn't had a date in 12 years, since I married my ex-husband. I can visualize myself standing in front of the museum, waiting for Gary to show up. I was cold but I didn't want to put my coat on because I wanted him to see my new outfit. I think being anxious made me feel even colder. So there I was, shivering, feeling like I could hardly breathe. Then this man walks by real close to me, looks me up and down, and keeps walking. I knew it was Gary because he told me what he looked like."

2. ***Experience the unhealthy negative emotions.*** As you vividly imagine the experience, let yourself feel any strong emotions that come up for you—the *C,* or emotional consequence of this experience. Really feel those feelings, get in touch with them, and for a few minutes fully experience them. Don't try to avoid the feelings or change them; just face them and feel them.

   Example
   "I felt sick to my stomach. I felt disgusted with myself. I just wanted to disappear into a hole in the ground. I felt so repulsive. I felt overwhelming shame. And then I felt rage at Gary. How could he have made me feel so bad?"

3. ***Changing the emotions.*** After you have allowed yourself to feel these disturbing emotions for a few minutes, push yourself to change those feelings so that you feel different inside. Change them so that instead of feeling unhealthy and inappropriate emotions such as rage, shame, and depression, you feel emotions such as disappointment or annoyance. You can do this. Keep pushing yourself and working at it until you start to experience a shift in your feelings, a new emotional consequence.

   Example
   "This is hard, but I'm sort of doing it. I do feel annoyed; I got this new dress and took time off work so I could get ready, and then this guy doesn't even speak to me. I feel disappointed too. He seemed so nice over the Internet. I thought maybe this would turn into a special relationship."

4. ***Examine the process.*** You are succeeding in changing your emotions from the self-destructive ones of shame and rage to new and appropriate feelings of disappointment and annoyance. When we look at how you made that happen, we will see that you have changed your belief system (*B*), which mediates between the activating event (*A*) and the emotional consequence (*C*). Let's identify the old and the new beliefs.

   Example
   "At first I was thinking, 'You really are a hopeless failure. It's unbearable that I was stood up like that—so humiliating.' And I felt so angry with Gary. We had an understanding, and he should not have treated me so badly. But then I started to think about it differently. Nobody

but me knew what was going on. It wasn't a public humiliation. And I sure learned something about Gary fast. It's a good thing I didn't really get interested in him and then discover what he was really like. I do still feel annoyed that I wasted all that time and effort, and I'm disappointed that things didn't work out. But I guess I just got carried away with my romantic fantasies. I think I'll find other ways to meet people besides the Internet."

5. ***Repetition and practice.*** Keep repeating the process. Imagine the scene, bring up the disturbing feelings, and then deliberately push yourself to change your feelings so that you feel displeased and disappointed but not disturbed. I encourage you to practice this exercise at least 10 minutes a day until you can easily bring up the activating event and the disturbing feelings and then, just as easily, change those into feelings that are not harmful to you.
6. ***Reinforcing the goal.*** It may take a few weeks, but before too long you will find that, when you bring up the activating event, you will automatically and easily experience the feelings of displeasure and disappointment rather than rage and shame.
7. ***Generalization of skills.*** Then you can use this same technique for other situations. If you find that an activating event brings up strong and disturbing emotions, imagine the event and then push yourself to change those feelings to ones that reflect displeasure rather than disturbance. Once you have done this, identify both the disturbing irrational belief and the rational belief that enabled you to change your emotions.

CASE ILLUSTRATION

In this case illustration, the clinician uses the *ABCDE* model with Ava, who expresses upsetting feelings about an interaction she recently had with her parents.

CLINICIAN: Ava, tell me about the situation or activating event [*A*] that led you to feel so disturbed.

AVA: This awful thing happened to me at school. I had P.E. class, and I was in such a hurry to get dressed and catch the bus that I forgot to zip up my skirt. I went out in the hall like that! Some kids were looking at me, but I did not know what was wrong. One boy started to sing, "Zip-a-dee-do-da." Then I got it. I was so ashamed. All I wanted to do was go home and tell my mother. But when I got home, she was on the phone with my grandmother and couldn't be bothered with me. "I'm busy now," she said. "Go out and play with your friends." That was the last thing I wanted to do. So I took the dog and went up to my room. I wanted to die so that I wouldn't ever have to go back to school.

CLINICIAN: Tell me some more about the feelings [emotional consequences/*C*] you had when all this happened.

AVA: Well, I told you I felt ashamed, like I was the big joke of the school. I bet all the kids will be talking about me tomorrow. It was so awful! And then when I got home, even my mother didn't care. I felt horrible, like nobody loved me, like I was just a hopeless mess.

CLINICIAN: You had some strong negative emotions, feeling ashamed and rejected and unlovable, that were really disturbing you. Ava, remember we talked about irrational beliefs last week. Let's take out that list I showed you of common irrational beliefs [*B*] and figure out if any of them reflect the thoughts you had in reaction to this incident.

AVA: I certainly had this thought: "I am a bad or worthless person when I act weakly or stupidly." And then when my mom was too busy to talk to me, I thought this one: "I need to be loved by someone who matters to me a lot," and this one: "I am a bad, unlovable person if I get rejected." I thought this one too: "It's awful or horrible when major things don't go my way." I also thought, "My mom doesn't really love or care about me."

CLINICIAN: Many of the thoughts on the list really hit home for you. It seems like you had two groups of thoughts: one about not being loved by your mother and another about feeling worthless and devastated when the kids teased you.

AVA: Yes, that's right.

CLINICIAN: Let's start with the first group, thoughts about your mom not loving you and your feeling unlovable. Have there been other times when you needed to talk to your mom and she *was* there for you?

AVA: Yes, lots of times.

CLINICIAN: Then just because your mom was in a phone conversation and couldn't talk to you this one time, does it logically follow that she doesn't love you [logical dispute]?

AVA: She should have known I really needed to talk to her!

CLINICIAN: How should she have known that [empirical dispute]?

AVA: I don't know. I guess I didn't really tell her that.

CLINICIAN: Then does it logically follow that if she didn't want to talk to you at that time, that she doesn't love you?

AVA: No, I know she loves me. I was just disappointed that she wasn't there for me. It made me *feel* like she didn't love me.

CLINICIAN: Does the thought that she doesn't love you help you or hurt you [functional dispute]?

AVA: Well, it's making me feel pretty bad, and it kept me from talking to her when she finally got off the phone, so I guess it's hurting me.

CLINICIAN: Could there be other explanations for her not wanting to talk to you at that time [rational alternative]?

AVA: Yes, she was on the phone with her mother. It sounded like Grandma's husband had wrecked her car. I guess my mom needed to help her.

CLINICIAN: So can you tell me a thought that seems to be a more accurate reflection of your interaction with your mother?

AVA: Yes. My mom loves me, but I can't expect her to read my mind or be there for me every minute. She does her best to help me when I'm upset, but Grandma needed her then [effective rational belief].

CLINICIAN: And how are you feeling now?

AVA: I still feel disappointed that my mom was on the phone when I needed to talk to her. I felt so hurt that I never did tell her what happened.

CLINICIAN: What can you do about that now?

AVA: I guess I could go home and tell her about it. I think that would help me to feel better [new feelings and behaviors].

This process helped Ava change her beliefs about the activating events, resulting in changes in her feelings and behaviors. Her level of disturbance and the absolute nature of her thoughts both have changed, and she is no longer devastated by her interaction with her mother. This allows her to take constructive action to communicate her concerns to her mother. Ava's second group of irrational thoughts are addressed in the exercises.

EXERCISES

Large-Group Exercises

1. Review Ava's second group of irrational beliefs, including "I am a bad or worthless person when I act weakly and stupidly" and "It's awful or horrible when major things don't go my way." Use the four strategies (logical, empirical, and functional disputes and rational alternative) to dispute her beliefs. Then formulate effective rational beliefs that might replace Ava's irrational ones and identify new feelings and behaviors that are likely to result from her new beliefs. Suggest homework that Ava might do to help reinforce these positive changes.
2. Drawing on your knowledge of diverse groups, discuss which cultural groups are likely to be favorably disposed to REBT and which are likely to be uncomfortable receiving treatment via this approach. What sort of screening would you do to determine people's suitability for treatment with REBT?

Small-Group Exercises

1. Form into your groups of four people in two dyads. If possible, each participant should have an opportunity to assume both the role of the clinician and the role of the client. Each dyad should engage in a role-play in which the client begins by describing a disturbing experience. The clinician should then follow the *ABCDE* model in counseling the client. Allow approximately 15 minutes for each role-play, followed by 5 to 10 minutes of feedback from the observing dyad. Feedback should focus on the use of the *ABCDE* format as well as the nature of the therapeutic alliance.
2. Using dyads as described in Exercise 1, engage in role-plays using rational emotive imagery (illustrated in the Skill Development section) to practice changing emotions.

Individual Exercises

1. Write briefly in your journal about a time during the past week when you felt very upset or disturbed. Identify and dispute your irrational thoughts using the *ABCDE* format. Write your responses to each step in the process.
2. Identify a personal goal you have for yourself this week. Drawing on the strategies used in REBT, assign yourself two or three homework tasks to help you reach your goal.

Summary

Rational emotive behavior therapy is the first form of cognitive–behavioral therapy. REBT was developed by Albert Ellis more than 50 years ago. REBT takes the position that people disturb themselves by their irrational beliefs and that changing those beliefs to rational ones will reduce people's levels of disturbance and lead to positive changes in emotions and behaviors. REBT emphasizes problem solving. Sessions typically focus on a process to modify cognitions: identifying the activating event

(*A*), identifying irrational beliefs (*B*), looking at the negative consequences (*C*) of those beliefs, disputing (*D*) the beliefs, and replacing them with effective rational beliefs (*E*) that lead to changes in feelings and behaviors. Clinicians practicing REBT typically adopt an active, directive, and vigorous style and make use of a broad range of strategies to effect rapid change.

Recommended Readings

Bernard, M. E. (2011). *Rationality and the pursuit of happiness: The legacy of Albert Ellis*. New York, NY: Wiley.

Dryden, W. (2011). *Dealing with emotional problems using rational emotive cognitive behavior therapy*. New York, NY: Routledge.

Dryden, W., DiGiuseppe, R., & Neenan, M. (2010). *A primer of rational emotive behavior therapy* (3rd ed.). Champaign, IL: Research Press.

Ellis, A. (2001). *Overcoming destructive beliefs, feelings, and behaviors: New directions for rational emotive behavior therapy*. Amherst, NY: Prometheus Books.

Ellis, A. (2009). *All Out! An Autobiography*. New York, NY: Prometheus Books.

Ellis, A., & Dryden, W. (2007). *The practice of rational emotive behavior therapy* (2nd ed.). New York, NY: Springer.

Ellis, A., & MacLaren, C. (2005). *Rational emotive behavior therapy: A therapist's guide* (2nd ed.). Atascadero, CA: Impact Publishers.

Additional Sources of Information

http://www.rebt.org—Website of the Albert Ellis Institute. Information on REBT, training on this approach, and Friday evening workshops, as well as relevant publications and other resources, can be obtained here.

http://www.rational.org.nz—This is the website for the New Zealand Centre for Rational Emotive Behaviour Therapy. It offers articles, resources, self-help information, training opportunities, and links to many REBT and CBT sites around the world.

http://www.smartrecovery.org—Website of Self-Management and Recovery Training, a nonreligious alternative to 12-step programs based on Albert Ellis's ABCs of REBT. Includes online meetings, facilitator information, a message board, and other resources and links to help support and maintain recovery.

http://www.arebt.org—The Association for REBT provides a training and certification program for REBT therapists.

CHAPTER 14
Aaron Beck and Cognitive Therapy

Cognitive therapy had its beginnings in the 1960s and has grown in importance in the past 50 years to become one of the leading approaches to counseling and psychotherapy in use today. Cognitive therapy was initially created by Aaron Beck to provide a structured treatment of depression.

As we have seen, cognitive therapy and Ellis's rational emotive behavior therapy evolved around the same time. Both theories focus on cognitions—the automatic thoughts that everyone has—and how these cognitions, and the meaning people give to them, can be either helpful or harmful. Helping people to recognize and change dysfunctional or unhealthy ways of thinking so they can lead happier lives is the goal of both theoretical orientations. But there are some differences as well. The difference between rational emotive behavior therapy and Beck's cognitive therapy is one of emphasis. Ellis was very directive and frequently focused on decatastrophizing. Beck's style was less colorful, and his interest was focused more on finding what worked to alleviate dysfunction. Beck and his colleagues fueled the growth of cognitive therapy through the use of empirical research to validate its effectiveness, first with depression, and later with most of the other major Axis I disorders (Kellogg & Young, 2008). Recent research indicates that cognitive therapy and schema therapy are also effective in the treatment of borderline and other personality disorders, with substance abuse, for pain management, and in the treatment of sexual disorders (Hofmann, 2012).

Cognitive therapy is a well-organized, powerful, usually short-term approach that has proven its effectiveness. As the health care industry has moved toward evidence-based practice, cognitive therapy has become even more widespread. Forty-five percent of respondents to an American Psychological Association survey considered themselves to be cognitive–behavioral in their theoretical orientation, making it the most popular of any treatment modality (Stewart & Chambless, 2007). Cognitive–behavioral therapy is also the most frequently taught treatment methodology in U.S. graduate schools (Norcross, 2011; *Psychotherapy Networker*, 2007).

It is important to note that while cognitive therapies today maintain the underlying structure of Ellis's and Beck's work, most practitioners now integrate behavioral techniques and other forms of therapy that make it a more active approach. We will learn more about these newer treatment models in Part 5 of this book, which focuses on actions. But now we turn to the history of the development of Beck's cognitive theory.

AARON BECK

Aaron T. Beck, the man behind the development of cognitive therapy, was born in New England in 1921. He was the fifth and youngest child of Harry Beck and Elizabeth Temkin Beck, Russian Jewish immigrants to the United States (Weishaar, 1993). Two of the five children born to this family died in infancy, apparently contributing to emotional problems in Beck's mother. He perceived her as depressed, unpredictable, and overprotective—very different from his calm father.

Beck himself had many difficulties during childhood. He was often ill, missing many days of school. As a result, he had to repeat a grade, leading him to develop negative views of his intellectual abilities. In addition, his illnesses left him with many apprehensions, including a blood/injury phobia and fears of public speaking and of suffocation. Beck used reasoning to alleviate his anxieties and apparently was successful since he studied surgery as part of his medical training and gave many presentations throughout his life. A connection seems probable between his early experiences with anxiety and depression and his subsequent work, focused on treating those symptoms.

Beck graduated from Brown University and Yale Medical School, where he studied psychiatry. Although he was trained in psychoanalysis, he had little faith in that approach, even early in his career. At the University of Pennsylvania Medical School, Beck, an assistant professor of psychiatry, engaged in research designed to substantiate psychoanalytic principles. Instead, his work led him to develop cognitive therapy, which has since been the focus of his teaching, research, writing, and clinical work. He has spent most of his professional career at the University of Pennsylvania, where he established the Beck Institute for Cognitive Therapy and Research.

THE DEVELOPMENT OF COGNITIVE THERAPY

According to Judith Beck (2011), the roots of her father's cognitive therapy lie in the ideas of the Stoic philosophers of ancient Greece and Rome. Epictetus's belief that people are disturbed not by things but by the view they take of them is particularly relevant. George Kelly's (1955) personal constructs psychology is a modern precursor of cognitive therapy. Kelly was one of the first theorists to recognize the role of beliefs in controlling and changing thoughts, emotions, and actions. He suggested that people each have a set of personal constructs that enables them to make sense of and categorize people and experiences. These constructs operate like scientific hypotheses, paving the way for people to make predictions about reality. When their predictions are not borne out or when people recognize that their personal constructs are harmful, they may seek alternative constructs (Hergenhahn & Olson, 2007).

Aaron Beck's carefully designed research and professional writing led to the current widespread use of cognitive therapy. Beck drew on the ideas of George Kelly, Alfred Adler, and Karen Horney as he sought efficient and effective ways to help people. Working at the University of Pennsylvania in the 1960s, Beck and his colleagues initially sought to develop a structured, short-term, present-oriented, problem-solving approach to the treatment of depression (Beck, 1995). The book, *Cognitive Therapy of Depression* (Beck, Rush, Shaw, & Emery, 1979), described the results of this work, which had a powerful impact on the field of psychotherapy. It offered a clear and structured approach to the treatment of depression, the symptom clinicians most often see in both inpatient and outpatient mental health settings. Beck and his colleagues provided evidence that cognitive therapy was more effective in treating depression than the antidepressant medications of that time.

Beck has acknowledged a strong debt to Albert Ellis's work (Weishaar, 1993). At the same time, Beck's personal style, as well as the development of his theory, differs from Ellis's. Beck enhanced the importance of his system of cognitive therapy through research, clinical application, and writing. In demonstrations and videotapes, he appears reserved and thoughtful, a researcher at least as much as a clinician. His books, articles, and inventories, including recent titles such as *Cognitive Therapy of Anxiety Disorders* (Clark & Beck, 2011), *Schizophrenia: Cognitive Theory, Research and Therapy* (Beck, Rector, Stolar, & Grant, 2008), and "The Empirical Status of Cognitive–Behavioral Therapy: A Review of Meta-Analyses" (Butler, Chapman, Forman, & Beck, 2006), continue to expand the application of cognitive therapy and validate its effectiveness.

Beck published his first outcome study in 1977. Since that time, he has published more than 500 articles, authored or coauthored 25 books, and lectured throughout the world. He is the only psychiatrist to receive research awards from both the American Psychological Association and the American Psychiatric Association. Beck is listed as "one of the five most influential psychotherapists of all time" (*American Psychologist,* 1989).

Many others should be mentioned for their contributions to cognitive therapy. Aaron Beck's daughter, Judith S. Beck, has been collaborating with him for many years. Now director of the Beck Institute for Cognitive Therapy and Research and professor at the University of Pennsylvania, she continues the development of cognitive therapy, most recently with the publication of the second edition of her book *Cognitive Behavior Therapy: The Basics and Beyond* (2011), which provides a solid overview of what is probably the most widely researched form of therapy. In addition, other therapists such as Donald Meichenbaum (1994), who was among the first to combine cognitive therapy with behavioral interventions, and Beck's colleagues (Beck, Freeman, & Davis, 2006; Scott & Freeman, 2010), and others have expanded the model of cognitive therapy during the past 30 years.

Cognitive therapy has provided a solid foundation on which postmodern constructivist interventions have been built. More will be said about these newer approaches in the coming chapters.

IMPORTANT THEORETICAL CONCEPTS

Judith Beck (2011) has summarized cognitive therapy: "In a nutshell, the *cognitive model* proposes that dysfunctional thinking (which influences the patient's mood and behavior) is common to all psychological disturbances. When people learn to evaluate their thinking in a more realistic and adaptive way, they experience improvement in their emotional state and in their behavior" (p. 3). The purpose of cognitive therapy is to teach people to identify, evaluate, and modify their own dysfunctional thoughts and beliefs.

Development of Cognitive Distortions

Cognitive therapists believe that many factors contribute to the development of dysfunctional cognitions, including people's biology and genetic predispositions, life experiences, and their accumulation of knowledge and learning. Distorted cognitions begin to take shape in childhood and are reflected in people's fundamental beliefs; this makes people more susceptible to problems. In considering a stress-vulnerability model, as more stress occurs, the more the person's automatic thoughts are at the mercy of underlying dysfunctional beliefs and schemas. Because the processing of thoughts is already biased, distorted cognitions result (Scott & Freeman, 2010).

Cognitive therapists value the importance of making an accurate diagnosis. An extensive intake interview is used to give clinicians a good understanding of their clients' history, development, and background. Cognitive theory suggests that each mental disorder is characterized by relatively predictable types of underlying cognitive distortions. For example, feelings of depression typically stem from thoughts of loss. An accurate diagnosis can therefore facilitate identification of those distortions and ways to change them. It also can guide clinicians' information gathering so that they can better understand their clients. For example, discussion of childhood experiences probably is important in treatment of people with personality disorders, whereas discussion of traumatic experiences is essential for people diagnosed with post-traumatic stress disorder (PTSD). However, discussion of past experiences is less likely to be important in the treatment of people with disorders that are mild, brief, transient, and recent, such as adjustment disorders.

Although cognitive theorists focus primarily on thoughts, they take a holistic view of people and believe that learning about and understanding their feelings and behaviors also is important. Particularly important—and related to positive outcome—is understanding the emotional responses people have to their faulty cognitions and the impact of those cognitions on mood (Leahy, Tirch, & Napolitano, 2011). Having a comprehensive understanding of people is particularly useful in helping clinicians develop interventions that target all three areas of functioning: thinking, feeling, and acting.

According to cognitive theory, psychologically healthy people are aware of their cognitions. They can systematically test their own hypotheses and, if they find they have dysfunctional and unwarranted assumptions, can replace them with healthier, more accurate, and more helpful beliefs that lead to more positive emotions and behaviors.

Principles of Cognitive Therapy

The following important principles characterize the practice of cognitive therapy (Beck, 1995, 2011; Beck et al., 2006):

- Cognitive therapy is based on the finding that changes in thinking lead to changes in feeling and acting.
- Treatment requires a sound and collaborative therapeutic alliance.
- Treatment is generally short term, problem focused, and goal oriented.
- Cognitive therapy is an active and structured approach to treatment.
- It focuses on the present, although attention is paid to the past when indicated.
- Careful assessment, diagnosis, and treatment planning are essential.
- Cognitive therapy uses a broad range of strategies and interventions to help people evaluate and change their cognitions.
- Inductive reasoning and Socratic questioning are particularly important strategies.
- This is a psychoeducational model that promotes emotional health and prevents relapse by teaching people to identify, evaluate, and modify their own cognitions.
- Task assignments, follow-up, and client feedback are important in ensuring the success of this approach.

Levels of Cognitions

Cognitions can be categorized according to four levels: automatic thoughts, intermediate beliefs, core beliefs, and schemas. In cognitive therapy, treatment typically begins with automatic thoughts and then proceeds to identification, evaluation, and modification of intermediate and core beliefs and finally to revision of schemas.

Automatic thoughts are the stream of cognitions that constantly flow through our minds. As we go through our day, situation-specific thoughts spontaneously arise in reaction to our experiences: "I don't think I'll ever be able to get all that work done," "I think I'll eat a healthy lunch today," "I don't think I should call my father yet," "I'm going to help Bill with his homework tonight," "That man makes me think of my brother," and on and on. When people pay attention to their thoughts, they become more accessible and people can articulate and evaluate them.

Automatic thoughts mediate between a situation and an emotion. Consider the following example:

> ***Situation:*** Michael learns that his sister has been in town but did not call him.
>
> ***Michael's automatic thought:*** She finds me unlikable and doesn't want to be with me.
>
> ***Michael's emotion:*** Sadness.

What caused the emotion, sadness, was not the situation itself but the man's automatic cognition, reflecting the meaning he made of the situation. Understanding people's automatic thoughts is important in helping them change their emotions.

Intermediate beliefs often reflect extreme and absolute rules and attitudes that shape people's automatic thoughts. In the previous example, Michael's intermediate beliefs might include "A sister should call her family when she is in town" and "Being ignored by your sister is a terrible thing."

Core beliefs are central ideas about ourselves that underlie many of our automatic cognitions and usually are reflected in our intermediate beliefs. Core beliefs can be described as "global, rigid, and overgeneralized" (Beck, 2011, p. 34). They typically stem from childhood experiences, are not necessarily true, and can be identified and modified. Core beliefs reflect our views of the world, other people, ourselves, and the future. They may be positive and helpful such as "I am likable," "I am a capable person," and "The world is full of interesting and exciting opportunities and people." However, they also can be negative, such as "People only care about themselves," "The world is a dangerous place," and "I make a mess of everything." Most negative core beliefs can be categorized as *helpless core beliefs* such as "I am weak" and "I am a failure" or as *unlovable core beliefs* such as "I am not good enough" and "I am bound to be abandoned" (Beck, 2011, p. 233). In this example, Michael seems to have unlovable core beliefs.

As clinicians get to know and understand a client and hear a series of automatic thoughts, they can formulate hypotheses about that client's core beliefs. At an appropriate time, clinicians can share this hypothesis with the client for confirmation or disconfirmation, along with information on the nature and development of core beliefs. Clients are encouraged to view their core beliefs as ideas rather than truths and to collaborate with the clinician to evaluate and, if indicated, change their core beliefs.

Schemas have been defined as a "hypothesized mental structure that organizes information" that encompass the core beliefs (Beck, 2011, p. 33). They go beyond core beliefs, in breadth and depth, and include thoughts, emotions, and actions. Schemas have content as well as structural qualities such as breadth, flexibility, and prominence.

Beck viewed schemas as "specific rules that govern information processing and behavior" (Beck et al., 2006, p. 8). Schemas lead us to have expectations about experiences, events, and roles and to amplify those with information contained in our schemas. Schemas can act as mental filters, affecting the way we perceive reality. Schemas are idiosyncratic and habitual ways of viewing ourselves, the world, and the future. Schemas can be personal, familial, cultural, religious, gender related, or occupational in origin and application (Beck et al., 2006). Examples of maladaptive schemas include dependence/incompetence and deprivation.

Schemas may be activated by a particular stimulus or lie dormant until triggered. For example, a person may have a danger schema that gives the message "The world is a dangerous place. Avoid any possible danger." This schema is usually latent but can be activated by threats to that person's safety.

When a schema has been activated, it readily incorporates any confirming information and tends to neglect contradictory information. For example, when people view themselves as incompetent, they accept negative information they receive about themselves and overlook or dispute anything positive. Tuckey and Brewer (2003) found that schemas influence retention and distortion of memories. We are more likely to recall observations that are consistent or inconsistent with our schemas, compared to observations that are irrelevant to our schemas; inaccuracies in recollections are particularly likely to be schema consistent.

The distinctions among automatic cognitions, intermediate beliefs, core beliefs, and schemas can be confusing. Consider the following example, illustrating each of these. After several disappointing relationships, Joshua has developed a rewarding relationship with Sharon; after living together for 2 years, Sharon suggests marriage and Joshua agrees. He has the following thoughts:

- ***Automatic thoughts:*** I can't be the sort of husband Sharon wants and our marriage will end.
- ***Intermediate beliefs:*** A good husband must be willing to sacrifice his own needs for those of his wife and children. Marriage is a difficult endeavor at which few succeed.
- ***Core belief:*** I am not able to love another person and have little to offer in my relationships.
- ***Schema:*** I am inadequate and am destined to fail, no matter how hard I try. This makes me feel discouraged about my upcoming marriage; I feel disaster and shame hanging over my head. What's the point of trying if I know I will fail at whatever I do.

Because of this maladaptive schema, Joshua will probably focus on information that confirms his beliefs and ignore or explain away disconfirming information. He will enter marriage with a negative attitude, accompanied by ineffective behaviors that will contribute to the destruction of his marriage and the substantiation of his beliefs.

Schemas become amenable to analysis and modification after people have experienced some change as a result of assessing and altering their automatic thoughts, intermediate beliefs, and core beliefs. Beck viewed schema work as the heart of the therapeutic process (Beck et al., 2006). More will be said about working with schemas later.

Cognitive therapy operates at several levels, seeking to elicit and change people's symptoms as well as their automatic thoughts, intermediate beliefs, core cognitions, and underlying schemas. Once healthy thinking has been restored, clinicians help people to develop the skills they need to monitor, assess, and respond to their own cognitions as well as lead their lives more successfully.

TREATMENT USING COGNITIVE THERAPY

Treatment via cognitive therapy usually is time limited, for example, 6 to 14 sessions long for relatively straightforward problems (Beck, 2011). Sessions are carefully planned and structured to maximize their impact and efficiency. People complete inventories and intake questionnaires before beginning treatment. Clinicians review these before the first session in order to be well prepared.

Each session has clear goals and an agenda. Judith Beck (2011, p. 60) recommends the following 10 procedures for an initial session:

1. Establish an agenda that is meaningful to the client.
2. Determine and measure the intensity of the person's mood.
3. Identify and review presenting problems.
4. Elicit the person's expectations for treatment.
5. Educate the person about cognitive therapy and the role of the client.
6. Provide information about the person's difficulties and diagnosis.
7. Establish goals.
8. Recommend tasks and homework between sessions.
9. Summarize the session.
10. Obtain the client's feedback on the session.

Throughout the session, clinicians promote development of the therapeutic alliance and build trust, rapport, and collaboration while encouraging realistic hope and optimism.

Subsequent sessions follow a similar structure. They typically begin with an assessment of the person's mood, focusing particularly on changes. Next, the foundation for the session is established by making a transition from the previous session to the current one; clinicians ask about clients' learning from and reactions to the previous session and obtain an overview of the clients' week, highlighting any important happenings. This facilitates establishment of an agenda for the session, which always includes reviewing homework. The central part of the session addresses items on that agenda, with clinicians eliciting and assessing thoughts as well as emotions and actions related to the identified issues. Each session concludes with new homework, a summary of the session, and feedback from clients on the session and the process of treatment. Ending the session on a positive note promotes optimism and motivation.

Cognitive therapists make sure to explain to clients the nature and purpose of the sessions' structure. Clients generally find that structure reassuring. They know what to expect and are optimistic that this plan will help them as it has helped others. Of course, an agenda may be modified if needed, perhaps if a crisis has occurred, but any changes are planned when the agenda is determined at the outset of each session.

Goals

Cognitive therapists carefully specify goals for their treatment, and they draw on a rich array of interventions to achieve them. The overall goal of cognitive therapy is to help people recognize and correct errors in their information-processing systems. To accomplish this, clinicians help people identify both their immediate (automatic) and underlying (intermediate, core, schema) thoughts and beliefs as well as associated emotions and behaviors; evaluate the validity of these thoughts; and modify them if indicated. Throughout treatment, people learn to use this process independently and also to develop the skills and attitudes they need to think more realistically and lead more rewarding lives.

Clinicians and clients collaborate on determining specific goals. Once identified, goals are written down, with copies made for both client and clinician. Goals are referred to regularly to assess progress. Having clear, specific, and measurable goals is an important component of cognitive therapy and increases the likelihood that clients and clinicians will collaborate to achieve a shared objective.

Therapeutic Alliance

"Cognitive behavioral therapy requires a sound therapeutic alliance" (Beck, 2011, p. 7). The cognitive therapist is active, collaborative, goal oriented, and problem focused.

Cognitive therapists strive to be nonjudgmental and help clients to develop the skills they need to make their own judgments and choices. As mentioned earlier, cognitive therapists use Socratic questioning to lead clients through what Scott and Freeman (2010) refer to as "guided discovery" (p. 35). By asking questions that clients can answer, focusing the clients' attention on information that is relevant but they may not be aware of, and moving from the concrete to the abstract, the client is guided toward new thoughts and ideas from which they can formulate their own conclusions.

The four stages of guided discovery are:

1. Socratic questioning to elicit the client's concerns
2. Active listening for clarification, inconsistencies, and emotional reactions
3. Summarization to provide feedback and enhance clarification
4. Synthesis or analytical questions that pull all of the information together, along with the client's original concern, and pose an analytical question (Scott & Freeman, 2010).

The therapeutic relationship is crucial to the success of this approach, and cognitive therapists maintain a great deal of role flexibility. Problems that arise within the therapeutic relationship need to be explored. Judith Beck (2011) suggests asking clients for feedback at the end of the session or any time a client's affect appears to become negative during the session. Especially when working with difficult clients, therapists need to identify when such problems occur, conceptualize the reason it occurred, and work toward correcting the problem to prevent a rupture in the therapeutic alliance.

Case Formulation

Before cognitive therapists move forward with interventions designed to modify cognitions, they take the time to develop a case formulation, reflecting in-depth understanding of the client. According to Persons (1989), a complete case formulation includes six elements:

1. List of problems and concerns
2. Hypothesis about the underlying mechanism (core belief or schema)
3. Relationship of this belief to current problems
4. Precipitants of current problems
5. Understanding of background relevant to development of underlying beliefs
6. Anticipated obstacles to treatment.

A thorough case formulation enables clinicians to develop treatment plans that are likely to be successful. When planning treatment, cognitive clinicians identify the best points for initial intervention, treatment strategies that are likely to be helpful, and ways to reduce anxiety and other obstacles to progress. Treatment usually focuses first on overt automatic cognitions related to clients' presenting problems and, as progress is made, shifts to identification and assessment of underlying core beliefs and schemas.

Eliciting and Rating Cognitions

Judith Beck (2011) suggests a basic question to elicit people's thoughts: "What was going through your mind just then?" (p. 83). Once one thought is presented, it often leads to production of other thoughts. Especially important are thoughts that appear repeatedly in conjunction with a variety of experiences and have a negative impact on the person. Beck uses what she calls a dysfunctional thought record to facilitate identification and modification of such thoughts (p. 95). This record includes six items:

1. The situation that elicited the thoughts and its accompanying physical responses
2. Date and time of the situation
3. Automatic thoughts and extent of belief in those thoughts rated on a 0% to 100% scale
4. Emotions and their intensity, rated on a 0% to 100% scale
5. Nature of distortion and ways of modifying the thoughts
6. Outcome, including revised beliefs, ratings of automatic and revised thoughts, current emotions and intensity ratings, and new actions.

The first four items are completed initially, as in the following example:

1. The school called to tell me that my son had been seen breaking into the school over the weekend. He was accused of vandalizing the computer room. I felt a knot in my stomach; I felt light-headed and tense all over.
2. This happened on Monday morning about 8:30 A.M.
3. I am a failure as a parent: 95% belief rating. My son is a hopeless criminal, and it's my fault: 90% belief rating.
4. Anxious: 95% intensity; sad: 85% intensity.

Determining the Validity of Cognitions

Once the cognitions have been elicited and placed in context, people can assess their validity. Especially important is clinicians' use of guided discovery (also called Socratic dialogue) via skillful questioning and experiments to help people test the reality of their thoughts. These are powerful techniques that must be used with care. Therapists should never act as though they know better than the client, should not debate or argue with clients, and should remain neutral on whether a thought is distorted. The clinician's role is to help clients find the truth.

The following dialogue illustrates the use of questioning to help the client in the previous example assess the logic and validity of her thoughts:

CLINICIAN: One thought you had was that your son was a hopeless criminal. What led you to have that thought?

CLIENT: Well, it sounds like he committed a crime.

CLINICIAN: Yes, he may have. Does he have a history of criminal behavior?

CLIENT: No, not at all. He's always been very well behaved.

CLINICIAN: So this is the first time he has been suspected of breaking the law?

CLIENT: Yes.

CLINICIAN: And what is your definition of a hopeless criminal?

CLIENT: I guess it's someone who repeatedly breaks the law, who can't be rehabilitated.

CLINICIAN: And does that sound like your son?

CLIENT: No. I guess I overreacted when I said he was a hopeless criminal.

CLINICIAN: And what about your thought that you are to blame for his behavior. What led you to think that?

CLIENT: I'm his parent. Aren't I the biggest influence in his life?

CLINICIAN: Yes, your role is certainly an important one. How might you have encouraged him to become a criminal?

CLIENT: I don't know what you mean.

CLINICIAN: I wonder if you have engaged in criminal behavior yourself.

CLIENT: No, of course not.

CLINICIAN: Perhaps you condoned criminal behavior or didn't try to teach him the difference between right and wrong?

CLIENT: No, just the opposite. I have very strong values, and I always tried to transmit them to my son. When he misbehaved, I would talk to him about what was wrong with his behavior and teach him how to act differently.

CLINICIAN: I'm confused then, about how you might have caused his criminal behavior.

CLIENT: I guess I was just feeling bad and wanted to find an explanation. But I can see that I certainly never taught him to break the law.

Experiments designed to test hypotheses stemming from faulty thinking are another important approach to helping people evaluate the reality of their cognitions. In the previous example, the client might use her statements "My son is a hopeless criminal" and "I am to blame for my son's criminal behavior" as hypotheses. Clinician and client then develop experiments or ways to test these hypotheses. The client might talk with her son about the reasons for his behavior, confer with school personnel about this incident as well as about her son's usual behavior at school, and read about criminal behavior.

A third approach is to use the three-question technique, a form of the Socratic method that helps clients to revise negative thinking. The therapist asks the client: (1) What evidence is there for the belief? (2) How else could the situation be interpreted? (3) If it is true, what would the implications be? Each of the three questions helps the client to delve deeper into the distorted belief, recognize the distortion, and adopt more objective thinking.

In our example, the boy might have been erroneously accused of breaking into the school. Even if he had committed the crime, mitigating factors might have played a part, such as his being forced or coerced to engage in the break-in.

Following are additional approaches that cognitive therapists use to help people evaluate the validity of their cognitions:

- Asking clients how another person whom they respect would think about the situation
- Asking them what they would say if their child or friend had the thoughts they have
- Using humor or exaggeration to take an idea to its extreme

- Helping people recognize their tendency to think negatively
- Encouraging people to imagine "what if" their worst fears came true and then think of ways to deal with them so the fears have less power over them
- Suggesting alternate explanations for a situation
- Helping people find a middle ground to counteract extreme ways of thinking
- Redefining or reconceptualizing a problem so that it is more amenable to change
- Decentering, or helping people see they are not the cause of the problem or the center of attention.

Labeling the Distortion

Evaluation of distorted cognitions can be facilitated by categorizing and labeling the distortions. This helps people see more clearly the nature of their unrealistic thinking, reminds them that other people have had similar distorted cognitions, and gives them a tool for assessing subsequent thoughts. Many lists of cognitive distortions have been published (Beck, 1976; Burns, 1999). Here these categories are illustrated with statements made by the previous client:

- ***All-or-nothing or polarized thinking:*** Viewing a situation in terms of extremes rather than on a continuum. "Either my son is innocent, or he is a hopeless criminal."
- ***Overgeneralization:*** Drawing sweeping conclusions that are not justified by the evidence. "I am a failure as a parent because my son was arrested."
- ***Mental filter (selective abstraction):*** Focusing selectively on negative details and failing to see the broad picture. "I know my son has been a good student and has not caused any problems in the past, but all I can think about is that he broke the law."
- ***Disqualifying the positive:*** Paying attention only to negative information. "What good are all my efforts to be a good mother if this is the result?"
- ***Jumping to conclusions (arbitrary inferences):*** Drawing hasty and unwarranted conclusions. "My son must be guilty. Someone saw him hanging around the school late that night."
- ***Magnification/minimization:*** Making too much of the negative, devaluing positive information. "My son stole a candy bar from another child when he was four. He was destined to become a criminal."
- ***Emotional reasoning:*** Believing that something is true because it feels that way; paying no attention to contradictory evidence. "I just feel like this is my fault, and no one can convince me it isn't."
- ***"Should" and "must" statements:*** Having definite and inflexible ideas about how we and others should behave and how life should be. "I should never have let Kevin get his driver's license. I should have made sure I met all his friends. I should have been a better mother to him."
- ***Labeling and mislabeling:*** Attaching an extreme, broad, and unjustified label to someone. "Kevin is a hopeless criminal."
- ***Personalization:*** Assuming inordinate responsibility for events or others' behaviors. "My son and I had an argument about his curfew three days before the school break-in. If I hadn't yelled at him, this probably never would have happened."
- ***Catastrophizing:*** Predicting a negative outcome without considering other possibilities. "I just know Kevin will be sent to prison for this."
- ***Mind reading:*** Attributing negative thoughts and reactions to others without checking if they are present. "My husband will never forgive Kevin for this. He'll disown him."
- ***Tunnel vision:*** Focusing only on the negative aspects of a situation. "I can't do anything right as a parent. There I was, eating dinner, while my son was breaking into the school. How could I not have known what was going on?"

Becoming familiar with these categories of cognitive distortions can help people identify, understand, and dispute their own cognitive distortions. In addition, reviewing this list can reassure clients that having cognitive distortions is common and that dysfunctional thinking can be changed. This reassurance can reduce self-blame and facilitate efforts to formulate healthier and more valid cognitions.

Assessment of Mood

Assessing mood is an important part of cognitive therapy for many reasons. Troubling emotions are often the reason people seek treatment. Upsetting emotions are likely to be close to the surface and presented early in treatment. Those feelings can point the way to distorted cognitions. In addition, monitoring the nature and intensity ratings of people's emotions can provide evidence of progress, while improvement in mood can enhance clients' motivation and optimism. Cognitive therapy was initially developed for the treatment of depression and anxiety and considerable research demonstrates the effectiveness of this approach in treating those emotional symptoms.

Cognitive therapists use structured approaches to assess emotions, as they do to assess thoughts. One of Aaron Beck's major contributions to psychotherapy is the development of brief, concise inventories that provide a quick measure of the nature and intensity of emotions that are most likely to be troubling to people. These inventories include the Beck Depression Inventory (BDI), the Beck Anxiety Inventory (BAI), the Beck Hopelessness Inventory, and the Beck Scale for Suicidal Ideation. Published by Psychological Corporation, these inventories each take only a few minutes to complete. Any or all of these might be administered to obtain an emotional baseline before a person begins treatment. If elevated scores are obtained on an inventory, administration of that inventory every few sessions enables client and clinician to track and quantify changes in emotions. An even more rapid assessment of emotion can be obtained using an informal 0 to 100 scale of severity or intensity of a specific mood such as anger, jealousy, or sadness. Clients can rate themselves on these scales at the beginning of each session.

Strategies for Modifying Cognitions

Clinicians work closely with clients to restructure their cognitions and help them find words to express their new cognitions accurately, realistically, and in ways that are compatible with their emotions. This process involves helping people deepen their beliefs in their revised cognitions and make those cognitions part of themselves.

Once again, cognitive therapists draw on a wealth of strategies to accomplish these goals. Although many of these techniques are primarily cognitive in nature, others are behavioral and will be addressed further in Part 5. Following are some of the strategies that enhance the work of cognitive therapists:

- *Challenging absolute statements.* Clients often use absolutes such as "never" and "always" when telling their stories. "My husband is never home for dinner" or "My boss is always late." By challenging the absolute nature of these statements (i.e., "Never? In the past month, your husband has never been home for dinner?" or "Always is pretty definitive"), the clinician gives the client an opportunity to retract the absolute statement and clarify the behavior more accurately.
- *Activity scheduling* encourages people to plan and try out new behaviors and ways of thinking as well as to remain active despite feelings of sadness or apprehension. Learning a new and interesting skill and having a good time can contribute to improved moods and clearer thinking.
- *Reattributing blame.* Clients often turn internally and blame themselves whenever something goes wrong in their lives. This false attribution of blame can start a cascade of negative

emotions and behaviors. Through the use of Socratic dialogue and asking questions that get to the heart of the problem, clinicians can help clients look at the situation more clearly, as illustrated in this brief dialogue:

CLIENT: A pipe burst at my parent's house while they were on vacation and now the whole condo is flooded. It's all my fault.

CLINICIAN: Were you watching your parent's house while they were gone?

CLIENT: No, I haven't been there in years. They live in Florida, but I should have had the water turned off before they left.

CLINICIAN: Did they ask you turn off the water?

CLIENT: No.

- *Cognitive rehearsal* is a strategy in which people mentally rehearse a new behavior and then create a cognitive model of themselves successfully performing that behavior. Some athletes use this technique to improve their skills in their sport. A woman married to a verbally abusive husband used this approach to rehearse asserting herself to her husband, making it easier for her to stand up to him when he spoke to her in a demeaning way. A variation is for people to imagine themselves as someone they admire and then tackle a challenging situation as if they were that person.
- *Diversions* or *distractions* also can help people reduce their negative thinking. A woman who was diagnosed with a life-threatening illness had a good prognosis but still experienced constant thoughts of death. To distract herself from these troubling thoughts, she mentally cataloged each item in her extensive wardrobe, beginning the mental list anew each time the negative thoughts returned.
- *Self-talk* is a technique in which people repeat to themselves many times a day positive and encouraging phrases that they have identified as helpful, such as "Don't let fear control you. You can do it." In essence, they are giving themselves a pep talk.
- *Affirmations* are closely related to self-talk. An affirmation is a sort of slogan that is positive and reinforcing. People can post these in prominent places such as the refrigerator or keep them in a three-ring binder of index cards where they can review them frequently and be reminded to shift their thinking. An adolescent girl chose as her affirmation "Someday you will realize your great potential." Keeping those words in mind helped her deal effectively with challenges.
- *Keeping diaries* of events, realistic and distorted cognitions, emotions, and efforts to make positive changes can increase people's awareness of their inner and outer experiences. These written records can provide important material for discussion in sessions and serve as a way to track both progress and difficulties.
- *Letter writing* provides another avenue for exploring and expressing thoughts and feelings. The woman whose son was accused of breaking into his school (discussed previously) might benefit from drafting a letter to her son expressing her reactions to his behavior. The letter need not be mailed but can be used as the focus of a session.
- *Systematic assessment of alternatives* (cost/benefit analysis) is an approach that can help people make wise decisions or choices. They first list their options, along with the pros and cons of each one. Then they assign numbers on a scale of 1 to 10, showing the importance of each advantage and disadvantage. Finally, they total the numbers assigned to the pros and cons of each option. A man considering a career change used this approach to help him decide whether to remain in his secure, well-paying position in computer technology or pursue his lifelong goal of becoming a counselor; the numerical totals strongly reflected a preference for becoming a counselor, whereas the list of cons pointed out obstacles to this goal.

- *Relabeling* or *reframing* experiences or perceptions can help people think differently about them. For example, a woman who had few dating experiences at age 35 stopped thinking of herself as a failure and instead viewed herself as a late bloomer.
- *Role-playing* can enable people to actualize some of the new thoughts they have about themselves. For example, a man who had developed a more positive view of his abilities role-played sharing his accomplishments with his friends, asking his supervisor for a raise, and inviting a colleague to join him for lunch.
- When *role-playing a dialogue between old and new thoughts,* clients can use two chairs (as described in Chapter 10) to represent both their old and their new thoughts. Moving from one chair to another, they engage in a dialogue between the two groups of thoughts. This can help people clarify changes in their thinking and solidify their rational thoughts.
- *Distancing* involves projecting into the future to put a problem in perspective and diminish its importance. A woman realized that getting a *B* in a college course would mean little to her in 10 years.
- *Bibliotherapy,* or the use of books in the counseling process, can help a person modify his or her thinking. Reading books about other people who have coped well with experiences similar to the client's, can be cathartic, providing emotional release, new ways of thinking and interacting, and help clients to solve problems.

One example of bibliotherapy involved the treatment of a 12-year-old boy who had lost his mother. The boy was sad, especially when he came home from school and she was not there. In therapy, after the female therapist conducted an assessment and recognized the client's need for catharsis, she gave him a copy of *Tear Soup,* a picture book about grief and loss in which a woman is cooking soup (tear soup) that helps her express her underlying feelings of grief. The boy began to identify with the person who was making the soup, and the recognition that it was okay to grieve. Other types of bibliotherapy include interactive bibliotherapy in which a workbook is used to help the client address the ongoing issue. Erford and colleagues (2010) provide the following recommendations in the use of bibliotherapy: (1) Therapists should only use books they have read; (2) the client's specific reality should be kept in mind during the process; (3) reading level and interest should be taken into account; and (4) not all clients will enjoy reading or have the time to complete the book. Movies and videos can also be used as a form of bibliotherapy.

- *Graded task assignments* are activities that clients complete between sessions. Starting with easy assignments that guarantee success, clinicians gradually increase the difficulty of the tasks, so that people continue to learn from them and feel a sense of mastery and accomplishment.

Termination and Relapse Prevention

Like the other phases of cognitive therapy, the concluding phase is carefully planned and structured to help people successfully apply what they have learned through treatment. Sessions are scheduled less frequently, typically shifting to every other week, then to once a month, then to every 3 months for at least a year (Beck, 2011). This gives people the opportunity to test their skills and cope with any setbacks while maintaining contact with their clinicians.

Normalizing setbacks and stressing the importance of ongoing learning can enable people to cope with future disappointments successfully. Life skills such as assertiveness, decision making, coping strategies, and communication skills, which have probably been taught throughout the treatment process, are reviewed and solidified. Progress also is reviewed, with every effort made to help clients accept credit for and take pride in their accomplishments. Clinicians address any concerns that clients have about termination and elicit feedback about the treatment process. Finally, clients and clinicians collaborate in developing goals and plans for clients to continue their progress on their own.

APPLICATION AND CURRENT USE OF COGNITIVE THERAPY

Cognitive therapy has established itself as a major treatment approach. Because Aaron Beck and his colleagues, as well as other cognitive therapists, have encouraged and engaged in extensive research on the impact of this approach, its effectiveness has been more clearly demonstrated in more than 500 outcome studies (Beck, 2011). Cognitive therapy is effective in a variety of populations and with an ever expanding range of applications.

Application to Diagnostic Groups

Originally developed for the treatment of depression, cognitive therapy has since been found to be effective for most of the major Axis I disorders, particularly mood disorders, anxiety disorders, and PTSD (Dobson, 2010). A recent study found sustained improvement at 5-year follow-up for the treatment of social phobias (Mortberg, Clark, & Bergerot, 2011). Cognitive therapy has been used successfully to treat insomnia and alcohol abuse, to alleviate stress and worry, to reduce suicidal thoughts, and for pain management (Dobson, 2010; Hofmann, 2012).

Because of its focus on changing cognitions, this type of therapy can provide an effective adjunct to medical treatment for disorders that are associated with high levels of stress, anxiety, or depression. Clients with infertility, epilepsy, erectile dysfunction, and breast cancer have all reported benefiting from adjunctive cognitive therapy to reduce negative cognitions. Cognitive treatment helps people manage chronic pain (Otis, 2007), lowers anxiety in gay clients recently diagnosed with HIV (Spiegler, 2008), helps people manage behavioral issues related to epilepsy, and increases relaxation and improves sleep in clients with restless leg syndrome (Hornyak et al., 2008).

Beck and colleagues (2008) combined neurobiology with psychology to show how a cognitive approach can be used to understand and treat schizophrenia. Delusions, hallucinations, negative symptoms, and formal thought disorder are conceptualized in terms of cognitive theory. Growing research in the area of severe mental disorders, such as bipolar disorder and schizophrenia, has found cognitive therapy to be an effective adjunct to medication in the treatment of delusions and hallucinations. Interventions include helping clients to recognize nonpsychotic misinterpretations and challenge their upsetting interpretations, behavioral experiments to help clients check out delusional misinterpretations, and treatment to reduce symptoms of depression and anxiety and reduce suicidal risk. Cognitive therapy has also been shown to improve insight and treatment adherence for people with schizophrenia (Kingdon, Rathod, Weiden, & Turkington, 2008). Cognitive therapy has become so popular, and its effectiveness so widespread, that manuals and workbooks are available for most Axis I and Axis II disorders.

Application to Multicultural Groups

Because cognitive therapy is respectful, addresses present concerns, and does not require disclosure of emotions and experiences that may feel very personal, this approach appeals to people from a wide variety of ages and backgrounds. It is especially useful in treating people for whom sharing thoughts is more comfortable and acceptable than sharing emotions. For example, the respectful stance of the cognitive clinician, as well as the emphasis on thoughts inherent in this approach, seems well suited for people from Asian backgrounds who often are reluctant to share deeply personal experiences and emotions with people who are not close family or friends.

However, if there is a research gap to be found anywhere in the cognitive therapy literature, it is in the area of cultural diversity. Certain groups are simply underrepresented in the treatment outcome literature. While a growing number of those seeking treatment in the United States are from an increasingly diverse array of cultural backgrounds, religions, sexual preferences, disabilities, and socioeconomic status, the providers of mental health services seem to be less diverse. In fact, the American Psychological Association reports that 94% of APA members are of European American background (Pantalone, Iwamasa, & Martell, 2010).

What should a therapist do? "Do CBT as you know it," according to Pantalone and colleagues (2010, p. 454). Logic, as well as empirical research in general, suggests the value of using cognitive therapy with people from diverse cultures. Of course, cognitive therapists must use culturally competent skills and communication styles, and not make assumptions about what is in the person's best interest. A collaborative approach that considers the client to be the expert on his or her own problems would be consistent with the cognitive therapy paradigm. In one study, Kubany et al. (2004) found that, in an adapted version of cognitive therapy used to treat "battered women" with PTSD, "white and ethnic minority women benefited equally" (p. 3) from treatment.

There is some evidence that cognitive therapy is an effective treatment approach for people of all ages. Cognitive therapy can be adapted in work with elderly adults to accommodate age-related cognitive decline (Gallagher-Thompson, Steffen, & Thompson, 2008). It is effective with play therapy, and in improving self-esteem in children (Seiler, 2008), and for childhood disorders such as ADHD, conduct disorder, oppositional defiant disorder, adolescent mood and anxiety disorders, eating disorders, and childhood trauma (Crawley, Podell, Beidas, Braswell, & Kendall, 2010; Hoch, 2009; Reinecke, Dattilio, & Freeman, 2006). Although components of each group will be specific to the age-range and the disorder, common elements usually include an education and problem-solving component, cognitive restructuring, education about affect, relaxation training, practice or role-playing, reinforcement, and some method to encourage transportability of lessons learned to other aspects of the child's life.

The following example provides an outline for a 10-session cognitive group therapy intervention for middle-school students with symptoms of PTSD (Stein et al., 2003, p. 605):

Session 1: Introductions, explanation of treatment using stories, information on types of stress and trauma

Session 2: Education about healthy responses to stress and trauma, relaxation training

Session 3: Introduction to cognitive therapy, explanation of the connection between thoughts and feelings, measuring fear, fighting off negative thoughts

Session 4: More about staving off negative thoughts

Session 5: Coping strategies, construction of a fear hierarchy

Session 6: Exposure to troubling memories through imagination, drawing, and writing

Session 7: Continuation of exposure-based treatment

Session 8: Social problem solving

Session 9: Practice using social problem solving via the hot seat

Session 10: Psychoeducation about relapse prevention and "graduation."

An increasing number of books, treatment manuals, meta-analyses, and research studies illustrate the populations and varieties of topics that can benefit from a cognitive group approach (Crawley et al., 2010).

Application to Other Groups

Increasing use has been made of cognitive therapy with psychiatric inpatients, in partial hospitalization programs, and through computer-assisted delivery methods. These modalities enable cognitive therapists to reach more people and to use cognitive therapy for preventive purposes.

A 4-year study on the effectiveness of cognitive–behavioral therapy with psychiatric inpatients showed that a manualized treatment approach to group therapy, as an adjunct to medication and other treatments, resulted in fewer readmissions for clients with schizophrenia and bipolar disorder (Veltro et al., 2008). Cognitive therapy has also been used successfully as an adjunct treatment in partial hospitalization settings (Witt-Browder, 2000).

Cognitive family therapy can also provide much-needed assistance. A study by Pavuluri (2004) illustrates the integration of medication management, cognitive therapy, behavior therapy, and family-focused therapy (FFT), along with psychoeducation to treat 34 children diagnosed with bipolar disorder. Interventions focused on increasing coping skills and empathy in family members, decreasing stress and expression of negative emotions, and improving family problem solving and communication. Treatment also included collaboration with the children's teachers and psychoeducation on bipolar disorders. Outcome measures found significant reductions in symptoms such as attention difficulties, aggression, mania, psychosis, depression, and sleep disturbance, along with improved overall functioning.

Psychoeducation, based on cognitive therapy, can be conducted with people experiencing problems or mental disorders, with people at risk, and with a general population. Cognitive psychoeducation presents the concept that thoughts underlie feelings and actions and describes strategies that people can use to monitor, assess, dispute, and modify their thoughts. Information on behavioral strategies further enhances the process.

Current Use of Cognitive Therapy

Although the fundamentals of Beck's cognitive therapy have changed little in the past 40 years since it first gained attention, cognitive therapy continues to evolve. Two relatively new uses of cognitive therapy that have provided greater depth and usefulness are schema therapy and emotion schema therapy. Of course, behavioral therapy is the treatment method most commonly integrated with cognitive therapy to create cognitive–behavioral therapy (CBT). But this treatment modality is so extensive, it is the subject of its own chapter. Much more will be said about CBT in Chapter 16.

SCHEMA THERAPY Schema therapy, developed by Jeffrey Young (1990/1999), goes beyond Beck's cognitive therapy and integrates interpersonal, attachment, and experiential techniques to achieve change at the emotional level. The approach goes deeper than most cognitive therapies, to recognize that core schemas have developed in childhood that can have lifelong implications. Schema therapy can be seamlessly integrated with CBT for Axis II or other disorders such as substance abuse, mood and anxiety disorders, or eating disorders (Rafaeli, Bernstein, & Young, 2011). The approach offers a bridge between regular CBT or brief forms of treatment and longer interventions that attempt to get at the root of more ingrained problems.

As discussed earlier, schema therapy was originally developed to work with clients with character disorders and those with chronic problems for whom focused interventions were not working. By looking at early childhood adaptive patterns, schema therapy helps clients understand how actions in the present trigger self-defeating emotional patterns from childhood. "Early maladaptive schemas are self-defeating emotional patterns that begin early in our development and repeat throughout life" (Young, Klosko, & Weishaar, 2006, p. 7).

Schema therapy helps clients to recognize their maladaptive patterns that fall within five schema domains:

1. ***Disconnection and rejection:*** Abandonment, defectiveness/shame, social isolation, emotional deprivation, mistrust/abuse

2. ***Impaired autonomy and performance:***
   a. Dependence/incompetence
   b. Vulnerability (to harm or illness)
   c. Enmeshment
   d. Failure
3. ***Impaired limits:*** Entitlement/grandiosity, lacking self-control or discipline
4. ***Other directedness:*** Approval- or recognition-seeking, subjugation, self-sacrificing
5. ***Overvigilance and inhibition:*** Negativity, emotional inhibition, punitiveness, unrelenting standards/criticalness.

When a schema is activated, a person responds in one of three ways: (1) overcompensation, (2) avoidance, or (3) surrender to the schema as if it were true (Ohanian & Rashed, 2012). All three of these responses could lead to problems in coping with life and relationships. For example, Suzanne is a divorced woman who has an attachment schema that causes her to fear abandonment. Her attachment schema is activated one Friday night when a man she has been seeing for 3 months does not show up at the restaurant at the agreed-upon time. When activated, Suzanne responds with emotions: anger that he does not respect her enough to be on time, sadness that he might not be the right man for her, and fear that she will always be alone. She responds by leaving the restaurant in a huff, avoiding his calls, and not responding to his text messages. Suzanne's method of coping (avoidance) was learned in childhood when she would avoid her mother's anger and wrath by leaving the house and going to the neighbor's. But the childhood method of coping does not work so well now that Suzanne is an adult. In this case, by actively avoiding the man's attempts to reach her, she prevented him from explaining that he had been in a car accident and was unable to keep the date. By resorting to her childhood pattern of avoidance, Suzanne unconsciously contributed to the creation of the very situation that she feared most—an end of the relationship and the result that she is alone once again.

The goal of schema therapy is to help people achieve and maintain a healthy adult mode of functioning (Ohanian & Rashed, 2012). The assessment phase may include the use of experiential exercises and schema inventories such as the *Young Schema Questionnaire* (Young, 2005), the *Young Compensation Inventory* (Young, 2003a), the *Young Parenting Inventory* (Sheffield et al., 2005; Young, 2003b), and the *Schema Mode Inventory* (Young et al., 2007). The therapist's own responses to the client also provide valuable information.

Interventions in schema therapy include the use of cognitive and experiential techniques, helping clients recognize and change self-defeating patterns, and the use of the power of the therapeutic alliance in an intervention known as limited reparenting (Kellogg & Young, 2008; Rafaeli et al., 2011). By recognizing that people develop maladaptive schemas because core needs were not met in childhood, the therapist works to create a therapeutic environment in which the client's needs can be met. Therapists also use empathic confrontation to challenge clients' maladaptive schemas (Edwards & Arntz, 2012).

People have a variety of schemas that they use in different situations, including emotional, decisional, relational, and physical schemas (Beck et al., 2006). Recent neurobiological research reinforces that a great deal of mental processing occurs at the unconscious or implicit level (Uhlmann, Pizarro, & Bloom, 2008). Temperament, biological predisposition, and life experience contribute to the development of coping styles. When working with schemas, the therapist must take care to balance empathic attunement with caring confrontation. The goal is to help clients develop and sustain a healthy adult schema so they have greater amounts of flexibility and freedom, and, ultimately, are happier.

Schema therapy has been found to be effective in treating people with borderline personality disorder (Farrell, Shaw, & Webber, 2009; Giesen-Bloo et al., 2006; Nadort et al., 2009), people with relational problems (Rafaeli et al., 2011), and people who are dually diagnosed with a co-occurring personality disorder and an Axis I disorder such as an anxiety, mood, or substance use disorder. Schema therapy can be brief, but is generally longer in duration, depending on the client's needs. It also differs from cognitive therapy in that it explores childhood origins of psychological problems.

INTEGRATION WITH OTHER TREATMENT APPROACHES Cognitive therapy has increasingly been combined with other approaches to create a powerful integrated treatment system. Clinicians currently practicing cognitive therapy also seem more cognizant of the importance of addressing emotions. Emotional schema therapy (EST), recently developed by Leahy and colleagues (2011), is an integrative approach that combines schema therapy and cognitive restructuring with a focus on emotion regulation. EST recognizes that emotion regulation is often a necessary precursor to being able to accomplish cognitive work with clients, and is built on the following principles:

- Emotions are universal and adaptive.
- Presuppositional beliefs and schemas about emotion lead to emotional expression that is either appropriate or escalated, much as anxiety is escalated in a panic attack.
- Schemas about emotion can include fear of expressing emotion, shame-based emotion, catastrophizing, and feeling that one's emotions are unique, permanent, or out of control.
- Strong emotions are viewed as intolerable feelings to be avoided, thus many people turn to drugs, alcohol, binge eating, and other impulse control disorders in an attempt to reduce strong emotions.
- Emotional understanding, expression, and validation help to normalize, universalize, and reduce shame, guilt, and fear associated with lack of emotional control (Leahy et al., 2011).

EST interventions incorporate psychoeducation about emotions, as well as emotional validation and regulation techniques such as mindfulness, self-compassion (loving kindness), and stress reduction. No research is currently available on the effectiveness of EST, but the combination of cognitive and affective interventions has been associated with positive outcomes. More research is necessary on this promising approach.

Cognitive therapy is also being used as a culturally sensitive method to help people with trauma. Hinton and colleagues (2012) have adapted cognitive therapy to help traumatized refugees and ethnic minorities. Their approach describes 12 components of culturally sensitive treatment for refugees who have been traumatized and outlines a model to improve emotional and cognitive flexibility in this population.

EVALUATION OF COGNITIVE THERAPY

Although cognitive therapy has a great deal to offer, it also has limitations. Keeping these in mind can help clinicians maximize the effectiveness of this approach.

Limitations

Cognitive therapy is, of course, not for everyone. It is a structured approach that requires people to assume an active and collaborative role in their treatment and to complete suggested tasks between sessions. In addition, cognitive therapy stresses present-oriented, relatively brief treatment. The goal of cognitive therapy is improved ability to think clearly and cope with life's challenges.

People seeking unstructured, long-term treatment that focuses on development of insight and exploration of background may view this therapy as ill suited to their needs. In addition, people who are reluctant to participate fully in their own treatment, are intellectually limited, or are unmotivated to make changes may not be good candidates. Careful screening of clients as well as discussion about the nature of cognitive therapy can help clinicians determine if a client is an appropriate candidate for treatment.

Cognitive therapy also is demanding of clinicians. Clinicians must be organized, comfortable with structure, and willing to use inventories and forms to elicit and assess clients' concerns and progress. They must be knowledgeable about human development, learning theory, behavior therapy, and diagnosis, and be able to skillfully use a broad range of interventions. Planning and effort are integral to the success of cognitive therapy. Both clients and clinicians should be aware of the commitment required by this approach.

Other potential limitations can result from therapist shortcomings. At its inception, some clinicians erroneously viewed cognitive therapy as a rapid solution to immediate concerns; they neglected to develop a strong therapeutic alliance, downplayed the importance of empathy, and even became critical and judgmental of what the clinicians perceived as people's dysfunctional thoughts. These views reflect a misunderstanding of cognitive therapy and would not be reflected in effective treatment. Readers should keep in mind that cognitive therapy has more depth and complexity than may be evident initially and care should be taken to fully understand this powerful approach.

Strengths and Contributions

Cognitive therapy has many strengths. Because this approach is effective at ameliorating the most common concerns presented for treatment—depression and anxiety—it is useful with a broad range of disorders and clients. It is well received by most people because it is clear and logical and is not intrusive. Cognitive therapy does not require people to share intimate details of their past or focus extensively on their emotions. It is an empowering and nonthreatening approach. As we have seen, cognitive therapy draws on a broad array of interventions and can be integrated with many other treatment approaches.

The clear and carefully planned structure of cognitive therapy facilitates both teaching and research on this treatment system. Its time-limited nature makes it efficient and appealing, while its use of long-term follow-up provides a safeguard against relapse. Its emphasis on building a collaborative client–clinician alliance, providing assignments between sessions, giving the client credit for progress, reinforcing positive changes, and teaching skills is empowering. This approach is designed not just to resolve immediate problems but to enable people to manage their lives successfully.

Although mastery of cognitive therapy is not as simple as it seems, with training and experience most clinicians can easily learn and use it effectively. All clinicians should be familiar with the powerful and important concepts of cognitive therapy.

Cognitive therapy has made important contributions to counseling and psychotherapy. Aaron Beck's work, in particular, has emphasized the importance of research and evidence of effectiveness. This has led to increased research throughout the helping professions as well as development of treatment manuals designed to provide some uniformity to treatment and facilitate assessment of efficacy. Cognitive therapy's use of case formulations and treatment planning is compatible with today's emphasis on goal setting and accountability in treatment and has established a standard that other treatment systems are expected to follow.

The field of cognitive assessment is more than 30 years old. During that time, Beck and others have promoted the development and use of many helpful inventories that illuminate cognitive processes, anxiety and mood disorders, phobias, schemas, and other constructs that had previously been difficult to measure. Beck's depression and anxiety inventories, and Young's schema questionnaires mentioned earlier, are just a few of the self-report questionnaires that have become the most frequently used tools for cognitive assessment available today (Dunkley, Blankstein, & Segal, 2010).

Perhaps the most important contribution of cognitive therapy is the message that analysis and modification of distorted cognitions are important ways to help people change. Although emotions, actions, and background should never be ignored in treatment, helping people develop more realistic cognitions is an effective and efficient way to help them reach their goals.

SKILL DEVELOPMENT: ANALYZING AND MODIFYING COGNITIONS

This Skill Development section focuses on analyzing and modifying cognitions. It draws heavily on Aaron Beck's work and provides an example of cognitive therapy. Although all cognitive theorists dispute irrational thoughts, they do not all do so in the same way or use the same terminology.

People have thoughts, emotions, and behaviors. When a person describes a problem or concern, one of these is likely to be more accessible or prominent than the other two. For example, Harold was very upset about an interaction with his wife Carol that occurred when Harold's younger brother Louis was dying of cancer. Review the following three ways in which Harold might describe the interaction with his wife:

> ***Description 1:*** We were supposed to take our vacation when I found out that Louis was dying. I talked to the doctors, who said he only had a few weeks to live. I tried to be there for Louis. I told Carol that I wanted to postpone the vacation, so we put it off for a month. Louis was failing but was still alive then, so I suggested we postpone the vacation again. Carol wouldn't consider it. So I went on the vacation even though it was not what I wanted to do. Louis died while we were in Spain. We flew right home for the funeral.
>
> ***Description 2:*** We were supposed to take our vacation when I found out that Louis was dying. I was devastated when I found out. I couldn't bear the idea of going on a vacation while he was dying. I felt enraged when Carol refused to postpone our vacation a second time, but I was afraid I would lose my marriage if I didn't comply with her wishes. Louis died while we were in Spain. I felt so guilty that I hadn't been there with him.
>
> ***Description 3:*** We were supposed to take our vacation when I found out that Louis was dying. All I could think of was that I needed to be with him when he died. When Carol refused to postpone our vacation the second time, I thought she didn't care anything about me and only thought about her own needs. But I believed that it would hurt my marriage if I didn't go on the trip with her. Louis died while we were in Spain. I thought that I would never be able to forgive myself for not being with him.

Eliciting Actions, Emotions, and Thoughts

Each of Harold's descriptions has a different focus. Description 1 focuses on actions, Description 2 on emotions, and Description 3 on thoughts. When eliciting and analyzing thoughts, obtain all three aspects of a person's reactions. Start with the most accessible of the three (thoughts, emotions, or actions) and then ask about the other two, writing them down concisely and checking with the client to make sure that important thoughts, feelings, and behaviors have been captured accurately.

Burns (1999) referred to this process as the *triple column technique*. This strategy involves eliciting people's actions, thoughts, and emotions in relation to a particular situation. A rating scale of 0 to 100 is then used to assess the strength of people's emotions and the extent of their belief in their thoughts. This approach provides a baseline for use later in determining whether people's thoughts and feelings have changed.

For Harold, his description of his actions, thoughts, and emotions and the accompanying rating of his thoughts and emotions looked like this:

Identifying Actions

CLINICIAN: Describe the actions you took in response to this situation.

HAROLD: I persuaded Carol to postpone our vacation once; but when I asked her to postpone the vacation a second time, she refused. I went to Spain with her.

Identifying and Rating Thoughts

CLINICIAN: Identify the thoughts you had in response to this situation. Then, on a 0 to 100 rating scale, with 100 representing absolute belief and 0 reflecting no belief, indicate how much you believe your thoughts.

HAROLD:
1. I thought Carol didn't care about my feelings when she wouldn't postpone the vacation: 95.
2. I believed it would cost me my marriage if I didn't go on a vacation with Carol: 90.
3. I think I am a terrible person for abandoning my brother: 99.

Identifying and Rating Feelings

CLINICIAN: Identify the emotions you had in response to this situation. Then, on a 0 to 100 rating scale, with 100 representing the strongest possible emotion, indicate how strongly you are experiencing the feelings you reported.

HAROLD:
1. Devastated by my brother's death: 99.
2. Fearful of losing my marriage: 95.
3. Guilty that I had left my brother: 92.

Assessing the Validity of the Cognitions

The next step is helping people determine whether their cognitions have validity and are healthy and helpful to them. The clinician's role is not to criticize or devalue the cognitions but to maintain an objective stance and help clients evaluate their cognitions. Below are examples of approaches to evaluating and modifying cognitions:

- ***Reality testing:*** Assess the accuracy of the thought, using past experiences, research, logic, experiments, and other sources of information. Harold might consider whether his wife's past behavior supports his cognition that she doesn't care about his feelings. He also might talk with his wife about his interpretation of her insistence on their taking a vacation while his brother was dying.
- ***Seeking alternative explanations:*** Clinician and client brainstorm other possible and usually more positive explanations. For example, Harold considered the possibility that his wife felt a strong need for a vacation and was afraid to travel without him, as well as the possibility that she believed a vacation would help him deal with his brother's dying.
- ***Decatastrophizing:*** This involves identifying the most negative possible outcome or interpretation of a cognition and then assessing its likelihood, probable impact, and possible solutions. For Harold, this would be the thought that his wife no longer loved him and that their marriage was over. Articulating the thought allowed him to see that he could survive the end of his marriage although it would be difficult for him.

Harold found the process of seeking alternative explanations to be, helpful. In addition, he decided to engage in some reality testing. Although Carol sometimes seemed insensitive to his needs, when he pointed them out to her, she usually showed concern for his feelings. Viewing her as indifferent to his feelings, then, was not consistent with their history. Assisted by the clinician, he planned a conversation with Carol to seek a better understanding of her insistence on a vacation and her perception of their marriage. Carol told Harold that she had been concerned about his health and believed that Louis would survive for at least another month. She thought that Harold, who had been with his brother night and day during his illness, needed to get away. When Louis died while they were on vacation, Carol realized that she had made a mistake but thought that she would only make matters worse if she told Harold that. She reassured him that, although they did have some difficulties in their marriage, she was not considering a divorce and was willing to seek help for their marriage.

Identifying a Core Cognition

A core cognition often underlies specific thoughts. This cognition is a general statement that serves as a sort of screen for how people view their world and themselves. Identifying core cognitions can help people apply their learning and see that their specific, automatic cognitions may not be valid.

One of Harold's core cognitions was "I must please other people or they will reject me, since I don't have much to offer them." After identifying this cognition, he could see that his inability to assert himself with his wife was related to his low self-esteem. He recognized how this core cognition colored many aspects of his life and often led him to make choices that he later regretted. It also prevented him from letting other people get to know him and curtailed the closeness and intimacy in his relationships.

Categorizing the Cognitive Distortions

Dysfunctional or distorted cognitions are, in some way, inconsistent with objective reality. Usually these are negative thoughts about the self, reflecting guilt and low self-esteem, or negative thoughts about people's relationships and context that exaggerate the likelihood of undesirable events and behaviors. Such thoughts typically lead to unhealthy emotions and unhelpful actions.

Distorted cognitions can be categorized (Beck, 2011; Burns, 1999). Following is a list of types of cognitive distortions, illustrated by statements that Harold might make:

- ***All-or-nothing thinking:*** If I don't do everything in my power to please my wife, she will leave me.
- ***Overgeneralization:*** Relationships just don't work out for me. My high school sweetheart dumped me. My first wife was unfaithful. My marriage to Carol is doomed too.
- ***Mental filter:*** I know that Carol said she wanted to work on our marriage and said that she loved me, but my first wife said those things too. I don't think I can trust Carol.
- ***Disqualifying the positive:*** Yes, it's true that I spent every day for a month with Louis when he was dying. I made sure he had good care; I brought hospice in to help him; I even got a lawyer to come to the hospital so he could have a will prepared. I know I made a difference for him. But the bottom line is I wasn't there when he died. What good is all the rest if I wasn't there when he needed me most?
- ***Jumping to conclusions:*** Carol and I had a big fight this morning, and now she's over an hour late coming home from work. I think she's left me.
- ***Magnification/minimization:*** Carol told me that she wanted diamond earrings for her birthday, but I forgot. Instead, I got her some pearls. She was really disappointed. How could I have forgotten something that was so important to my wife? Why would she want to stay married to me?
- ***Emotional reasoning:*** My sister told me she made sure Louis was comfortable when he was dying, and she was with him until he died. She said Louis understood why I left. But I still feel awful. We were so close; it must have been harder for him without me there. No matter what my family says to me, I still feel guilty for leaving Louis.
- ***"Should" and "must" statements:*** A good husband should do everything he can to please his wife. I must be exactly the sort of husband that Carol wants.

- ***Labeling and mislabeling:*** I'm a loser. Nothing I do works out. No matter how hard I try, I'm just a failure.
- ***Personalization:*** Maybe Louis would have lived longer if I had been there. I think I gave him a reason to go on. He had already lived longer than the doctors expected, and who knows how long he could have kept going. It's my fault that he died when he did.
- ***Catastrophizing:*** If Carol leaves me, my life is not worth living. I couldn't go on.
- ***Mind reading:*** I know Carol doesn't understand my concern for my family. She probably just thinks I can't stand up for myself.
- ***Tunnel vision:*** I can't do anything to please Carol.

Harold's original cognitive distortions can be categorized as follows:

1. I thought Carol didn't care about my feelings when she wouldn't postpone the vacation: *Jumping to conclusions.*
2. I believed it would cost me my marriage if I didn't go on a vacation with Carol: *All-or-nothing thinking.*
3. I am a terrible person for abandoning my brother: *Mislabeling and magnification.*

Disputing and Replacing Cognitions

Once the distorted cognitions have been identified, examined, and categorized, they can be disputed. Client and clinician collaborate in finding alternate cognitions that have more validity and are likely to be more helpful to the client. These are written down as replacements for the original cognitions. Harold's revised thoughts follow, along with the ratings of his belief in these new thoughts:

1. "I thought Carol didn't care about my feelings when she wouldn't postpone the vacation" was replaced with "Although I felt hurt when Carol refused to postpone our vacation, I can see that she was doing what she thought was best for both of us." (65)
2. "I believed it would cost me my marriage if I didn't go on a vacation with Carol" was replaced with "Although I believed that I had to go on a vacation with Carol to save my marriage, my marriage is stronger than I thought. We do have problems but we are committed to our marriage and willing to work on the problems." (80)
3. "I am a terrible person for abandoning my brother" was replaced with "I still regret deeply that I was not there when my brother died, but I can see that I did a great deal for him throughout his life, especially after he got sick. I had no way of knowing that he would die while we were away. If I had known that, I would not have left him." (95)

Rerating Thoughts and Feelings and Modifying Actions

The final steps include:

- Rerating the original thoughts
- Rerating the original emotions
- Identifying and rating new emotions
- Revising actions.

Harold's Reratings of His Original Thoughts

1. I thought Carol didn't care about my feelings when she wouldn't postpone the vacation: 30.
2. I believed it would cost me my marriage if I didn't go on a vacation with Carol: 15.
3. I am a terrible person for abandoning my brother: 45.

Harold's Reratings of His Original Feelings

1. Devastated by my brother's death: 75.
2. Fearful of losing my marriage: 40.
3. Guilty that I left my brother: 50.

Harold's Ratings of His New Feelings

1. Sad about the loss of my brother: 100
2. Hopeful about the future of my marriage: 65
3. Regretful that I wasn't with my brother when he died: 90

Harold's New Actions

1. Carol and I have agreed to enter marital counseling.
2. My brother had been on the police force and volunteered considerable time to help children whose parents had been on the force and were killed in the line of duty. I will continue his work in honor of his memory.

Harold has experienced considerable change. Although he is, of course, still grieving the death of his brother and regrets that he was not present when Louis died, he is beginning to forgive himself and to come to terms with his brother's death. Significant change is evident in his perceptions of both his wife's feelings and the stability of his marriage. Success in collaborating with his wife to improve their marriage should help him feel even more secure in his marriage and more positively about himself and his relationship with his wife. The volunteer work he plans to undertake is a meaningful way to honor his brother's values and advance his brother's goals; it also should bring personal rewards to Harold.

Review of Steps in Analyzing and Modifying Cognitions

1. Elicit and write down actions, emotions, and thoughts related to a troubling experience.
2. Rate the belief in the thoughts and the intensity of the emotions on a 0 to 100 scale.
3. Assess the validity of the cognitions.
4. Identify any accessible core cognitions.
5. Categorize the cognitive distortions.
6. Dispute and replace dysfunctional cognitions with healthier and more valid cognitions.
7. Rate the revised cognitions.
8. Rerate the intensity of original thoughts and emotions.
9. Identify and rate new emotions.
10. Identify new actions.

CASE ILLUSTRATION

The case of Harold has already illustrated the process of eliciting, identifying, assessing, disputing, and modifying cognitive distortions. Consequently, what we consider here is only the first part of a case illustration; the exercises that follow will enable you to complete the picture.

The following dialogue with Edie is designed to elicit cognitive distortions. Look for them as you read.

EDIE: I'm really glad we had an appointment today. I've been so worried. I think Roberto may be involved with another woman.

CLINICIAN: What led you to think that?

EDIE: He always has his cell phone on. But yesterday I tried to call him for hours, and it was turned off. And then he put on a sports jacket and tie today when he left for work. He never dresses up like that. I started to think that maybe he's trying to impress someone.

CLINICIAN: Those thoughts must have been upsetting. What other thoughts did you have about this?

EDIE: You know that my father was unfaithful to my mother. I thought, here we go again. It's happening to me now. I'm just like my mother. I can't make my marriage work.

CLINICIAN: So it seemed like the past was repeating itself. How have you and Roberto been getting along lately?

EDIE: Actually, pretty well, but that makes me suspicious too. He gave me a beautiful gift for Mother's Day. He's probably just feeling guilty. But who would want to stay married to me? All I do is complain. I'm not much of a wife. And forget about sex. . . .

CLINICIAN: What feelings do all these thoughts bring up for you?

EDIE: I feel pretty discouraged. Here we've been seeing you for months, and I thought there was some hope of keeping our family together, but it doesn't look that way. I feel scared. How will I manage without Roberto?

CLINICIAN: This situation must be very frightening. What actions are you going to take?

EDIE: What can I do? If I ask Roberto about it, it might just bring the situation to a head and he'll decide to leave. Maybe if I just pretend I don't notice what's going on, he'll stay married to me . . . until the next woman comes along.

CLINICIAN: Do you know for sure of extramarital relationships that Roberto has had?

EDIE: No, he must hide them pretty well.

EXERCISES

Large-Group Exercises

Using the dialogue with Edie, go through the following steps of cognitive therapy:

1. List Edie's prominent thoughts, emotions, and planned actions. Try to home in on her central thoughts, summarizing them in three to five cognitions.
2. From what you know about Edie, rate the probable belief in her thoughts and the intensity of her feelings on the 0 to 100 scale.
3. Using the list of cognitive distortions presented in the Skill Development section, identify the nature of each of the distorted cognitions you identified.
4. Develop a plan to help Edie assess the validity of her cognitions. Draw on the suggestions presented previously in this chapter as well as your own ideas.

5. Assume that your work with Edie has been successful. Write rational responses or restatements to replace each of the cognitive distortions you identified. Be sure to use language that is likely to be acceptable to Edie.
6. Identify new emotions and actions that might characterize Edie's responses after you have helped her replace her distorted cognitions with healthy thoughts.

Small-Group Exercises

1. Identify the type (or types) of cognitive distortion reflected in each of the following examples. As a group, discuss ways you would help each of the following people assess the validity of his or her statement then come up with at least two alternative interpretations:

   Person A: My physician didn't call to tell me the test results. She probably has bad news and doesn't want to tell me.

   Person B: My agency didn't get the grant we had applied for. My colleagues did such a good job writing the proposal. It was probably the budget I prepared that ruined it for them. I thought I was asking for too much money, but I wanted to be sure the project would succeed.

   Person C: I was doing great on my diet, but then I went to Gary's wedding and made a pig of myself. I just know I'll gain back all the weight I lost. It's hopeless for me to even try to get myself in shape.

   Person D: I really should visit my mother every day. It's hard for me because she has dementia and doesn't recognize me, but a daughter should see her mother as often as she possibly can, no matter what.

   Person E: I was having a great time on my date with Nur until I made a fool of myself. We were at an amusement park, and she wanted to go on this ride that went up and down and around and around. I didn't really want to, but I thought, "If she wants to go, I should go too." I started to feel sick on the ride; and as soon as we got off, I had to run for the bathroom. You can imagine the rest. I was so humiliated. She'll never go out with me again. She's probably telling everyone how weak I am.

   Person F: The other girls avoid me because they know that my mother works in the school cafeteria. I know she needs a job and wanted one that would let her be home with me when I'm not at school, but she's ruining my life. I'll never be popular or have lots of friends like Jessica. Her mother doesn't have to work at all and drives a Mercedes when she picks her up after school.

Individual Exercises

1. Select a recent experience during which you had strong emotions. Identify at least three emotions, one action, and two thoughts that accompanied the experience. Try to identify at least one cognitive distortion that you had in relation to the experience. Write down the distortion in your journal. Then, in writing, go through the steps of rating, assessing, classifying, disputing, replacing, and rerating your cognition(s). What new emotions and actions now seem available to you?
2. We all have thoughts, emotions, and actions. Observe yourself as you go through the day. Which of these categories is most accessible to you? Are you most likely to discuss thoughts, feelings, or actions with other people? Which of the three is most likely to worry you and stay in your mind? Write your answers in your journal.

Summary

Cognitive therapists believe that the most effective way to help people make positive changes is by enabling them to identify, evaluate, and, if indicated, modify their thoughts. While attention is also paid to emotions and actions, dysfunctional thoughts are the target of treatment. Developed by Aaron Beck and his associates, cognitive therapy is a relatively brief, structured approach that offers specific plans for change, gives people clear explanations of all steps in the treatment process, and teaches skills that empower people and promote their emotional well-being. Clients and clinicians work collaboratively, with clinicians drawing on an extensive array of creative interventions to promote and reinforce positive change. Task assignments and inventories are used and contribute to the clarity and impact of cognitive therapy. Research has proven the effectiveness of cognitive therapy with a broad range of mental disorders and clients. It is especially effective in treating depression and anxiety.

Recommended Readings

Beck, A. T., Freeman, A., & Davis, D. D. (2006). *Cognitive therapy of personality disorders* (2nd ed.). New York, NY: Guilford Press.

Beck, J. S. (2005). *Cognitive therapy for challenging problems: What to do when the basics don't work.* New York, NY: Guilford Press.

Beck, J. S. (2011). *Cognitive behavioral therapy: Basics and beyond* (2nd ed.). New York, NY: Guilford.

Clark, D. A., & Beck, A. T. (2011). *Cognitive therapy of anxiety disorders.* New York, NY: Guilford.

Crane, N. (2009). *Mindfulness-based cognitive therapy.* New York, NY: Routledge.

Gallagher-Thompson, D., Steffen, A. M., & Thompson, L. W. (Eds.). (2008). *Handbook of behavioral and cognitive therapies with older adults.* New York, NY: Springer.

Hofmann, S. G. (2012). *An introduction to modern CBT.* New York, NY: Wiley.

Leahy, R. L., Tirch, D., & Napolitano, L. A. (2011). *Emotion regulation in psychotherapy: A practitioner's guide.* New York, NY: Guilford Press.

Rafaeli, E., Bernstein, D. P., & Young, J. (2011). *Schema therapy.* New York, NY: Routledge.

Zarb, J. M. (2007). *Developmental cognitive behavioral therapy with adults.* New York, NY: Routledge.

Additional Sources of Information

Although many journals in psychology and counseling include articles on cognitive therapy, two focus specifically on treatment via this approach: the *Journal of Cognitive Psychotherapy* and the *International Cognitive Therapy Newsletter.*

Training in and information on cognitive therapy is widely available. The following is a good place to begin gathering additional information on education and resources:

http://www.beckinstitute.org—This is the website for the Beck Institute for Cognitive Therapy and Research. The Beck Institute offers weekend and weeklong training opportunities as well as extended training, videoconferences, distance learning, recommended readings, and books and inventories.

http://www.cognitivetherapynyc.com—This is the website of the American Institute for Cognitive Therapy in New York. This organization of researchers and psychotherapists provides cognitive–behavioral treatment as well as information. The affiliated Foundation for the Advancement of Cognitive Therapy (FACT) conducts research and provides training on CBT.

http://www.academyofct.org—The Academy of Cognitive Therapy, founded in 1999, is an organization of clinicians, educators, and researchers in cognitive therapy. The academy supports continuing education and research and also serves as a certifying organization for CBT. Blogs by Aaron Beck and Robert Leahy are featured.

Inventories developed by Aaron Beck and others and used in cognitive therapy can be ordered from:

The Psychological Corporation
555 Academic Court
San Antonio, TX 78204
(800) 211-8378

http://www.schematherapy.com—This website developed by Jeffrey Young includes inventories, publications, a bibliography, outcome studies, and training opportunities on schema therapy.

CHAPTER 15

Overview of Action-Focused Treatment Systems

Actions, the fourth component in the BETA model (background, emotions, thoughts, actions), are the focus of Part 5 of this book. Throughout the book, the terms *actions* and *behaviors* are used interchangeably. Actions are usually overt, observable, and measurable. Actions affect and are intertwined with our thoughts and emotions. Treatment focused on modifying behaviors often leads to clear and rapid changes.

Each of us may be the only one who is aware of our feelings and thoughts; they can be kept private, and any given thought or emotion may not have an impact on our lives. That is not the case with behaviors. Once we take action—choose which road to travel—we make an irrevocable move in a certain direction. In addition, the potentially public and observable nature of behaviors intensifies their impact. Although background, emotions, and thoughts may underlie our behaviors, the actions we take are most likely to determine the direction of our lives as well as our relationships with others and their perceptions of us. Even a small act such as leaving for work early has a profound impact if it enables a person to avoid an accident, meet a new friend in the cafeteria, or make a positive impression on a supervisor.

Sometimes people feel overwhelmed and immobilized when they consider the possible impact of their behaviors, so they avoid making choices and taking action. However, inaction is an action in itself and does have consequences.

THE IMPORTANCE OF ACTIONS IN COUNSELING AND PSYCHOTHERAPY

Focusing on behavior change has many advantages in treatment, most of which are similar to the advantages of focusing on cognitions. However, an emphasis on actions has additional advantages as well as some drawbacks.

The Advantages of Focusing on Actions

Most clinicians recognize that emotions, thoughts, and actions have reciprocal relationships. Whether or not clinicians focus primarily on behaviors, they should be aware of the potential benefits of paying attention to clients' actions.

BEHAVIORS AS PRESENTING PROBLEMS Clients' presenting problems often focus on behaviors. People rarely seek treatment because of dysfunctional thoughts, although they do sometimes seek help for negative emotions such as depression and anxiety. Usually, however, what impels them to seek help is an upsetting behavior, either their own or someone else's. Common behavioral concerns include overeating, unhealthy use of drugs or alcohol, poor impulse control, difficulty finding a rewarding job, and problems in developing rewarding relationships. Because behaviors often prompt treatment, people are more likely to feel heard and to believe that treatment will be helpful if, at least initially, it addresses those concerns.

Attending to unrewarding or self-destructive behavior is particularly important in treatment of people who are not self-referred for help. For example, people who are fulfilling court-mandated treatment requirements, who have been encouraged to meet with an employee-assistance counselor at work, or who have been brought for help by a concerned parent or dissatisfied partner usually are in treatment because their behaviors have violated the law or been unsatisfactory or troubling to others.

THE ACCESSIBILITY OF BEHAVIORS Behaviors usually are more accessible than either thoughts or emotions. Think back to yesterday at this same time. You may have difficulty recalling your thoughts and feelings, but you can probably remember where you were and what you were doing. You may have been listening to a lecture, driving home from work, or taking a nap. Because behaviors are linked to the structure of our days, we can usually remember them, whereas thoughts and emotions are more difficult to recall.

COMFORT IN DISCUSSION OF BEHAVIORS Discussion of people's behaviors is likely to be less threatening than discussion of their early childhood experiences or their troubling emotions and somewhat less uncomfortable than discussion of their cognitions. People are used to talking about their activities with others but are less likely to talk with others about thoughts and emotions.

In addition, most actions are overt and observable, whereas thoughts and emotions are covert and often not obvious. Thus, questions about behaviors seem less intrusive than questions about emotions and cognitions. Few people, for example, would be uncomfortable with questions such as "What time did you get up this morning?" and "What did you say to your child when you learned he lied to you?" but they might experience discomfort responding to questions such as "What thoughts led you to stay in bed all day?" and "How did you feel when your child lied to you?"

ACCURACY OF INFORMATION Discussion of actions is socially acceptable, even among casual acquaintances, and people seem more able to present accurate information about their behaviors than about their emotions and cognitions. Having clear and valid information, especially at the beginning of treatment, is essential in formulating realistic goals and a viable treatment plan, as well as in developing a positive therapeutic alliance. (Of course, keep in mind that some people will deliberately present inaccurate information about their behaviors, especially those that are socially and legally unacceptable such as excessive use of drugs or aggressive expressions of anger.)

EASE OF MEASUREMENT Actions are amenable to measurement. People can determine the baseline frequency of a behavior and then assess change in such variables as how many beers they drink each day, how often they exercise, how many hours they devote to work, and how much time they spend with friends. Because even small changes can readily be identified, people trying to modify their actions often have rapid evidence of improvement. This can be empowering and promote motivation, optimism, and further change.

At the same time, if an incorrect diagnosis, case formulation, or treatment plan has been made, that probably will be reflected in a lack of behavior change in response to treatment. This alerts the clinician to the need for a revised and more effective treatment approach.

THE AVAILABILITY OF BEHAVIOR CHANGE STRATEGIES A broad range of behavior change strategies has been developed. This enables clinicians to individualize treatment plans, bring creativity to their work, and maximize the likelihood of success by tailoring treatment to a particular person and behavior.

EXTENSIVE RESEARCH SUPPORT Because the impact of behavior change strategies usually is easy to assess and because most behaviorally oriented clinicians are favorably disposed toward empirical research, an extensive body of literature describes and affirms the effectiveness of behavior and cognitive–behavioral therapy. These treatment approaches have received more support than other approaches, not because behavior and cognitive–behavioral therapy are superior, but because of the extensive research conducted on these approaches.

The Limitations of Focusing on Actions

Although treatment systems that focus on behavior change have many advantages, they also have some shortcomings. An exclusive focus on actions can lead clinicians and clients to ignore thoughts and feelings that need attention and are important in solidifying change. This can lead to superficial treatment and limited results.

For example, Lily sought counseling for help with time management; she expressed a wish to have more involvement with her husband and children. Underlying her presenting problem were feelings of self-doubt and low self-esteem, disappointment with her marriage, and fear that her husband was having an affair. Lily's marital concerns were exacerbated by feelings of betrayal stemming from childhood sexual abuse by her father. Neglect of Lily's thoughts, emotions, and background would have done her a disservice and probably led to treatment that at best would have had limited success.

Several safeguards can reduce the possibility that clinicians focusing on actions will miss important underlying concerns. First, they should conduct a comprehensive assessment of their clients via a thorough intake interview and appropriate inventories. This helps provide a full picture of clients and facilitates development of a treatment plan that is broad enough to address both presenting problems and relevant underlying concerns. Second, clinicians should closely monitor the progress of treatment; if rapid change is not evident, clinicians may not have accurately conceptualized a case and may need additional information and a revised treatment plan. Third, behavior counseling should usually not be used alone. Combining behavior treatment strategies with cognitive approaches, in particular, enhances the power of behavior therapy and enables clinicians to successfully address a broad range of concerns.

IMPORTANT THEORETICAL CONCEPTS

The application of behavior therapy varies, depending on clinician, client, concern, and setting. Most approaches to behavior therapy can be described by one or more of the following five models, each of which will be introduced in this chapter and discussed in greater depth in the chapters to come (Wilson, 1995):

1. ***Applied behavioral analysis.*** Derived from B. F. Skinner's theory of operant conditioning, this approach looks at the impact of environmental events on behavior. It takes a scientific approach and focuses on observable, measurable behavior.
2. ***Neo-behaviorism.*** Drawing on Pavlov's classical conditioning as well as stimulus–response theories, this focuses on the process of conditioning or learning responses.
3. ***Social learning theory.*** Based on the research of Albert Bandura, this approach seeks to understand the interaction of cognitive, behavioral, and environmental factors in shaping behavior. Many strategies that clinicians use to enhance self-efficacy and reduce learned helplessness reflect an understanding of social learning (Bandura, 2006).
4. ***Cognitive–behavioral therapy.*** Reflected in the work of Meichenbaum, Ellis, and Beck, this approach looks at how cognitions shape behaviors and emotions. This treatment system makes use of both cognitive and behavioral strategies to effect change.
5. ***Multimodal therapy.*** Multimodal therapy, developed by Arnold Lazarus, is based on principles of behavior therapy. Multimodal therapy integrates strategies from a wide range of treatment methodologies into a holistic systematic approach to assessment and treatment planning.

Basic Assumptions Shared by Action-Focused Therapies

Regardless of their specific approach to behavior therapy, all action-focused therapies generally subscribe to the following commonalities (Antony & Roemer, 2011):

- Although genetics plays a role, individual differences are derived primarily from different experiences.
- Behavior is learned and acquired largely through modeling, conditioning, and reinforcement.
- Behavior has a purpose.
- Behavior therapy seeks to understand and change behavior.
- Therapy should be based on the scientific method and be systematic, empirical, and experimental. Goals should be stated in behavioral, specific, and measurable terms, with progress assessed regularly.

- The focus of treatment should generally be on the present. Even if behaviors are long-standing, they are maintained by factors in the current environment.
- Behaviors must be viewed in the context in which they occur.
- A client's environment can be manipulated to increase appropriate behaviors and decrease harmful behaviors.
- Education—promoting new learning and transfer of learning—is an important aspect of behavior therapy.
- People need to take an active part in their treatment to successfully change their behaviors. Clients have primary responsibility for defining their goals and completing homework tasks. The treatment plan is formulated collaboratively, with both client and clinician participating actively in that process.

Therapeutic Relationship

Like cognitive therapists, those who practice behavioral, cognitive–behavioral, and reality therapy are more directive and focused than the therapists who use the other approaches we have discussed in this book. Behavior therapists are far more likely to develop and focus on treatment plans, set goals and objectives, and monitor homework assignments in their efforts to help their clients effect behavioral change. Behavior therapists recognize the importance of a collaborative and positive therapeutic relationship and the communication of encouragement as important in promoting learning and motivation. They tend to take a holistic approach—interpreting behavior broadly as anything an organism does, including thinking and feeling—and are interested in the total person. Although objectivity and the scientific method are valued, behavior therapists also recognize the importance of understanding and respecting individual differences.

THE EARLY HISTORY OF BEHAVIOR THERAPY: THE FIRST WAVE

Behavior therapy, initiated during the 1950s and 1960s, presented a powerful challenge to the principles of psychoanalysis. Behavior therapy's focus on observable behaviors rather than the unconscious; on the present rather than the past; and on short-term treatment, clear goals, and rapid change had considerable appeal.

As its name implies, behavior therapy focuses entirely on specific behavior with the goal of changing or modifying that behavior. Health-related behaviors such as smoking, obesity, and sedentary lifestyle have become the focus of increased interest in the United States because these unhealthy behaviors have been linked to illness and preventable deaths. Similarly, childhood behaviors such as bullying, tantrums, or poor sleep habits can become the focus of clinical attention. Adult behaviors such as road rage, drinking, phobias, and others can be modified as well. In fact, almost any human behavior can be the subject of behavior therapy.

Unlike many of the theories discussed in this book, behavior therapy is not strongly associated with one or two names. Instead, many people contributed to the evolution of this approach. Some, like Skinner, Harlow, and Pavlov, used principles of behavior change to shape the actions and reactions of animals. Others, including Eysenck, Lazarus, Wolpe, Dollard and Miller, Krumboltz, and Bandura, applied behavior therapy and learning theory to people.

The development of learning theory presupposed that all psychological disorders were the result of faulty learning in childhood. Skinner's theories, which used reinforcements to assist learning, were followed by Wolpe's theory of systematic desensitization in which people were gradually introduced to a fear-producing object while being taught relaxation techniques. Later, Bandura discovered the role of social learning in the reinforcement of behavior.

Ivan Pavlov

In the early 1900s, Ivan Pavlov (1927), a Russian physiologist, identified and described a type of learning that now is known as *classical conditioning.* His study of conditioning dogs' responses is well known. Pavlov demonstrated that, by simultaneously presenting an unconditioned stimulus (meat paste) and a conditioned stimulus (the sound of a tuning fork), researchers could elicit the dogs' salivation using only the conditioned stimulus (the sound) because the dogs learned to associate the sound with the meat.

Pavlov also studied the process of *extinction.* For a while, the dogs in his study salivated to the sound of the tuning fork, even when the sound was no longer accompanied by the meat. However, over time, the salivating response diminished and eventually disappeared in response to the tuning fork alone.

John W. Watson

John W. Watson, an American psychologist, used Pavlov's principles of classical conditioning and *stimulus generalization,* along with concepts of learning theory, to change human behavior. Rejecting psychoanalysis, then the prevailing treatment approach, Watson (1925) proposed what he called *behaviorism.* Watson demonstrated that an unconditioned stimulus (a loud bell), paired with a conditioned stimulus (a white rat), could lead a child to emit a conditioned response (startle) in reaction not only to a white rat but also to white cotton and Watson's white hair.

B. F. Skinner

Building on the work of Pavlov and Watson, B. F. Skinner developed a theory of behavior that has become the foundation on which behavior modification is based (Martin & Pear, 2007). His ideas, known as operant reinforcement theory, postulate that how often a behavior will be emitted is largely determined by the events that follow that behavior. Drawing on the principles of operant conditioning in one of his studies, Skinner used rewards to gradually shape the behavior of pigeons until they learned to peck at a red disk. Similarly, children's behavior can be shaped through parental reinforcement; for example, parents who attend primarily to children's misbehavior inadvertently reinforce that behavior.

Skinner called this *operant* behavior because the behavior "operated" on the environment and was controlled by its effects. Operant conditioning refers to the schedules of reinforcement responsible for producing the new behavior. Based on the effect of consequences, schedules of reinforcement may be continuous, fixed ratio, fixed interval, or variable rate. Shaping refers to the manner in which more complicated behaviors are reinforced. For example, Skinner was able to reinforce a pigeon to turn in a circle by reinforcing small successive approximations of the desired behavior until the pigeon was able to complete an entire turn with only one reinforcement. The results of these early studies in operant conditioning were published in his first book *The Behavior of Organisms* (1938).

Other terms related to behavior therapy include the following:

- ***Positive reinforcement:*** A behavior followed by a positive reinforcement has an increased probability of being repeated. Positive reinforcement involves providing a "reward" to a client upon completion of a desired behavior (at the schedule of reinforcement that has been determined). Positive reinforcement encourages a behavior to be repeated, much as a parent's smiles and excitement reinforce a baby to smile.
- ***Aversive stimulus:*** The opposite of positive reinforcement, an aversive stimulus is something that might be found to be unpleasant, such as shocking a mouse. A behavior followed by an

aversive stimulus results in a decreased probability of the behavior occurring in the future. This both defines an aversive stimulus and describes the form of conditioning known as *punishment*. If you shock a mouse for doing *x*, it will do less of *x*.

- ***Negative reinforcement:*** Negative reinforcement involves the removal of an already active aversive stimulus (e.g., turning off the electricity when the mouse stands on its hind legs will result in the mouse standing more). Therefore, behavior followed by the removal of an aversive stimulus results in an increased probability of that behavior occurring in the future. Negative reinforcement is often mistaken for punishment, when in fact the two are separate, and important, concepts in behavioral theory. Operant learning can be used to shape behavior. Skinner compared this learning with the way children learn to talk—they are rewarded for making a sound that is similar to a word until in fact they can say the word.

Skinner was a strict behaviorist who believed that the only scientific approach to psychology was one that studied behaviors, not internal (subjective) mental processes. He believed that who we are and everything we do is shaped by our experiences of punishment and reward. The best summary of his theories is contained in his book *About Behaviorism* (1974). Skinner continued to write (*Walden II,* 1948/2005; *Beyond Freedom and Dignity,* 1971; and a three-part autobiography), lecture, and receive numerous awards for his contributions to psychology until his death from leukemia in 1990. His principles are still incorporated within treatments of phobias, addictive behaviors, and in the enhancement of classroom performance (as well as in computer-based self-instruction).

John Dollard and Neal Miller

Subsequent work by John Dollard and Neal Miller (1950) contributed greatly to our understanding of learning theory and paved the way for behaviorists to move into the arena of psychotherapy. Dollard and Miller identified four important elements in behavior: drive, cue, response, and reinforcement. In *Social Learning and Imitation* (Miller & Dollard, 1941), they wrote:

> What, then, is learning theory? In its simplest form, it is the study of the circumstances under which a response and a cue stimulus become connected. After learning has been completed, response and cue are bound together in such a way that the appearance of the cue evokes the response. . . . The connection between a cue and a response can be strengthened under certain conditions. The learner must be driven to make the response and rewarded for having responded in the presence of the cue. (p. 1)

The more frequently a stimulus and a response coincide, with the response being rewarded, the stronger is the tendency to emit the response when that stimulus occurs, leading to the development of a habit or habitual response. This is the essence of the *stimulus–response (S-R)* concept, which, according to behavior theorists, determines the behaviors that people learn.

For example, Jamila was the third child in a family of seven children. Both parents worked outside of the home and had little time for positive interactions with their children. Whenever one of the children was sick, however, the parents gave them extra time and attention. Jamila learned that illness was the best way to elicit her parents' attention and so exaggerated even minor physical symptoms for the nurturance that would bring her. She continued this behavior into adulthood, even though it had a deleterious effect on her relationships, her employment, and eventually on her marriage.

Dollard and Miller found that *counterconditioning* could reverse habits. This involves pairing the behavior to be changed with a strong incompatible response to the same cue. For example, Jamila's behavior gradually changed as her employer, friends, and partner became annoyed with her frequent complaints of physical discomfort and withdrew from her when she reported feeling ill.

Joseph Wolpe

Joseph Wolpe (1969) described a similar process, *reciprocal inhibition,* in which eliciting a novel response brings about a decrease in the strength of a concurrent habitual response. A parent who makes a silly face to cheer up a child who is crying after a minor fall is a simple example; the silly face elicits amusement, which automatically reduces the sad emotions associated with the fall. Wolpe's ideas led to the development of *systematic desensitization,* a powerful tool that pairs relaxation with controlled exposure to a feared stimulus such as heights or dogs. This technique still is widely used, especially in the treatment of phobias. Wolpe also developed strategies to promote assertive behavior.

Wolpe's work reflects the concept of *stimulus generalization.* When people learn to respond in a particular way to one stimulus, they often behave in that same way when presented with similar cues. For example, a child who is taught to be respectful of teachers is likely to behave respectfully toward other authority figures. Sometimes behavior is overgeneralized and becomes inappropriate or unhealthy. Then people need to learn *stimulus discrimination*—the ability to distinguish among similar cues. For example, most of us have learned to confide in a small number of close friends but recognize that it is inappropriate to share many details of our personal lives at work (stimulus discrimination). However, some people share intimate details of their lives not only with close friends but with casual associates, perhaps reflecting inappropriate stimulus generalization.

UNDERSTANDING TERMINOLOGY

The terminology of behavior therapy can be confusing. However, becoming familiar with terminology facilitates understanding of this approach as well as of personality development. Following is a review of important terms, illustrated by the experiences of Theresa, a 33-year-old woman receiving chemotherapy for breast cancer. Although we discussed some of these terms previously, we review them here for clarification.

Theresa presented many issues related to her diagnosis of cancer. She had always been fearful of injections and found blood tests and intravenous chemotherapy difficult. She had anticipatory nausea associated with her chemotherapy, becoming queasy when driving into the parking lot of the clinic where she received treatment, whether or not she was scheduled for chemotherapy. In addition, although her prognosis was encouraging, Theresa constantly ruminated about the likelihood of her death.

Theresa's anticipatory nausea can be explained by *classical conditioning.* The *unconditioned stimulus,* the chemotherapy, elicited the *response* of nausea. Because that stimulus was paired with the *conditioned stimulus* of driving to the clinic, entering the parking lot became a stimulus that also elicited the response of nausea whether or not the chemotherapy also was present.

Theresa, like all of us, had an innate *drive* to avoid pain. When she received inoculations as a child, her parents reinforced her fears by paying special attention to her when she became fearful. As a result of this *operant conditioning,* her fear of injections became *habitual* and evolved into a *phobia.* In fact, through the process of *stimulus generalization,* Theresa experienced inordinate anxiety in reaction to any medical appointment, whether or not it necessitated an injection. Her *learned behavior* reflected a *stimulus–response model;* because her fearful behavior was rewarded in childhood, Theresa demonstrated fear and avoidance *(response)* to the *stimulus* of any medical visit.

Her therapist used several behavioral approaches to modify Theresa's responses. *Systematic desensitization* was used in the hope of *extinguishing* Theresa's excessive fear of medical visits and inoculations. An *anxiety hierarchy* was created, listing her fears in ascending order from the mildest fear (a visit to a dermatologist that would not involve any physical discomfort) to the most frightening (a visit to the oncologist for chemotherapy). Beginning with the mildest fear, the therapist helped Theresa to relax and feel empowered while visualizing the frightening stimulus. This process of *reciprocal inhibition* paired relaxation and positive feelings with an *aversive stimulus* (a frightening image) to decrease the strength of the fear response. Theresa also learned to use both relaxation and *stimulus discrimination* to reduce her fears; she learned to relax when approaching medical visits and driving into the parking lot at the oncology clinic and reminded herself that not all medical appointments involved discomfort.

Counterconditioning was used to help Theresa further reduce her fears; when she began to ruminate or felt anxious, she visualized herself triumphantly completing her chemotherapy and setting off on a trip to Bali that she was planning. The feelings of pride and optimism elicited by that image counteracted and reduced her apprehension. To make sure she could readily access this positive image, the therapist led Theresa through a process of *covert modeling* in which she mentally rehearsed dealing effectively with her fears about chemotherapy. Joining a support group of other women diagnosed with breast cancer also provided Theresa with an experience in *social learning and reinforcement* and gave her additional *role models.*

INTRODUCTION TO THEORETICAL MODELS

The first wave of behaviorism provided a basis on which behavioral psychology was built. Behavioral approaches can be used alone, or integrated with cognitive therapies (as discussed in Part 4 of this book) such as REBT and Beck's cognitive therapy. As we shall read in Chapter 16, when interwoven, cognitive–behavioral treatment systems can have a powerful impact on behavioral change. Clients learn, through the process of cognitive restructuring, to replace their faulty thinking with healthy, positive, and constructive thoughts that help them also to change their behavior. Chapter 16 describes many other useful strategies including cognitive–behavior modification and stress inoculation training developed by Donald Meichenbaum, and the newer approaches that incorporate mindfulness and acceptance.

Readers should keep in mind that the demarcation between cognitive and behavioral approaches is not always clear. Cognitive approaches focus on changing thoughts; behavioral approaches concentrate on modifying actions; and cognitive–behavioral approaches attend to both thoughts and actions. The differences are primarily those of emphasis.

Reality therapy is a type of behavioral therapy based on choice theory, which was developed in the 1960s by William Glasser. Choice theory focuses on total behavior, which is based on four interacting needs present from birth until death—acting, feeling, thinking, and physiology. Glasser believes that most actions are chosen, and therefore we create our lives through the choices that we make. Consequently, Glasser believes that people must take responsibility and be accountable for their actions. Reality therapy is particularly useful in settings such as schools, correctional institutions, and substance use treatment programs that emphasize changing behavior. Chapter 17 focuses on reality therapy and the WDEP system developed by Robert Wubbolding (2007b) as part of a practical, cross-cultural, theory of behavior that is founded on universal human principles and is applicable to everyone.

Summary

This chapter discussed the importance of focusing on actions in counseling and psychotherapy as well as some of the advantages and disadvantages of emphasizing behaviors in treatment. Behavioral terminology was introduced along with a case vignette to help readers understand the application of behavior therapy. The chapter also provided a brief look at the history of behavior therapy, and a short introduction to the discussion of the second wave of behavioral theories—cognitive–behavioral therapy, and the so-called third wave—newer approaches that focus on emotions as well as behaviors and cognitions.

CHAPTER 16

Behavior Therapy and Cognitive–Behavioral Therapy

In the writing of this chapter I was constantly reminded of the old television commercial for Reese's peanut butter cups, in which two people—one carrying a chocolate bar, and the other eating peanut butter—bump into each other.

The first person remarks, "Hey, you got peanut butter on my chocolate."

The second person responds, "No, you got chocolate on my peanut butter."

The end result, of course, is a delicious combination of both peanut butter and chocolate that is much more satisfying than either one alone.

The same could be said for cognitive and behavioral therapies. Strictly behavioral therapies do not include much cognitive analysis, and strictly cognitive therapies do not include much behavioral therapy. But when the two are combined, like peanut butter and chocolate, they become better than either one alone.

In Chapter 15 we read about the historical roots of behavior therapy, or what might be called the first generation of behavior therapy. By the 1980s, behavior therapy had established its place in psychotherapy, and its effectiveness was well substantiated by research. However, many clinicians were dissatisfied with traditional behavior therapy, which de-emphasized the therapeutic alliance, viewed the clinician as the authority, and sometimes seemed dehumanizing. As a result, the shape of behavior therapy began to evolve through the influence of Bandura and social learning theory and the move toward integration of behavior therapy with cognitive therapy reflected in the work of Meichenbaum, Lazarus, Ellis, Beck, and others. During the past 30 years the application of this approach has broadened and made it less mechanical and more sensitive to individual needs. A positive and collaborative therapeutic alliance is now an essential element of treatment. And the incorporation of mindfulness and other concepts has provided an entirely new focus for behavioral therapy.

Readers should keep in mind that the differences among cognitive therapy, behavior therapy, and cognitive–behavioral treatment are primarily those of emphasis. Cognitive approaches focus on changing thoughts; behavioral approaches concentrate on modifying actions; and cognitive–behavioral approaches attend to both thoughts and actions.

THE DEVELOPMENT OF SOCIAL LEARNING THEORY

Our discussion turns now to the biography of Albert Bandura, the developer of social cognitive theory, which emphasizes how individuals learn by observing and modeling others (Bandura, 2006), followed by a broader look at behavior strategies and interventions.

Albert Bandura and Social Learning Theory

One of the most influential social learning theorists, Albert Bandura (1925–) was born in Canada and received his PhD from the University of Iowa. He later moved to Stanford University where he is now a distinguished professor emeritus. Bandura applied the principles of both classical and operant conditioning to social learning (1969, 1977, 1986). He found that in addition to direct experience, learning and subsequent behavior change could occur vicariously through observation of other people's behavior. The process, which Bandura called *modeling*, can elicit both positive and negative behaviors.

Modeling often has a beneficial impact, as when a parent models appropriate behavior. On the other hand, as Bandura's famous Bobo doll experiments suggest, children who observed an adult acting aggressively and hitting the Bobo doll were more likely to manifest aggressive behavior than children who had not been exposed to the aggressive behavior.

Not only do others influence our behavior, but through *reciprocal determinism,* our behavior influences our environment. Thus, cognitions, behaviors, and environment become intertwined in creating the human experience.

In his seminal work on social learning theory, Bandura (1969) found that modeling has more than just an impact on behavior. Modeling can actually change our cognitions about our abilities and improve our *self-efficacy*. Observing someone we admire undertake a challenging task can reduce our fears and facilitate our own efforts to perform the task. People with strong beliefs in their own efficacy are more likely to face problems as challenges to be reckoned with rather than threats to be avoided. Bandura found that self-efficacy impacts how a person thinks, feels, motivates himself, and behaves. More will be said about modeling in the discussion of behavior strategies and interventions in a later section.

Self-efficacy theory posits that a person will be able to perform a certain task based on her beliefs about how well she will perform (her competencies), as well as the consequences that come from doing it (environmental reinforcement). Over time, people develop a sense of their own competency at a given task. This sense of competency shapes their future attempts (Bandura, 1977). Many behavioral treatments, such as behavior activation therapy and exposure-based treatments, are based on the premise that self-efficacy increases as people increase time spent on behaviors at which they feel competent. Social cognitive theory expands on behavior theory and cognitive–behavioral theory by recognizing that not only reinforced behaviors or faulty thoughts are responsible for human behavior, but a complicated cognitive mediational process that includes cognitive, affective, motivational, and selection processes.

A threefold process involving self-observation, self-judgment, and how we attribute success or failure in our lives contributes to our self-regulatory process. Ultimately, the goal of social cognitive therapy is to assist and strengthen the human capacity for self-regulation. Psychological dysfunction or maladjustment is considered to be the result of learning; maladaptive behavior persists because there is some reward for that behavior, not because it results from sexual or aggressive impulses. Bandura (1973) has written extensively on aggression, violence, and adolescence and has testified repeatedly before Congress about the causes and possible solutions to aggressive behavior. As a result of his theories, most behavioral treatments (including exposure therapy and social skills training) now include a modeling component (Antony & Roemer, 2011).

Albert Bandura has been honored by the American Psychological Association with a lifetime achievement award. He has written seven books and published innumerable articles in scholarly journals. Now in his 80s, he continues to conduct research and teach at Stanford University, where he has worked since 1953.

TREATMENT USING BEHAVIOR THERAPY

Goals

Behavior therapy, as its name implies, seeks to extinguish maladaptive behaviors and help people learn new adaptive ones. The following is a partial list of goals that can be achieved through behavior therapy:

- Reduction in use of, or abstinence from, drugs and alcohol
- Reduction of undesirable habits such as nail biting and pulling out one's own hair
- Improvement in social skills such as assertiveness and conversation
- Amelioration of fears and phobias such as fear of flying, apprehension about public speaking, and excessive fear of snakes
- Improvement in concentration and organization
- Reduction in undesirable behaviors in children such as tantrums, disobedience, acting out, aggressiveness, and difficulty going to bed
- Improvement in health and fitness habits such as more nutritious eating, increased exercise, and more regular sleep patterns.

In addition to specific goals such as these, behavior therapists also have the general goal of teaching people skills that will help them improve their lives. Skills such as decision making, problem analysis and resolution, time management, assertiveness, and relaxation often are incorporated into behavior therapy.

Behavioral Strategies and Interventions

Clinicians can implement many different strategies to help clients begin to change their behavior. Some of the most useful interventions are listed here.

ACTING AS IF This strategy was first developed by Alfred Adler (discussed in Chapter 4), whose ideas can be viewed as an early version of cognitive–behavioral therapy (CBT). When confronting a challenging situation, people "act as if" they are someone whom they view as capable of handling the situation effectively. Children undergoing medical treatments, for example, have coped more successfully when they pretended to be their favorite superhero. Adults, too, can benefit from this empowering approach by acting as if they are an admired friend or colleague.

ACTIVITY SCHEDULING Planning activities that are rewarding and provide a sense of accomplishment can help people in many ways. Having a schedule provides focus and direction, which can counteract inertia, confusion, and problems in decision making. It can limit excessive sleeping or television watching and prevent isolation. It increases optimism and reduces depression by helping people realize that they can enjoy their lives and have successes.

Activities designed to accomplish treatment goals are particularly valuable. For example, the person who is overwhelmed by a recent job loss can benefit from preparing a realistic schedule of activities to find another job. The schedule should list the activities, when they will be performed, and how much time will be spent on each task.

Exercise and other forms of physical activity also can be very helpful. Research has shown that physical exercise can reduce depression and increase the secretion of endorphins that improve feelings of well-being (Ratey & Hagerman, 2008).

AVERSION THERAPY Rewards rather than punishments or negative consequences are usually favored in therapy because they enhance self-esteem, optimism, and relationships. However, sometimes linking undesirable behaviors with negative experiences motivates change. Readers should bear in mind that aversion therapy is a risky intervention. Care must be exercised when planning and implementing aversion therapy to be sure it does not have a negative emotional or physical impact and is respectful of people's rights and choices. Done poorly, aversion therapy can cause people to leave therapy prematurely, to feel exploited and traumatized, and to develop even more severe symptoms.

Antabuse, an emetic used to discourage people from consuming alcohol, is an example of aversion therapy. Time-outs, used to modify children's behavior, are another form of aversion therapy, although their primary purpose is to give a child an opportunity to calm down and reflect.

Visual imagery sometimes entails aversion therapy. For example, a woman who wants to stop smoking might imagine herself having severe difficulty breathing or coping with a smoking-related disease. A young man who is contemplating suicide so that his girlfriend will feel guilty about ending their relationship may change his mind after imagining himself lying in his grave while she goes on to have a full and rewarding life.

Satiation—giving people excessive exposure to a negative stimulus or behavior—is a type of aversion therapy. For example, the woman who wants to stop smoking might smoke a large number of cigarettes in rapid succession until she feels ill.

BEHAVIORAL REHEARSAL This strategy gives people an opportunity to practice a challenging task. The rehearsal might involve a role-play with the clinician or a practice session with a friend. Tape-recording the rehearsal or observing oneself in the mirror while practicing the desired behavior offers opportunities for feedback and improvement.

Behavioral rehearsal can be used for a wide variety of experiences. Making or refusing requests and sharing positive and negative feelings with others lend themselves particularly well to behavioral rehearsal. Behavioral rehearsal also can help people improve their social skills—for example, by practicing ways to initiate and maintain conversations or invite other people to join them in social activities.

BIOFEEDBACK Biofeedback involves the use of instruments that monitor bodily functions such as heart rate, sweat gland activity, skin temperature, and pulse rate and give people feedback on those functions via a tone or light. Biofeedback can promote reductions in tension and anxiety and increased relaxation. It also can have physical and medical benefits such as lowering blood pressure and improving pain control. It has been used to treat brain injuries, sleep disorders, ADHD, and depression (Myers & Young, 2012). Neurofeedback, a subset of biofeedback, allows people to monitor and regulate brain wave patterns and change behavior as a result.

CONTRACTING Establishing a clear agreement between client and clinician about the goals of treatment and the roles of both participants is an important component of CBT and behavior therapy. Contracting is usually done early in the treatment process. However, each time a new problem area is targeted for change, client and clinician can expand their contract to include additional objectives and procedures. This provides direction and motivation and can increase client cooperation with the treatment process.

DIAPHRAGMATIC BREATHING Taking slow, deep breaths and focusing on breathing can be calming and even induce sleep. This sort of breathing supplies the body with more oxygen, focuses concentration, and has been associated with increased self-control and mindfulness. Abdominal, or diaphragmatic, breathing is particularly helpful; people breathe in through the nose, expanding the diaphragm, and then expel the air through the mouth.

EXPOSURE Research has found that repeated contact with a feared or avoided stimulus will result in adaptation. In other words, the more exposure one has to a fearful object (for example, a snake, tarantula, or tall building), the less fear one will experience. In contrast, avoidance of the feared object serves to reinforce the fear and actually increases the resulting anxiety. More will be said about exposure-based therapies later in this chapter.

EXPRESSIVE AND CREATIVE ACTIVITIES Although art therapy, dance therapy, and music therapy are professions in their own right, clinicians with other areas of specialization sometimes incorporate these and other forms of creative self-expression into their work. This can enable people to become more aware of and give form to their emotions. Expressive techniques can be particularly successful with people who have difficulty verbalizing their feelings and concerns or who may feel stuck or blocked. These approaches can be freeing and empowering and are useful with both adults and children. Of course, they should be used cautiously by clinicians who do not have specialized training in therapeutic use of the arts.

EXTINCTION Extinction involves withdrawing the payoff of an undesirable behavior in hopes of reducing or eliminating it. For example, parents who give their children extra attention whenever they misbehave may be inadvertently reinforcing the undesirable behavior. Coaching the parents to pay attention to positive behavior and ignore misbehavior as much as possible is likely to reduce negative behavior.

FLOODING Flooding, like aversion therapy, is a high-risk intervention that must be used with caution, and only by clinicians who are well versed in the appropriate use of this strategy. In flooding, people are exposed to high doses of a feared stimulus in the expectation that this will desensitize them to the feared stimulus. An example is putting a person with a fear of balloons in a room full of balloons. The person must remain in the feared situation long enough for the fear to peak and then diminish. If the person leaves the situation prematurely, the fear may worsen and the person may learn to fear those who staged the flooding. In addition, the fear may lead the person to act in unsafe ways.

Some people believe that pushing a child into a swimming pool is a way to cure a fear of water. This misguided belief can endanger the child's life, create a traumatic experience, and impair the child's trust in others. Flooding should rarely be used, and then only after the client is fully informed about the procedure and consents to the procedure.

MODELING Modeling can be an adjunct to treatments such as assertiveness training; relationship training; social skills for children, adolescents, or adults; or any other situations in which people would like to improve their performance. People are most likely to be influenced by models who are similar to them in terms of gender, age, race, and beliefs; perceived as attractive and admirable in realistic ways; and viewed as competent and warm (Bandura, 1969). Five types of modeling are available:

1. Clinicians can serve as models, demonstrating target behaviors including social skills training or negotiation skills.
2. Clients can observe others engaged in behaviors or activities that they would like to emulate, such as public speaking, conversing at social gatherings, or offering suggestions at a meeting with their clients.
3. Covert or imaginal modeling involves the therapist describing a situation for the client to visualize. An example of covert modeling would be asking a 14-year-old boy to imagine saying "no" to a friend who was trying to get him to drink a beer.
4. Symbolic modeling via movies or books is a common approach to teaching children and young adults appropriate behavior. Bill Cosby's (2009) *Little Bill* young readers series helps children overcome their fears of going to bed, visiting the dentist, and playing with others.
5. Self-modeling is also an option. Clients can serve as their own models by making audio or video recordings of themselves engaged in positive and desired behaviors (Bandura, 1969).

REASONABLE (NATURAL) CONSEQUENCES Reasonable consequences are the logical, and usually unpleasant, outcomes of undesirable behavior. For example, the child who does not pick up her toys before dinner is required to clean her room after dinner instead of watching her favorite television program. Getting fired for repeatedly coming to work late is another example of such a consequence. Although reasonable consequences can be viewed as punishment, they are preferable to arbitrary and contrived punishments because they have a logical connection to the undesirable behavior and give people a strong message about the implications of their behavior.

REINFORCEMENTS Reinforcements and rewards encourage behavior change, enhance learning, and solidify gains. Reinforcements should be carefully selected and planned; they should be meaningful and worthwhile to the person so that they are motivating and should be realistic and reasonable. For example, giving a child a video game for cleaning his room once is not realistic, but setting aside $3 toward the purchase of a video game each week the child cleans his room 5 out of 7 days probably is.

Adults can create their own reinforcement plans. One woman who had difficulty paying bills on time set aside 1 hour twice a week for organizing her finances. Each time she completed the hour of financial planning, she rewarded herself by going to the bookstore to buy a new mystery and spending the rest of the evening reading her book.

Rewards need not be material. Social reinforcement, such as parental approval, a positive rating at work, and admiration from friends, can be at least as powerful. In addition, clients can reward themselves through positive affirmations and reminders of their success such as the declining balance on their credit bill and their improved grades. Reinforcements usually are most powerful if they are provided shortly after the success and are clearly linked to the accomplishment. Such reinforcers are particularly likely to solidify the desired change in behavior and contribute to either further change or maintenance of goal achievement.

RELAXATION Relaxation is often combined with other techniques such as systematic desensitization, abdominal breathing, hypnosis, and visual imagery. Teaching relaxation strategies in a treatment session and encouraging practice between sessions can facilitate people's efforts to reduce stress and anxiety and make behavioral changes. Several well-established relaxation strategies are available, including progressive muscle relaxation (sequentially tensing and relaxing each muscle group in the body); a body scan (each part of the body is systematically assessed and relaxed); and simple exercises such as head rolls, shoulder shrugs, and shaking one's body until it feels loose and relaxed.

SHAPING This technique is used to effect a gradual change in behaviors. People make successive approximations of desired behaviors, eventually leading to new patterns of behavior. For example, the following steps might help people with social anxiety improve their interactions with others:

- Spend 5 to 10 minutes at a social gathering. Do not initiate any conversations.
- Spend 5 to 10 minutes at a social gathering and greet at least two people.
- Spend 15 to 20 minutes at a social gathering, greet at least two people, introduce yourself to at least one person, and ask a question of one other person.
- Follow the previous step and, in addition, have a brief conversation about the weather and compliment the host on the food.

SKILL TRAINING An important component of promoting positive change is teaching people the skills they need to effect that change. Clinicians can teach clients both general skills (e.g., assertiveness training, decision making, problem solving, communication skills) and those serving the needs of a particular person (e.g., interviewing, anger management). Parents often benefit from learning to use behavior change strategies with their children. Bibliotherapy, or relevant readings, can supplement clinicians' efforts to teach new skills. Many books are available, for example, on assertiveness, time management, parenting, and other positive behaviors.

TOKEN ECONOMIES Particularly useful in group settings such as schools, day treatment programs, hospitals, prisons, and even families, token economies are an effective and efficient way to change a broad range of behaviors in a group of people. Behavioral rules or guidelines first must be established and then understood and learned by all participants. These guidelines are generally written out and posted to maintain awareness. Then a system of rapidly identifying and recording each person's performance of the desired behaviors is developed. Staff members in a group home, for example, might place stars or marks on a chart or distribute a poker chip as soon as possible after a desired behavior is emitted.

Finally, a system of rewards is developed. The rewards should be clear, realistic, and meaningful to the participants and be given in ways that are fair and consistent. In a typical token economy, the stars, points, or poker chips are used like trading stamps to earn privileges. For example, 2 points might be exchanged for television time or a telephone call, 5 points might merit a trip to the movies, and 15 points might be exchanged for a new CD. Opportunities should be provided for frequent redemption of rewards to provide reinforcement. In addition, social reinforcement (praise, appropriate physical affection) should be paired with the material rewards to develop intrinsic motivation and internalization of the desired behaviors. Generalization of the behaviors outside of the therapeutic setting promotes their establishment.

Current Developments

Today, clinicians practicing behavior therapy recognize that problems must be viewed in context. Clinicians explore the historical roots and antecedents of people's concerns, are sensitive to individual differences, develop positive and collaborative therapeutic alliances, and seek to know and understand their clients as individuals. Clinicians help to empower clients so that they can not only deal with immediate presenting concerns but also develop skills and strategies they can use in the future to lead healthier and more rewarding lives.

Some clinicians at first dismissed behavior therapy strategies, viewing them as superficial and likely to worsen or shift symptoms from one problem area to another (symptom substitution). However, extensive research has dispelled these concerns. The positive outcomes of behavior therapy tend to be enduring. Rather than leading to symptom substitution, these approaches often lead to a generalization of positive change in which people spontaneously apply the skills they have learned to many areas of concern.

Behavior therapy has made important contributions to counseling and psychotherapy. Behavior therapy has emphasized the importance of research on treatment effectiveness. The emphasis on goal setting, accountability, and outcome is very much in keeping with the requirements of managed care for treatment plans and progress reports, as well as clients' demands for efficient and effective treatment, Behavior therapy has also provided a foundation for the development of numerous other approaches—for example, reality therapy (discussed in Chapter 17) and multimodal therapy (discussed in Chapter 19).

The overriding goal of behavior therapy is to help clients become more flexible and sensitive in their reactions to the changes in their environment and to establish tools that are effective for the individual's needs (Antony & Roemer, 2011). We look now at the process of goal setting, an important part of treatment with behavior therapy.

GOAL SETTING IN BEHAVIOR THERAPY

Developing a Plan to Change Behavior

Once behavior therapists believe they have obtained enough information to have at least a basic understanding of their clients and to put their concerns in context, clinicians and clients collaborate to develop a plan, generally characterized by the following eight steps:

1. Describe the problem behavior.
    - Review the nature of the problem and its history.
    - Explore the context of the target (unwanted) behaviors.
2. Establish a baseline, reflecting the current frequency, duration, and severity of the target behaviors.

3. Determine goals.
   - Make sure that goals are realistic, clear, specific, and measurable.
   - Make sure that goals are meaningful to the client.
   - State goals positively. "Arrive at work on time at least twice this week" is a more appealing goal than "Avoid being late to work at least twice this week."
4. Develop strategies to facilitate change.
   - Change precipitating conditions that trigger undesirable behaviors.
   - Teach skills and provide information that contribute to the desired change.
   - Review and enhance impulse-control strategies.
   - Use additional strategies such as modeling, rehearsal, and systematic desensitization to facilitate positive change.
   - Formulate appropriate reinforcement contingencies and, if indicated, meaningful consequences.
   - Carefully plan implementation of the change process as well as ways to monitor and record the outcomes of that process.
   - Client and clinician make a written contract; clinician encourages the client to share the commitment to change with others.
5. Implement the plan.
6. Assess progress and evaluate the success of the plan.
   - Monitor and review the results of the implementation.
   - Emphasize successes.
   - Identify and address any obstacles to change.
   - If necessary, revise the plan.
7. Reinforce successes to promote empowerment and continue progressing and making positive changes.
8. Continue the process by making plans to promote maintenance of gains and prevent relapse.

PLANNING AND IMPLEMENTING BEHAVIOR CHANGE

We have looked at the steps involved in helping people change behaviors. These steps can, of course, be adapted to meet the needs of a particular person or problem. We review these steps here, illustrating them with the example of Izaak, whose supervisor reprimanded him for getting to work late. By learning and reviewing these steps, readers can both incorporate them into their work and apply them to themselves. These steps facilitate change in a variety of undesirable behaviors, including overeating, substance misuse, poor time management, unsatisfactory performance at work or school, inappropriate expressions of anger, children's misbehavior, insufficient exercise, smoking, unwanted personal habits such as nail biting, and deficiencies in social skills.

Step 1: Describing the Behavior

The first step in changing actions is describing the target behavior in specific and measurable terms. Both the undesirable behavior and the desirable change should be specified.

Izaak's presenting concern was arriving late to work. First the undesirable behavior was explored in detail. Izaak worked full time and had a wife and three children. His days were full and demanding. Because he had little time to unwind, Izaak would stay up until about 2:00 A.M. watching television so that he could have some time to himself. In the morning, he was tired and had difficulty rising early enough to help his wife get the children ready for school. As a result, mornings were usually very hectic. The children sometimes missed the school bus, requiring Izaak to drive them to school. Even when the children caught the bus, Izaak was usually at least 30 minutes late to work. Obtaining a full description of the undesirable behaviors made it clear that Izaak's lateness was a complicated situation with many contributing factors.

Izaak excused his lateness by explaining that he often worked through his lunch hour and stayed late at work. However, he recognized that his job description stated his working hours as 9:00 A.M. to 5:30 P.M. and that he was not adhering to those hours. The desirable change he sought was clear: arriving at work on time on a regular basis. Izaak also hoped to better manage the needs of his family while having more time for himself.

Step 2: Establishing a Baseline

Once the problem behaviors have been clearly described, a baseline can be obtained, reflecting the severity and frequency of the behaviors at the inception of treatment. To determine the baseline, client and clinician must agree on the following:

- ***Ways to measure the behavior.*** The two most common dimensions for measuring behavior are *frequency* (e.g., how many glasses of wine a person drinks daily, how many times in 1 hour a child got out of her seat at school, how many times a week a man yelled at his wife) and *severity* (e.g., how late the homework assignment was, how much damage was caused by the nail biting, how much clutter resulted from a person's hoarding behavior). Describing the behavior in clear and specific terms facilitates its measurement. For example, the problem of a messy house is difficult to assess unless it is described as including a floor piled with clothes, six boxes that remain unpacked, and a mildewed shower.
- ***Ways to record the measurement.*** People in treatment generally keep a record of their behaviors. They can use a checklist, a diary, or another written record of desirable and undesirable behaviors. Izaak used his date book to record his schedule for 5 days. He listed the times when the alarm went off, when he got out of bed, when he arrived at work, when he left work, and when he went to bed. For each day, he also wrote a brief description of what he did between rising and arriving at work.

In his next session, Izaak reviewed his records with the clinician. Izaak set his alarm for 6:00 A.M. each morning, but he rarely arose before 6:30. He was 30 to 45 minutes late to work each day—twice because he had to drive his children to school, once because he was delayed by his daughter who had misplaced her homework, once because the dog required attention, and once because Izaak slept until 7:00 A.M. He left work between 6:00 and 6:30 P.M. Four out of five nights he watched television until nearly 2:00 A.M.

Step 3: Determining Goals

Goals should be meaningful, clear, specific, measurable, and achievable. They should be logical outgrowths of the baseline information. Both clinician and client should understand and have a record of the goals, and both should agree that the client could accomplish the goals without extreme difficulty. Success in reaching goals is reinforcing and it encourages people to tackle more challenging goals, but failure to achieve goals can be discouraging, leading people to doubt themselves and their abilities. Consequently, goals should be designed to facilitate accomplishment rather than frustration.

Although Izaak was eager to make changes so that he could get to work on time each day, the complexity of the problem as well as its severity, as reflected by the baseline, suggested that goals should be approached gradually and incrementally. Izaak established an initial goal of getting to work by 9:00 A.M. at least once during the next week and getting to bed by 1:00 A.M. at least three times during the week.

Step 4: Developing Strategies

The next step in the process of changing behavior is identifying strategies to help people achieve their goals. The most effective interventions are those that help people to understand their problem behavior, develop skills specific to their needs, control impulsivity, and reinforce efforts made. Clinicians should consider several categories of strategies when helping people move toward their goals.

SKILL DEVELOPMENT AND EDUCATION People often need to develop new skills and learn new information to help them change problem behaviors. These might include assertiveness and communication skills, parenting skills, time management, decision making, and others.

IMPULSE CONTROL Problems with impulse control are often a key element in undesirable behaviors. Izaak, for example, described himself as "addicted to late-night television" and had difficulty curtailing that behavior. Teaching people impulse-control strategies such as relaxation, distraction, and avoidance of triggers can facilitate change.

REINFORCEMENT Rewards can motivate people to achieve their goals, help them take pride in their accomplishments, and encourage them to take on more challenging goals. Rewards can be *social,* such as encouragement and compliments from friends and family; *intrinsic,* such as the good feelings and improved health benefits a person experiences after losing weight or giving up smoking; or *extrinsic,* such as going out to dinner to celebrate purchasing a desired object. Extrinsic rewards can most easily be planned and controlled; they are most likely to be motivating if they are identified in advance and made contingent on the person's performance. As with goal setting, plans should be formulated so that the person is likely to receive a reward.

Reinforcements can be delivered regularly (each time the desired behavior is emitted) or intermittently. Lundin (1977) described four schedules of reinforcement:

1. *Fixed-interval reinforcement* occurs on a regular schedule, such as a weekly paycheck or quarterly report card.
2. *Variable-interval reinforcement* occurs at irregular intervals that average out to a specified time. For example, a pet receives five treats in 75 minutes or an average of one every 15 minutes, but the intervals between the treats vary from 5 to 30 minutes.
3. *Fixed-ratio reinforcements* are provided at a specified rate that depends on the number of responses made. People working on an assembly line may be paid for the number of parts they put together rather than for the hours they work.
4. *Variable-ratio reinforcements* usually seem random and unpredictable to the recipient, although they are controlled or planned by the provider. Winning at slot machines is an example. Variable-ratio reinforcements are powerful in encouraging responses because each response holds the promise of a reward.

Although penalties or punishments are sometimes used instead of rewards to shape behavior, rewards are generally more effective. They make the process of change a positive and empowering experience and promote motivation. In addition, if other people are dispensing the consequences, those people are likely to be perceived positively if they are giving rewards but viewed negatively if they are providing punishments.

However, punishments can provide a powerful and immediate message and do have a place in behavior change. Arrest of people guilty of domestic abuse, for example, can break through their denial, leading them to enter treatment and make positive changes.

Reasonable (or natural) consequences (discussed earlier in this chapter) avoid some of the potentially harmful consequences of other types of punishment but still give a strong message. Reasonable consequences are designed to grow logically out of an undesirable behavior; for example, a boy who neglects his homework is required to keep a notebook in which his teachers write down daily homework assignments for parent follow-up. The girl who uses six towels each time she bathes is made responsible for doing the laundry.

PLANNING Planning is almost always an essential element of behavioral change. Planning enables people to specify exactly how and when they will modify their behaviors and can help them anticipate and overcome obstacles to their efforts.

COMMITMENT Clinicians should help their clients invest themselves in the process of change and give it their best effort. Making a commitment to change, as well as a public declaration of the intent to change, encourages people to follow through on their plans. Their resolve can be further solidified through a written contract with the clinician and by talking about their goals and plans with friends or family members who can give them support and encouragement. Having a partner in a behavior change program, perhaps a friend who also wants to stop smoking or exercise regularly, can be reinforcing.

IZAAK'S STRATEGIES Izaak and his counselor identified the following helpful strategies:

1. ***Skill development.*** Izaak had little knowledge of time management. Before he began his program of change, his counselor reviewed principles of time management with him and suggested a book he might read on the subject. Izaak also received information on the cumulative effects of inadequate sleep so that he could realize the part that fatigue played in his difficulties.
2. ***Impulse control.*** Izaak needed help in controlling his impulse to watch television. He reported that he typically drowsed in front of the television and lost track of time. He decided to set a timer to go off at 12:30 A.M., reminding him that it was time to shut off the television and get ready for bed.
3. ***Planning.*** Planning was important in helping Izaak change his behavior. Izaak determined that he needed to rise by 6:15 A.M. to get to work on time. He set two alarms, one next to the bed for 6:00 A.M. and one across the room for 6:15 A.M. This allowed him a few welcome minutes to gradually awaken but made it likely that he would get out of bed at 6:15 A.M. to shut off the second alarm.

   Although some of the morning crises at Izaak's house were unavoidable, some could be averted by careful planning. Izaak and his wife agreed that, before their children went to bed, they would organize their clothes, books, homework, and lunch money to streamline the morning routine. The two older children were asked to assume responsibility for setting the table and putting out the breakfast food.

   To help Izaak shift some of his relaxation time to an earlier hour, he and his wife agreed that they would alternate taking responsibility for the children each evening. While one person was in charge of baths and homework, the other had an hour of quiet time to relax, read, or watch television.
4. ***Reinforcement.*** Izaak expected to receive some automatic reinforcement for his behavioral change. He anticipated getting better evaluations from his supervisor, feeling more relaxed, and having a less harried home environment. In addition, Izaak decided that, once during each

week in which he achieved his goals, he and his wife would hire a sitter so they could go out to dinner. This extrinsic reinforcer enhanced Izaak's sense of relaxation and positive feelings about his family.

5. ***Commitment.*** Izaak and his counselor wrote up a contract, including goals and strategies. Izaak shared this with his wife and asked her to help with his change efforts.

Step 5: Implementing Interventions

Once goals have been established and strategies determined, the plans for behavior change are implemented. People should keep a record of their progress as they did when determining the baseline of their undesirable behaviors. They also should make notes about anything that facilitates or hinders the implementation.

Izaak found that he did well with the parts of his plan that were under his control, but had difficulty persuading his children to help out in the morning and prepare for school the night before. He planned to ask the counselor for some help with this situation.

Step 6: Assessing Functioning

At regular intervals, clients and clinician monitor progress to maintain and reinforce successes and address difficulties in the plan. Prolonged experiences of failure should be avoided. When discussing the outcome of clients' behavior change plans, clinicians should be encouraging and optimistic but not judgmental, critical, or blaming. People often do not fully achieve their goals. This should be viewed as an opportunity for learning and for refining the plan rather than as a failure. Rather than focusing on excuses and disappointments, clinicians should help clients congratulate themselves on their efforts and any successes they had.

The initial assessment of Izaak's efforts indicated that Izaak got to work on time two days out of five and was less than 30 minutes late on other days. He arose by 6:15 A.M. every day and went to bed by 1:00 A.M. on four out of five nights; he felt that he could get to bed even earlier in the future without much difficulty. Izaak had enjoyed the hour of quiet time in the evening, even though he and his wife implemented that change on only two evenings. The children made progress in organizing themselves but were reluctant to accept new responsibilities.

Step 7: Reinforcing Gains

Assuming rewards have been built into the change plan and some success has been achieved, people can now reward themselves. Clinicians also can cautiously provide some social reinforcement, congratulating clients on their efforts and helping them to take pride in their accomplishments. However, clinicians should place more emphasis on encouraging clients to praise themselves. Clinicians who make positive as well as negative judgments of their clients risk imposing their values on clients and can detract from clients' self-direction and self-esteem.

Izaak experienced both intrinsic and extrinsic rewards for his efforts. He felt proud of his success and also felt less fatigued. In addition, his wife had complimented him for reducing some of the morning chaos. Izaak hired a sitter and made dinner reservations so he and his wife could celebrate his success.

Step 8: Continuing the Process

This last stage of a behavioral change plan takes one of three directions:

1. If the plan had some shortcomings and clients did not reach their goals, client and clinician consider what revisions in goals and strategies are likely to lead to greater success.

Considerable attention may be paid to the strengths and weaknesses of the original plan to determine how it needs to be improved.

2. If the plan was successful but the client has additional goals or wants to build on the accomplishments of the initial plan, client and clinician agree on new objectives and develop strategies to facilitate their accomplishment.
3. If clients are satisfied with their accomplishments, they work with their clinicians to solidify those gains and prevent relapse. Strategies such as involvement in a peer support group, ongoing self-monitoring, stress management, and periodic follow-up sessions are common elements in a relapse-prevention plan.

Izaak thought he had made a good start toward accomplishing his goals, but recognized that he had only begun to make a significant change in his behavior. He and his counselor developed additional goals and strategies to help him continue his efforts. In addition, the counselor suggested strategies Izaak could use to facilitate change in his children's behavior such as modeling, using praise and reinforcement, letting them choose their chores from a list, and reframing their new responsibilities as reflecting their maturity.

We turn now to the second generation of behavior therapy, which began with the integration of cognitive and behavior therapy, paying particular attention to cognitive–behavior modification and stress inoculation training developed by Donald Meichenbaum.

THE DEVELOPMENT OF COGNITIVE–BEHAVIORAL THERAPY

CBT evolved from cognitive therapy through incorporation of components of behavior therapy (Parker, Roy, & Eyers, 2003). Descriptions of CBT emphasize cognitions over behaviors, but do integrate guidelines and strategies for the two approaches in a synergistic way. With the creation of the discipline of affective neuroscience, Hofmann (2012) writes "a biological framework" is now available "to explain why CBT strategies are effective for regulating emotions—and how to further improve them" (p. 11).

Cognitive–behavioral therapy is not one specific approach, but a term applied to a coherent model that is open to and integrates new empirical findings about a pathological disorder into a new model of treatment for that disorder (Hofmann, 2012). As a result, CBT combines myriad treatments and techniques that all share a common principle that thoughts, rather than external circumstances, cause feelings and behaviors. CBT is a brief and time-limited approach that recognizes the importance of a sound and collaborative therapeutic alliance. CBT is structured and directive, relying heavily on the cognitive tools of psychoeducation, Socratic questioning, and the inductive method. These strategies are not intended to tell people how to think, act, or feel, but rather to help them test their hypotheses and think, act, and feel in ways that are helpful to them and consistent with reality. As in behavioral therapy, homework is an essential ingredient of CBT, and is used to help people make progress between sessions and apply what they have learned.

Donald Meichenbaum

Donald Meichenbaum, a founder of cognitive–behavioral therapy, is distinguished professor emeritus at the University of Waterloo, Ontario, Canada. Meichenbaum was raised in New York City before moving to the Midwest to get his PhD, and then to the University of Waterloo where he worked for more than 30 years. Since his retirement in 1998, he has spent winters in Miami, Florida, where he is research director of the Melissa Institute—a think tank for preventing violence in schools. Meichenbaum has been named one of the 10 most influential psychotherapists of the century. He has written numerous books and articles, including *Stress Inoculation Training* (1985). His book *Cognitive–Behavior Modification* (1977) is considered a classic in the field. He continues to lecture, write and present on topics from spirituality in psychology to post-traumatic stress disorder (PTSD), the educational potential of children, and inner dialogue.

During his doctoral dissertation research, Meichenbaum (1969) began to notice that people with schizophrenia who were taught healthy self-talk responded better on a variety of other measures and were less distracted. This led him to conduct additional research on the role of cognitive factors in behavior modification (1974, 1977). Influenced by Vygotsky (1967) and the recognition that behavioral control comes about first through external regulation (by parents or significant others) and later through self-regulation (via internalized self-instruction), Meichenbaum created a self-instructional training (SIT) program for impulsive children (Dobson & Dozois, 2010). His method of self-instruction teaches a person to respond with positive self-talk in the face of stressors or negative thinking.

Meichenbaum's theory combines cognitive strategies designed to modify maladaptive self-talk with knowledge of the developmental manner in which children learn by modeling behavior. In using SIT with a child with emotion dysregulation, for example, the clinician would model appropriate language such as "It's okay. I don't have to get upset. I will take some deep breaths and everything will be okay." After repeating the self-instruction several times, the child might be given a cue card to help remember or a tape recording of the session to take home, listen to, and practice between sessions. In self-instruction training, internal dialogue is monitored and changed to include coping statements that help the client when faced with stressors.

SIT is a self-management tool that provides a way for people to overcome negative self-talk, encourage themselves with more positive words, and teach themselves how to effectively cope in situations that had previously been difficult for them. In general, the therapist models behavior and the client practices the behavior by repeating it back. SIT can be used with all ages, and for many behaviors (anger, overeating, substance use) as well as specific disorders (depression, anxiety, phobia).

Cognitive–Behavior Modification

Probably the best-known treatment approach that is considered a form of CBT is Meichenbaum's cognitive–behavior modification. That approach is discussed here to illustrate CBT.

Meichenbaum (1993) developed cognitive–behavior modification (CBM) in an effort to integrate psychodynamic and cognitive treatment systems with the "technology of behavior therapists" (p. 202). He believed that no one of these treatment systems alone was sufficient to explain psychopathology and promote behavior change but that the combination could accomplish both goals.

Three assumptions of CBM clarify how Meichenbaum (1993) integrates cognitive and behavior theory:

1. ***Constructive narrative.*** People actively construct their own reality; "reality is a product of personal meanings" (p. 203).
2. ***Information processing.*** An activating event taps into a person's core cognitions, leading to an unhelpful, inaccurate, and distorted thought. People experience negative emotions and engage in unwise and harmful behaviors because they distort reality as a result of cognitive errors and misperceptions.
3. ***Conditioning.*** Cognitions are viewed as covert behaviors that have been conditioned. Correspondingly, they can be deconditioned and modified through both external and internal contingencies (rewards or negative consequences), thereby strengthening new and healthier cognitions. Modeling, mental rehearsal, and other strategies are important in effecting cognitive change.

According to Meichenbaum (1993), the role of the therapist is that of co-constructivist: helping people alter their stories and cognitions so they can build "new assumptive worlds" (p. 203). To accomplish this, treatment via CBM entails the use of cognitive interventions, such as Socratic dialogue (questions designed to promote clearer perceptions and thoughts) and reframing (changing terminology in an effort to change perceptions).

To illustrate these strategies, let's consider Telly, who believed that, following an argument, his daughter was enraged with him because she had not returned his telephone calls. The clinician might ask the following Socratic questions, of course pausing for responses between questions: "What leads you to assume that her silence reflects rage? Is she prone to react with rage? Is it possible that she is hurt or needs time to sort out her reactions to the argument? How can you determine what she is really feeling?" Using reframing, the clinician might refer to the daughter's decision to "take a break" or "take some time to cool off," rather than using Telly's language that describes her as "ending their relationship."

Although clinicians practicing CBM draw on a broad range of treatment strategies, they generally believe that treatment should be demystified and techniques de-emphasized. Learning and self-help are encouraged, and feedback from the client is welcomed. Clients become active, knowledgeable, and responsible partners in their own treatment.

Cognitive–Behavioral Strategies and Interventions

Cognitive–behavioral therapists draw from both behavioral and cognitive strategies to create new treatment approaches specific to the client's needs. As the evolution of cognitive–behavioral models suggests, there are a large number of different CBT approaches and techniques that can all be blended into "a family of approaches" (Hofmann, Sawyer, & Fang, 2010). We will not duplicate the behavioral strategies listed earlier in this chapter, but instead cover only those that have not yet been discussed. All of the techniques include the core element of cognitive restructuring as developed by Ellis and Beck. In addition, what follows is a brief discussion of other techniques or strategies that can be incorporated into treatment based on empirical evidence of their effectiveness. (See Hofmann, 2012, for a complete list of empirically supported treatments for specific disorders.)

STRESS INOCULATION TRAINING Meichenbaum developed one of the earliest, most useful, and most effective cognitive–behavioral treatment procedures: stress inoculation training. People typically experience stress because of a perception that their life circumstances exceed their capacity to cope, or to effectively use "behavioral and cognitive efforts to master, reduce, or tolerate the internal and/or external demands that are created by stressful transactions" (p. 3). Stress inoculation training is an approach to reduce stress. It assumes that if people can successfully cope with relatively mild stressors, they will be able to tolerate and successfully cope with more severe ones. In other words, as its name implies, stress inoculation training seeks to immunize people against the adverse impact of stress by helping them successfully handle increasing levels of stress. Treatment usually consists of 12 to 15 weekly sessions plus additional follow-up sessions over 6 to 12 months.

Stress inoculation training has three phases (Meichenbaum, 1985):

1. ***Conceptualization.*** Clients and clinicians develop a collaborative relationship. People are taught about stress; the relationship between stress and coping; and the roles that thoughts, actions, and emotions play in engendering and maintaining stress. Once people have an understanding of stress and the factors that promote it, their stressful thoughts and experiences (as well as the antecedents and consequences of those thoughts and experiences) are explored. Particular attention is paid to stress-inducing and stress-reducing self-statements

and self-talk. Initial goals of treatment include translating stress into specific fears and problems that are amenable to solution and helping people achieve some control over their lives.

2. ***Skills acquisition and rehearsal phase.*** Treatment during this phase teaches people to cope effectively with mild stressors by gathering information, using coping self-statements, learning relaxation strategies, changing their behaviors, or using other strategies to reduce those fears. In addition, people learn to apply problem solving to their fears according to the following five steps:
   - Problem identification
   - Goal selection, focusing on small manageable units of stress
   - Development of alternatives
   - Evaluation of each possible solution and its probable consequences
   - Decision making and rehearsal of coping strategies.
3. ***Application and follow-through.*** In phase 3, people implement their plans to solve problems and reduce stress. Increasingly distressing stressors are tackled as people become able to modify their dysfunctional thoughts, effectively use coping skills, and apply what they learned in phase 2. For example, a person might initially use self-talk to address a minor stressor such as being kept waiting for an appointment, and gradually work up to addressing major stressors such as a verbally abusive partner. Stress inoculation uses a subjective units of distress scale (SUDS) to help clients rate their stressors in hierarchical order. Before treatment begins, the client is asked to assign a number from 0 to 100 that accurately represents the distress he or she experiences in a given situation. Following treatment, the client is asked to reevaluate his or her stress level. The SUDS rating is used to represent the impact of stressors and then later to track clients' progress in coping with them.

Treatment includes continuous reinforcement and assessment of people's efforts and accomplishments. Strategies such as coping imagery and cognitive rehearsal are used to solidify gains, generalize learning to more significant fears, and help people to prevent or cope with relapses. Learning ways to reduce their fears, along with increased confidence from initial successes in managing stress, facilitates people's efforts to address other fears and problems successfully. Taking one step at a time and building on successes can make challenging situations manageable and foster self-esteem and more desirable cognitions and behaviors. In addition, encouraging people to have a sense of responsibility for their futures rather than their pasts during this phase of treatment can be very empowering.

BEHAVIORAL ACTIVATION THERAPY This mode of therapy involves increasing activity on a daily basis to help motivate people with depression who may experience low energy and may have withdrawn from life to such an extent that they are not capable of participating in cognitive therapy, do not have enough energy to recognize or discuss cognitive distortions, or cannot seem to overcome what may be keeping them stuck in their depression. Behavior activation therapy (BAT) is compatible with most cognitive and behavioral treatment strategies.

BAT is usually started at the beginning of treatment for depression, to help people increase their activity levels, improve their mood, and provide a source of pleasure on which they can build. By scheduling pleasant activities throughout the day, and creating regular times for sleep and meals, clients can keep track of their initial activity levels and chart their progress.

The most frequently used strategies in behavior activation therapy include establishing a list of pleasant activities; scheduling, monitoring, and charting activities; relaxation and skills training; recognizing aversive and avoidant behaviors; and confronting cognitive distortions. Sources of positive reinforcement seem to work best if they are pleasant, stable, repeatable, and diverse (Curran, Ekers, McMillan, & Houghton, 2012; Kanter, Busch, & Rusch, 2009).

Behavior activation has been around since Skinner first created behavior modification and has recently been expanded into a stand-alone treatment program that is easily administered, is generally well received by clients, and its efficacy is similar to that of cognitive therapies (Hayes, Strosahl, & Wilson, 2012). Dimidjian and colleagues (2006) found that BAT was comparable to medication and cognitive therapy in the treatment of all types of depression.

HABIT REVERSAL TRAINING Habit reversal training (HRT) uses reinforcement and other behavior techniques to help people recognize tics before they happen, monitor their own behavior during stressful situations, use relaxation techniques, and perform alternative behaviors that are incompatible with the behavior they are trying to extinguish, such as tics, trichotillomania, skin scratching, and skin picking (Adams, Adams, & Miltenberger, 2008; Veale & Neziroglu, 2010). HRT has been shown to be effective in reducing tics (Deckersbach, Rauch, Buhlmann, & Wilhem, 2006) and sometimes results in a reduction in the need for medication as well. Self-monitoring, behavioral techniques, relaxation training, and other adjunctive techniques are helpful.

EXPOSURE Exposure is one of the most important components of cognitive or cognitive–behavioral therapy for anxiety disorders. Through the use of exposure, the person learns to identify his or her fear responses; recognize maladaptive cognitions; confront or "sit with" the uncomfortable feelings without avoiding, running away, or otherwise modifying the experience; and achieve a certain amount of self-efficacy or control over the feelings of distress. As a result the person learns new methods of coping and handling emotions, rather than giving in to the fear (Bandura, 1977).

Flooding, graduated exposure, and systematic desensitization are all elements of exposure-based therapies. Most exposure-based treatments also include a cognitive component, usually cognitive restructuring, to help increase the client's positive coping statements, and reduce thought distortions, self-blame, and anxiety.

Pacing is another important consideration in exposure-based treatments. Some treatments are designed to take place within one session. *Flooding* or implosion, for example, usually provides intensive exposure over 30 minutes to 8 hours. Because of the intense emotions, flooding can be overwhelming and is not appropriate for use in the treatment of phobias in which it might be dangerous, such as phobias of driving over bridges or on highways.

Graduated exposure involves having the person confront the fear for a short period of time, and then gradually increasing the length of exposure with each session. An example of graduated exposure for an elevator phobia would involve taking the elevator to more floors with each successive treatment session.

Systematic desensitization, as created by Wolpe and discussed in Chapter 15, is a powerful strategy that is useful in reducing fears, phobias, obsessions, compulsions, and anxiety. Initial fears are generally worsened when the person avoids the feared stimulus and the avoidance is reinforced by the relief that follows. Systematic desensitization is designed to reverse this process by gradually exposing a person to the disturbing stimulus in ways that reduce rather than increase fear.

Treatment with systematic desensitization generally begins with one or two sessions of relaxation techniques, followed by the creation of an anxiety hierarchy. The least frightening presentation of the feared object (a picture of a spider, for example) is shown as the client conducts relaxation techniques. As clients becomes more comfortable with the spider picture, they might be shown a picture of multiple spiders, gradually moving up their hierarchy to watching a video of spiders, watching a spider in a terrarium, and eventually handling a spider. Systematic desensitization can be conducted in the imagination (imaginal), *in vivo* (in context), or a combination of both.

A third type of exposure, interoceptive exposure, is a structured treatment approach that encourages people to experience feared bodily sensations (such as shortness of breath or heart flutters) in the safe environment of a therapy session without engaging in avoidance or escape strategies. Treatment continues until adaptation occurs and the feelings are no longer frightening. An example of interoceptive exposure is spinning in a chair to achieve dizziness. Interoceptive exposure is used most frequently in the treatment of panic disorder (Forsyth, Fuse, & Acheson, 2009).

Virtual reality therapy uses technology to provide another delivery method for exposure-based treatments. By creating a human/computer interaction that imitates *in vivo exposure,* virtual reality can be particularly helpful for anxiety disorders including social anxiety, phobias, OCD, PTSD, and the fear of public speaking (Powers & Emmelkamp, 2008; Wallach, Safir, & Bar-Zvi, 2009). Interactions can be via video or 3D technology, and may include use of a joystick, glove, or similar device to provide interactive feedback between the person and the computer. A distinct advantage of virtual reality over other approaches is the ability to be able to adjust the level of stimuli the person receives.

One example of the use of virtual reality paired 33 people with height phobia with virtual 3D graphics designed to simulate the feeling of taking an elevator and performing tasks on a scaffold outside a 15-story building. In another study, a virtual environment was created that led 31 people with snake phobia to believe the environment was filled with dangerous hidden snakes. In both cases, use of virtual reality was shown to be as effective as other types of exposure-based therapies that did not use virtual reality (Klinger et al., 2005). Sensitivity and judgment must be used when incorporating virtual reality into treatment plans, and the technique should never be used as a substitute for therapy (Rothbaum, 2005).

Other elements that add to the effectiveness of exposure-based treatments include behavioral strategies such as relaxation training, deep-breathing instruction, paradoxical intention, rehearsal, hypnosis, role-playing, and modeling. Exposure-based therapies have been shown to be effective for a wide range of anxiety disorders including specific phobias (such as animals, thunderstorms, public speaking, and flying), PTSD and trauma, panic, and claustrophobia. They can also be adapted for use with children to help them overcome a fear of the dark or other frightening situations (Seligman & Reichenberg, 2012).

There are many different types of exposure-based therapies and they can be individualized for each client's needs. The Skill Development section at the end of this chapter provides a more detailed look at exposure-based therapy.

EYE MOVEMENT DESENSITIZATION AND REPROCESSING Eye movement desensitization and reprocessing (EMDR) is a form of exposure therapy that combines bilateral stimulation (eye movements, alternating sounds, and tapping), behavioral desensitization, and cognitive restructuring in a structured eight-phase process. EMDR was discovered in 1987 by Francine Shapiro (2001), a senior research fellow at the Mental Research Institute in Palo Alto, California. EMDR originally focused on people who had had traumatic experiences, including rape, molestation, and war experiences, by helping them to reduce negative images and emotions related to those images and modify self-destructive cognitions. To date, more than 50,000 clinicians have been trained to administer EMDR, which is an empirically supported treatment for trauma (Benish, Imel, & Wampold, 2008; Chambless et al., 1998) by the American Psychological Association, the American Psychiatric Association (2004), and the Department of Veterans Affairs (2004). EMDR also shows promise in the treatment of anxiety and mood disorders, specific phobias, eating, and conduct disorders (Davidson & Parker, 2001; Gauvreau & Bouchard, 2008; Shapiro, 2005).

PROBLEM-SOLVING THERAPY Originally developed by D'Zurilla and Goldfried (1971), problem-solving therapy (PST) provides a positive intervention that focuses on the acquisition of constructive problem-solving skills to address increased stress, relationship conflict, anxiety, mood disorders, and a variety of other issues that arise in daily life (Nezu, Nezu, & D'Zurilla, 2010). PST consists of a four-step process: (1) identifying the problem, (2) brainstorming alternatives, (3) conducting a cost/benefit analysis of possible solutions, and (4) monitoring and evaluating outcomes. Through the use of PST, clients reduce impulsive decisions, minimize conflict, and decrease the use of maladaptive coping skills such as avoidance, passivity, or emotion dysregulation. Visualization can be used to help clients imagine achieving the goal successfully.

Nezu and colleagues (2010) recommend a reverse-advocacy role-play in which the clinician espouses a problem and the client provides reasons why the clinician's thinking is maladaptive, illogical, unreasonable, or negative. During the alternative finding phase, they brainstorm as many different solutions as possible. Successful application of problem-solving skills increases self-efficacy, helps clients to visualize successful outcomes, and results in the development of new skills that can be transferred to other areas of their lives. PST has been used successfully for relational problem solving, compliance with behavior change (for clients with diabetes, obesity, substance abuse), with physical illness (recurrent headaches, cancer, pain), and with increased stress due to caregiving (D'Zurilla & Nezu, 2007, 2010). PST may also be useful as a preventive intervention for reducing excess stress, adolescent/parent conflict, and the spread of HIV (Nezu et al., 2010).

THE THIRD GENERATION OF BEHAVIOR THERAPY

The third generation refers to the introduction of acceptance-based therapies such as dialectical behavior therapy, acceptance and commitment therapy, and mindfulness into the cognitive–behavioral tradition (Dobson & Dozois, 2010; Herbert & Forman, 2011).

These approaches to behavioral therapy combine experiential and mindfulness techniques with cognitive and behavioral approaches. Mindfulness-based interventions have become extremely popular, with nearly 300 scholarly articles published about the topic in 2009 alone (Crane, Kuyken, Hastings, Rothwell, & Williams, 2010). The empirical success of mindfulness-based interventions has resulted in their integration into treatment for all sorts of medical and psychiatric conditions including pain management, heart conditions, head injury, and nearly all behavioral disorders (Crane et al., 2010).

These approaches share important traits with other CBT approaches; specifically, their ultimate goal is to change behavior (Dobson & Dozois, 2010). Most of these approaches incorporate similar actions: acceptance of what is happening, nonjudgment of thoughts, and present-moment awareness. As readers will learn, the following approaches—dialectical behavior therapy, acceptance and commitment therapy, and mindfulness-based cognitive therapy—are very different from the traditional CBT treatments discussed so far.

Dialectical Behavior Therapy

Marcia Linehan (1993) and her colleagues developed dialectical behavior therapy (DBT), a form of behavior therapy, primarily to treat people with borderline personality disorder who were chronically suicidal. They found that clients treated with DBT were less likely to drop out of treatment and had fewer hospitalizations and better overall treatment outcomes. Based on its initial success, DBT has since been adapted for use with couples, children, and adolescents and as a tool for anyone needing help with emotion regulation.

THE DEVELOPMENT OF DBT Since its initial development, the dialectical perspective and DBT techniques have been applied to other disorders including substance use disorders, impulse control disorders, anxiety and mood disorders, and other personality disorders (Marra, 2005). DBT is appropriate for any clients who experience intense emotions, especially those who attempt to escape from such emotions through dissociation, distraction, and participation in harmful behaviors such as substance use, cutting, eating disorders, and other impulse control disorders.

DBT THEORIES AND STRATEGIES DBT is based on a dialectical philosophy, a biopsychosocial view of disorders, and the integration of behavioral therapy with the Eastern beliefs and attitudes of mindfulness, acceptance, and compassion. The goal of DBT is to develop dialectical thinking and practice skills that result in emotion regulation, reduce suffering, and improve relationships.

Dialectics. The philosophy of dialectics is a way of looking at reality. As we have seen in Chapter 11 in the discussion of narrative and constructivist approaches, within every person's story there is "an alternative story (a dialectic pole). A person who tells us how she has failed in life can tell a success story, too" (Almagor, 2011, p. 33).

According to Almagor (2011), the use of dialectics helps clients to

1. Develop a broader perspective on their problem
2. Learn to look for the dialectic pole
3. Consider more options as a result
4. Get unstuck and develop competence.

For example, a common dialectic between married couples revolves around the use of free time. Frequently, one person wants to spend more time with their partner, while the other is comfortable with the current situation. The issue is one of independence and dependence. When couples begin to realize the dialectic pole between the two ideals, they begin to understand the other person's perspective. "Erin is at work all day, and just wants to relax when she comes home" or "Even though I sometimes feel pressured, it's really a *good* thing that he wants to spend more time with me."

When the couple can consider the problem from a different angle, more creative and egalitarian solutions become available to them. In dialectics, the clinician helps the client to see the dialectic pole inherent in the problem, consider all of the options, and then make a choice that leads toward change.

Worldview. An underlying assumption in DBT is that clients are experiencing a dialectical conflict between themselves and their environment. From a dialectical perspective, everyone is right. All behavior is functional. DBT therapists work hard to understand the worldview of the client, to validate their feelings, and then to help them consider alternative possibilities.

Biopsychosocial view. Borderline personality disorder is considered to have both biological and environmental causes (Linehan, McDavid, Brown, Sayrs, & Gallop, 2008). Emotion dysregulation may be the result of attachment wounds, traumatic experiences, loss, the competition between wants and needs, or genetic or other causes (Marra, 2005). DBT assumes that "emotions themselves (their intensity, duration, and perceived nonspecific manifestation) are the primary causative factor in psychopathology" (Marra, 2005, p. 7). The emotions precede the development of thoughts. Once these neural networks begin to fire, they continue as a result of a "kindling effect." Once a pattern has been established, similar events may set off "triggers" that result in repeated incidents of intense emotion, feelings of abandonment, or a need to take action to stop the unpleasant emotions.

Linehan believes borderline personality disorder results from the combination of emotional vulnerability and an invalidating environment. One of the ways in which DBT helps in this situation is to recognize that there is an assertion, and there is an opposite to that assertion. Helping the client to create a synthesis between the assertion and the argument can help them to see choices and possible resolutions to the problem. The client is helped to find solutions that are consistent with their goals. For example, a young woman named Ashura with four children repeatedly erupts in explosive rages aimed at her mother-in-law, who watches her children.

ASHURA: When my mother-in-law brought the kids back to my house late after the weekend, I was so angry with her that I told her off, slammed the door in her face, and locked it! That will teach her to bring them back late!

CLINICIAN: So, you really showed her. Maybe you should really show her and just keep the kids yourself, and not let them go with her if she's going to bring them back late.

ASHURA: No! I would never do that.

CLINICIAN: Why not?

ASHURA: Because the kids love going to her house. She plays with them and makes cookies. Sometimes she even makes them dinner. Plus, then I wouldn't have anyone to watch the kids while I work.

CLINICIAN: Those are all positive things. It sounds like you have a win–win situation. Is there any other way to get your needs met?

CLIENT: I could ask her to call me if she's going to be late. Or I could go to her house and pick them up myself.

This dialogue illustrates the inconsistencies between the client's behavior (yelling and slamming the door) and her goals (child care in a loving and safe environment so she can work) without confronting the client's behavior directly.

DBT helps clients to recognize how their attempts to deny, avoid, and escape strong emotions paradoxically make those emotions more intense. By helping clients to accept their feelings, providing tools for emotion recognition and regulation, and decreasing emotional avoidance (through psychoeducation and exposure), DBT empowers clients to increase their tolerance of distress and use coping skills such as meditation and mindfulness to regulate their emotions.

The use of DBT is guided by seven assumptions (Smith & Peck, 2004, pp. 30–31):

1. Clients are doing the best they can.
2. Clients want to improve.
3. Clients must learn their new behaviors in all relevant contexts.
4. Clients cannot fail in DBT; any effort is progress.
5. Clients may not have caused all of their problems, but they have to solve them anyway.
6. Clients need to do better, try harder, or be more motivated to change.
7. Clients' lives are currently unbearable as they are being lived.

DBT TREATMENT DBT is characterized by four stages:

1. Clinicians help people make a commitment to treatment and facilitate their attainment of basic competencies such as keeping themselves safe, reducing self-destructive behaviors (e.g., drug and alcohol use, unwise sexual activity, self-injury), and teaching relevant skills such as interpersonal effectiveness, self-care, and emotion regulation.
2. Desensitization and other strategies help people deal with traumatic experiences and the impact of past messages and events.
3. Self-respect, problems of living, and individual goals are the focus of this stage, as clients begin to look to the future and apply what they are learning.

4. The final stage promotes synthesis and generalization of gains; integration of past, present, and future; development of spirituality; acceptance of self and reality; increased self-respect; achievement of individual goals; better coping skills; and a greater capacity for happiness.

The role of the therapist is an important factor in the success of DBT, which considers the relationship between client and clinician to be reciprocal. Clients are changed; clinicians are changed too. Similarly, behaviors that interfere with therapy may spawn from either the client or the clinician (Swales, 2012). DBT is an active therapy, with clinicians participating in the dialectical process as well as providing psychoeducation, skills training, coaching, and group work.

Similar to the other approaches in this chapter, DBT incorporates mindfulness as well as considerable support for clients. Clients receive at least 1 year of 1-hour weekly individual therapy sessions and 2-hour weekly group therapy, emphasizing skill training and problem solving.

CURRENT STATUS Initial empirical research on DBT yielded positive results. People treated with at least 1 year of DBT achieved considerable reductions in suicidal ideation, hospitalization, anxiety, and anger and increases in occupational and social adjustment (Linehan & Kehrer, 1993). Subsequent research indicates DBT is also effective in reducing other nonsuicidal self-injurious behaviors (McMain et al., 2009). These and other studies indicated that common symptoms accompanying borderline personality disorder, including substance misuse and dysfunctional eating, were also alleviated.

DBT can be a demanding, and yet rewarding, treatment modality. Changes that take place as the result of a dialectic process have been shown to be long lasting (Conoley & Garber, 1985; Samai & Algamor, 2011).

Acceptance and Commitment Therapy

Acceptance and commitment therapy (ACT) has much in common with dialectical behavior therapy. Both are considered to be behavior therapies, both attend to cognitions, and both help clients learn that they do not have to act on their thoughts or emotions.

THE DEVELOPMENT OF ACT Stephen Hayes is the name most widely associated with the development of acceptance and commitment therapy. ACT shares common philosophical roots with constructivism, narrative, and feminist psychology. It is considered to be part of the third wave of behavioral and cognitive therapies that add an experiential element to the approach. Also in keeping with behavioral therapies, ACT is committed to empirical research, and a number of controlled studies have been published to document its effectiveness in the treatment of anxiety, depression, and chronic pain (Hayes et al., 2012; Morris & Oliver, 2012).

THEORIES AND STRATEGIES ACT is based on relational frame theory, a behavioral theory of human language and cognition that helps people recognize how they become entangled in thoughts and words and how those entanglements result in internal struggles against themselves. Hayes writes that "fusion with verbal content can lead to suffering" (Hayes et al., 2012 p. 243) so he recommends the use of defusion whenever a client becomes "mindy" or perseverating. Through the use of metaphor, paradox, and experiential exercises, clients learn how to break up fused thoughts and make healthy contact with their cognitions, feelings, memories, and physical sensations. Rather than challenging their thoughts, as in traditional cognitive therapy, clients gain the skills necessary to accept their thoughts, develop greater clarity about personal values, and commit to needed behavioral change.

The major goals of acceptance and commitment therapy are to help clients accept cognitions and emotions that are outside of their control and to encourage clients to make a commitment to creating a life that they value. Mindfulness practices, including present-moment awareness, staying centered in the body, and acceptance, are also employed. The acronym, ACT, captures the core concepts of acceptance and commitment therapy quite well:

A = Accept and embrace thoughts and feelings, especially difficult feelings such as anxiety or pain.

C = Choose a direction in life that reflects who the client truly is.

T = Take steps toward action.

In ACT, the therapeutic alliance is "strong, open, accepting, responsible, and loving" (Morris & Oliver, 2012, p. 71). It is also bidirectional, with clinicians impacting clients, but clients also impacting clinicians. The therapist is more experiential than cognitive, providing empathic encouragement and reassurance. ACT therapists are also respectful of cultural differences, honor diversity and community, and may be open to spirituality.

CURRENT STATUS ACT can be applied to a wide range of problems and disorders, with change strategies being tailored to meet the needs of the client. Acceptance and commitment therapy seems particularly well suited for the treatment of anxiety disorders. Phobias, PTSD, obsessive-compulsive disorder, panic, and other types of anxieties that are reinforced by avoidance tend to respond well to the experiential exercises of ACT such as externalization, exposure to the avoided feelings, and acceptance (Hayes et al., 2012). According to Hayes, acceptance is an alternative to avoidance. Acceptance is "voluntary, open and receptive," and it involves a willingness to interact with the feared object or feelings (p. 272). Hayes notes that acceptance can sometimes have a negative connotation as in giving up or defeat. But in the context of ACT, acceptance is a positive emotional response.

Randomized controlled studies have shown the effectiveness of ACT to treat depression, psychosis, heroin addiction, substance abuse, chronic pain, and borderline personality disorders (Morris & Oliver, 2012). Three meta-analytic reviews supporting ACT have now been published (Hayes, Luoma, Bond, Masuda, & Lillis, 2006; Ost, 2008; Powers, Zum Vorde Sive Vording, & Emmelkamp, 2009). This, combined with the publication of treatment manuals and practitioner's guides, has helped ACT wind its way into mainstream practice. Clearly, ACT is a promising new approach that adds an element of experiential theory to the traditional cognitive and behavioral milieu.

Mindfulness-Based Cognitive Therapy

Mindfulness-based cognitive therapy (MBCT) is an experiential cognitive therapy treatment approach that was originally created as a relapse-prevention treatment for depression, based on Jon Kabat-Zinn's (1982) mindfulness-based stress reduction (MBSR). MBCT, however, focuses on cognitive change while it incorporates mindfulness meditation practice.

THE DEVELOPMENT OF MBCT The success of MBSR in Massachusetts in the 1980s captured the attention of cognitive scientists in the United Kingdom and Canada—Zindel Segal, Mark Williams, and John Teasdale—who were conducting research on the cognitive vulnerability process that triggers and maintains depression (Crane, 2012). In conjunction with Kabat-Zinn, the trio developed a manualized version of MBCT that is closely aligned with MBSR but emphasizes cognitive processes as well. Two randomized controlled trials have since provided the evidence base to support MBCT's effectiveness (Ma & Teasdale, 2004; Teasdale et al., 2000).

MBCT THEORIES AND STRATEGIES New research indicates that MBCT is more effective than maintenance with antidepressant medication in the treatment of relapse in depression (Chase, 2012).

It has recently been found, through research using functional MRIs, that the mechanism by which mindfulness and acceptance strategies are effective is that of exposure and response prevention (Holzel et al., 2011). "Acceptance leads to change in situations of prior non-acceptance" and reduces the need to escape, avoid, or experience severe emotional reactivity to a triggering event. "As exposure operates arousal is reduced, and this change leads to further acceptance" (Fruzzetti & Erikson, 2008, p. 351).

An understanding of the mechanism by which depression is reactivated is one of the beneficial side effects of the development of MBCT. Human brains are hard-wired to react to threat, and once those neural pathways have been developed, they are more likely to be activated by another event that the brain perceives as threatening. MBCT reduces the threat by helping to break the cycle in which ruminative thoughts erupt in an effort to problem solve a given situation to be deemed unacceptable by the person. Through mindfulness meditation and the practice of acceptance, the aversive or avoidant feelings that keep the negative thoughts in the mind are eliminated (Hayes et al., 1999). A fallacy arises in the brain that instinctively wants to be "doing" something to solve the problem, return to equilibrium, and make the negative feelings go away, but Williams (2010) notes that the more a person tries to analyze, ruminate, and problem solve, the more he is triggering the very cycle from which the he is trying to escape. Thus, the wisdom of no escape (Chodron, 1991).

The alternative response to "doing" is "being," a paradigm shift that Crane and colleagues (2010) refer to as the "doing and being mode of mind." The doing mode, as previously mentioned, is what the brain does. It creates thoughts, whereas the being mode is in touch with direct experience, moment by moment, recognizing bodily sensations as they arise, without agendas or judgments, and letting go of thoughts. The result is an openness to new experience, rather than ruminating on how to achieve an objective or solve a problem. In mindfulness meditation whatever thoughts come up are okay, but the person does not have to follow that story line.

In an investigation into how mindfulness meditation works, Holzel and colleagues (2011) identified the following components of mindfulness meditation that create a process of self-regulation: (1) attention regulation, (2) body awareness, (3) emotion regulation, and (4) change in perspective of self.

MBCT TREATMENT Generally, MBCT is conducted in eight group sessions of 2 to 2.5 hours in length. One all-day session is included. Follow-up sessions may be scheduled randomly in the following year to reinforce practice. Group size is usually limited to 10 or 12 participants, and each person is interviewed in advance to determine their readiness for treatment. The treatment protocol is similar to the following (Crane, 2012):

Weeks 1–4 Developing skills, mindfulness meditation training, present-moment awareness, recognition of thoughts, emotions, bodily sensations, and behaviors

Weeks 5–8 Shift toward recognition of more challenging thoughts and feelings, working on acceptance

People who practice mindfulness meditation are expected to set aside a certain amount of time daily for practice. They learn to conduct a body scan, to pay attention to their breathing, how to meditate, and how to bring their mind back to the present moment when it wanders. Instruction on mindful movement and walking meditation are also taught as part of the repertoire of skills. Therapists who conduct mindfulness meditation classes also embody the spirit of mindfulness (Crane, 2012). This provides attendees with the opportunity to learn from someone who has shared the same experiences and struggled with the same problems. Dialogues in class are conducted from the position of fellow voyager.

Using mindfulness, people learn to stay in the moment using a decentering approach that reduces "black and white" either/or thinking and encourages an accepting attitude. As the person focuses on the breath, thoughts become like clouds floating through the client's mind, without judgment and without getting stuck. Hofmann and colleagues (2010) describe decentering as being similar to the process of distancing in CBT in which client's gain objectivity over thoughts. However, instead of changing troublesome thoughts, or avoiding them, a decentered attitude is one of accepting things exactly as they are, in the moment.

CURRENT STATUS Meditation has been shown to change the way in which the brain functions. It reduces emotions, improves rational decision making, and prevents relapse in depression by reducing or altering the brain's neural response to sad mood. This neural response can trigger a cascade of ruminative and avoidant behavior in people with a prior history of depression (Coelho, Canter, & Ernst, 2007; Farber & Metzger, 2009; Kirk, Downar, & Montague, 2011).

The practice of mindfulness has been found helpful for many other purposes and with a variety of people. Mindfulness is helpful in the prevention of relapse for drug and alcohol addiction, to reduce gambling, and in the treatment of children with ADHD and emotion dysregulation (Vallejo & Amaro, 2009). It may also have implications for couples counseling, suicide prevention, and as an adjunct to medication management in the treatment of bipolar disorder (Miklowitz, 2010; Williams et al., 2008).

Research is ongoing to differentiate between the various aspects of mindfulness to determine what exactly produces the changed effect. Aspects of mindfulness such as body scan, focus on breathing, acceptance of thoughts, and present-moment awareness, may be at work individually or may be found to work together to generate a synergistic effect (Vallejo & Amaro, 2009).

Mindfulness meditation can also be part of a spiritual practice or it can be part of behavioral or psychological practice. MBCT can be integrated with REBT or another treatment modality, or used as a stand-alone treatment.

Some authors (Harrington & Pickles, 2009) have questioned whether treatment approaches that include mindfulness should be classified as cognitive therapy, since the focus of mindfulness techniques varies from the cognitive goal of identifying and changing dysfunctional thoughts, to instead recognize and accept thoughts, and then let them pass without judgment or action.

TREATMENT USING COGNITIVE–BEHAVIORAL THERAPIES

Behavior therapy, CBT, and acceptance therapies make substantial use of specific strategies and interventions. Although these are important treatment ingredients, they should not overshadow the broad goals of treatment and the importance of the therapeutic alliance.

Goals

CBT encompasses goals similar to those of behavior therapy, but also entails additional goals related to modification of thoughts. These might include enabling people to recognize, assess, and modify their dysfunctional cognitions; changing persistent underlying cognitions such as "I must be perfect" and "I am unlovable"; and helping people make positive changes in their self-talk and sense of empowerment.

In CBT, cognitive goals and behavioral goals are usually complementary and often intertwined. For example, Megan has been unable to locate employment because of a combination of her self-defeating thoughts (e.g., I can't do anything right; no one would want to hire me) and impairment in her skills (e.g., writing a resume, presenting herself well in an interview, initiating conversations, time management). Although Megan's primary goal is to locate rewarding employment, many small goals along the way would focus on changing both thoughts and behaviors to help her achieve that goal.

Therapeutic Alliance

Behavior and cognitive–behavioral therapists believe that establishment of a positive and collaborative therapeutic alliance is essential. Clinicians practicing CBT assume many roles: teacher, consultant, adviser, devil's advocate, supporter, role model, encourager, and facilitator. Active listening, understanding, caring, respect, and concern are all part of the therapist's repertoire as is helping clients to understand and make use of the principles of CBT. Although therapists encourage and reinforce positive change, they also value genuineness and professionalism. Clinicians practicing CBT are cautious about giving advice and praise. They want clients to take credit for their positive changes rather than attribute them to the therapists.

Clients are expected to participate fully in the process of behavior or cognitive–behavioral therapy and take responsibility for presenting their concerns, identifying their goals, and implementing plans for change. Clinicians typically encourage clients to try out new behaviors, complete tasks between sessions, self-monitor, and provide feedback to the clinicians.

APPLICATION AND CURRENT USE OF COGNITIVE–BEHAVIORAL THERAPIES

The family of cognitive–behavioral therapies has a broad range of applications. Used either alone or in combination with other treatment systems, their principles and strategies can be applied in almost any treatment setting and with almost any client or problem.

Application to Diagnostic Groups

Many empirical studies support the use of behavior therapy with the most prevalent mental disorders. These include mood disorders, anxiety disorders, some personality disorders, eating disorders, and substance use disorders. In addition, behavior therapy can relieve both emotional and physical symptoms associated with medical conditions.

MOOD DISORDERS Especially when combined with cognitive therapy, behavioral therapy has demonstrated strong effectiveness in the treatment of mood disorders (Seligman & Reichenberg, 2012). Cognitive interventions can modify dysfunctional thoughts that maintain depression, hopelessness, and low self-esteem. Similarly, behavior change strategies such as activity scheduling and systematic decision making can reduce the severity of depression, counteract the inertia and confusion often associated with depression, and promote feelings of mastery and competence. The use of MBCT to prevent relapse of major depressive disorder has been well documented in the literature. The collaborative nature of this approach, as well as its clear rationale and its use of structure and achievable goals, also enhances its effect in treating depression.

ANXIETY DISORDERS CBT is also effective in treating many types of anxiety disorders. People diagnosed with social phobias often benefit from training in social skills involving instruction in assertiveness and communication, modeling, role-playing, and practice. Reduction in the level of self-criticism via CBT also can enhance treatment of people with social phobias. Substitution of positive activities for negative ones and distraction can help people cope with obsessive-compulsive disorder (OCD). Aversion therapy, satiation, and flooding, used with great care, also can be useful in the treatment of OCD.

Trauma-based concerns, including acute stress disorder and PTSD, also respond well to CBT (Hofmann, 2012). Strategies such as education about PTSD, cognitive restructuring, breathing retraining, imaginal desensitization, and confrontation of feared situations have been shown to give people a greater sense of control and alleviate symptoms.

OTHER MENTAL DISORDERS Cognitive–behavioral therapies also have demonstrated effectiveness with many other mental disorders and health problems. Token economies and reasonable consequences have been used successfully to treat children and adolescents diagnosed with conduct disorders. Relaxation, activity scheduling, and time management all can be helpful to people with attention-deficit disorders. Behavior therapy has demonstrated effectiveness in helping people diagnosed with mental retardation, impulse-control disorders, sexual dysfunctions, sleep disorders, and paraphilias (Hofmann, 2012). Behavior therapy plays a major role in the treatment of eating disorders, including bulimia nervosa and anorexia nervosa (Pike, Walsh, Vitousek, Wilson, & Bauer, 2003), as well as disorders that involve unhealthy use of drugs or alcohol (Hofmann, 2012). Research also supports the use of CBT in the treatment of people with sexual dysfunctions or assaultive behavior (Lanza et al., 2002).

Application to Multicultural Groups

Behavior therapy and CBT have wide appeal and are easily integrated into treatment with people from a variety of backgrounds and situations. These approaches are easily understood and logical, respect individual differences, and offer a large repertoire of interventions to address almost any concern. Behavior therapy and CBT encourage people to play an active and informed role in their treatment, promote learning and competence, and can produce rapid and positive results that are reinforcing

Hays (2009) defines evidence-based practices in psychology as a combination of best available research and clinical expertise in the context of client characteristics, culture, and preferences. As we have seen, CBT has become the most widely researched evidence-based psychotherapy, and the most widely practiced treatment modality among clinicians. In her work, Hays provides 10 suggestions for integrating multicultural considerations into CBT, beginning with a complete assessment of the needs of the person and his or her family. Culturally competent counselors recognize clients' culturally related personal strengths including pride in abilities, culture, and language; interpersonal supports, including extended families and religion; and environmental supports. Verifying if a client's presenting problem is primarily cognitive (internal) or environmental (external) and validating any reported experiences of bias or oppression are also components of culturally competent practice (Hays, 2009).

Hays also emphasizes the importance of culturally respectful behavior. Given that rapport appears to be the main focus of research on building relationships among European Americans, the concept of respect tends to be more highly valued among Asian, Native American, African, African American, Latin, and Middle Eastern cultures, especially with relationships involving authority figures. For a complete discussion, interested readers are referred to "Evidence-Based Practice, Cognitive–Behavior Therapy, and Multicultural Therapy: Ten Steps for Culturally Competent Practice" (Hays, 2009).

CBT, along with medication, has been found to reduce depression in low-income young African American and Latina women. Treatment was enhanced when combined with encouragement, intensive outreach, and direct services such as child care and transportation (Miranda et al., 2003). CBT may be well suited to Latino clients given its transparency, its consistency with the culture's traditional directness, and its problem-solving approach (Organista, 2007). A study of Mexican American women with binge eating disorder emphasized the importance for counselors not to assume that even though many Latinas are collectivist and enjoy a lot of support from their community, food and body image go along with cultural expectations influenced by the same community (Shea et al., 2012).

Current Use

The use of behavior therapy and CBT extends far beyond treatment of individuals with mental disorders. Relaxation, hypnosis, and visual imagery have been used in behavioral medicine to reduce pain and help people cope with cancer, heart disease, and other chronic and life-threatening illnesses. Schools and correctional institutions, as well as day treatment and inpatient treatment programs, rely heavily on behavior therapy to teach and establish positive behaviors.

In addition, behavior therapy and CBT can be used in family and group counseling, as well as individual therapy. The reinforcement and modeling provided by the other group members make the group setting especially well suited for CBT. Cognitive–behavioral group counseling enables people to learn and experiment with new behaviors, while receiving information and feedback from multiple sources. Hearing other people's thoughts also can help people to broaden their perspectives, identify and modify their own dysfunctional thoughts, and reinforce their valid and reasonable thoughts and feelings.

Parents can benefit from learning behavior change strategies and using those to shape their children's behavior. Such common parental interventions as time-out, rewards, consequences, and limit-setting reflect behavior therapy. Meditation, mindfulness, and DBT have also been adapted for use with children and adolescents, especially in the area of emotion regulation.

Most of us use behavior change strategies in our everyday lives. When we reward ourselves with a snack after finishing a difficult chore, give a chronically late friend a message by deciding not to wait more than 15 minutes, or embark on a plan to improve our diet and exercise, we are using behavior change strategies. These approaches have been around for decades, and have a great deal to offer. They are also easily integrated with a broad range of other approaches, including psychodynamic therapy, Gestalt therapy, and person-centered counseling. Such combinations can deepen the impact of treatment and ensure that resulting changes are meaningful and enduring.

EVALUATION OF COGNITIVE–BEHAVIORAL THERAPY

More than any other treatment approach, extensive research has been conducted on CBT. The literature suggests that treatment focused on cognitions and behavior can be very powerful and effective. Of course, it also has limitations.

Limitations

Despite, or perhaps because of, the evidence-based approach of CBT, most of the criticisms of this approach focus on the following:

1. The possibility exists that treatment will accomplish only superficial and temporary gains.
2. Emotions and insight may not receive the attention they merit in treatment.
3. Clinicians may home in too quickly on behaviors, without sufficiently exploring their underlying antecedents and dynamics. For example, a clinician may emphasize development of social skills in a woman who is fearful of dating and neglect her history of abuse.

In addition, clinicians may become so caught up in the need to follow protocol for evidence-based practice that they fail to address changes occurring in real time. As a result, people may feel manipulated and powerless rather than experience the growth in self-worth and competence that should result from treatment.

Comorbidity also causes difficulty for evidence-based approaches. Most people do not fit neatly into one category of diagnosis, but overlap, as in mixed anxiety and depression, or people dually diagnosed with substance use disorders and another Axis I or II disorder (Emmelkamp,

Ehring, & Powers, 2010). Clearly treatment manuals that focus on one diagnosis or the other will not do justice to the totality of the problem.

Treatment limited to CBT is not the ideal approach for all clients. Indeed, as many as 30% to 40% of people treated with current CBT treatments are not successfully helped, and this figure has not improved in the past 25 years (Emmelkamp, 2004; Emmelkamp et al., 2010).

While an initial focus on cognitions and behavior might promote change and enhance motivation, people with long-standing and deep-seated problems will probably need other approaches or medication combined with CBT. This combination can help clients develop insight and allow them to work through past concerns, while also helping them make cognitive and behavioral changes. In addition, although CBT can help people with psychotic and other severe disorders, medication and other interventions also are needed. Behavior therapy and CBT are useful with almost all clients but often need to be combined with other treatment modalities to maximize their effectiveness.

Some concern has also been raised over the spiritual aspects of mindfulness-based treatments, and concern has also been expressed about the opposite, efforts to remove traditional Eastern spirituality from mindfulness practice (Fruzzetti & Erikson, 2010). Mindfulness-based cognitive therapy is not considered to be religion based, but rather a tool for staying present in the moment.

Strengths and Contributions

Cognitive–behavioral therapies offer a choice of empirically supported treatments, they lend themselves to the development of guidelines that can be followed by other mental health professions based on what works, and they offer a straightforward approach to treatment that has both face and empirical validity. These approaches emphasize goal setting, accountability, and results. They are respectful and collaborative, encouraging people to take responsibility for themselves. Although improved behaviors and thinking are the targets, treatment also seeks to improve emotional health. Emmelkamp and colleagues (2010) add that manualized treatments are also easy to disseminate and transport to community and academic settings for training.

SKILL DEVELOPMENT: EXPOSURE-BASED CBT FOR HOARDING

Cognitive–behavioral therapy is one of the most powerful interventions in the treatment of anxiety disorders. It is particularly effective in the treatment of OCD, phobias, and excessive fears of certain situations such as socializing, flying, and public speaking. It also is useful in addressing other apprehensions and anxieties. For example, it can help to reduce stress and anxiety in people who have a difficult time parting with objects or throwing things away, even when failure to do so results in clutter to such an extent that it ultimately results in the inability to use a room for its intended purpose. For example, the kitchen becomes so cluttered the homeowner cannot cook in it anymore; or boxes and papers are piled so high in the bedroom that the door cannot be opened. Symptoms of this level of clinical significance occur in 2% to 5% of the population (Mueller, Mitchell, Crosby, Glaesmer, & de Zwaan, 2009). Strong negative emotions (feelings of loss, grief, or depression) may occur when a person thinks about giving away some of their possessions. Conversely, positive emotions are likely to result when acquiring and saving items. As a result, the person begins a cycle of behavior in which cleaning or sorting clutter makes them feel bad, so they avoid those negative feelings that accompany their thoughts, and instead seek to shop or acquire more to make themselves feel better.

Recent research indicates that excessive acquisition and difficulty discarding items to the extent that results in hoarding may stem from information processing deficits, problematic beliefs and behaviors, and emotional distress and avoidance (Steketee, Frost, Tolin, Rasmussen, & Brown, 2010). Treatment, therefore, must address the faulty cognitions. Steketee and colleagues recommend a combined CBT approach that uses habituation (exposure to the avoided situation to reduce anxiety), direct exposure to sorting, and cognitive strategies to challenge errors in thinking and beliefs that contribute to hoarding behavior.

Relaxation and fear are incompatible responses; as a result, fear of a stimulus typically diminishes if relaxation can be achieved and maintained during exposure to that stimulus. However, this treatment can have a reverse effect if not well planned; premature, or too intense, exposure (in this case to overwhelming and uncomfortable feelings of letting go of objects) can result in the client quitting treatment or refusing to participate. Consequently, careful pacing is essential to successful treatment using exposure-based therapies.

As mentioned earlier, exposure to the frightening stimulus may occur in the imagination (imaginal desensitization) or the real world (*in vivo* desensitization). One is not clearly more effective than the other. The choice of whether to use imaginal desensitization, *in vivo* desensitization, or a combination of the two is determined primarily by the nature of the feared stimulus and the ease of creating a situation of controlled exposure to that stimulus. In the case of hoarding, a therapist can work with a client on location, or in the office with the use of guided imagery, to help the client re-create the distressful feelings that occur when they attempt to dispose of objects. As the action is moved forward, the client is asked to describe and rate his or her feelings or thoughts on a hierarchy of discomfort every 5 to 10 minutes. A simple 0-to-10 scale can be used to rate feelings of anxiety or discomfort.

After one or more sessions have been spent on developing the therapeutic alliance, exploring the antecedents and symptoms of the fear, and discussing the person's history and present life situation so that the symptoms can be viewed in context, exposure-based therapy typically follows a series of steps. These steps are illustrated by the case of Judy, a 48-year-old woman who could not part with things and as a result has developed a hoarding problem that prevents her from inviting people over to her house because of the shame and embarrassment she feels. It is also, beginning to cause tensions at home with her husband.

1. ***Teach an effective relaxation strategy.*** Judy was taught to relax by shifting her breathing to a pattern of slow diaphragmatic breaths while focusing on her breathing. She also was taught to relax her body progressively, by gradually moving her attention down from her head to her toes until her entire body felt relaxed.
2. ***Help the client identify cognitive distortions that reinforce the hoarding behaviors.*** *Cognitive restructuring* is an important element of treatment for hoarding. Following several sessions with Judy, her therapist was able to identify the following distortions underpinning Judy's hoarding behavior:
   - ***All-or-nothing thinking:*** "If I give the blender away, even though I haven't used it in years, I won't be able to make margaritas." (even though Judy never invites anyone to her house)
   - ***Moral reasoning:*** This type of reasoning is seen in "should" statements: "I should be able to clean up this room. What is wrong with me?"
   - ***Emotional reasoning:*** "I can't give away that vase. It was a wedding present from my Aunt Jayne."
   - ***Discounting the positive:*** "Even if I clean off the bed so I can sleep in it, the rest of the room is still a mess."

Steketee (2011) noted that thoughts that lead to hoarding behavior are different for everyone. What is difficult for one person may be easy for another. When working with people who cannot get rid of clutter, some of the most difficult feelings arise surrounding perfectionism ("I can't do it perfectly, so why even bother?"), money ("It might be valuable some day"), or personal identity. One woman could not throw out boxes of shells, feathers, and other detritus she and her daughter had collected on trips to the beach over the years, even though her daughter was now in graduate school.

The next step in cognitive restructuring is for the therapist to help Judy create a list of statements to refute her beliefs, such as:

- "I'm giving away the clothes that don't fit. If I lose weight, I'll treat myself and buy some new ones!"
- "I can do this. I will feel the anxiety, and do it anyway."

3. ***Establish an anxiety hierarchy.*** Judy was asked to create a list of anxiety-provoking stimuli ranked according to the amount of anxiety or fear each elicits. A 0-to-100 SUDS scale could be used, or in this case, the therapist simply asked Judy to rate her anxiety on a scale of 1 to 10, with 10 being the strongest negative emotion. Judy decided that a 10 rating would be the overwhelming process of cleaning out the storage unit she rents. She experiences near panic whenever she thinks about it. Judy gave a rating of 5 to going through her clothes closet and donating items to charity. A much easier task, rated a 1 on Judy's hierarchy scale, is sorting through the mail that had piled up and throwing out unnecessary items.
4. ***Provide controlled exposure.*** Judy's counselor used *in vivo* desensitization and went on location to Judy's house for the first few sessions to help her confront her avoidance. The more a person avoids something associated with negative feelings, the more the feelings are reinforced. Multiple types of avoidance responses have been identified in association with hoarding behavior—not having people over to the house because of the clutter, for example, or starting to sort through a box of clutter, feeling anxious, then becoming overwhelmed and quitting. Strong negative feelings trigger the urge to avoid the feelings, and set the stage for the development of anxiety problems.

After helping Judy relax as fully as possible, the counselor asked Judy to complete the least stressful task on her list—sort through the box of mail that had accumulated. Judy went through the mail without too much anxiety until she came upon some birthday cards from friends that she could not bring herself to throw away. The counselor encouraged Judy to hold the cards and think about the people who had sent them. After a few minutes, Judy relaxed and smiled. She was able to think of the people without needing to hold on to the cards. The therapist suggested Judy take a picture of her cards with her iPhone so she could look at them again whenever she wanted to. But Judy decided she was still having problems throwing the cards away.

Using Socratic questioning and the downward arrow technique to ask deeper levels of questions can help the therapist to get the client to see the absurdity of his or her thinking (Steketee, 2011). If Judy had wanted to keep the birthday cards, the therapist might have asked:

THERAPIST: "Why are they so important to you?"

JUDY: "They were the only birthday cards I got this year."

THERAPIST: "What does that signify to you?"

JUDY: "These are my friends. They are the only people who love me."

THERAPIST: "What would happen if you threw the cards away?"

JUDY: "Well, they would still love me!"

After this discussion, she could let them go. In the next session, Judy was able to move to the next item on her list. The exposure and desensitization process must be carefully planned so that it does not raise anxiety but instead promotes feelings of self-confidence, optimism, and control.

Eventually, Judy learned to tolerate some discomfort and develop new skills for discarding items and experiencing the anxiety as it arises. As we have seen, combining cognitive methods with behavioral exposure is more effective than either technique alone for reducing hoarding behavior (Steketee et al., 2010).

During the next session at Judy's house, the therapist helped her create a three-pile sorting system in which she would sort items for trash or donation, items she wanted to keep, and those that she would box up and decide what to do with later. Helping clients to develop a list of guidelines beforehand helps the process run smoother and confronts avoidance. Judy decided to endorse the following: "I will donate clothing that isn't flattering" and "I will give away any books that I have two copies of."

Judy began to categorize, sort, remove, and repeat (Beck, 2011; Steketee, 2011). Her discomfort was then rated every 5 to 10 minutes, so the therapist could control the level of exposure to ensure Judy would not become overwhelmed and quit. Habituation helped Judy recognize the anxious feelings, but continue sorting and cleaning anyway, recognizing that although her anxiety and emotional thinking made her uncomfortable, those feelings would not hurt her.

After Judy had successfully decluttered an area, the therapist helped her to create a new set of rules related to acquisition, so that the problem would not occur again. Acquisition rules might include "I won't buy any more books unless I pay cash" or "Even if it's on sale, I won't buy anything that won't be used in the next thirty days."

Continuing the desensitization between sessions, with the help of a friend or a family member who has been coached by the clinician, is one option that can also accelerate progress, as long as the person is never exposed to more than she had successfully handled in her counseling sessions. In Judy's case, after multiple sessions on location, she was able to continue the process in the therapist's office. She took a picture of the closet she needed to clean and brought it in to the session. After five more sessions, she brought in another picture that showed the progress she had made.

Although Judy was able to deal with some of the items on her list, she continues to have intense feelings of being overwhelmed whenever she thinks about the storage unit. However, she has made much progress inside her house, enough so that she was able to celebrate her success by inviting friends over for dinner (and making margaritas!).

CASE ILLUSTRATION

As treatment of Edie, Roberto, and Ava Diaz progressed, the clinician realized that Edie's self-consciousness, her apprehensions about socialization, and her weak interpersonal skills had an impact not only on Edie but on the rest of the family. Because of her social discomfort, Edie avoided talking to Ava's teachers and the parents of Ava's friends and was reluctant to accompany Roberto to office parties or on business trips. Her avoidance of these and similar situations had relieved Edie of considerable stress and anxiety; however, negative reinforcement had occurred. The rewards she experienced from social avoidance had further entrenched this behavior, so that Edie's apprehension about and avoidance of interpersonal contact had worsened over the years.

Edie and her therapist decided to use Meichenbaum's (1985) stress inoculation training (SIT) to address her social difficulties. This approach integrates both cognitive and behavior change strategies. The process of using SIT with Edie had three phases:

1. ***Conceptualization:*** First, the clinician explained SIT to Edie, reviewing the interventions that would probably be used and describing how SIT was likely to help her. Once Edie's questions and concerns were discussed, she felt ready to cooperate with the process and was optimistic that it might alleviate her long-standing social discomfort.

Edie and her therapist then clarified the nature of the problem and established realistic goals. Edie believed that people generally found her unappealing and uninteresting. She feared that if she risked exposure to social situations, she would experience painful rejection and humiliation. Using the SUDS scale, the extent of Edie's fears was assessed. Specific goals were identified that focused on reducing her fears of rejection and humiliation in social situations and increasing her participation in social conversations and activities.

2. ***Skills acquisition and rehearsal:*** Several techniques were used to help Edie overcome her fears:
   - At work, where Edie felt competent and her professional role was clear, she experienced little social anxiety and interacted well with others. Edie identified communication skills that served her well in her role as librarian and identified ways to transfer them to other interpersonal arenas.
   - The therapist helped Edie dispute her belief that she would certainly be rejected and humiliated in social situations. This had not happened to her since adolescence, and she could report only two instances of ever having seen other people rejected and embarrassed in a social setting.
   - Edie further developed her social skills. Her therapist provided readings and exercises on assertiveness and communication and helped Edie to identify and practice skills that seemed useful to her. She and the therapist paid particular attention to role-playing ways to initiate and develop conversations.
   - Because she enjoyed reading, Edie sought out literature on shyness, as well as biographies of people who viewed themselves as having had social difficulties, so that she could learn more about ways to cope with her social discomfort.
   - Edie identified a coworker whose social skills she admired. She observed that person in order to identify her social strengths and use her as a role model. In addition, Edie tried to act as if she were that person when she role-played conversations in her treatment sessions.
3. ***Application and follow-through:*** Edie and her clinician generated some small steps for Edie to take in order to apply her developing social skills and increased self-confidence. Edie considered volunteering at Ava's school, accompanying Roberto on a business trip, and throwing a small party. Although she anticipated engaging in all of these activities eventually, she decided to begin by inviting the mother of one of Ava's friends to have tea with her after they dropped their daughters off at ballet class. Edie felt relatively safe with this woman and believed that meeting one person at a time with readily available topics of discussion (tea, the ballet class, their daughters) would provide a successful experience. A role-play of social conversation over tea helped Edie feel well prepared for this venture.

After the tea, Edie processed the experience with her therapist, focusing on what she did well and identifying a few ways in which she might have improved on the experience. For example, she had gotten flustered when it was time to pay the check and saw that she needed to develop more comfortable strategies for dealing with that. Edie rewarded herself for her efforts, as well as for her success, and began to plan the next steps to improve her social skills.

EXERCISES

Large-Group Exercises

1. Although the value of CBT has clearly been substantiated by research, some clinicians view it as less powerful than psychodynamic therapy. Discuss what thoughts and feelings might underlie this perception and then discuss your reactions to and perceptions of CBT.

2. Using your class as the target group, plan implementation of a token economy that might be useful in promoting learning in the class. Identify the behavioral goals, the system for tracking and recording performance, and the rewards for positive behavior.
3. Ava is troubled by fears of the dark and of being alone. Plan her treatment, using behavioral strategies. Be sure to view her presenting problems in the context of what you already know about Ava and her family. The treatment plan should include, but not necessarily be limited to, determining how to establish a baseline, setting specific goals, identifying treatment strategies, establishing rewards or reinforcements, and specifying ways to track progress. In addition, consider whether to integrate other approaches with the behavioral interventions.

Small-Group Exercises

1. Following the guidelines presented in Large-Group Exercise 3, plan treatment for the following behavioral difficulties:
   - A 4-year-old refuses to go to bed on time and delays his bedtime by several hours each evening with requests for stories, drinks of water, and other attention.
   - A 33-year-old man reports family conflict as a result of his nightly consumption of 8 to 10 cans of beer.
2. Divide into your groups of four, composed of two dyads. Each dyad should engage in a 15-minute role-played counseling interview in which the person playing the client talks about a behavior he or she would like to change while the person in the clinician role gathers information on the nature of the concern, its context, and its frequency or severity. If you have time, begin to identify realistic goals and procedures to effect behavioral change. Spend 10 minutes processing each role-play after it is completed, providing feedback to both client and clinician on strengths and areas needing improvement.
3. Divide into your groups of four. Using problem-solving therapy (PST), role-play a scenario of your own choice or the following: A family of four seeks therapy to help their 23-year-old son who has bipolar disorder and continues to smoke marijuana. Be sure to consider all four steps (defining the problem, generating alternatives, decision making, and monitoring the outcome). Be sure the therapist uses at least one reverse-advocacy role-play. Spend 10 minutes processing each role-play after it is completed.

Individual Exercises

1. Identify a fear or source of apprehension in your life. Following the guidelines presented in the Skill Development section of this chapter, develop a plan to use exposure therapy to help yourself reduce this fear. Write down the plan in your journal and then try to implement it.
2. Consider a behavior that you would like to increase, decrease, or change. Develop a written treatment plan to help yourself make that change. The treatment plan should include, but not necessarily be limited to, determining how to establish a baseline, setting specific goals, identifying treatment strategies, establishing rewards or reinforcements, and specifying ways to track progress. Continue your learning by actually implementing the plan you have developed. Write in your journal about the successes and challenges you experience as you try to implement this plan.
3. Mindfulness-based stress reduction often begins with a body scan to help focus breathing and present-moment awareness. When you are alone, stretch out into a comfortable position, and take several deep, cleansing breaths. Begin by focusing your attention on the toes of your right foot. Notice how your toes feel; they might be tingling, or you might not notice any

sensation at all, in which case just notice a lack of sensation. Continue focusing on the various parts of your body, slowly working your way from your toes to the top of your head. If your mind wanders (which it will!) just gently bring it back to focus on your body, without criticism or judgment. When you have finished, write about your experience in your journal. Was it easy to focus your awareness on your body, or was it difficult? If thoughts or restlessness prevented you from completing the body scan, you might want to try a mindfulness exercise that is more active, such as walking meditation.

Summary

Behavior therapy evolved during the 20th century from the research of B. F. Skinner, Ivan Pavlov, John W. Watson, Joseph Wolpe, Albert Bandura, and others. This treatment approach takes the stance that behavior is learned and consequently can be unlearned. Behavior therapists are concerned about results; so they take the time to establish a baseline, develop interventions that facilitate behavioral change, use reinforcements to solidify gains, carefully plan implementation, and monitor progress.

Today, behavior therapy and cognitive therapy are more likely to be combined rather than used alone. Their merger into cognitive–behavioral therapy, promoted by Donald Meichenbaum and others, expanded the application of cognitive and behavioral strategies and created a powerful treatment approach. Although practitioners of CBT focus on improving thoughts and behaviors, they also pay attention to the whole person; recognize the importance of history, background, and context; explore emotions; and take steps to develop a positive and collaborative therapeutic alliance. Behavior therapy and CBT have demonstrated strong effectiveness with a wide range of people and problems. These concepts and interventions should be incorporated into the work of all clinicians.

Recommended Readings

Baer, R. A. (Ed.). (2006). *Mindfulness-based treatment approaches: Clinician's guide to evidence base and applications*. Burlington, MA: Elsevier.

Dimeff, L. A., & Koerner, K. (Eds.). (2008). *Dialectical behavior therapy in clinical practice: Applications across disorders and settings*. New York, NY: Guilford.

Hayes, S. C., Strosahl, K. D., & Wilson, K. G. (2012). *Acceptance and commitment therapy: The process and practice of mindful change* (2nd ed.). New York, NY: Guilford.

Hick, S. F., & Bien, T. (Eds.). (2008). *Mindfulness and the therapeutic relationship*. New York, NY: Guilford Press.

Hofmann, S. G. (2012). *An introduction to modern CBT: Psychological solutions to mental health problems*. Malden, MA: Wiley-Blackwell.

Kabat-Zinn, J. (1990). *Full catastrophe living: Using the wisdom of your body and mind to face stress, pain, and illness*. New York, NY: Delacorte.

Linehan, M. (1993). *Skills training manual for treating borderline personality disorder*. New York, NY: Guilford.

Martin, G., & Pear, J. (2007). *Behavior modification: What it is and how to do it* (8th ed.). Upper Saddle River, NJ: Pearson/Prentice Hall.

Meichenbaum, D. H. (2007). Stress inoculation training: A preventative and treatment approach. In P. M. Lehrer, R. L. Woolfolk, & W. E. Sime (Eds.), *Principles and practice of stress management* (3rd ed., pp. 497–516). New York, NY: Guilford.

Spriegler, M. D., & Guevremont, D. C. (2010). *Contemporary behavior therapy* (5th ed.). Belmont, CA: Wadsworth.

Numerous journals focus on CBT and behavior therapy, including *Behavior Therapy, Cognitive and Behavioral Practice, Advances in Behaviour Research and Therapy, Child and Family Behavior Therapy, Cognitive Therapy and Research,* and *Journal of Behavior Therapy and Experimental Psychiatry.*

Additional Sources of Information

http://www.abainternational.org/—Website of the Association for Behavior Analysis.

http://www.nacbt.org—The National Association of Cognitive–Behavioral Therapists is dedicated to the teaching and practice of CBT. It offers seminars and other educational opportunities, literature on CBT, and certification for practitioners.

http://www.nyicbt.org—Website of the New York Institute for Cognitive and Behavioral Therapies.

http://www.ibh.com/html/meichenbaum.html—The Institute for the Advancement of Human Behavior provides information on Donald Meichenbaum's stress inoculation training.

http://www.abct.org—The website of the Association for Behavioral and Cognitive Therapies offers webinars and podcasts. The association holds an annual convention, provides training and continuing education, and publishes three journals: *Behavior Therapy, Cognitive and Behavioral Practice,* and the *Behavioral Therapist.*

http://www.emdr.com—The EMDR Institute, established by Francine Shapiro, conducts training and research on EMDR. The website contains efficacy research, training information, a bibliography, and links to other EMDR-related organizations worldwide.

http://www.umassmed.edu—The Center for Mindfulness in Medicine, Health Care and Society at the University of Massachusetts Medical Center provides mindfulness-based stress reduction programs, training, research, and publications.

http://www.contextualpsychology.org—The Association for Contextual and Behavioral Science provides information on relational frame theory and acceptance and commitment therapy, along with training and an annual conference.

http://www.behavioraltech.org—This website, developed by Marcia Linehan, includes information, training, workshops, and other resources related to mindfulness and dialectical behavior therapy.

CHAPTER 17

Reality Therapy

Reality therapy, initially developed by William Glasser in the 1960s, is solidly grounded in cognitive and behavioral theory and interventions. Like other cognitive–behavioral approaches to treatment, reality therapy focuses on the present and helps people change their thoughts and actions so they can lead more rewarding lives.

However, reality therapy is more philosophical than other cognitive–behavioral approaches and emphasizes self-determination and process more than results. This no-excuses approach encourages people to take responsibility for both their difficulties and their joys. While acknowledging that environment, heredity, and culture play a role in a person's development, reality therapy believes that people always have the ability to make choices in their behavior. They do not need to be a victim or feel trapped by these influences (Wubbolding, 2011). As Glasser (1998a) stated, "We choose *everything* we do, including the misery we feel" (p. 3). Helping people make choices that increase their happiness and meet their needs without harming others is the essence of reality therapy.

Drawing heavily on cognitive and behavioral strategies, reality therapists guide people through a process of change that helps them become aware of their needs, recognize the ingredients of a rewarding life, and establish goals and procedures to improve their lives. Through this process, people gain more control over their lives and assume responsible and rewarding roles in society.

Reality therapy has been used in many mental health settings. Schools and substance abuse treatment programs are particularly suited to this approach. According to Glasser, reality therapy can be effective with almost anyone, regardless of diagnosis or background. Although not all clinicians agree, reality therapy does have much to offer.

WILLIAM GLASSER

William Glasser was born in 1925 and grew up in Ohio. His early years were difficult; Glasser (1998a) reports that his father was occasionally violent, while his mother was overly controlling. Even as a child, he recognized the incompatibility in his parents' relationship. This history is telling in light of Glasser's later emphasis on personal responsibility, not harming others, and the marital or partner relationship.

Glasser became a chemical engineer but later changed his career goals and entered medical school. He received his medical degree from Case Western Reserve University in 1953 and then trained to become a psychiatrist.

Between 1956 and 1967, Glasser was a psychiatrist for the Ventura School for Girls, a prison school operated by the California Youth Authority, housing 400 adolescents. This experience had a profound impact on Glasser's views of mental health and psychotherapy. He concluded that traditional psychoanalysis offered little to help the young women at the Ventura School and began to develop what would become reality therapy.

Glasser concluded that many of the difficulties of the adolescents at the Ventura School stemmed from their failure to take responsibility for themselves and their lives and to act in ways that truly met their needs. Although they might have believed that they were seeking to meet their needs, the result—their involuntary stay at the Ventura School—was not their desired outcome. By helping the girls think more clearly about their present needs, holding them responsible for their behavior, and playing an active and involved role in treatment, Glasser became much more effective. Implementation of his ideas for change resulted in an 80% success rate.

Glasser's first book, *Mental Health or Mental Illness?* (1961), laid the groundwork for reality therapy. His *Reality Therapy* (1965) spelled out the principles that continue to be fundamental to this approach: that people who take responsibility for themselves and their behaviors and are aware of and able to meet their basic needs without harming others are likely to lead happy and fulfilling lives. Glasser's work emphasizes the importance of relationships as well as responsibility. He believes that a warm, accepting clinician is essential to the success of treatment, just as he believes that close and positive relationships are essential to mental health and happiness.

Relationships have been important in Glasser's own life. His first wife, Naomi Glasser, shared in the development of reality therapy. That marriage ended after 46 years, with his wife's death from cancer. Glasser said he married his present wife, Carleen, after they checked their needs to ensure they were compatible. Together they have written several books on relationships (1999, 2000, 2007). Glasser's three children also play a significant role in his life.

Since the 1960s, Glasser has developed and expanded the scope of reality therapy. Focusing his writings and lectures on the application of reality therapy in treatment as well as its use in school and business settings, he has succeeded in establishing its importance. Currently based at the William Glasser Institute in Chatsworth, California, Glasser continues to play an active role in the development of reality therapy.

ROBERT WUBBOLDING

Reality therapy found another important spokesperson in Robert E. Wubbolding, director of the Center for Reality Therapy in Cincinnati, Ohio; training director at the William Glasser Institute; and professor emeritus of counseling at Xavier University in Cincinnati. Wubbolding has played an important role in the development and promotion of reality therapy and has lectured and taught reality therapy on five continents. He is a prolific author who has written more than 10 books including *Reality Therapy* (2011) for the American Psychological Association's Theories of Counseling Series. His writings facilitate implementation of reality therapy through case studies, exercises, and treatment protocols.

THE DEVELOPMENT OF REALITY THERAPY

Reality therapy began in the 1960s with three relatively straightforward concepts that Glasser (1965) labeled *reality, responsibility,* and *right and wrong.* He believed that all people have two basic and intertwined human needs: relatedness (to love and be loved) and respect (to feel worthwhile to oneself and others). Behavior that shows appreciation for our own needs and those of others leads to feelings of self-worth and to rewarding relationships, thereby meeting the two basic needs. Desirable behavior also reflects awareness of reality, responsibility for oneself, and understanding of right and wrong.

Some aspects of Glasser's initial ideas have stayed the same while others have changed. His early writings placed considerable emphasis on ethical issues and de-emphasized individual differences. However, recent writings sound less judgmental and imply, rather than insist on, the importance of right and wrong in the therapeutic process. In addition, his writings now convey greater appreciation of individual differences, although reality therapy generalizes about the causes and appropriate treatment of emotional difficulties.

Early writings identified eight steps for clinicians to follow in using reality therapy (Evans, 1982): (1) Build rapport with clients. (2) Ask "What are *you* doing?" (3) Collaborate with clients in evaluating their behavior. (4) Help people make a plan to do better. (5) Help clients commit to the plan. (6) Do not accept excuses. (7) Do not interfere with reasonable consequences. (8) Do not give up! Although current writing rarely includes these steps, they still are relevant to reality therapy.

In addition, Glasser's list of basic needs has expanded, as have treatment procedures. (We discuss these points later in this chapter.) Glasser's emphasis on responsibility, relationships, and making choices and taking actions that fulfill our needs has changed little. These concepts form the foundation of reality therapy.

With the publication of his book *Warning: Psychiatry Can Be Hazardous to Your Mental Health* in 2003, Glasser raised concerns about the psychiatric profession's dependence on psychotropic drugs for the management of mental health. He has since developed a format for choice theory focus groups to help people with conditions that are traditionally treated with medication (e.g., fibromyalgia, severe mental illness), and as a preventive measure for symptoms of mental disorders.

Control Theory

In the 1970s, Glasser discovered the writings of Powers (1973) and others on control theory or control system theory. Glasser incorporated concepts of control theory into reality therapy. He conceptualized people as driven by inner control systems in the brain that guide behaviors and emotions so that they are instrumental in moving people in directions that seem likely to fulfill their needs. According to Glasser (1984), "A control system acts upon the world and itself as part of the world to attempt to get the picture that it wants" (p. 39). Unfortunately, people's control systems sometimes cause difficulties by misdirecting their efforts and leading them to try to control others.

For Glasser, awareness and assessment are the keys to modifying our control systems and improving our lives. He believed that the first step is to become cognizant of the pictures in our heads that reflect our needs and wants. We then can become aware of what we are doing to reach our goals. By assessing the impact and success of our behaviors, we can determine whether change is warranted and, if so, use creative strategies to modify our thoughts, emotions, and behaviors. Although Glasser (1984) recognizes that immediate, intense, short-term feelings can emerge spontaneously at times of frustration or satisfaction, he is convinced that people can choose and control their long-term feelings.

Choice Theory

For many years, this treatment system was known as reality therapy/control theory. However, in 1996, Glasser determined that underlying reality therapy was choice theory rather than control theory. Choice theory postulates that people's choices of thoughts, feelings, and actions largely determine the quality of their lives. Glasser's view of the brain as a control system "aligning the external world to what we want as well as closing the gap between what we want and what we have" continues to be part of reality therapy (Wubbolding, 2000, p. xiii). However, choice theory, underlying reality therapy, is more important in helping people improve their lives (Glasser, 1998a).

IMPORTANT THEORETICAL CONCEPTS

Reality therapy has evolved considerably over the years and has expanded its applications. At present, it is a well-developed treatment system that is used successfully in a broad range of settings.

Human Development

According to Glasser (1998a), problems originate during early childhood when we encounter people who believe they know what is right for us. Because of our youth, inexperience, and self-doubts, we accept this external control and come to believe that others make us feel or act as we do. However, "external control harms everyone, both the controllers and the controlled" (p. 7).

Instead, according to reality therapy, the way to rear emotionally healthy children is to surround them with loving and supportive people who enable them to experience freedom, power, and fun in responsible ways. Children's belief in themselves as well as their ability to identify and meet their needs in positive ways should be fostered, instilling attitudes and behaviors that will serve them well as they mature.

Despite this emphasis on childhood development, reality therapy views people as basically self-determining and able to overcome their early difficulties. According to Glasser (1998a), "We are rarely the victims of what happened to us in the past" (p. 3). However, if people have not learned to satisfy their needs during the early years, they may require help in developing new ways of feeling, thinking, and behaving.

Reality therapists pay little attention to the past. Instead, they believe that past issues are expressed in present unsatisfying relationships and behaviors. Treatment is most likely to succeed by focusing on those present manifestations. According to Wubbolding (1991), "People are motivated to fulfill a current force inside of them . . . early childhood conflicts, unconscious reasons, and external stimuli do not cause present behavior" (p. 21).

Five Basic Needs

Human needs are "at the core of human existence as the engines of human choice" (Wubbolding & Brickell, 2008, p. 30). Reality therapy holds that all people are born with the following five basic needs that are fixed at birth (Glasser, 1998a). The relative strengths of these five needs give people their different personalities (Wubbolding, 1991):

1. *Belonging:* Loving and being loved; having contact, connections, interactions, and relationships with people
2. *Power/achievement:* Feelings of accomplishment and competence, self-esteem, success, and control over one's own life
3. *Fun/enjoyment:* Pleasure; the ability to laugh, play, and appreciate being human
4. *Freedom/independence:* The ability to make choices; to live without excessive and unnecessary limits or constraints
5. *Survival:* The essentials of life, including good health, food, air, shelter, safety, security, and physical comfort.

Because these needs overlap, fulfillment of one may speed fulfillment of others. For example, people with positive relationships probably have greater enjoyment of life. However, these needs also can conflict. People who channel great effort into achieving power or independence may have difficulty forming rewarding relationships.

Reality therapy takes the position that all human behavior is purposeful and directed at meeting one or more of the fundamental needs (Wubbolding, 2011). Although the five needs are universal, the specific wants that people pursue in an effort to meet their needs are particular to the individual. For example, having a family may be a want that satisfies one person's need for belonging, whereas another person may satisfy that need with an involvement in team sports. People are motivated to bridge the gaps between what they have and what they want to meet their needs. However, feelings such as loneliness and deprivation can limit people's motivation. Reality therapists seek to change those feelings, not by directly addressing emotions, but by changing thoughts about wants and needs as well as corresponding purposeful behaviors.

Concept of Mental Illness

Although trained as a medical doctor and psychiatrist, Glasser does not ascribe to the disease model of mental illness. He accepts that people have symptoms, but does not believe there is anything wrong with their brains that cannot be changed through the synergistic effects of supportive relationships and changed actions. Glasser believes that choice theory is superior to medication in the treatment of symptoms, even in the treatment of severe mental disorders. Glasser accepts that several brain disorders exist (e.g., Parkinson's disease, Alzheimer's), but he believes that these disorders should be treated by neurologists.

Mental illness, according to reality therapy, is actually people's failure to meet their five needs in responsible and effective ways—overemphasizing some needs while neglecting others. According to

Glasser (1998a), people engaged in antisocial behavior, for example, generally focus on their needs for power and freedom and do not satisfactorily address their needs for love and enjoyment. Glasser believes that even people with psychotic disorders and depression choose their symptoms. Symptoms are chosen by people because they have little control over the real world and thus decide to use "crazy creativity" (Glasser, 1984) in the form of hallucinations and delusions over which they do have control. Conventional diagnostic terminology is not central to reality therapy; instead, mental illness is conceptualized as problems in choices, need satisfaction, and responsibility. Common symptoms of emotional difficulties include loneliness (rather than belonging); loss of control (rather than empowerment); boredom and depression (rather than fun); frustration, inhibition, or rebelliousness (rather than freedom); and illness or deprivation (rather than safety and security). Glasser (2003) writes that "severe unhappiness can lead to bipolar disorder, schizophrenia, and chronic excruciating pain with no pathology to explain it, as in the condition called fibromyalgia" (p. 57). Instead of treating these disorders with medication, Glasser believes that using reality therapy to help people choose to connect with others in their quality world can relieve their symptoms and help people overcome their unhappiness. Reality therapy and choice theory do no harm, whereas antidepressant and antipsychotic medications have documented side effects and have not been tested for long-term effects on the brain (Glasser, 2003).

Concept of Mental Health

Reality therapy has a clear vision of emotionally healthy people: those who are successful in meeting their five basic needs. Emotionally healthy people choose thoughts, feelings, and behaviors wisely and responsibly. Their choices help them meet their needs while respecting the rights of other people to fulfill their own needs. They do not view setbacks and suffering as an inevitable part of life, but rather as an early warning sign that they need to look at their behavior and relationships and make better choices. Furthermore, emotionally healthy people not only seek to improve their own lives but take steps to help others and to make the world a better place (Wubbolding, 1991). Such people have a success identity rather than a failure identity. They have a clear and positive sense of themselves that reflects their own internal frames of reference; they do not derive their sense of themselves from the perceptions of others.

Total Behavior and Motivation

As Glasser (1998a) observed, all people can do at birth is behave. All aspects of functioning are linked to behavior. He calls people's overall functioning *total behavior,* which is composed of four inseparable components: acting, thinking, feeling, and physiology. Reality therapists believe that all behavior is chosen, that people can directly control the acting and thinking components and thereby gain indirect control over feelings and physiology. Glasser compared the four elements in total behavior to the four wheels of a car, with acting and thinking represented by the front wheels. When the car moves, all four wheels move. The direction of the car cannot be changed by the movement of only one wheel. Neither can a person's actions be separated from the other components of thinking, emotion, and physiology. When a person swings a golf club, the action cannot be separated from the total behavior. Similarly, when a person chooses to depress, the entire being is involved.

As in Adlerian therapy, reality therapists believe all behavior is intentional and has a purpose. To continue the car metaphor, change may occur in overall direction, in specific actions (the two front wheels), or by altering the person's wants (Wubbolding, 2011). Regardless of the specific concern, reality therapy believes in changing actions first; thoughts or self-talk will follow. Eventually, changes in feelings and physiology will happen as well, just like the back wheels of the car must follow the direction of the front wheels. Of course the vehicle must be driven with intentionality, otherwise erratic driving (behavior) will result.

When a person wants to change behavior, it is best to start with the most easily changed component—actions. We have more direct control over actions and thinking than we do over emotions and physiology. As in the car analogy, the front wheels move first, and steer where the vehicle goes, while the rear wheels follow. By changing the action or behavior, the total behavior is changed. As in other cognitive therapies, feelings and emotions are secondary. Feelings are considered, but are seen as analogous to the lights on the dashboard of the car. "Feelings and emotions indicate a healthy or unhealthy life direction" (Wubbolding & Brickell, 2008, p. 46). This emphasis on thoughts and behaviors is what makes reality therapy a cognitive–behavioral approach to treatment.

Quality Worlds

According to Glasser (1998a), people have quality worlds formed of pictures or images of the sort of life they would like to have, the people they want to be with, the possessions or experiences they would like to have, and the ideas and beliefs they value. These pictures guide people's efforts to satisfy their needs and are linked to the success they have in meeting those needs. For example, if a woman with good work skills puts a promotion into her quality world, representing a way for her to meet her need for achievement, she has made responsible picture choices, and her related behaviors will probably be successful. However, if her way to satisfy her need for love is represented in her quality world by a picture of her best friend's husband, she is not making responsible choices and is unlikely to meet her needs.

Reality therapists believe that people can choose the pictures they put in their quality worlds. If they choose pictures that are unattainable or unlikely to meet their needs, they probably will experience frustration and disappointment. By becoming aware of their needs, as well as the pictures in their quality world, people can make better, wiser, and more realistic choices; have greater control over their lives; and fulfill their needs.

WDEP System

The procedures involved in reality therapy are represented by the acronym WDEP, which includes four main elements: wants, direction and doing, evaluation, and planning. These can be applied in whatever order seems most likely to be helpful.

W: WANTS Reality therapists explore clients' wants and the pictures in their quality world, focusing on what they want that they *are* getting, what they want that they *are not* getting, and what they are getting that they *do not want* (Wubbolding, 2011). Keeping in mind that wants are linked to needs, clinicians also encourage clients to look at that connection by asking questions such as "How do you perceive your wanting to drop out of high school as meeting your needs?" In work with adolescents or adults with alcohol or substance abuse problems, reality therapists help the client to recognize that some wants are better off being delayed. Helping people to realize that some wants are unrealistic or unreasonable, while others can be helpful to the establishment of interpersonal relationships, and the recovery process, is an important role of the reality therapy counselor (Wubbolding, 2011).

Reality therapy, a phenomenological approach, recognizes the role that perceptions have in behavior. It helps people become aware of their perceptions so that they can modify them if appropriate. According to Wubbolding (1991, 1995), perceptions pass through two filters. The lower-level filter, called the *total knowledge filter,* recognizes and labels perceptions; the upper-level filter, the *valuing filter,* evaluates perceptions. Reality therapists facilitate this evaluation by suggesting that people distinguish among positive or need-satisfying perceptions, negative perceptions, and neutral perceptions. For example, "That is an attractive piece of jewelry" is a neutral perception. "I deserve that diamond more than she does" is a negative perception that can lead to relationship difficulties, whereas "I share my friend's happiness about receiving a beautiful engagement ring" is a positive perception because it enhances feelings of love and belonging. Becoming aware of and evaluating their perceptions can help people meet their needs.

An aspect of the *W* in WDEP is helping people choose to make positive changes. Wubbolding (2007b, p. 303) identified five levels of client commitment to change:

1. I don't want to be here.
2. I want the outcome but not the effort.
3. I'll try; I might.
4. I will do my best.
5. I will do whatever it takes.

If people begin treatment at the first or second level, an important goal of treatment is to help them see how they can benefit from changing their choices so that they move on to higher levels of commitment.

D: DIRECTION AND DOING Reality therapists devote considerable attention to exploring people's total behavior, including actions, thoughts, emotions, and physiology. Helping people describe their total behavior as specifically as possible, as well as the goals and impact of those behaviors, is integral to treatment. The focus of reality therapy is on what people are doing, not on why they are acting in certain ways.

E: EVALUATION Clinicians encourage clients to evaluate their goals, their actions, their perceptions, and the consequences of all these. Evaluation does not involve a judgment about the goodness or badness of these dimensions. Instead, evaluation is based on whether behaviors and perceptions are realistic and helpful to clients as well as to others. Clinicians might facilitate the process by asking thought-provoking questions such as "How realistic is it to expect that your daughter will never misbehave?" and "What success have you had in using drugs to build relationships?"

Both the discussion of doing and the evaluation process focus primarily on the present and emphasize positive and successful aspects of people's lives. The past is discussed only in terms of its impact on the present. Helping clients conduct evaluations is the main focus of the WDEP process (Wubbolding, 2011).

P: PLANNING Reality therapists view planning as essential and encourage people to have long-range plans and goals that are subdivided into a series of short-term, realistic plans. As Wubbolding (1991) put it, "To fail to plan is to plan to fail" (p. 95). Plans should evolve from self-evaluation and reflect desired changes in wants and total behavior. Wubbolding (2007b, p. 305) listed the following eight qualities of viable plans, represented by the acronym SAMI^{2}C^3. Plans should be:

- *Simple,* clear, and understandable
- *Attainable;* able to be accomplished by the client
- *Measurable* via inventories, diaries, and other methods of recording progress
- *Immediate;* implementation can start right away
- *Involving* the clinician in appropriate ways such as giving feedback, serving as a sounding board
- *Controlled* by the client rather than someone else
- In keeping with the client's *commitment* to change and recognition that this change is important
- Reflecting *consistent* and repeated changes in behavior.

Usually, planning focuses on modifying and improving actions because that is the aspect of total behavior over which people have the greatest control. However, focusing on thoughts may provide a point of entry, enabling people to believe that choosing different actions will be beneficial. According to reality therapy, feelings do not need to be addressed directly, although they can be important sources of information on wants and perceptions; if actions change, emotions will correspondingly change.

Planning and choice go hand in hand. The primary goals of planning are to help people make better choices and take more control of their lives. According to Glasser (1998a), if people can make bad choices, they can make better ones.

In his 2011 book on reality therapy, Wubbolding notes that religion and spirituality are behaviors chosen by some people to satisfy wants and needs, but these are not part of Glasser's choice theory. He quotes Glasser as saying that "anyone instructing others about choice theory is free to add needs to the basic five, but it should be emphasized that the additional needs are beyond the original theory" (Wubbolding, 2011, p. 39).

Unlike some other approaches to cognitive and behavior therapy, reality therapy focuses more on process than outcome, more on the behaviors that are used to achieve desired results than on the achievement of the results themselves. This perspective offers two advantages: It encourages people to develop behaviors they can generalize to other situations and reduces the risk that people will view themselves as failures if they make better choices in their behaviors but do not immediately obtain their desired outcomes.

Importance of Relationships

Since its inception, reality therapy has viewed relationships as key to both development of difficulties and achievement of a more rewarding life. According to Glasser (1998a), "People who have no close relationships are almost always lonely and feel bad" (p. 30).

Glasser (1998a, 2000) is particularly interested in the partner relationship and suggests that the best marriages are between people with similar personalities. In addition, he believes that marriages are most likely to be successful if both people are low in power and freedom needs and high in their needs for fun, love, and belonging.

Parenting is, of course, another important role in relationships. Glasser advocates loving children no matter what, but suggests that parents may dislike how children behave and can let them know that some behaviors make loving them difficult. He cautions parents to avoid being punitive and judgmental, although he believes they do need to establish guidelines, rules, and limits for their children. Encouragement and acceptance are seen as far more helpful than censure. Like Adlerian therapists, reality therapists maintain that an essential element in good parenting is helping children learn from their mistakes, thereby turning disappointments into successes rather than promoting feelings of failure.

TREATMENT USING REALITY THERAPY

As a cognitive–behavioral approach, reality therapy uses many of the same strategies that have been discussed in Parts 4 and 5 of this book. However, reality therapy also is characterized by its own set of goals, relationships, and strategies.

Goals

The fundamental goal of reality therapy is to enable people to have greater control over their lives by making better choices. Wise choices are perceived as those that meet the following three criteria:

1. They help people meet their innate needs and their specific wants, reflected by the pictures in their quality world.
2. The choices are responsible; they not only help the person making the choices but also respect the rights of other people and contribute to their efforts to make wise choices.
3. The choices are realistic and are likely to be attained through sound planning.

The following goals are also important:

- People form and sustain positive, mutually rewarding, respectful relationships.
- They develop a success identity rather than a failure identity.
- They have a consistent repertoire of healthy actions that enhances their total behavior by helping them think clearly, experience happiness and other positive emotions, and take steps to maintain their physical health.

Therapeutic Alliance

Reality therapists view a positive client–clinician relationship as essential to treatment. As Glasser (1975) stated, "The ability of the therapist to get involved is the major skill of doing reality therapy" (p. 22).

Reality therapists are very much human beings in the treatment process. They share their perceptions and experiences and frequently ask for feedback. They pay little attention to transference and countertransference. Instead, they present themselves as people with skills and information they can use responsibly to help others. They are warm, friendly, caring, respectful, optimistic, attentive, and authentic with clients. Although reality therapists maintain ethical and professional behavior, they may talk about a sports event or give a person advice about what to wear to a meeting if such interactions promote rapport and help people achieve their goals.

Clients and clinicians form a collaborative team to help clients explore, evaluate, and revise their choices. Clinicians do not assume responsibility for telling clients what choices to make or for evaluating clients' behaviors. However, they do take considerable responsibility for the direction and success of treatment. They promote motivation and commitment, provide support and encouragement, guide the WDEP process, teach planning and other skills, and use creativity, imagination, and humor to motivate clients and provide new perspectives.

Clinicians help people formulate realistic and viable plans. As part of this process, they negotiate clear commitments and contracts with their clients. They avoid wasting time on excuses and strive to move forward rather than backward. Reality therapists are firm and determined to help people. They never give up.

Language is important in this approach. Reality therapists consciously establish a positive environment free from criticism, fault finding, or blaming. Problems are referred to in the past tense and solutions in the present or future tense. Therapists ask about wants and needs and reduce the time clients spend "venting" or complaining. Feelings, according to Wubbolding (2011) must be attached to actions. Reality therapists make extensive use of the first-person pronouns *I* and *we* to emphasize the collaborative nature of the treatment process. They ask *what* rather than *why* questions. Clinician self-disclosure sometimes facilitates involvement.

Clinicians use compassionate confrontations, when necessary, to highlight a discrepancy in the client's thoughts or actions. Confrontations are handled sensitively and nonjudgmentally, using questions that invite exploration and feedback. According to Bratter, Esparat, Kaufman, and Sinsheimer (2008), awareness is the ultimate goal of these compassionate confrontations. They also represent the voice of society, reminding people of the reality of moral, legal, and ethical standards. The Skill Development section later in this chapter focuses on caring confrontations.

Strategies

Reality therapists value creativity as well as understanding, appreciating, and motivating each person. As a result, they draw on a broad range of interventions to promote clients' involvement in treatment and bring energy and interest into the sessions. Included in reality therapists' repertoire are a broad range of cognitive and behavioral interventions, many of which are discussed next.

METAPHORS Reality therapists use metaphors, similes, images, analogies, and anecdotes to give clients a powerful message in a creative way (Wubbolding, 2011). Clinicians also listen for and use metaphors and themes that clients present. For example, a therapist told a client whose hobby was fishing that his efforts to meet his goals seemed like fishing without bait in a lake with few fish.

RELATIONSHIPS Reality therapists view relationships as essential to a rewarding life. They encourage clients to form relationships and coach them on ways to make them rewarding. According to Wubbolding (1991, pp. 55–57), the foundation of a strong relationship is time spent together with the following characteristics: It is effortful, valued by each person, enjoyable, focused on the positive, noncritical and nonargumentative, regular and repetitive, but time limited, and promotes awareness of each other. As an example, he suggests taking frequent and regular walks with a friend as a way to build closeness.

QUESTIONS Although reality therapists advocate evaluation of total behavior, they want that assessment to come from the clients. Reality therapists avoid telling people what is not working for them or how they should change. Rather, they use carefully structured questions to help people take a close look at their lives and determine what does and does not need change (Wubbolding, 2011). Examples of such questions include "What did you do yesterday to satisfy your need for belonging?" "Is what you are doing helping you?" "Is the plan you have made the most effective plan you are capable of formulating?" Reality therapy can be easily adapted, via language and word change, for people from different cultures. For example, people from Japan may be put off by such a direct question as "What do you want?" but may be more comfortable being asked "What are you looking for?" or "What are you seeking?" (Wubbolding, 2011, p. 113).

WDEP AND SAMI^{2}C^3 As we have discussed, the concepts represented by these acronyms play an important part in keeping both clients and treatment focused and productive. WDEP reflects the process of moving toward change by *evaluating wants* and *direction* and formulating *plans.* SAMI^{2}C^3 represents the elements that maximize the success of plans: simple, attainable, measurable, immediate, involving, controlled, consistent, and committed.

POSITIVE ADDICTIONS According to Glasser (1976), negative addictions or repetitive self-destructive behaviors, such as misuse of substances, acting out, and depressing oneself, reflect giving up. Such behaviors characterize people who either have never learned to meet their needs in effective and responsible ways or have lost that ability.

Glasser suggests that people can reduce negative behaviors by developing positive addictions. These are behaviors that provide mental strength and alertness, creativity, energy, confidence, and focus, but do not dominate or control people's lives. Examples include regular exercise, journal writing, playing music, yoga, and meditation. Acquiring a positive addiction generally takes

6 months to 2 years of regular practice, usually 45 to 60 minutes at a time. Glasser (1976) suggests the following guidelines for choosing and nurturing positive behavioral patterns:

- The behavior should be noncompetitive and capable of being done alone.
- The behavior can be accomplished without inordinate mental or physical effort.
- The behavior should have value to you.
- The behavior should be one that you believe will lead you to improve in some way if you persist in it.
- The behavior should be one that you can perform without criticizing yourself.

USING VERBS AND "ING" WORDS Because reality therapists want people to realize that they have considerable control over their lives and can choose their total behavior, clinicians deliberately make extensive use of active verbs and "ing" words. Rather than describing people as *angry, depressed, phobic,* or *anxious,* they describe them as *angering, depressing, phobicking,* or *anxiety-ing*. This implies that these emotions are not fixed states but instead are actions that can be changed.

REASONABLE CONSEQUENCES Reality therapists believe that people should be responsible and therefore should experience the consequences of their behaviors. For example, the adolescent who returns home after curfew may have to be grounded for the next weekend, and the woman who is never ready when her carpool arrives may need to be dropped from the carpool. Reality therapists do not advocate making excuses or special exceptions. At the same time, they are not punitive; rather than focusing on what people did wrong, they focus on what people can choose to do differently so that they do not suffer the negative consequences of irresponsible and unrealistic behaviors.

RENEGOTIATION Client progress in counseling and psychotherapy is rarely smooth; occasional lapses or backsliding are the norm. When this occurs in reality therapy, clinicians use renegotiation to help people do something different. Emphasis is on developing new or revised plans with a high likelihood of success and identifying and rehearsing ways to cope with temptations to diverge from agreed-on plans and goals.

PARADOXICAL INTERVENTIONS Reality therapists use paradoxical interventions, initially developed by Viktor Frankl, an existential therapist discussed in Chapter 9. These creative interventions encourage people to take responsibility for themselves. Paradoxical interventions typically take two forms (Wubbolding, 1988):

1. They *relabel* or *reframe* to promote choice and control. People might be viewed as lacking in skills rather than psychotic. Disappointments might be referred to as learning experiences rather than failures.
2. They involve *paradoxical prescriptions.* Reality therapists might encourage people to imagine the worst that could happen and find ways to cope with that, to choose their symptoms rather than fight them, to do the opposite of what is not working, or to schedule a relapse. Of course, suggestions always reflect accepted ethical standards.

SKILL DEVELOPMENT Education is an important aspect of reality therapy. Clinicians help people develop skills to help them fulfill their needs and wants in responsible ways. Reality therapists might teach people assertiveness, rational thinking, development of positive addictions, planning, and other skills that promote growth and responsibility.

APPLICATION AND CURRENT USE OF REALITY THERAPY

Reality therapy is a flexible approach that has been used for individual, group, and family therapy and for a great variety of people and problems. It is widely used in schools, correctional institutions, and rehabilitation programs and probably is the most popular approach to treating problems with drug and alcohol use. Reality therapy also has been used in both inpatient and outpatient mental health settings.

Application to Diagnostic Groups

The literature suggests that reality therapists view their approach as useful with almost everyone, regardless of the nature of their backgrounds, problems, or mental health. Although this perspective is questionable, assessing the effectiveness of reality therapy with particular diagnostic groups is difficult. Reality therapists avoid using common diagnostic nomenclature and view the concept of mental illness as invalid and harmful. Instead, reality therapists view people with mental disorders as lacking the skills necessary to meet their needs.

As a result of this stance, few empirical studies describe the use of reality therapy with people diagnosed with specific mental disorders. Glasser (1998a), Wubbolding (2000), and others (Carey, 2003; Howatt, 2003; Mottern, 2002) do present case studies of people presenting concerns that suggest the presence of mental disorders. For example, Wubbolding describes the successful use of reality therapy with adults and adolescents who are incarcerated, with people who misuse substances, and with those experiencing depression and low self-esteem. He also provides examples of the effective use of reality therapy with people who experience bullying, domestic violence, and family conflict. Recent research indicates reality therapy is also effective for treating children who have been sexually abused as well as for people with impulse control disorders and Internet addiction. Ellsworth (2007) integrated reality therapy in her work with children who had been sexually abused. By focusing on strengths and weaving in humor and creativity, abused children were helped to make decisions about the healing process that empowered them to choose to be healthy and positive rather than allowing themselves to continue to feel like victims. Kim (2007) outlined the use of control theory and reality therapy in a 10-session group therapy program for Internet-addicted college students in Korea. The program seems promising. Future outcome research will be necessary to document treatment effectiveness.

Although reality therapy may well be effective in treating many disorders, the limited empirical research on the use of reality therapy with people diagnosed with severe mental disorders is a concern. Kim (2005), for example, reported on a controlled study of the effectiveness of reality therapy for 30 inpatients with schizophrenia. The results show positive changes in self-esteem, internal locus of control, and problem-focused stress coping. However, the positive symptoms of schizophrenia (e.g., hallucinations, delusions) were not studied. Anecdotal evidence suggests that reality therapy is best suited for treatment of people with mild to moderately severe mental disorders, including eating disorders, elective mutism, self-esteem, and career satisfaction (Wubbolding, 2011). With severe disorders such as bipolar and psychotic disorders, as well as with long-standing disorders such as personality disorders, reality therapy should be used with caution, if at all, and will probably need to be combined with medication and other treatment approaches.

Application to Multicultural Groups

Reality therapy seems well suited to a diverse and multicultural population. Reality therapy is phenomenological and is interested in getting to know people and understanding their worldviews and quality world. It helps people identify their wants, evaluate them, and develop responsible plans to achieve their wants. It is a respectful and humanistic approach. It advocates treating each person as an individual, recognizes the importance of relationships, and encourages people to help each other. Although reality therapy promotes self-evaluation, therapists do not make judgments or impose their values on others. The positive and action-oriented nature of reality therapy makes it especially appropriate for people who might find a psychodynamic approach to be intrusive and inappropriate.

The reality therapy literature since 2000, particularly the *International Journal of Reality Therapy,* has focused heavily on the use of this approach with multicultural clients. Wubbolding (2011) taught reality therapy in Asia, Australia, Europe, and the Middle East and has described ways to adapt this treatment system to other cultures. For example, he emphasizes the importance of looking at the particular balance of basic needs in each culture and suggests that "I'll try" should be viewed as a firm commitment for people from Asian cultures.

Barr (2009) discusses reality therapy from a Jewish perspective, comparing the tenets of choice theory with the Talmud. He found that choice theory is consistent with the idea of freewill, which is pivotal to Judaism. In an exploration of Jewish ethnic identity, Altman and colleagues (2010) indicated that a person's Jewish identity plays an important role in relationships with others (e.g., friends, family, non-Jews) and is a critical aspect of his or her being. Many articles, both theoretical and applied, describe the successful application of reality therapy in a variety of cultures, for example, in Korean (Kim & Hwang, 2006), Chinese (Li,1998), and Islamic cultures (Jusoh & Ahmad, 2009).

Sanchez and Garriga (1996), however, raised concerns about the application of reality therapy to some cultural groups. They point out, for example, that fatalism (the idea that some things are meant to happen regardless of what people do) is an important belief in Hispanic culture. Clinicians should exercise particular caution and sensitivity when using reality therapy with people whose belief system emphasizes a higher power, predestination and predetermination, and the value of an external locus of control. Sanchez and Garriga suggest speaking of a dual control framework with such clients, sharing action and responsibility with a higher power but still striving for an improved quality world and better need satisfaction. Overall, "Implementing reality therapy is an artful process that takes into consideration the worldview of clients as well as empowering them by offering choices and presenting alternatives" (Wubbolding & Brickell, 2008, p. 48).

Reality therapy may be helpful to people coping with physical disabilities and illness. Its encouragement of a success identity and emphasis on responsibility, autonomy, and self-efficacy are likely to be empowering. Several studies support this conclusion. Glasser (2001), for example, applied choice theory to aid people with fibromyalgia. Rapport (2007) incorporated the five basic needs of choice theory (survival, belonging/love, power, freedom, and fun) to assess and counsel people with disabilities and sexual, romantic, or intimacy issues. Weisler (2006) found that patients with cancer believed reality therapy to be a helpful coping strategy. Kelsch (2002) used choice theory to help people with multiple sclerosis gain more control over their illness.

Application to Schools

In light of reality therapy's origins in a correctional school, it is not surprising that Glasser and Wubbolding (Wubbolding, 2007a, 2011) have maintained a strong interest in the use of reality therapy in schools. Reality therapy has sought to replace the punitive and judgmental atmosphere of many schools with an environment that is encouraging and reinforcing: "A good school could be defined as a place where almost all students believe that if they do some work, they will be able to satisfy their needs enough so that it makes sense to keep working" (Glasser, 1986, p. 15).

Glasser has suggested several approaches to effecting positive change in schools:

- ***Learning teams.*** Groups of two to five students of varying ability levels study and learn cooperatively, motivated by feelings of belonging in the group. Their goals include both learning new material and convincing their teachers that they have mastered the material. Teams are changed regularly to promote interaction.

- ***Quality School Model.*** This model reconceptualizes the school environment to eliminate coercion and promote cooperation, safety, and consideration (Glasser, 1998b; Schwartz, 1995). Teachers strive to make course work useful and meaningful and to teach in a way that meets students' basic needs and contributes to their sense of fulfillment. Features of this model include year-round education to promote continuity, parent action teams to increase involvement, teachers and students sharing lunch and other activities, partnerships with businesses, elimination of bells to signal times, elimination of grading, peer tutoring in multi-age learning groups, open classrooms, computer-aided learning, student portfolios, student-led conferences and businesses, and daily self-evaluations for staff and students. The model recognizes the importance of both psychological and academic growth and emphasizes a win–win perspective.

Although a relatively small number of schools have fully implemented the Quality School Model, many have incorporated facets of reality therapy into their teaching and counseling programs. Murphy (1997) reviewed six studies of reality therapy used with varied student populations, including students with learning disabilities, students at risk, and Mexican American students. Programs were 4 to 12 weeks long. All studies yielded some positive results. However, the diversity of the studies and the weak design of some studies led Murphy to conclude that, although reality therapy seems to enhance behavior and interest in school, more research is needed before firm conclusions can be drawn.

Passaro, Moon, Wiest, and Wong (2004) suggested ways for schools to apply reality therapy to in-school discipline with the use of a time-out room for students with ADHD and conduct disorder. Out-of-school suspensions decreased, daily behavior ratings improved by as much as 42%, and participation in general education classes also improved. The authors noted that reality therapy is a "highly effective" treatment methodology for this difficult to treat population (Wubbolding, 2011, p. 118).

Stehno (1995) suggested ways for school counselors and other clinicians to apply reality therapy to the classroom. Rather than assuming the role of expert or diagnostician, counselors engage in process or collaborative consultation with teachers, forming a partnership to identify and resolve problems. This sort of consultation is characterized by five steps: (1) becoming involved, (2) identifying wants, (3) identifying and evaluating the success of current behaviors, (4) making a plan, and (5) following up.

Glasser's WDEP model can be used to create a classroom environment in which students' basic five needs are met, and teachers are content. By minimizing fear and coercion, and focusing instead on the need for freedom, power, love and belonging, survival, and fun, students learn to develop an internal locus of control rather than seeking external sources of rewards. The teacher uses the principles of choice theory to develop a customized classroom environment in which students learn to monitor and motivate themselves. The focus is always on behavior and choice. Erwin (2004) writes that the choice school approach integrates with any planning approach or curriculum.

With growing educational applications of choice theory, and the continuing need for individual assessment and the development of appropriate interventions, Burns and colleagues (2006) developed the Student Needs Survey. The 25-item questionnaire assesses the five basic needs for physiological and psychological health (connection, freedom, fun, power, and security) to help document children's unmet needs and to help develop intervention plans for use in Quality Schools. Additional information on Quality Schools is available online at http://www.wgai.net.

Current Use of Reality Therapy

Reality therapy continues to have a strong following among mental health professionals. Glasser, Wubbolding, and others continue to lecture and write in support of their approach. In addition to its well-established use in schools and substance use treatment programs, reality therapy also is used in a broad range of other settings.

Particularly important in recent years are efforts to combine reality therapy with other approaches that will broaden and deepen its use. Examples include Schoo's (2008) use of a combination of choice theory and motivational interviewing with clients who are chronically ill; Fulkerson's (2003) integration of transactional analysis, psychoanalysis, and reality therapy to help families become aware of and change dysfunctional patterns; Pierce's (2003) development of mindfulness-based reality therapy, which integrates Buddhist philosophy and interventions such as relaxation and meditation with reality therapy; and Mottern's (2003) effort to combine choice therapy with a multicultural perspective based on Native American stories and viewpoints.

EVALUATION OF REALITY THERAPY

Like the other cognitive–behavioral approaches to treatment, reality therapy has a great deal to offer clients and clinicians. However, it also has limitations.

Limitations

Reality therapy has some important shortcomings that clinicians should bear in mind. It pays only limited attention to helping people understand and deal with their environments and minimizes the importance of the past in people's development and difficulties. As a result, reality therapists may overlook some of the barriers and experiences that limit people's choices, and they may focus too much on symptoms.

In addition, reality therapists' disregard of the importance of diagnosis is inconsistent with current professional guidelines. Equating mental illness with lack of knowledge about responsible ways to meet one's needs is highly questionable and may lead to inadequate treatment and neglect of important areas of concern. Many clinicians also disagree with Glasser's (1998a) doubts about the existence of repressed memories and the diagnosis of post-traumatic stress disorder.

In addition, reality therapy minimizes the value of psychotropic medication (Glasser 1998a, 2003). Glasser writes: "Good psychotherapy precludes the need for [brain] drugs" (1998a, p. 88). Glasser believes that medication is dangerous to people's health and undermines their ability to help themselves (Lennon, 2003).

The John Dewey Academy (JDA) in Great Barrington, Massachusetts, uses a learning-centered variation of reality-based therapy with angry adolescents, many of whom have previously been hospitalized for psychiatric disorders such as ADHD, conduct disorder, and self-destructive behavior (Bratter, 2010). No psychotropic medications are allowed, only education and compassionate, caring confrontation in a residential treatment setting. The study's authors write: "Personality and affective disorders are rarely cured by medicinal approaches. There is no pill that teaches self-respect and cures noxious narcissism, dishonesty and anti-social attitudes. Therefore we eschew the use of psychotropic medications at JDA and view drug-free as a viable treatment goal" (Bratter et al., 2008, p. 22). The study cites a 28% graduation rate, with 100% of those students going on to higher education. More research is needed to substantiate the effectiveness of this nontraditional treatment on dually diagnosed and self-destructive adolescents.

Although effectiveness research on choice theory has yet to support his claims, changes in our understanding of the dynamics of the brain have been in line with some of Glasser's beliefs. Specifically, neurological research during the past 20 years has revealed the neuroplasticity of the brain. That is, the brain is capable of changing across the life span and some portions can be regenerated. Social interactions and learning have been shown to contribute to those changes at a cellular level. Barber (2008) wrote, "Neuroplasticity supports the efficacy of old-fashioned psychotherapy. . . . Who would have thought neuroscience would show that psychotherapy is a robust treatment capable of working at a biological level?" (p. 198). In fact, those changes are not additive, but synergistic, with the interactions changing brain function, which in turn improves interactions (Barber, 2008; Kandel, 2008). No doubt the additional positive impacts of psychotherapy will continue to be documented as neurobiological research continues to evolve.

Strengths and Contributions

Nevertheless, reality therapy has many strengths. It is a clear, positive, straightforward approach to treatment that makes sense to most people. It is respectful, empowering, and encouraging and addresses fundamental issues in people's lives such as motivation, need satisfaction, and control. Reality therapists become involved with their clients in appropriate professional ways. Reality therapy's emphasis on the importance of both relationships and responsibility in people's lives is relevant and timely in light of prevalent problems of violence and family disruption. Also relevant is its emphasis on choice at a time when many people feel overcommitted and overprogrammed. In addition, reality therapy has a strong preventive component and offers sound and hopeful ideas for changes in schools and other institutions.

Research documents positive outcomes for reality therapy, particularly in schools and therapeutic communities (Wubbolding, 2007a). In addition, many published case studies describe the successful use of reality therapy with a variety of clients (Wubbolding, 2000). However, continued research is needed on the application of reality therapy to specific client groups so that clinicians have a clearer idea of its appropriate use.

Reality therapy has made important contributions to counseling and psychotherapy. It provides a clear and structured approach to treatment that is widely used in schools and rehabilitation programs. It emphasizes the importance of values in treatment and reminds clinicians not to neglect relationships and responsibility. Its appreciation and description of the collaborative therapeutic relationship have broadened the appropriate role of the clinician. It can be easily integrated with other treatment approaches, such as Gendlin's focusing technique, to create a powerful tool (Burdenski & Wubbolding, 2011). Finally, it focuses attention on the need to help people engage in honest self-evaluation and make wise and responsible choices and plans.

Wubbolding (2011) noted that Glasser's greatest contribution may be in developing a system (reality therapy) of mental health rather than a system to treat mental dysfunction.

SKILL DEVELOPMENT: CARING CONFRONTATION

Confrontation is a highly charged word that may seem incompatible with the supportive and encouraging role of the clinician. However, when done with care and sensitivity, confrontations can help people more honestly and accurately evaluate their behaviors, acquire a better grasp of reality, and act in more responsible ways.

Confrontation can be defined as the process of noting discrepancies, usually in a person's words and behaviors, and reflecting those discrepancies back to the person. Confrontation should never involve shaming, belittling, or attacking, and should not precipitate a debate between client and clinician about who is right.

A confrontation typically has three parts:

1. An introduction, which identifies the client statements, actions, or thoughts that prompted the intervention.

2. The body of the confrontation, which points out the issues or discrepancies. In keeping with reality therapy, this statement should be tentative, gentle, and respectful.
3. An invitation for the client to respond. Questions such as "What do you make of that?" and "Would you be willing to explore that with me?" usually are used. They prompt people to reflect and self-evaluate and are unlikely to lead them to feel judged. Questions also offer people the opportunity to choose not to discuss the confrontation or to disagree with the clinician. These responses suggest that the clinician probably should not pursue the topic at present. However, it has been mentioned and is likely to arise again.

Consider the following example of a caring confrontation:

CLINICIAN: Ronnie, several weeks ago, you told me that you and your fiancé are on a limited budget and are saving to buy a house. Today, you told me that you are buying a wedding gown that costs five thousand dollars. I wonder if buying the wedding gown will help you meet your need for your own home. Would you be willing to take a look at that with me?

The clinician has identified a discrepancy in the information that Ronnie has presented. This is reflected back to her in an unemotional and nonjudgmental way, with an invitation for Ronnie to explore this discrepancy.

Ronnie may respond in a variety of ways. She may have information that resolves the discrepancy: "I didn't tell you that my aunt gave me five thousand dollars specifically to buy a wedding dress." She may open the door to further clarification of her values and choices: "This is the most important event in my life, and I want it to be as special as possible." Or she may reflect on her choices and make a self-evaluation: "I never put those two pieces together. Maybe it isn't a good idea for me to spend so much on a dress that's only important for one day, but the house will mean something to us for years." Whether or not Ronnie sees the situation as her clinician does is not important; what does matter is that she has an opportunity to reflect on, clarify, evaluate, and possibly change her choices so that they better meet her needs. The exercises later in this chapter will give you an opportunity to develop some caring confrontations.

CASE ILLUSTRATION

Roberto consulted his therapist a few weeks before Thanksgiving because of family difficulties during the previous year's Thanksgiving holiday. His therapist applied the WDEP and SAMI^{2}C^3 formats in the context of reality therapy to help Roberto plan to make the holiday more rewarding this year.

ROBERTO: Thanksgiving last year was a disaster. I don't want a repeat of that.

CLINICIAN: What did you do?

ROBERTO: Well, I came home early on the day before Thanksgiving to have some extra time with Edie and Ava. I did have to bring some work home, and I wanted to get that done first, so I just said hello and headed over to the room where we have the computer. Before I know it, Edie flings the door open and is in my face about how I never help and am not really part of the family. I could not calm her down, so I just picked up my stuff and went back to the office. Who needs that! Of course, this spoiled Thanksgiving Day; Edie and I just glared at each other for most of the day.

CLINICIAN: So even though you came home early and were thinking of your family, somehow your actions backfired and wound up not meeting either your needs or your family's. When you think about the five basic needs that we have discussed, how do you evaluate your efforts?

ROBERTO: You know, I can see that my thoughts and actions were at cross-purposes. In coming home early, I was focused on my needs for love and fun; I really wanted to have a close, enjoyable time with my family. But I did not give them that message. When I went right to the computer, all Edie saw was me trying to meet my need for achievement. She didn't know I just had a little work to do and then was going to spend time with the family. I guess I really didn't try to see things from her perspective.

CLINICIAN: So you have some new thoughts about what happened last year. What are the needs you want to focus on this Thanksgiving?

ROBERTO: Definitely fun and love and belonging.

CLINICIAN: And what pictures do you have in your head about what that would look like?

ROBERTO: We would all get along. We'd all pitch in to cook dinner. We'd have some good food and good conversation. I'd make a fire in the fireplace. Then maybe we could do something fun like taking a walk or going to a movie.

CLINICIAN: Let's develop a plan to help you make those pictures real. We've reviewed the eight steps in the SAMI^{2}C^3 model for making successful plans: simple, attainable, measurable, immediate, involving, controlled, consistent, and committed. What plan comes into your mind?

ROBERTO: I could come home early again on the day before Thanksgiving but not bring any work home. I could ask Edie if she needs any help. And I could suggest something fun to do after Thanksgiving dinner.

CLINICIAN: How does that plan fit the criteria?

ROBERTO: It seems simple and attainable. I guess it's measurable; I can tell if I'm doing what I planned or not. I'm certainly committed to changing our holiday experience. But I'm not sure the plan is immediate; and I don't know how I could make it more involving, controlled by me, or consistent.

CLINICIAN: So you've made a start at planning, but how could you modify the plan so that it meets more of the criteria?

ROBERTO: I could make it immediate by starting right now. I'll write down the plan and tell Edie about it when I get home. I could even ask her now if there are ways I could help, like shopping or cleaning the house. If I offer specific ways to help, I have more control over the plan, and I'm taking more initiative. Edie complains that I leave everything at home up to her, so taking the initiative seems like a good idea.

CLINICIAN: So you see ways to make the plan more immediate and consistent as well as more under your control. Are there ways I could be involved in helping you?

ROBERTO: Maybe you could touch base with me sometime during the week to help me stay on track. I really want to, but sometimes I get so caught up with work . . . .

CLINICIAN: How about if I telephone you on Tuesday to see how things are going?

ROBERTO: That would be great.

CLINICIAN: Now let's look at the plan again to evaluate how well it promises to fulfill your needs and wants in realistic and responsible ways. Then you can write down the specifics.

EXERCISES

Large-Group Exercises

1. Although reality therapy has many strengths, it also presents some potential pitfalls, notably the risks that clinicians will ignore important diagnostic information and will fail to refer clients for medication when research suggests that is necessary to treat their difficulties. Discuss the potential negative impact of these risks on the treatment process and then develop ways to minimize those risks while practicing reality therapy.
2. Reality therapy takes the stance that nearly all aspects of people's lives are under their control. Discuss whether this belief is realistic and responsible, especially as applied to people in groups who often have experienced discrimination such as African Americans, people with visible disabilities, and people who are gay, lesbian, bisexual, or transgendered. In what ways is this stance likely to be helpful to people? Hurtful to them?
3. Review the Case Illustration in this chapter. Identify in the dialogue the elements of the WDEP and $SAMI^2C^3$ formats.

Small-Group Exercises

1. Divide into your groups of four, composed of two dyads. Each dyad should engage in a 15-minute, role-played counseling interview in which the person playing the client presents a behavior he or she would like to change and the person in the clinician role uses the $SAMI^2C^3$ format to facilitate development of a plan to effect change. Feedback should focus on the use of the $SAMI^2C^3$ format as well as overall strengths and areas needing improvement in the role-play.
2. Divide into your groups of four, composed of two dyads. Each dyad should engage in a 15-minute, role-played counseling interview in which the person in the clinician role helps the client discuss the balance of his or her five basic needs and identify at least one important way in which he or she is fulfilling each of the five needs. Feedback should focus on how well the clinician helped the client to explore balance and implementation of the five basic needs as well as overall strengths and areas needing improvement in the role-play.
3. In your small groups, develop caring confrontations in response to the following client statements. Your statements should reflect the format for caring confrontations presented in the Skill Development section. Each group member should write out his or her responses individually before discussing and refining them in the group. Evaluate the responses in terms of whether they are likely to facilitate client awareness and self-evaluation without sounding judgmental or negative.

   Client A: My coworkers have been giving me grief because I get to work late. They say they need my input on our project each morning. They don't understand that I'm a night person. I like to stay up late, and it's hard for me to get up in the morning. My job is important to me, but I don't think it should matter so much when I get there.

   Client B: My mother is just impossible. You know, she's nearly 80 years old and really can't live alone anymore. I offered to come up and help her move into one of those continuing care places. I suppose they're all awful, smelly and depressing . . . I've never been inside one . . .

but what choice does she have? So, no, she doesn't want to do that. She didn't say it, but I bet she wants to move in with me.

Client C: I can't believe what my stepfather did. When I was out, he went through my backpack and found some drugs I had in there. I told him I was just keeping the stuff for a friend; but of course, he didn't buy that. Now he's saying I need to go into a drug rehab program. What does he think I am . . . a drug addict? I just smoke some marijuana once in a while. At least I don't go nosing around in people's personal possessions.

Client D: My supervisor said some things that upset me. She said that people who get public assistance are "ripping off the government" and "taking advantage of the middle class" and "getting a free ride." She doesn't know that I had to go on public assistance when my husband left me with three young children. She's so wrong about what it's like. I wish I could straighten her out; but if I tell her about my background, she'll just write me off as one of those "welfare cheats." She's usually caring and understanding, so I know she didn't mean to hurt me. I'll just keep quiet about my reaction.

Individual Exercises

1. Identify a positive addiction that you would like to make part of your life. Write out a plan, following the $SAMI^2C^3$ format, to establish that positive behavior in your life.
2. Reality therapy stresses the key role that relationships play in both people's happiness and their misery. Write one or two pages in your journal about ways in which relationships have had an impact on your feelings of well-being. Then identify two small and specific changes you would like to make in the way you relate to others. Write them down and consider making a commitment to implementing those changes.
3. Draw a picture of the images in your quality world. Write a paragraph about what your drawing represents and means to you.

Summary

Reality therapy, initiated by William Glasser in the 1960s and developed primarily by Glasser and Robert Wubbolding, is an optimistic and encouraging treatment approach. It focuses on present thoughts and behaviors and helps people meet their basic needs more successfully by making better choices. Responsibility (fulfilling one's own needs in ways that respect other people's rights to meet their needs) is key to this approach as are positive relationships. Clinicians play an active and involved role, promoting client self-evaluation and realistic and viable planning. Glasser (2003) summed up the essence of reality therapy: "Accepting that everything you do is a choice is a cornerstone of mental health" (p. 50).

Recommended Readings

Ellsworth, L. (2007). *Choosing to heal: Using reality therapy in treatment with sexually abused children.* New York, NY: Routledge.

Erwin, J. C. (2004). *The classroom of choice: Giving students what they need and getting what you want.* Alexandria, VA: Association for Supervision and Curriculum Development.

Glasser, W. (1965). *Reality therapy.* New York, NY: Harper & Row.

Glasser, W. (1986). *Control theory in the classroom*. New York, NY: Harper & Row.

Glasser, W. (2000). *Counseling with choice theory*. New York, NY: HarperCollins.

Glasser, W., & Glasser, C. (2007). *Eight lessons for a happier marriage*. New York, NY: HarperCollins.

Wubbolding, R. E. (1991). *Understanding reality therapy*. New York, NY: HarperCollins.

Wubbolding, R. E. (2009). *Reality therapy training manual* (15th rev.). Cincinnati, OH: Center for Reality Therapy.

Additional Sources of Information

http://www.wglasser.com—The William Glasser Institute, founded in 1967, offers training, certification, and resources on reality therapy, as well as information and consultation on the Quality School Model.

http://www.realitytherapy.org.uk—The Institute for Reality Therapy UK offers training in choice theory, reality therapy, and the Quality School Program in the United Kingdom.

http://www.wgai.net—William Glasser Association International provides an international conference, training programs, and a list of Quality Schools.

http://www.journalofrealitytherapy.com—Information on the *International Journal of Reality Therapy* can be found at this website.

http://www.realitytherapywub.com—This is Robert Wubbolding's website.

CHAPTER 18

Family Systems Approaches

Family. The word itself conjures up all types of memories, feelings, and thoughts. We are influenced tremendously by our families of origin. From the time we are born, we begin to develop early attachments to our primary caregivers. Even as we grow and become independent, the need for connection and attachment to others continues. Our families shape us, influence our development, and model appropriate or inappropriate behavior. It is only within the context of the larger family system that the individual can be fully understood.

Family therapy, its history and development, is the focus of this chapter. We begin with an overview of general systems theory before moving to a discussion of specific family systems theories. Family therapy is often indicated for problems with family dynamics, communication, or to adjust to transitions, loss, or illness. The changing nature of families can also be a source of stress. As of 2010, 4.4 million U.S. homes held three generations or more under one roof, a 15% increase from 2008 (U.S. Bureau of Labor Statistics, 2012). Given the increase in the number of families experiencing economic difficulties, behavioral therapy with couples, families, and children is expected to increase.

The Skill Development section at the end of the chapter is based on Monica McGoldrick's work diagramming the family system through the use of genograms. The information, examples, and exercises in this chapter will introduce you to some of the skills that are essential in helping clinicians work with couples and families. Readers should keep in mind that the goal of this chapter is to provide a survey, an overview, of the breadth of theories related to the BETA format. An in-depth discussion of the topic would require several semesters of course work. Therefore, readers are encouraged to review related chapters for applicable background information on theories and theorists and refer to the suggested readings and resources at the end of this chapter if you are interested in more details about the theories or techniques discussed here.

OVERVIEW OF FAMILY SYSTEMS THEORY

Most families seeking therapy need help in finding a solution to a problem the family is experiencing. Single-parent, blended, multigenerational, and multinuclear families present unique concerns to be addressed. All family therapy, regardless of structure or theoretical orientation, is:

- Brief
- Solution focused (or crisis focused)
- Action oriented
- Focused on here-and-now interactions among family members
- Focused on how the family creates, contributes to, and continues the problem.

As with all types of counseling and psychotherapy, therapists who work with families must first begin by creating a therapeutic alliance. The relationship between the therapist and the family members begins even before the first session, with the very first telephone call or contact with the family. A challenge for family and couples therapists is to be constantly aware of who they are aligning themselves with to ensure the creation of an equal alliance with each family member. This requires vigilance on the part of the therapist to recognize any ruptures in the alliance that need mending.

Therapists who work with couples and families take on many different roles: coach, consultant, model, teacher, or collaborator who works with the family to facilitate change. Certainly there are times, however, when the family therapist must also be the expert, especially when establishing behavior modification plans for children or when prescribing particular interventions. In postmodern family therapies, such as solution-focused brief family therapy and narrative therapy, the therapist is decidedly a nonexpert. The therapist views problems as distressing to the family and, therefore, helps the family eradicate them by working collaboratively to find solutions to the problems.

Family therapists address many of the same ethical issues as individual or group therapists. However, many more issues arise when a therapist works out of a systemic perspective. Therapists are reminded that they may not ethically practice in areas in which they have not been trained and supervised. Additional specifications are contained in the ethical guidelines of the American Association for Marriage and Family Therapy (http://www.aamft.org) and in the ethical codes of each of the major counseling and psychological organizations.

DEVELOPMENT OF FAMILY SYSTEMS THEORY

Individual therapy puts the person in the limelight while the influence of the family recedes into the background. In the family systems perspective, the family is in the limelight and individuals are seen as subunits, or parts of the whole.

General systems theory was first proposed by Ludwig von Bertalanffy in the 1920s, and later adopted by family therapists. The biologist created a theory that provided one holistic organizational system for understanding living organisms and social groups (von Bertalanffy, 1968/1976). Within this framework he found that general system laws apply to any type of system, that each organism is an open system that experiences continuous input and output, and that a system can be defined by the interrelationships among the subunits. Each participating unit not only contributes to the whole, but also has an effect on the other participating units. Thus, to understand how a system works, we must first understand the interactional process that takes place between each of its subunits.

In the family system, each person is a part of multiple subsystems, all of which interact in various ways. For instance, in our example family of Roberto, Edie, and Ava, Edie is a wife and partner to Roberto, a mother to Ava, and a daughter to her mother and stepfather. We can consider Edie to be a member of four independent and functioning subsystems. She is a participant in the partner subsystem, the parent subsystem, the child subsystem, and even the subsystem of women in the family. Each of these subsystems functions autonomously (as when Edie and Roberto, working from the parental subsystem, establish and enforce bedtime rules for their daughter Ava), and yet is also a part of the overall interactional system.

General systems theory provided a new and holistic way of thinking. Rather than viewing organizations on a linear progression, von Bertalanffy's theory described a type of circular causality in which each of the interactions between the component parts has an effect on the other. Putting it in terms of an equation, it is not A causes B and B causes C and C causes D and so on in a linear progression. Rather "A does not cause B, nor does B cause A; both cause each other" (Goldenberg & Goldenberg, 2008, p. 18) in circular causality. In this manner, every subunit of a system has an impact on, and is impacted by, the other subunits. Additionally, patterns form and persist over time as parts of a process as well as a structure.

Von Bertalanffy's theory illustrates that nothing and no one exists in isolation. For example, the family member with bipolar disorder not only affects family functioning, but is also impacted by the family's reaction to the effect bipolar disorder has on the family member. From a family systems perspective, dysfunction is not considered to be pathology that occurred to one individual within a family, but the result of various dysfunctions that were both cause and effect of the current situation. If no one and nothing exists in isolation, then the boundaries of pathology become blurred beyond the point of recognition. In family systems theory, the focus is on multiple causality at all different levels. The focus has shifted away from a study of the mind of the individual to a focus on the behavioral consequences of interpersonal relationships.

HISTORY OF FAMILY THERAPY

Marital counseling and child guidance were practiced for decades before family therapy was born. In 1929, the Marriage Consultation Center was opened in New York City, and in 1941, the American Association of Marriage Counselors was formed. AAMC changed its name in the 1970s to the American Association of Marriage and Family Counselors, in recognition of the growth of family therapy.

Most marriage counseling is brief, solution focused, and sought in response to a crisis such as an increase in frequency or level of arguments, marital infidelity, threat of divorce, or serious disagreements over child rearing, money, sexual frequency, ineffective communication patterns, power, and control. Indeed, more people report seeking counseling for problems within their marriage than for any other reason.

Conjoint family therapy first occurred after World War II as a result of the increased need for family therapy. Much of the early research and development was in the area of helping families who had a member with severe mental illness such as schizophrenia (Lebow, 2008). In the 20 years marked by 1950 to 1970, most of the major theoretical orientations in psychology developed a family-focused component. Through the pioneering work of Murray Bowen, Jay Haley, Virginia Satir, Carl Whitaker, Salvador Minuchin, and others, each of these early family theories incorporated general systems theory as well as first-order cybernetics—looking at the communication patterns and feedback loops within the family system from an outside perspective.

In the past two decades, newer types of family therapies have emerged that address what was lacking in previous theories. The influence of postmodern thought can be seen in the development of constructivist and narrative approaches; second-order cybernetics; cultural, sexual orientation, and gender-sensitive theories; and eclectic and integrated approaches to family therapy. Research has also emerged to support the effectiveness of marital and family therapy in general, as well as the improved efficiency of specific approaches to particular family-related problems (such as emotionally focused therapy for couples and cognitive–behavioral family therapy). The past 20 years have also seen the emergence of couples therapy as a separate entity from family therapy. Throughout this book we have followed the BETA format, and we will continue that structure as we examine how background, emotions, thoughts, and actions impact the family system.

FAMILY THERAPIES THAT FOCUS ON BACKGROUND

Adlerian Family Therapy

Alfred Adler was the first psychoanalyst to adopt a holistic view that considered the importance of family relationships in the creation of the individual. By 1922, Adler was involving the entire family in the counseling process. In later years, he helped to create child guidance clinics where teachers, parents, and schools worked together to help children develop better self-esteem, overcome feelings of inferiority, and create more positive child development processes.

Adlerian constructs such as birth order, sibling rivalry, inferiority, and social interest implied that the individual could only be understood in relation to the whole. Adler's holistic approach introduced the following concepts to psychotherapy, which had, until that time, been largely influenced by Freud's theories of drives:

- The effect of the family constellation on individual and family functioning
- The idea that people must be viewed in their family, social, and cultural contexts
- The importance of establishing a collaborative therapeutic alliance
- A positive focus that emphasizes strengths, encouragement, empowerment, and support

- A focus away from pathology (i.e., problems are a normal part of life that provide opportunities for growth)
- Psychoeducation as part of the therapeutic process.

APPLICATION TO CHILDREN Adler's Individual Psychology (see Chapter 4) is well suited for use with children and has been adopted by many school counselors as well as clinicians who treat children. Adler's approach offers counselors a flexible yet structured approach that lends itself well to treatment of both immediate and long-standing concerns of young people. His emphasis on cooperation, character building, and development of self-esteem (overcoming inferiority, according to Adler) is compatible with current emphases in the treatment of children and adolescents.

Nicoll (1994) developed classroom guidance programs based on Adler's theories. Nicoll proposed the following five-stage model for classroom use:

- Increase awareness and appreciation of individual differences.
- Teach about the range of human emotions, promote awareness of our own feelings, clarify the impact our actions have on other people's feelings, and encourage the development of empathy.
- Foster good communication skills.
- Promote cooperation and collaboration skills.
- Encourage responsibility and use natural consequences.

Rudolf Dreikurs, a therapist and writer, spread awareness of Adler's ideas among educators and parents. Dreikurs drew on Adler's ideas in his writings on effective parenting. *Children: The Challenge* (Dreikurs & Soltz, 1991) and *Discipline Without Tears* (Dreikurs, Cassell, & Ferguson, 2004), originally published in 1972, have become classics and are still used in parenting classes. Dreikurs suggested that children's misbehavior is a reflection of their goals and lifestyle. All behavior has a purpose, and he identified four possible motives behind childhood misbehavior (Dreikurs et al., 2004):

- Attention getting
- Power
- Revenge
- Withdrawal (displays of inadequacy).

Teachers and parents typically have negative responses to these behaviors. However, their automatic reactions often reinforce an undesirable behavior. For example, they may engage in a power struggle with the child who wants to be in charge or may reprimand an attention-seeking child, inadvertently providing the desired attention. Dreikurs suggested that, by understanding the goal of a child's misbehavior, people can address it more successfully. For example, teachers and parents should attend to and reinforce only the positive behaviors of an attention-seeking child and acknowledge the power of a child who wants to be in charge, encouraging cooperation and responsibility as part of his or her leadership role.

Adlerian play therapy is yet another extension of Adler's work. According to Menassa (2009), its purpose is to build relationships with children that "(a) enhance their social interest; (b) overcome or reduce their feelings of inferiority; and (c) make changes in their life goals and mistaken beliefs about self, others, and the world" (p. 22). Adlerian play therapists use a four-stage process that includes (1) relationship building and exploration; (2) lifestyle assessment to gather information; (3) insight; and (4) reorientation to help the child make positive changes in thoughts, feelings, and behavior. Specific interventions include:

- Encouragement
- Play and stories used as therapeutic metaphors
- Limit setting
- Analysis of early recollections and lifestyle
- Discussion of family constellation and atmosphere
- Verbal tracking
- Sharing of hypotheses to promote self-awareness
- Teaching new behaviors.

APPLICATION TO PARENTING Adler's ideas, especially as interpreted by Dreikurs, Dinkmeyer, and others, can provide a solid foundation for teaching parenting skills, improving family functioning, and helping parents to raise healthy children. Dreikurs had a vision of families that emphasized communication, respect, encouragement, teaching, the use of natural and logical consequences, and the expectation that children should assume age-appropriate responsibilities. He also recognized the importance of families having fun together, an aspect of family life often forgotten in our busy society. Dreikurs advocated the use of a family council in which all family members convene at the same time each week to talk about their family and address any concerns or difficulties. Even young children should be involved in these meetings and should have the opportunity to express themselves. This fosters a sense of belonging, responsibility, cooperation, and participation. It also teaches children to solve problems in relation to the whole family and not just the individual, which is consistent with the Adlerian focus on social interest (Shifron, 2010). For a child, improving the family connection and feelings of belonging can also reduce feelings of inferiority.

Several structured parent education programs, including Active Parenting and Systematic Training for Effective Parenting (STEP), evolved from Adler's ideas. Developed by Dinkmeyer and McKay (1997), the STEP system offers guidelines on motivating, disciplining, understanding, communicating with, and encouraging children. This educational program emphasizes the use of natural and reasonable consequences, teaches reflective listening, and presents tools to promote better understanding of children.

Adlerian family therapy is a positive, empowering approach for working with children and their families. Parent training programs continue to be popular and are taught at schools and other locations across the country.

Interest in Adlerian family and couples therapy continues to grow. Research on the application of Adlerian therapy to children, classroom management, behavioral and substance abuse problems in adolescence, in marriage counseling, and across cultural, socioeconomic, sexual orientation, and genders is frequently published in the *Journal of Individual Psychology* and other professional journals (Curlette & Kern, 2010). It also lends itself to integration with other types of therapies (Carlson & Robey, 2011) and can be adapted as a resilience-focused brief family therapy (Nicoll, 2007).

Multigenerational Family Therapy

In the 1940s, Murray Bowen was among the first to combine psychoanalysis with systems theory. Bowen conceptualized the family as "an emotional unit, a network of interlocking relationships best understood when analyzed within a multigenerational or historical framework" (Goldenberg & Goldenberg, 2008, p. 175). Bowen's approach provided a bridge between psychodynamic approaches that focused on the individual and the development of family systems theory with its emphasis on the family unit as a whole.

Over the course of his lifetime, Bowen created the first comprehensive theory of family development. His theory includes new language to explain complex family interactions (e.g., emotional cutoff, multigenerational transmission process, differentiation of self), as well as a deliberate and systematic method of treatment. Following years of clinical experience and research, Bowen established the Georgetown University Family Center where he taught his multigenerational theory for 30 years. Later work by his former student Monica McGoldrick expanded family therapy across gender and cultural domains (McGoldrick, Giordano, & Garcia-Preto, 2005; McGoldrick & Hardy, 2008), and expanded Bowen's work on multigenerational genograms into several comprehensive volumes (McGoldrick, 1998; McGoldrick, Gerson, & Petry, 2008). More will be said about genograms in the Skill Development section at the end of this chapter.

DEVELOPMENT OF MULTIGENERATIONAL FAMILY THERAPY Murray Bowen was born in 1913 and raised in Tennessee. He was the oldest of five children. After medical school, he became a psychiatrist specializing in childhood schizophrenia and began applying Freudian principles to the treatment of severe mental illness. Bowen worked at the Meninger Clinic and later at the National Institute of Mental Health where he conducted research on his theory of treating family members together rather than individually. In 1959, he moved to Georgetown University where he worked until his death in 1990. He was the founder and first president of the American Family Therapy Association.

IMPORTANT THEORETICAL CONCEPTS Theory and practice in Bowenian family therapy are intertwined. Bowen was a psychiatrist who was psychodynamically trained. He believed that theory provided the frame for working with families and children, and was confident that if the theory was strong enough, it could stand alone without the need for techniques. To Bowen, not only was the nuclear family important, but the extended family also provided a rich source of background, values, culture, and emotional systems that is passed from generation to generation.

Bowen developed eight key concepts to explain the emotional relationship system within the family. Each of these concepts is described briefly below. For a more detailed discussion, see Bowen's *Family Therapy in Clinical Practice* (1978):

1. ***Differentiation of self.*** Bowen's concept of differentiation of self has been credited by some as being the personality variable most critical to mature development and psychological health (Licht & Chabot, 2006). The balance between appropriate connectedness to others and autonomous functioning is the key to psychological health. Those who are able to distinguish between feeling and thinking function at a higher level. Separating emotions from reason results in differentiation, or a person's ability to work through his or her own emotional and rational processes to make decisions. The opposite of differentiation is fusion, in which emotions tend to rule a person's decision making. The more differentiated a person is, the higher that person's level of functioning. A fully differentiated person is able to use both thoughts and emotions in determining his or her own best course of action.
2. ***Triangulation.*** Triangulation results when uncontrolled anxiety between any two members in the family system causes one person to team up with a third family member. The two people unite and blame the third person for the family dysfunction. This alignment with another person relieves individual anxiety, but the resulting triangulation ultimately causes problems in the family system.
3. ***Nuclear family emotional system.*** Bowen believed that the nuclear family emotional system was a multigenerational phenomenon that included not only the nuclear family that physically lived together, but also the effect of the extended family regardless of where family members reside or even if they are living or dead. In Bowenian theory, the only way to resolve current family problems is to differentiate from the family of origin and change interactional patterns.

Diffusion results when boundaries develop and individual family members can think in terms of "I" rather than "we." The greater the stress, the more likely the family is to fuse to seek security. Dysfunction and pathology result when individuals are unable to differentiate themselves from their family (Bowen, 1976, 1978).

4. ***Family projection process.*** Within the mother–father–child triangle, parents have a tendency to select the most vulnerable child, the one who has the least differentiation of self and the most fusion with one of the parents, to project their own problems onto. The undifferentiated parent is often the mother. For example, the child responds to the mother's anxiety and becomes anxious himself. The mother, being the primary caregiver, responds to the child's anxiety and the father (providing the third side of the triangle) becomes supportive of the mother in efforts to deal with the child. The child then becomes identified as having the problem, the triangle is established, and the family projection process has been created.
5. ***Emotional cutoff.*** One or more of the children in a family, especially those who are least involved in the family projection process, are likely to escape from the family dysfunction by putting geographic or emotional distance between themselves and their families. Bowen noted that such a cutoff is a person's attempt to deny attachments and unresolved conflicts that exist. Kerr (1981) wrote that an emotional cutoff reflects a problem (unresolved fusion), solves a problem (reduces anxiety by limiting contact), and creates a problem (isolates family members). Subsequent contact with family members may be perfunctory and brief. Cutoffs tend to occur in families in which a high level of anxiety and dependence is present (Bowen, 1978). In Bowenian family systems theory, genograms are an important tool in helping to identify intergenerational family patterns such as cutoffs and fusion, and helping to prevent them from affecting the next generation (McGoldrick et al., 2008).

   Bowen believed that where cutoffs existed, work needed to be done to mend emotional attachments to the family of origin. Clients were frequently sent back to their family of origin to observe and work on their own differentiation of self. Bowen also believed that all family therapists needed to work out their emotional ties to their own family of origin prior to working with clients. He believed such work was necessary so that the therapist's own family issues did not seep into the therapist's work with a family.
6. ***Multigenerational transmission process.*** Newly formed nuclear families unconsciously repeat the behavior patterns of their parents. In Bowen's multigenerational model, basic patterns are passed down through modeled behavior and family assumptions about gender roles, finances, family responsibility, work ethics, coping skills, and ways of dealing with stress. In this way, family systems become models of expectations and form replicas of past generations. People either try to emulate their family of origin or do the opposite—even choosing a partner who is similar to, or decidedly different from, their opposite sex parent. Bowen believed it was only through an awareness of this multigenerational transmission process that clinicians could truly understand the family system and the individual. How families cope with stress and anxiety is a key consideration. If the stress level is high, several patterns are likely to reoccur based on how previous generations handled stress.
7. ***Sibling position.*** Like Adler, Bowen believed birth order shaped a person's future relationships. Specifically, children develop certain traits based on their relationship within the family. For example, a woman who was the oldest child would be more suited to marrying a man who had an older sister. Affiliated with sibling position are certain assumptions and interactive patterns that are learned in the family of origin.
8. ***Societal regression.*** Bowen added the concept of societal regression to his later work, thus the concept is less well developed and integrated into his theory. Basically, societal regression means that problems of differentiation and individuation are reflected in society as a

whole. Under conditions of chronic stress (e.g., economic, societal), society as a whole reacts the same way that individual families would—experiencing more anxiety, regression, and less differentiation between the intellect and emotion.

GOALS The goal in Bowenian family therapy is to reduce anxiety, increase differentiation of the self, and establish healthy emotional boundaries between family members. This can only come about through an understanding of how the family system, going back through several generations, has influenced the current family dynamics.

TREATMENT PROCESS Bowenian therapy is a process that looks at patterns, especially as they relate to emotion, structure, and triangulation. During the assessment stage of treatment, a genogram of at least three generations of a client's family tree is constructed. The genogram delineates structural relationships (marriages, births, deaths) and emotional relationships (fusion, cutoffs, triangulation) in conjunction with the family. The genogram serves as a tracking tool throughout the therapy process and provides an outline of family interactional patterns. The genogram also illuminates patterns such as substance abuse, depression, physical or emotional abuse, and other patterns in behavior, relationships, and family structure that are transmitted from generation to generation (McGoldrick et al., 2008). Figure 18.1 is a genogram of the Diaz family. Genograms are discussed in greater detail in the Skill Development section at the end of this chapter.

Bowen did not necessarily involve children in the therapy process; he believed that parents were responsible for their children's problems. Instead, Bowen preferred to work with parents on their own self-differentiation with the hope that those efforts would trickle down into increased insight and reduced anxiety in the family as a whole (Becvar & Becvar, 2006). Bowen worked with the parents conjointly and asked them to accept his premise that the basic problem in the family was between the two of them. He would then help the couple to improve their insight on self-differentiation and detriangulation—always taking care, of course, not to be drawn into the triangle himself.

Through therapist coaching, couples gradually become diffused. Their new interactional patterns have positive effects on other family members until a new equilibrium is reached. This might require as few as 5 to 10 sessions for some families, and as many as 20 to 40 sessions in others

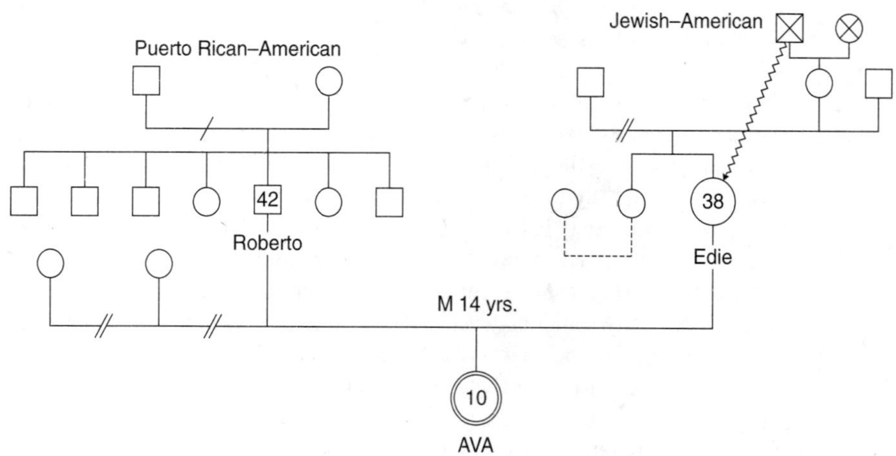

FIGURE 18.1 Genogram of the Diaz Family.

(Goldenberg & Goldenberg, 2012). Sometimes only one member of the couple, usually the most differentiated, would be seen in therapy for a period of time until the person was sufficiently differentiated for the couple to be able to work together as a team to address dysfunction in the family and begin to function more cognitively and less emotionally.

THERAPEUTIC ALLIANCE In Bowenian systems theory, the therapist remains objective and takes a neutral stance. The therapist does not join with the family but, rather, remains differentiated and curious about patterns, beliefs, and assumptions that led the family to its particular problem or dysfunction. The therapist serves as a catalyst to help families gain insight into the impact of multigenerational influences.

Bowen believed that before clinicians can help families differentiate, they must first address their own family dynamics. Therefore, training in this method involves extensive personal work so that the therapist becomes fully differentiated (Lebow, 2008). Within sessions, therapists avoid becoming triangulated with the families, and model calm impartiality instead.

LIMITATIONS As with other psychoanalytic theories, Bowenian therapy can be lengthy, time consuming, and costly, and may not be practical. It shows a cultural gender bias by valuing reason and rationality—a commonly accepted male trait—over emotion, a traditionally female trait. In Bowenian theory, mothers are frequently viewed as overly involved, while fathers are often absent. Families in crisis may have more immediate needs that must be attended to before delving into past patterns of behavior.

CURRENT STATUS Bowenian therapy should be considered in the broader scope of relational work. Recent research on differentiation of self seems to indicate that people are likely to select partners with similar levels of differentiation, and that levels of differentiation may impact the quality of the relationship as well as expectations about family life (Spencer & Brown, 2007). The theory also has implications for work with aging families, caregivers, and adult children (Piercy, 2010). One recent longitudinal study of 50 nuclear families found that higher functioning nuclear families had more balance and pursued more goals (Klever, 2009). The theory is also culturally inclusive. McGoldrick and colleagues' (2008) work on culture and gender has added much to Bowen's original theory.

Structural Family Therapy

Structural family therapy, developed by Salvador Minuchin, was the dominant form of family therapy in the 1970s (Becvar & Becvar, 2006). Structural family therapy is based on general systems theory. Organizational structures, rules, and communication and behavior among family members are the focus of clinical attention.

DEVELOPMENT OF STRUCTURAL FAMILY THERAPY Born and raised in Argentina, Salvador Minuchin began his career as a family therapist in the early 1960s. In his classic text, *Families and Family Therapy* (1974), Minuchin identified family subsystems with boundaries that were often invisible to family members. Minuchin specified two patterns that are common to troubled families: some become enmeshed, chaotic, and tightly interconnected, whereas others remain disengaged, isolated, and seemingly unrelated.

IMPORTANT THEORETICAL CONCEPTS Every family consists of multiple subsystems. By recognizing and identifying how the family is organized, the therapist becomes familiar with how the family functions as a whole. Boundaries between the family subsystems are delineated, and diagrams or family maps are sometimes drawn to illustrate the family structure. The main concepts of structural family therapy as described by Minuchin are discussed next.

Subsystems. Three subsystems are of particular interest to structural family therapists: parental (those who are responsible for the children), spousal (may be different than parental), and sibling (all related children). Generally, the spousal subsystem is the first to develop. It is composed of the original partners. How these two people support each other impacts the way in which the family is structured and how well it will function. Once children come along, a parental subsystem develops based on those responsible for the care and raising of the children. A healthy and cohesive parental subsystem is necessary for the development of a functioning family system, yet the parental subsystem must be flexible enough to change as the children's needs change. As a team, parents define appropriate boundaries that distinguish among subsystems but do not cause enmeshment, disenfranchisement, or inappropriate cross-generational interactions. These terms are discussed in more detail below.

Minuchin believes that membership in one subsystem should not interfere with membership in another. For example, the intimacy of a husband and wife should not interfere with their ability to parent their children.

Boundaries between systems. Boundaries provide a way to look at who is involved in each subsystem. Boundaries exist on a continuum from rigid to loose. Rigid boundaries result in disengagement of family members, whereas extremely loose, permeable boundaries are likely to lead to a lack of any boundaries at all, or what Minuchin refers to as enmeshment. Structural family therapy works to move families away from either extreme and toward more flexible boundaries that function effectively within the family.

Family boundaries change over time depending on environment, culture, developmental stages, and relationship styles (Rigazio-DiGilio & McDowell, 2008). Boundaries are unhealthy when they become too rigid or exclude particular family members. For example, if the two older sisters in a family form a coalition that continually excludes their 4-year-old brother, the child who is left out may begin to expect the mother to provide more time for activity and comfort. This may in turn put more stress on the mother who is already busy taking care of a newborn baby. The result is disruption and a negative impact on the functioning of the entire family system.

Family hierarchy. Each family has a hierarchy that determines power and control within the family. Questions of how decisions are made, what role each family member plays, and where authority and status reside all contribute to the family hierarchy. In some families the mother is the ultimate arbiter of decisions; in others decisions may be made by both parents, the grandparents, or the father. Different hierarchies exist in different families; as long as they are fulfilling the needs of all family members and are clearly delineated, the family's hierarchy can work well. Problems arise, however, when families develop alliances and coalitions. Alliances that form across generations can be especially problematic. Structural family therapists identify alliances, coalitions, and triangulation in families and work toward creating functional alliances (e.g., mother and father supporting each other) that are also flexible and allow for a range of interactions within the family.

A coalition between a parent and a child can result in a parentified child—one who is given responsibilities within the family that are inconsistent with the child's role or age (Minuchin, 1974). However, coalitions are not always unhealthy. A coalition can be helpful if its formation leads to treatment, as when several family members form a coalition to help a son with a substance abuse problem.

TREATMENT PROCESS The goal of structural family therapy is to restructure the family transactional system so that more effective and healthy interactions are established among family members, and the family as a whole becomes better able to cope with stress. In treatment, the family's hierarchy is established, appropriate boundaries between subsystems are delineated, and outgrown rules are brought up to date to reflect the family's current development. For structural family therapists, the easiest way to improve dysfunctional family behavior and improve symptoms is to eliminate or change the family's transactional patterns that maintain the dysfunctional behaviors (Goldenberg & Goldenberg, 2008).

The process of change consists of three phases as outlined by Minuchin (1974). In the first phase, the therapist joins with the family and assumes a leadership position. In the second phase the therapist determines the family's structure, and in the third phase the therapist works to change that structure. Toward that end, structural family therapists use multiple techniques, alone or sequentially, either to form a therapeutic system (as in joining) or to disrupt the current system and facilitate change. We look at some of these techniques next.

Joining. Minuchin (1974) describes how he sometimes becomes like a distant uncle, and joins with the family system by accommodating to the family's style, using their language and terminology, respectfully joining with them in their myths and stories, and adopting their affective style (if they are demonstrative, he becomes demonstrative, too; if detached, he remains aloof). As the therapist blends into the family, the hierarchy, boundaries, and coalitions become apparent. Through the joining process, the structure of the family system is revealed to the therapist.

Reframing. Reframing places the original event or situation into a different context. The goal is to relabel the event, giving it a more positive slant. Reframing is used to change family perceptions and, as a result, provide more options and explanations based on a new way of looking at the situation.

Enactment. Through the process of enactment, the therapist brings an issue of family conflict into the here and now of the therapy session so that hierarchies and family dynamics can be mapped and alternative transactional patterns can be introduced. By reenacting a problem, family members learn that the problem is not the fault of the individual, but of the entire family system that continues to perpetuate the same behaviors.

Family maps. Structural family therapists use family mapping as a tool to illustrate the family relationships listed above. Maps, similar to genograms, visually represent family subsystems, boundaries, hierarchies, and alliances. Maps can also be used to set goals and to assess the progress of counseling.

EVALUATION Structural family therapy has been found helpful in a variety of settings and with different family problems. Minuchin has applied structural family therapy in his work with families with anorexia, diabetes, asthma, and other chronic disorders (Minuchin, Rosman, & Baker, 1978).

Structural family therapy is open to family structures that differ from the traditional model. Minuchin recognized that a family does not always consist of the traditional two parents and their biological children. He believes that holding all families up to this model is harmful. Families may be one-parent families, gay or lesbian families, step-parent and blended families, or three-generation families. Families, regardless of their makeup, go through change; Minuchin believes the role of the therapist should be to help families through the inevitable transitions and stressors that come along.

FAMILY THERAPIES THAT FOCUS ON EMOTIONS

Experiential family therapy grew out of the humanistic-existential tradition and incorporates elements of person-centered, Gestalt, and process-experiential theories that emphasize affect and expression of feelings (refer to the chapters in Part 3). The focus is on the here-and-now experiences and the manner in which sharing and processing emotions can help to improve the quality of interactions within the family. As in existential therapy, process, growth, and action are emphasized, while background and historical information are considered less important. Experiential family therapy focuses on process more than content. In other words, the content of the presenting problem is viewed as less important than the process of what is happening in the here and now.

Emotions are important in experiential therapies and the therapist focuses a great deal of attention on exploring and empathizing with feelings. Clients are encouraged to recognize, express, and accept their feelings. Toward that end, experiential family therapy may incorporate the following interventions:

- In-session and between-session experiments that help to improve the connections between people
- Exploration of the quality of interactions in the family
- Expression of feelings in the moment
- Discussion of the patterns of interpersonal interactions that lead the family into difficulties.

Dysfunction is considered to result from lack of connection or failure to take emotional risks.

Virginia Satir and Carl Whitaker are regarded to be early pioneers in experiential family therapy. More recently, Leslie Greenberg and Susan Johnson have combined attachment theory with process-experiential theory in the development of emotionally focused couples therapy. Their theory provides an exciting new way to work with couples that is both theoretically sound and shown by the research to be effective. Each of these theories is outlined below.

Virginia Satir

Virginia Satir was a leader in the early development of family therapy. Born on a farm in Wisconsin in 1916, she first became a schoolteacher before obtaining an advanced degree in psychiatric social work from the University of Chicago. After nearly a decade as an agency clinician, she opened a private practice in Chicago. Satir was an international lecturer, trainer, and family therapist, and helped to establish the Mental Research Institute (MRI) in Palo Alto, California, where she was known to frequently begin training workshops with a meditation (Banmen & Banmen, 1991). In 1964, she first published *Conjoint Family Therapy* (1975), a groundbreaking work that is considered to be a classic in family therapy literature.

Over her lifetime, Satir worked with more than 5,000 families, sometimes providing group family therapy to multiple families at a time. Until her death in 1988, Satir remained at the forefront of the family therapy movement. Her work continues through the Virginia Satir Global Network.

DEVELOPMENT OF THEORY An important part of emotional expression results from good communication, and Satir was instrumental in establishing the importance of congruent communication patterns in family relationships. Satir noted that people speak with their entire bodies. More than just an expression of words, communication includes body language, tone, posture, facial expressions, and other subtle indications of affect. Frequently, words and body language are in conflict when people say one thing while their facial expressions and body language reveal something completely different. Such incongruence sends out mixed messages. Like Carl Rogers, Satir underscored the importance of congruence in all communications. Today, her model is referred to as Satir Transformational Systemic Therapy, which is a strengths-based, change-directed approach to family therapy (Andreas, 2012; Banmen, 2008).

IMPORTANT THEORETICAL CONCEPTS Several important concepts underscore Virginia Satir's model of family therapy.

Humanistic. As a humanistic psychotherapist, Virginia Satir believed in building self-esteem and self-worth in all individuals, as well as self-actualization. She implemented Carl Rogers's core conditions of empathy, unconditional positive regard, and congruence. Satir believed people have the answers within themselves and that after they learn effective communication skills, they are able to create solutions to their own problems. She has been quoted as saying "Life is not what it's supposed to be. It is what it is."

Process/experiential. After establishing trust, development of awareness through the experiential process is necessary for change to occur. In other words, it is not enough for the therapist to point out how the client is acting; the client must experience it within the session. As a process-experiential therapist, Satir used what she termed *reconstruction* to help families reenact and clarify their dysfunctional communications.

Communication. Satir believed that healthy families are more emotionally open and expressive in their feelings, and their affect tends to be congruent with their communications. Unless raised in a healthy environment, however, children do not usually learn how to express their feelings. In fact, children are often told to suppress their feelings, or deny them, when parents give them messages such as "Always be polite," "Don't let them see you cry," and "Put on your game face." Such statements give children a mixed message, or double bind, which often confuses them and prevents effective communication.

All relationships are built on trust, and Virginia Satir believed that when that trust is threatened, stress results. Under stress, a person retreats into survival mode and will communicate from one of five survival strategies: placating, blaming, super-reasonable, irrelevant, or congruent (Satir, 1975). Following is a brief definition of each survival strategy:

1. ***Placating.*** The placator's survival strategy is to get along. Regardless of their true feelings, under threat or stress, placators will agree with the other person, even at the expense of their own true opinion. For example, a child who has learned to placate his parents is likely as an adult to always agree with his wife when she becomes angry. "Yes, dear, you're right. I shouldn't work so many hours. From now on I'll be home every night at 5:00."
2. ***Blaming.*** Regardless of who is right or wrong, the blamer will always take on an angry "I am the boss" stance, whenever he or she feels threatened or stressed. The underlying need is for power and for the other person to back down. The blamer is often critical, demoralizing, and domineering, and can sometimes become a dictator or become physically aggressive in the family.
3. ***Super-reasonable.*** The super-reasonable person will respond under stress as impassive, logical, and correct. Interacting only on a cognitive level, this person will never give away his or her true feelings. When asked how they feel, super-reasonable people are likely to respond with what they think. Of course, a price is paid for shutting off their emotions, and these types of people often become loners, removing themselves from social interactions.

4. ***Irrelevant.*** Under stress, some people will respond with communication that is unrelated to the context of what is going on around them. This extraneous communication is designed to change the subject, to avoid conflict, or deny that anything is wrong. For example, in the midst of a discussion about fidelity, the "irrelevant" person may leave the room to get a cup of coffee. An extreme form of shutting out reality and disconnecting from what is going on around them can lead to fantasy or florid psychosis.
5. ***Congruent.*** The final form of communication identified by Satir is congruence. People who respond congruently have no discrepancy between what they are feeling and what they say. Satir (1975) explained, "A nice straight message. Nothing is crossed out. It is all there: Self, Other, and Context. There is total congruence with the situation" (p. 47).

Of these five communication stances, only the congruent stance is healthy and leads to improved communication and connections between people. One technique used by Satir in family therapy was to ask each family member to exaggerate his or her own communication stance. In doing so, the blaming father might point his finger and furrow his brow in an expression of anger, the "irrelevant" son might look out the window and hum a silly song, and the placating mother might implore everyone to just get along.

Satir stressed that all communication stances are learned behaviors and can be changed. She believed that symptoms signal that something is wrong in the family's communication patterns or that family rules are interfering with a family member's growth. She believed the problem is never the problem—it is how people cope that becomes the problem. Under stress, people will fall back on their survival communication stance as their best attempt to cope with a situation. By improving communication skills, helping family members to be more congruent in their interactions, and focusing on the process, not the problem, Satir believed that each family member would become more aware of him- or herself and others in the family, become more congruent and authentic, and increase self-esteem.

THERAPEUTIC ALLIANCE Satir was reported to be a warm, humorous therapist who did not believe a cognitive approach was sufficient. Rather than rely on techniques or intellectualization, she believed change occurs only through experiential moments. "It is simply a question of life reaching out to life. As a therapist, I am a companion. I try to help people tune in to their own wisdom. Of course, all this doesn't fit much with psychotherapeutic theory!" Even so, she was named by her peers as one of the four most influential counselors of all time (*Psychotherapy Networker,* 2007).

Satir identified her approach as a process model in which the therapist and family worked together to effect change. The therapist is responsible for creating a safe environment in which family members can risk looking at themselves and their interactions. Establishing trust with every member of the group is essential for change to take place. She included all family members in the process, took a family history that included a chronology of family events, and practiced flexibility in time and place of therapy. Satir was so flexible that she once met a family at the airport for a 3-hour session when she was on a layover between flights.

TREATMENT PROCESS The role of the therapist in Satir Transformational Systemic Therapy is to help family members to experience and communicate their emotions and to recognize the communications they leave out. Satir was an active and directive therapist, who believed in equality among family members. She would often stand a child on a chair so he could communicate at the same level with other members of the family. She believed in giving people an experiential change in the therapy hour and frequently used metaphors, like the self-esteem pot, to help make a point (Springer & Wheeler, 2012).

This type of therapy includes a blend of Gestalt, psychodrama, role-plays, modeling, family sculpting, videotapes, or other exercises or games to reenact old wounds and help family members develop new awareness, change misperceptions, and foster empathy for each other. Satir (1975) believed that "through the development of new awareness comes new understanding" (p. 135).

Following the new understanding is the realization of multiple options and choices for change. For Satir (1975), the goal of family therapy is not to heal people, but for the therapist to serve as a change agent and facilitator to "work until enlightenment occurs for the group" (p. 210). As people become more aware of their dysfunctional communication styles, they learn to express themselves on a deeper emotional level. For example, rather than expressing anger that her husband went out with his friends after work without her, a wife might express her underlying feeling of how hurt she felt. Expressions of primary emotions such as hurt or sadness are more likely to elicit empathy and understanding in the other partner and result in supportive and caring communicative overtures, rather than defensive and angry ones.

Several of Satir's innovative methods include:

- Experiential exercises used in and between sessions
- Techniques to establish effective communication patterns
- Family sculpting and choreography
- Humor
- Group therapy for families.

CURRENT STATUS As an early pioneer, Satir had an incredible influence on the development of family systems therapy. Her insistence on open and direct communication, her recognition of the importance of language, and her belief in family resilience were vital contributions in the early years of family therapy's development and have been instrumental in the development of dynamic, nonlinear systems of therapy. The Satir model continues to be a popular way to work with families and is being taught worldwide, especially in China, where the need for mental health counseling is outpacing availability (Li & Vivien, 2010). Satir's influence continues to be seen in the development of holistic, experiential, systemic theories such as Susan Johnson's work on emotion-focused couples therapy and in the work of the Satir Institute of the Pacific (http://www.Satirpacific.org), which provides worldwide training in Virginia Satir's growth model and publishes the *Satir Journal*.

Carl Whitaker

Carl Whitaker (1912–1995) was a psychiatrist who became an influential pioneer in the development of family therapy. Even more than Virginia Satir, Carl Whitaker used his personality in the service of psychotherapy. Whitaker was spontaneous and personable, and often shared his own stories with his clients. He used his intuition and timing to make effective interventions with families.

One can see the influence of Kierkegaard, Nietzsche, and other existential philosophers in his theory. He believed that fear of loss, either real or imagined, is the primary driving force in families. He identified three types of loss: (1) loss of order and meaning, (2) loss of family spirit, and (3) ultimately, the fear of death (Keith, Connell, & Whitaker, 1992).

Whitaker believed that all family members should attend counseling sessions, including grandparents and even ex-spouses. Multigenerational support was necessary, he believed, to the effectiveness of counseling. As do other experiential therapists, Whitaker emphasized increasing affect in the family, modeling good communication skills, and focusing on what is happening in the moment rather than on past or future concerns. He focused more on humanness instead of pathology, and believed families had a built-in drive to solve their own problems. The therapist's role was to activate this potential (Connell, 1996).

Whitaker was convinced that more than insight was necessary. For change to occur, insight had to be accompanied by meaningful experience. In particular, two types of experiences seemed to be most effective—when a family risks being separate or more individual or angry than usual, and when a family risks being more intimate.

Consistent with most humanistic therapists, Whitaker worked in the here and now, unconcerned with the past or why problems occurred. Instead, he focused on the process—on what occurred during the family session—rather than the presenting problem. Whitaker was often creative in his interventions; he thought that creativity could foster new outlooks and perspectives.

THERAPEUTIC ALLIANCE Whitaker believed that "the therapeutic alliance is sacred" (Connell, 1996) and is based on what he called "bilateral caring" (Whitaker & Napier, 1977). In other words, the therapist connects with the client on what Satir has termed "the level of being" and the client, too, sees fragments of him- or herself in the therapist. In general, therapists should be nondirective and let families work out their own solutions to problems. However, the therapist should be very directive within the session and become an authority figure to the family, which allows the family to act out their dysfunctional communication patterns. Early in therapy, even with the first phone call, Whitaker began to tip the balance of power and assert his authority. Within sessions, his humor, spontaneity, and even absurdity were reflected in interventions that helped the family to recognize and express feelings that had previously been outside their awareness (Whitaker, Warkentin, & Malone, 2011).

Whitaker worked almost exclusively with a cotherapist. Early in his career, he developed the cotherapy model to prevent therapists from becoming enmeshed in the powerful family system. The two therapists were agents of the family as a whole, not just an individual family member. He assumed that therapy "is a symbolic parenting experience" (Napier & Whitaker, 1978, p. 91), but did not believe that cotherapists need necessarily be of opposite genders.

According to Walsh (1998), Whitaker stressed the need for playfulness and family humor in fostering family resilience, but avoided humor that was sarcastic, cruel, or had the potential to be destructive. Whitaker believed loyalty, commitment, and accountability are necessary foundations for relational permanence and a sense of wholeness and will help families weather the inevitable stress storms that arise.

Because Whitaker's style was so personal, spontaneous, and intuitive it did not lend itself to structured training. Students of his theory were required to conduct internships with him as a condition of training. Neither did Whitaker's work with families lend itself to research, so little empirical research exists on the effectiveness of his methods.

Emotionally Focused Couples Therapy

Emotionally focused therapy was developed in the 1980s by Susan Johnson and Leslie Greenberg (1985, 1987) and was named emotionally focused therapy (EFT) to draw attention to the importance of emotion as a powerful agent of change. As research into couples therapy has advanced, emotion has become much more accepted for playing a role not only in relationship distress, but also as a motivator for positive change. Twenty years of outcome and process research, including a meta-analysis, indicate that EFT is one of the most effective models of couples therapy. Nearly 90% of couples who participate in emotionally focused couples therapy make positive changes to their relationships (Jencius & West, 2003; Johnson, 2008).

DEVELOPMENT OF EMOTIONALLY FOCUSED COUPLES THERAPY Susan M. Johnson is a clinical psychologist who was born in England in the middle of the last century. She later moved to Canada and worked with children in a therapeutic treatment center. Johnson was influenced by Carl Rogers's client-centered therapy and Fritz Perls's Gestalt approach. She also became interested in John Bowlby's work with attachment theory, especially as it related to adult relationships. Johnson is credited with creating emotionally focused couples therapy. This experiential form of therapy has become one of the most researched and validated approaches to addressing distress in couples (Johnson & Woolley, 2009). Johnson is currently a professor of clinical psychology and psychiatry at the University of Ottawa, director of the Ottawa Couple and Family Institute, and director of the International Centre for Excellence in Emotionally Focused Therapy. She conducts international training and certification programs on emotionally focused couples therapy, has authored numerous articles and chapters on emotionally focused therapy, and has written several books, including *The Practice of Emotionally Focused Couple Therapy* (2004) and *Hold Me Tight* (2008), that focus on the importance of emotional connection to the success of committed relationships.

IMPORTANT THEORETICAL CONCEPTS EFT is a systemic theory that synchronizes a humanistic-experiential approach with theories of adult attachment, using emotion as the language of change. These four important concepts are outlined below:

1. ***Systemic.*** EFT is a systems theory founded on von Bertalanffy's early works and based more specifically on Minuchin's structural approach (Johnson & Woolley, 2009). Individual behavior can only be considered as part of the whole. The focus is on patterns of behavior. Change must not only occur in the individual's behavior (a level one change), but in the pattern of the couple as a whole (level two change).
2. ***Humanistic-experiential.*** EFT follows in the humanistic tradition of belief in the basic goodness of people, their innate desire to self-actualize, and the importance of unconditional positive regard, congruence, and empathy. The creation of a positive therapeutic alliance is a necessary condition for change to take place. As in all experiential therapies, EFT therapists believe that new behavior and new insight come about only as a result of reprocessing emotions in the here and now of the session.
3. ***Attachment.*** EFT is also grounded in attachment theory. "The basic tenet of attachment theory is that a safe emotional connection to a few loved ones is a fundamental survival need wired in by millions of years of evolution" (Johnson & Greenman, 2006, p. 3). Bowlby (1988) referred to this as a "safe haven." Johnson clarifies that a safe haven is not a place, but a way of being with another person. Securely attached couples are emotionally accessible and responsive to each other. They reach for and find that safe connection in their partner, in what Johnson refers to as "effective dependency" (2007, p. 9). However, when partners experience disconnection, a predictable process begins to unfold. Initial anxiety results in protest and anger, which is followed by clinging and seeking behavior. If the attachment figure does not respond, depression and despair set in. Attachment theory offers couples therapists a map to the key moves that shape a love relationship.
4. ***Emotion.*** EFT focuses on emotion as the prime mover in couples therapy. Emotion is accessed and unpacked in the therapy session. It is not enough to develop insight; emotions must be reenacted in the presence of the partner. The partner will then experience empathy, or a softening of his or her feelings. It is only then that a "new corrective emotional experience of engagement with one's partner" can occur. This "is the essence of change in EFT" (Johnson, 2004, p. 13).

"Emotion is the music of the attachment relationship. To ignore it, as many couple and family therapies have done, is to leave the onion out of the onion soup" (Johnson, 2007, p. 6). EFT therapists focus "on the core emotions identified as universal: anger, fear, surprise, shame, joy, sadness, and hurt/anguish" (Johnson & Greenman, 2006, p. 3), and use their listening skills and reflective interventions to enhance and reduce expressed emotion.

Emotionally focused therapy integrates attachment theory with an experiential and systemic approach. The primary assumptions of EFT include the following:

1. The main issue in marital conflict is the security of the emotional bond between partners.
2. Emotion underlies all attachment behavior and is the prime mover behind interpersonal change.
3. In relationships, problems are maintained by the dominant emotions of each of the partners.
4. The attachment needs of the partners are generally healthy and adaptive. It is how these attachment needs are played out when insecure attachment is perceived that becomes the problem.
5. Change does not occur as a result of negotiation, emotional catharsis, or insight. Change only occurs as a result of reprocessing "the emotional experience underlying each partner's position in the relationship" (Johnson, 2004, p. 52).

THERAPEUTIC ALLIANCE The therapist provides a safe environment in which emotions, both positive and negative, can be explored. To do so, the therapist must establish and maintain a positive therapeutic alliance with both partners. As in other humanistic theories, the therapist takes on a collaborative role, is respectful of each person, and focuses on the moment-by-moment processes. Rather than a coach, diagnostician, or teacher, the EFT therapist is a process consultant, a choreographer, and a collaborator.

TREATMENT PROCESS In EFT, the focus is always on the emotional connection between partners. "The goal of EFT is to reprocess experience and reorganize interactions to create a secure bond between the partners, a sense of secure connectedness" (Johnson, 2004, p. 12). The presenting problem is never the problem, rather it is the lack of connection between the partners that is the problem. After the couple is more securely attached, they are able to work out their problems with less rancor and free from attachment insecurity.

In emotionally focused therapy for couples, the change process has been divided into nine steps that are designed to be implemented in 8 to 20 sessions (Johnson, 2004). These nine steps take place in three distinct phases: de-escalation, change in interactional positions, and consolidation and integration of gains and progress made. Each of the nine steps is outlined in further detail in a comprehensive workbook (Johnson et al., 2005). What follows is a brief description of the three phases of treatment in which these steps would unfold:

1. ***Phase 1: De-escalation*** (Steps 1–4). The first four steps involve assessment and determination of problematic cycles and the emotional states that go along with them. In this phase of treatment, the couple is encouraged to express their emotions. Negative cycles are identified and couples are helped to recognize the primary feelings (e.g., sadness, anger, hurt) underlying their reactive secondary emotions (e.g., resentment, withdrawal). At the end of phase 1, couples begin to detach from their negative patterns and the relationship becomes more stable. At this stage of treatment the presenting problem is no longer the problem, rather the negative cycle becomes the problem.
2. ***Phase 2: Change in interactional positions*** (Steps 5–7). The couple recognizes and unites to overcome the negative interactional cycle that has developed between them. The second

phase of treatment is when the bulk of the work of emotionally focused therapy unfolds. Here each partner is encouraged to express, first individually, and later together, the deeper emotions behind their feelings. The therapist choreographs emotional reenactments. Partners are no longer overwhelmed by their emotions, but are able to hear and accept their partner's needs and integrate their own needs into new interactional behavior. Withdrawn partners become more emotionally involved and more hostile partners begin to express their fears and take new risks.

3. ***Phase 3: Consolidation and integration*** (Steps 8 and 9). By now, couples have developed a new, secure attachment to each other. The old distress has been relieved, they can communicate effectively about problem areas, and they become capable of solving ongoing problems in the relationship. In the final phase of treatment, the couple's gains are solidified; they are reminded of their old negative interactional cycle and encouraged to maintain the positive interactions they have developed so that both members of the couple continue to communicate effectively and get their emotional needs met.

INTERVENTIONS Emotionally focused therapy is a simple, yet revolutionary method of couples counseling. Couples are not taught how to communicate more effectively. Nor are Bowenian techniques, such as genograms, or behavioral exercises and homework prescribed. Instead, the EFT therapist uses empathy and reflection to track emotion and uses those emotions to produce alternative feelings in the partner through enactments during the session. This is the underlying cause of change in EFT.

By using Rogerian reflective listening skills to reflect and track emotions, the EFT therapist can help each partner express the pain they have kept to themselves and experience catharsis. When one partner hears the other's pain, he or she is apt to "soften" or empathize with the partner, thus reducing his or her own negative, angry, or resentful feelings.

EFT therapists use both interactive and structural techniques such as enactments to help couples access and express their emotions. As negative feelings are reduced, the couple is more likely to rebuild their connection based on expressed emotion, empathy, and a secure attachment bond.

Specific interventions used by emotionally focused therapists include:

- Asking evocative questions
- Reflecting emotional responses
- Reframing patterns in terms of attachment and negative cycles
- Tracking and replaying key moments
- Creating enactments in which the couple makes their patterns explicit
- Slowly encouraging new ways of connecting
- Validating and normalizing responses.

APPLICATION The EFT model is increasingly being used throughout the world. It appeals to people from a variety of cultures and backgrounds because it focuses on issues that are universal—attachment and connection—and uses interventions that are respectful and collaborative (Greenman, Young, & Johnson, 2009). EFT is used with all types of couples including older couples, gay and lesbian couples, couples struggling with chronic illnesses such as cancer or depression, and military couples (Rheem, Woolley, & Weissman, 2012). EFT has been found to be particularly effective for couples in which one member has experienced severe trauma or PTSD (Greenman & Johnson, 2012; Johnson, 2002).

CURRENT STATUS Emotionally focused therapy has grown in popularity. EFT and behavioral couples therapy are the only two empirically validated treatments for couples (Johnson & Woolley,

2009). Perhaps because of its solid grounding in attachment theory, a lack of pathologizing, and a focus on the healing powers of emotion, EFT has even been found to be effective with inexpressive partners, with traditionally avoidant male partners, and with issues that are difficult to address, such as infidelity, sexual disorders, and sexual abuse trauma (Johnson & Woolley, 2009; MacIntosh & Johnson, 2008). It provides a structured, experiential, attachment-intervention model for helping couples communicate on a deeper level. However, EFT is not appropriate for working with couples who have different agendas such as a separating couple, a couple in which one person seeks to maintain an affair, or in clearly abusive relationships.

EFT has been adapted for use with families and is frequently used to treat adolescents who have depression or are suicidal (Johnson & Lee, 2000). Research indicates that attachment insecurity and disconnection often are at the core of childhood and adolescent behavior problems (Diamond & Stern, 2003; Moretti & Holland, 2003).

EVALUATION EFT has entered the mainstream of treatment for couples therapy, in large part due to its empirically validated support and its focus on love and connection. This is the first relational theory of adult love to be synchronistic with other research on the nature of emotion and attachment and to provide a road map for therapists. EFT is also consistent with new developments in the field of neuroscience that relate to health and emotion, stress, and bonding. Clearly, emotionally focused therapy has much to offer therapists who work with couples. Future research is expected to support its effectiveness in working with families as well.

FAMILY THERAPIES THAT FOCUS ON THOUGHTS AND ACTIONS

As we have seen in the previous chapters on thought-oriented treatment approaches (refer to Part 4 of this book) and those that focus on actions (see Part 5), much overlap exists between behavioral and cognitive theoretical orientations. This is even more true when cognitive and behavioral therapies are applied to family systems interventions. Therefore, the two theories are combined in our discussion of theories that focus on both thoughts and actions.

Behavioral and Cognitive–Behavioral Family Therapy

Behavioral and cognitive–behavioral family therapies provide the most diversity in terms of type and scope of treatment options. Following are just a few of the different modalities that reside under the cognitive–behavioral and behavioral umbrella of treatment approaches:

- Functional family therapy
- Cognitive–behavioral family therapy
- Behavior modification
- Behavioral parent training and parent skills training
- Behavioral treatment of sexual dysfunctions
- Cognitive–behavioral couples therapy
- Family-focused therapy
- Behavioral family systems therapy
- Dialectical behavior therapy for children and adolescents
- Rational emotive behavior therapy for childhood behavior problems.

A discussion of each of these treatment modalities is beyond the scope of this chapter. What follows is a look at one of the most prevalent and effective forms of behavioral therapy: behavioral parent training.

BEHAVIORAL PARENT TRAINING Behavioral therapy has been a useful intervention for troubled families for more than 30 years. Building on the earlier work of B. F. Skinner, the creator of behavior therapy, and Albert Bandura, who developed social learning theory, Gerald Patterson created a variety of interventions that can be used by parents to improve children's behavior and reduce family stress and dysfunction. Patterson is often recognized as one of the first behavioral family therapists. He operationalized many of the theoretical concepts found in Bandura's social learning theory.

In the 1950s, Patterson conducted behavioral parent training and developed workbooks for parents. By using interventions such as contingency contracting, token economies, modeling, and time-out, parents learned to improve their children's positive behaviors and extinguish the negative behaviors. (A complete review of behavior modification techniques is included in Chapter 16.)

Also referred to as parent skills training, behavioral parent training teaches parents to socialize and manage children. Behavioral parent training is based on classical behavior therapy and follows the premise that behavior is encouraged by what happens afterward to reinforce the specific behavior. Consistent with other action-focused theories, the focus of therapy is on changing current behavior, not on determining underlying causes of the behavior.

Rather than working with the entire family, behaviorists are more likely to work with one family member (most often a parent) individually. Through didactic instruction and the use of written materials, the therapist teaches the parent specific skills to manage the child's problem behavior. The therapist may also use interventions such as role-playing, rehearsal, modeling, and prompting to improve the parent's interactions with the child. Regardless of which methods are used, progress is charted over the course of treatment and success is rewarded with positive reinforcement.

Behaviorists do not see the problem as embedded in the family system. However, as social learning theorists, behaviorists believe that the child's behavior, although disruptive to the family, has actually been learned and reinforced by parental actions. To change behavior, parents learn to change the consequences.

In most cases, one parent attends behavioral parent training to focus on increasing the child's positive behaviors while decreasing negative ones. Operant conditioning is most frequently used and parents are trained in shaping behavior, how to set up and maintain token economies, and the appropriate use of time-out. The goal of behavioral parent training is to increase the rate of rewarding experiences while decreasing the rate of negative experiences and to teach parents communication and problem-solving skills.

Therapeutic alliance. The therapist in behavioral parent training serves as a teacher, instructing the individual or dyad on how to effect behavioral change. The therapist is also a collaborator, a coach, and an expert. Therapists model good behavior and provide feedback. As in all behavioral therapies, therapists play an active role in helping clients determine what behavior needs to be changed and then help the family set up behavior management programs.

Interventions. The following steps would be included in a typical parent training program (Becvar & Becvar, 2006):

1. Explain relevant social learning theory principles.
2. Clearly define target behaviors to change.
3. Assess the antecedents and reinforcing behaviors currently in place.
4. Establish a baseline to chart the frequency of the behavior.
5. Train the parent in the specific process for changing the problem behavior.

Prior to implementing behavioral parent training, therapists should consider four factors: (1) Is environmental control of the problem behavior possible? (2) Do any problems exist in the parental relationship that would prohibit the parents from working together as a team to implement the plan? (3) Does the parent have any problems (e.g., severe anxiety, depression) that would prohibit him or her from learning behavioral parent training? (4) How can the particular child best be helped to develop self-control? (Becvar & Becvar, 2006).

Evaluation of Behavioral and Cognitive–Behavioral Family Therapies

Behavioral therapy is helpful in working with children with conduct disorder, in families with schizophrenia, to decrease marital conflict, and in sex therapy (Nichols, 2010). A cognitive–behavioral approach has been found to be particularly effective as an intervention for at-risk parenting behavior (Gladding, 2007). Family-focused therapy has been shown to be effective for working with families in which a family member has bipolar disorder (Miklowitz, 2008).

Behavioral and cognitive–behavioral treatments for individual and family problems lend themselves to research and measurement. Therefore, it is not surprising that they are consistently among the treatment modalities most likely to be found effective. Research on parent training programs for children and adolescents with problem behaviors has shown a 75% improvement rate in the child's behavior. Research indicates that when a key family member changes dysfunctional behavior, the entire family is likely to benefit. However, in families in which only one person changes while the family system remains the same, those benefits are likely to be short lived.

Behavioral and cognitive–behavioral approaches to family therapy are frequently integrated with other treatment modalities, or used as an adjunct to other family therapy approaches (Dattilio, 2005).

POSTMODERN APPROACHES TO FAMILY THERAPY

In a postmodern approach to family treatment, therapists no longer look at one perspective or search to find the best solution; rather, they consider the perspectives of everyone in the family as equally correct. Solutions, rather than right or wrong, are ideas to be considered, approaches to be tried, and a way to integrate multiple perspectives. There are few clear-cut answers, lots of ambiguity, and a variety of choices that could lead to change.

The therapist's role in postmodern family therapy is as an information gatherer and an agent of change. Through skillful listening, information gathering from all family members, and acting as a participant-observer, the therapist works with the family in an interactive process to come up with alternatives to their current problems.

Evolving out of systems theory and cybernetics, strategic family therapy dominated family systems theory in the 1970s. Several models of strategic family therapy developed: the Mental Research Institute brief therapy model, the problem-solving model (also known as the communication model) developed by Jay Haley and Cloe Madanes, and Milan systemic therapy. Each of these models presents a pragmatic, problem-solving approach, which considers how families often contribute to, and maintain, their own problems. We will look at each theory briefly.

Mental Research Institute Model

Strategic family therapy had its beginnings in the 1950s in Palo Alto, California, in conjunction with the development of the Mental Research Institute (MRI). It was there that Gregory Bateson, Jay Haley, John Weakland, Paul Watzlawick, Don Jackson, and others influenced by Milton Erickson and his work with hypnotherapy became interested in applying paradoxical techniques in their work with families.

IMPORTANT THEORETICAL CONCEPTS In the MRI approach, families are considered basically healthy and capable of solving their own problems. However when they become stuck (defined as doing more of the same), professional help becomes necessary to get them through the impasse. Therapy begins by identifying ways in which the system maintains the problem, identifying the rules and family communication patterns that contribute to the problem, and then changing the rules.

APPLICATION, TREATMENT PROCESS, AND TECHNIQUES Treatment using the MRI model follows a six-step process:

1. Introducing the treatment
2. Clarifying the problem
3. Identifying behaviors that maintain the problem
4. Setting goals
5. Developing and implementing interventions
6. Terminating therapy.

After the problem has been identified, the strategic family therapist explores the family's history of trying to solve the problem, efforts that the therapist believes might actually be contributing to the family dysfunction and the continuation of the pattern. Solutions that perpetuate problems tend to fall into three categories: (1) denial that a problem exists, and therefore nothing is done to solve it; (2) the family focuses on solving a different, unrelated problem, and thus action is taken when it is not needed; and (3) hierarchical (action is taken but it is taken at the wrong level). After surveying the family's unsuccessful efforts, the therapist develops interventions specific to the family's problems and convinces the family to implement the interventions, thereby interrupting the family's problem-perpetuating pattern.

Rather than thinking of symptoms as uncontrollable, strategic family therapy looks behind the symptoms to explore any secondary gain that might be reinforcing the symptom. Haley (1963) described symptoms as strategies that were adaptive for a particular situation that also served the purpose of controlling or manipulating the behavior of others. For example, a husband who always works late at the office and complains that he has no control over the situation may actually be benefiting from the underlying "payoff" of not having to help with the household responsibilities when he gets home late.

Interventions in strategic family therapy take the form of directives prescribed by the therapist. These directives often run counter to common sense. According to Madanes (1991), directives are to strategic therapy "what interpretation is to psychoanalysis. It is the basic tool of the approach" (p. 397). These powerful interventions serve to encourage the family to change, unite the family (even if it becomes united against the therapist), and promote feedback that the therapist can use to help solve the family's problems.

Directives are not intended to harm but may sometimes seem to be punishing or even absurd. For example, ordeal therapy, developed by Haley (1984), consists of therapist directives to the client to perform an unpleasant event after the problem behavior has occurred. For example, a man who has repetitive nights of insomnia is given a directive to get up and clean the house every time he can't sleep. Another directive that Haley once made involved a contract with a married couple with alcohol use problems. Under the terms of the contract, the first person who had a drink and broke the contract agreed to walk around the house naked the following day. In ordeal therapy, the "ordeal" is generally more unpleasant than the symptom. However, for ordeal therapy to be effective, the client must have a willingness to solve the problem and a commitment to following the therapist's directives, no matter how ridiculous or punitive such actions might seem.

Directives in strategic family therapy are generally paradoxical and serve to create a double bind. For example, a teenage daughter whose behavior of staying out all night is causing problems in the family might be directed by the therapist to stay out every night and only come home once a week. This sets up a double bind for the daughter who now feels she is being told she can't stay in her own house. If she complies, she is letting the therapist control her; if she doesn't comply with the directive, she is changing her behavior in the direction her parents want. Such double binds are intended to overcome any resistance to change. Haley believed the real issue in families was often one of power and control.

Examples of other types of paradoxical directives used in strategic family therapy include:

- ***Reframing:*** defining the problem differently using language that positions it in a more favorable light
- ***Restraining:*** directing clients not to change too quickly, or not to change at all
- ***Prescribing the symptoms:*** telling someone who worries a lot to spend the entire weekend worrying
- ***Declaring hopelessness:*** agreeing with clients that their situation is hopeless and there is nothing that can be done.

Such paradoxical techniques create double binds that help the family to overcome resistance and bring about change quickly (Nichols, 2009). Therapy using the MRI model is brief and focused, with therapists taking a detached stance (Lebow, 2008).

Problem-Solving Therapy

Problem-solving therapy evolved through the work of Jay Haley after he left the Palo Alto group to join Salvador Minuchin at the Philadelphia Child Guidance Clinic. In 1976, Haley and Cloe Madanes, a therapist and former MRI colleague, moved to Washington, DC, where they developed the Family Therapy Institute.

Problem-solving therapy focuses on family member communication patterns. Specifically, Haley noted that the functionality of a family system could be determined by the manner in which individuals within the family communicate with one another and the alliances they form with other family members. Haley's model was influenced by Salvador Minuchin and hypnotherapist Milton Erickson and includes communication approaches to therapy.

Haley was a student of Milton Erickson, whose hypnotic techniques required the therapist to assume full charge of the treatment and to set directives and goals to help clients change. Haley became interested in issues of power and control in interpersonal relationships. His classic text *Strategies of Psychotherapy* (1963) underscores his view that symptoms can be seen as a pathological control strategy. While Haley's work became popular in the 1980s, many seasoned therapists expressed concern about his unconventional techniques. For example, in working with a family to solve their child's bed-wetting problem, Haley and Richeport-Haley (2007) instructed the parents to tell their child to wet the bed on certain nights, with increasingly longer periods of time in between.

In problem-solving family therapy, neither insight nor multigenerational information is important. Instead, the therapist focuses on the present, and is responsible for setting behavior-oriented goals for the family to achieve. Change occurs through the process of the family carrying out the therapist's directives (Goldenberg & Goldenberg, 2012). Haley strategized closely with families to develop unique interventions that would work for their particular problems.

THERAPEUTIC ALLIANCE Problem-solving counseling is directive and concrete. Counselors take the role of educators and directors, providing homework, setting up assignments, teaching new skills, and offering advice. Therapists focus on the here and now of control struggles and communication patterns within the family. Haley wrote that "my most significant contribution is breaking therapy down to a practice of specific skills—of simple ideas, skills, and techniques. This is quite different from the non-directive ideology the field had when I first got into it" (Haley & Richeport-Haley, 2007, p. B-7).

Haley made several notable contributions to family therapy. He developed unique tools and "experiments" to help families overcome resistance; he is credited with developing the concept of seeding; he used directives to create experiential moments that facilitated change; and he recognized that problems in families often occur at transition points in the life cycle. Overall, Haley's strategic family therapy was much more directive than any therapy had been heretofore. The therapist assumed responsibility for directing and influencing family change. Haley was one of the many innovators in strategic family therapy worldwide. We next take a look at Italy's Milan School.

Milan Systemic Therapy

The classic Milan model was developed in Italy by Mara Selvini Palazzoli, Luigi Boscolo, Gianfranco Cecchin, and Giuliana Prata. The Milan group of psychiatrists shifted the focus away from Haley's philosophy of behavioral change without insight to a more cognitive version of strategic family therapy. The Milan group developed interventions such as circular interviewing and positive connotations to help families view themselves in a less dysfunctional manner. For example, a teenager's substance use problem might be reframed as behavior she continues in order to bring her otherwise distracted and busy parents closer together. Such reframes are often more acceptable to family members and serve to plant the seeds that perhaps others in the family may be contributing to the problem as well.

Circular questioning is a fundamental strategy developed by the Milan School that has since been adapted by many other models of therapy (Fleuridas, Nelson, & Rosenthal, 1986). Through circular questioning the family is encouraged to become more expansive and consider a broader perspective. Relational questions, such as "What does your wife do when you start drinking?" or "What does your mother say to your father when she finds your bed empty in the morning?" put the client into a relational context. Instead of seeing the problem merely from their own perspective, circular questioning puts their behavior in the context of the larger family system. Circular questioning helps families to think in more systemic terms rather than thinking of behavior as a linear process. Gerson (1996) found that circular questions, asked out of genuine curiosity, elicit spontaneous responses that help the family to think in a more interdependent manner.

Other innovations developed by the Milan group include the manner in which therapy is conducted. A team of therapists is frequently positioned behind a one-way mirror to provide suggestions and advice. And, in what Tomm (1984) has termed "long brief therapy," sessions are often held once a month for a period of 10 or 12 months.

Evaluation of Strategic Family Therapy

Overall, strategic family therapy provides a brief, directive, problem-focused approach that addresses the family's presenting problem. Several concepts, particularly the idea that the family is contributing to the problem through its unsuccessful attempts at solution, and the idea that many symptoms are reinforced by secondary gains (e.g., controlling others' actions, avoidance of responsibility) were first suggested by Milton Erickson and became an important part of strategic family therapy. Interventions such as paradoxical directives, guaranteeing therapeutic success, and the use of absurd directives are several of the unconventional techniques to come out of strategic family therapy. The Milan School, through its development of circular questioning, positive connotation, and other less directive and confrontational techniques, has also produced effective interventions that have been adopted by other therapeutic approaches.

Brief strategic therapy has been empirically validated for use with children and adolescents with behavior problems and drug abuse (Robbins et al., 2010). More research is needed on strategic family therapy or the Milan approach with other types of clients and different problems. Some critics of the strategic approach question whether focusing on change without psychological assessment or a full history of the presenting problem could be harmful, or at best only result in first-order change. Many of the paradoxical interventions developed by Haley are viewed by some as absurd, punitive, or even manipulative. According to Nichols (2009), it was this manipulative aspect of the theory that eventually "turned family therapists against strategic family therapy" (p. 108). The Milan School and more contemporary strategic family therapists have moved toward developing a more positive, collaborative, and congruent relationship with clients.

Solution-Focused Brief Family Therapy

With the development of solution-focused brief family therapy, Steve de Shazer and Insoo Kim Berg shifted the focus of therapy from problems to finding solutions. This postmodern, constructionist theory believes that reality is defined by both time and culture. Therefore, therapeutic treatment of families must include their social, historical, and cultural contexts.

Similar to solution-focused brief therapy (SFBT) for individuals (discussed earlier in Chapter 11), solution-focused brief family therapy (SFBFT) helps families to set workable goals that incorporate new behaviors and use solution-focused language to effect change. Interventions from SFBFT therapists might include the miracle question, as well as other standard interventions such as "Do one thing different" or "Pay attention to what you do when ________ happens." Rather than focusing on changing problem behavior, SFBFT focuses on stopping the dysfunctional pattern that has resulted. Simple, small changes are likely to be successful and open doors to increasingly more positive changes.

SFBFT emphasizes short-term treatment of between 5 and 12 sessions, believes that families really want to change, and that only a small amount of change is necessary to increase confidence and create enthusiasm. Focusing on coping skills, asking for exceptions, and fostering resilience are solution-focused brief interventions that are used in individual and family therapy alike.

LIMITATIONS Limitations of this approach are similar to those expressed about SFBT: It is too simplistic, there is not enough supporting research, and it relies too much on repetition of the same interventions.

Narrative Therapy with Families

Despite the fact that narrative therapy is not a family systems theory, does not consider psychological symptoms to be related to family conflict, nor does it view some problems as interactional (Nichols, 2010), White and Epston's narrative approach to individual therapy has application for child, adolescent, and family therapy as well.

IMPORTANT THEORETICAL CONCEPTS Narrative therapy (see Chapter 11) views problems as stories to be deconstructed. In the process, therapists help parents and children to give voice to their stories, examine them through new eyes, and challenge assumptions, so that new and more hopeful stories can be written.

Narrative family therapists use the intervention of externalization to distance people from the problem, reduce or eliminate blame and defensiveness, and allow family members to focus on the impact of the problem on their lives. A symptom such as depression, for example, is not considered to be an individual problem, but to have an impact on the entire family. The family is asked how depression negatively affects the family. Then the family is asked how they could join forces to solve the problem. By separating the problem from the individual, families are better able to create new narratives that help, rather than harm, the family.

THERAPEUTIC ALLIANCE Narrative therapists avoid judgments and categorizations, and help the family look for exceptions and times in the past in which the problem did not occur. Planning for setbacks is frequently done ahead of time by asking families what they would do if their problem reappeared. Positive affirmations such as celebrations and certificates are methods frequently used by narrative therapists to encourage, acknowledge, and document progress (White & Epston, 1990). At the conclusion of therapy, many narrative therapists write thoughtful letters delineating the family's progress. Such letters are a means of helping the family to maintain the changes they have made, as well as carrying on the connection between the therapist and the family.

EVALUATION Even problematic parental behavior can be externalized so that parents can look at their own behavior in the context of good intentions. By honoring the uniqueness of the individual, eliminating blame, and helping families to deconstruct old stories and create hopeful new stories, narrative therapy has developed its own place as a family therapy. Narrative therapy for children and families has been used to help children with attention-deficit/hyperactivity disorder (ADHD) (Looyeh, Kamali, & Shafieian, 2012), eating disorders, attachment issues, and trauma (Dallos, 2006; Freeman, Epston, & Lebovitz, 1997; White & Morgan, 2006) and to help parents put an end to negative multigenerational patterns such as alcohol misuse and abusive anger. It has been used in play therapy with children, with adolescents individually, and with their families.

INTEGRATIVE MODELS OF FAMILY SYSTEMS THEORY

To date, the research literature has not identified one single approach to family therapy that is more effective than all of the others. Certainly some family therapies have been shown to be more efficient for specific populations or in treating certain disorders, but no theoretical orientation has been found to be the most effective overall. Prochaska and Norcross (2009) report that most family therapists today use an integrated or eclectic approach to treatment.

People are complicated. Relationships are even more complicated, with each person comprising an array of backgrounds, emotions, thoughts, and actions. To be effective, any theory of family therapy must address all of the biopsychosocial influences that impact the family. As we will discuss in Chapter 19, rather than following one pure theoretical orientation, seasoned therapists often supplement their preferred orientations with interventions from other treatment modalities. That is not to say that chaos reigns and therapists erratically switch from one orientation to another, but that they have developed an integrated approach that allows them to draw from more than one theory. In the words of Pinsof and Wynne (2000), "Good therapy is fundamentally disciplined improvisation" (p. 1).

Technical Eclecticism

This approach borrows techniques from many different theoretical schools, without adhering to the theoretical positions that created them. Although eclecticism draws from a variety of methodologies, the techniques still must be integrated in a systematic way into the therapist's currently existing theoretical framework to avoid clinical inconsistency or a lack of focus. In other words, there must be a reason why the therapist chooses and uses techniques from other theoretical orientations.

Most therapists have a primary theoretical stance and borrow selectively from other orientations. A therapist's original selection of theoretical orientation might be influenced by the graduate school they attended, by a particular professor's orientation, or by their supervisor's orientation. Other elements also come into play including how well the theory fits with their philosophy of life, comfort in using the techniques, and the availability of advanced training. Some family theories are closer in nature and therefore make an easier fit, whereas others work less well together.

Integrative Models

Some therapists combine two distinct orientations to create a third. For example, Les Greenberg and Susan Johnson integrated experiential and family systems theory into emotionally focused couples therapy (Greenberg & Johnson, 1988; Johnson, 2004). Most models of family therapy have been empirically validated to be effective. Integration would seem to be appropriate, and yet caution must be taken to avoid combining too many theories into an ineffective muddle.

Common Factors

The common factors approach also applies to family systems theory. Because no one theory best explains the broad range of family problems and dysfunctions, no one approach could possibly address the complex array of client symptoms, backgrounds, cultures, and populations. Families may best be served by an approach that focuses on the aspects most family theories have in common. These common factors have been found to be at least as important, if not more important, than theoretical orientation (refer to Chapter 20 for a complete list of common factors).

APPLICATION OF FAMILY THERAPY

Froma Walsh, in the fourth edition of her book *Normal Family Processes* (2012), talks about the new "normal" 21st-century family. She notes that what had previously been considered unconventional arrangements are now the most commonplace in the United States. Nuclear families consisting of a mother and father, in which the father works and the mother stays home with the children and runs the household, are not the norm. Today's families are multinuclear, multiracial, multigenerational, and have diverse economic and spiritual needs. Even so, all families rely on systems and support networks outside of the immediate family, regardless of how the immediate family is defined. Walsh notes that the new normal may actually be the most optimal for addressing the challenges and needs faced by today's families.

Application to Culturally Diverse Families

Along with the changing family comes the need for culturally competent clinicians and those who can adopt a strengths-based perspective. All therapists should be culturally competent and sensitive to race, gender roles, ethnicity, socioeconomic status, and sexual orientation. They should be capable of developing a sound therapeutic alliance with people whose cultural backgrounds differ from their own. Gladding (2007) notes that when family therapists do not understand or value cultural diversity or the importance of specific traditions or beliefs in a particular family, the therapist is likely to misunderstand, stereotype, or even pathologize the family. Many therapists now focus on resilience, solutions, and choice, rather than pathology or family dysfunction. Most managed care providers, however, still need to designate a particular client for reimbursement purposes.

Application to Specific Types of Families

Remarried, blended, multinuclear, or multigenerational families share many of the same problems that most families face, but also present with concerns specific to their unique situation. For example, Waites (2009) provides a multigenerational model for working with African American families in which intergenerational kinship is a source of support and care for relatives and nonbiological family members alike. This support often continues across the life span. Waite's intergenerational solidarity model provides an Afrocentric worldview that helps counselors to build on the family's strengths and incorporate culturally relevant issues, questions, and empowerment-oriented strategies.

Healthy adjustment for remarried or blended families often involves solidifying the bond between the couple while simultaneously adjusting to the differing developmental needs of the children. Stepfamilies often come to counseling in crisis or after problems have strained the relationship. Experiential and structural family therapy can be particularly helpful in working with these families. Virginia Satir's family sculpting techniques can help blended family members become more aware of interpersonal connections. Similarly, Susan Johnson's emotionally focused therapy can help them become more emotionally connected. Minuchin's structural family therapy with its goal of establishing a clearly defined hierarchy can help families to form new boundaries after the blended family is created. Developing a multigenerational genogram can also help families to recognize patterns of behavior in their families of origin and to avoid prior mistakes (Gladding, 2007).

Lesbian and gay families comprise 10% of cases seen in marriage and family therapy (Alonzo, 2005); perhaps these couples are more likely to address problems head-on and to seek professional help (Means-Christensen, Snyder, & Negy, 2003). Issues of role conflict, extended family support, and levels of satisfaction in the relationship are common presenting problems. Lack of complementary role models and social support, as well as continuing discrimination in many areas of life, can also cause additional stress that contributes to problems in daily living.

Marriage and family counselors who work with gay and lesbian couples should be able to address issues of cultural discrimination and homophobia related to being gay, understand intergenerational dynamics that may contribute stress to the family, and be familiar with community resources, state and local laws, and the diversity of gay and lesbian lifestyles (Alonzo, 2005; Gladding, 2007). In addition, when working with families with adolescents coming out as lesbian, gay, or bisexual, narrative therapy has been shown to provide a framework that can help families reauthor their stories and revise individual member identities as they work on becoming families with lesbian or gay members. Narrative therapy is recognized for incorporating elements and techniques that are culturally sensitive and recognizing the roles of power and privilege in society and their effect on what it means to be lesbian and gay (Saltzburg, 2007).

Application to Diagnostic Populations

Bountiful research supports the use of family therapy in the treatment of addictions, eating disorders, adolescent mood and anxiety disorders, ADHD, childhood conduct disorder, and autism spectrum disorders (Kaslow, Broth, Smith, & Collins, 2012). Psychoeducation for families in which a child has schizophrenia is also effective and has been shown to reduce the incidence of rehospitalization (Lieberman & Murray, 2012; McFarlane, Dixon, Lukens, & Lucksted, 2003).

EVALUATION OF FAMILY THERAPY

Overall, improvement rates in marriage and family therapy are comparable to improvement rates in individual therapy, and all types of family therapy have been found to be more effective than no treatment at all (Gladding, 2007). Taking a systemic approach to treatment was found to be more effective than individual treatment in cases of substance abuse, anorexia, and severe mental illness (Seligman & Reichenberg, 2012).

The latest findings summarize the overall research on family therapy as follows:

1. A variety of family therapy modalities have been found to be more effective than individual therapy in treatment of family-related issues.
2. In all types of couples therapy, successful outcomes appear to be related to improvements in communication. In general, in heterosexual couples, treatment outcome is more closely related to the man's attitude toward therapy (Symonds & Horvath, 2004).
3. Although people frequently work on marital issues individually, conjoint couples therapy is more effective than individual psychotherapy. In fact, negative outcomes are twice as likely to occur if marital problems are treated in individual therapy instead of conjoint therapy.
4. Short-term premarital couples counseling is effective in improving interpersonal skills and relationship quality (Carroll & Doherty, 2003). Long-term results are not available.
5. It is not surprising that positive outcomes in family therapy are related to treatment attendance (Norcross, 2011). However, retention is more difficult when working with multiple people.

Research also seems to indicate that improvement rates, as well as deterioration rates in family therapy, are similar to improvement and deterioration rates in individual therapy. In family therapy, deterioration can occur for a variety of reasons related to the therapist, including these: The therapist does not handle emotion-laden content well; the therapist moves too quickly over difficult subject matter; the therapist does not have a structure for de-escalating family conflict; or the therapist does not support family members (Fenell & Weinhold, 2003).

Most family therapy is of short duration (1 to 20 sessions) and the research bears out that this is as effective as long-term therapy. Therapy conducted with a cotherapist is no more effective than therapy conducted by one therapist. One criticism of family therapy is that it is sometimes viewed as a field unto itself, with a separate language all its own (see the Glossary of Terms section at the end of this chapter). Other criticisms include administrative issues such as the difficulty of scheduling appointments with multiple people, increased record keeping, and concerns about confidentiality. Most clinicians who choose to work with families find it to be a rewarding and effective way to help people.

SKILL DEVELOPMENT: GENOGRAMS

Therapists who work with families use many different techniques to gather and organize family information. Murray Bowen was the first to develop genograms—graphic depictions of several generations of a family—as an information-gathering and assessment tool in therapy. Genograms are a concise and practical tool for maintaining a great deal of information about the family, its interrelationships, and patterns.

Typically, genograms are created in the first session, with additional information being added as it becomes known. Most genograms include at least three generations. Family patterns are often transmitted from generation to generation, and the genogram provides a graphic illustration through which such patterns can be identified. Repetitive patterns in behavior, relationships, and family structure can be seen both horizontally and vertically across generations.

Gathering Information

When eliciting information for a genogram, the therapist either works with one family member individually or with the family as a whole. Gathering a family's history should always be done respectfully, and, as with all other session documents, confidentiality of information should be maintained (McGoldrick & Hardy, 2008).

Drawing a Genogram

Most genograms begin with the index person (IP) at the bottom of the page. The index person is designated by a double box. The IP's parents are documented on the row above, and the top row illustrates grandparents. Births, deaths, marriages, divorces, siblings, parents, and grandparents are documented. Adoptions, foster children, abortions, and miscarriages can also be included. When known, dates of birth, marriage, and death are listed.

After the initial family has been drawn, the genogram can be expanded to identify the relationships between people. Closeness, enmeshment, disengagement, and family cutoffs are indicated by the appropriate type of line (see Figure 18.2). Physical and sexual abuse is designated by a zigzag line attached to an arrow to indicate who was abused:

Disorders such as substance abuse, depression, or severe mental illness can also be shown on the genogram by shading in a portion of the circle or square. Addictions are indicated by shading in the bottom half of the symbol. Serious mental or physical illnesses are shown by filling in the left half of the circle or square. The type of disorder should be written near the symbol.

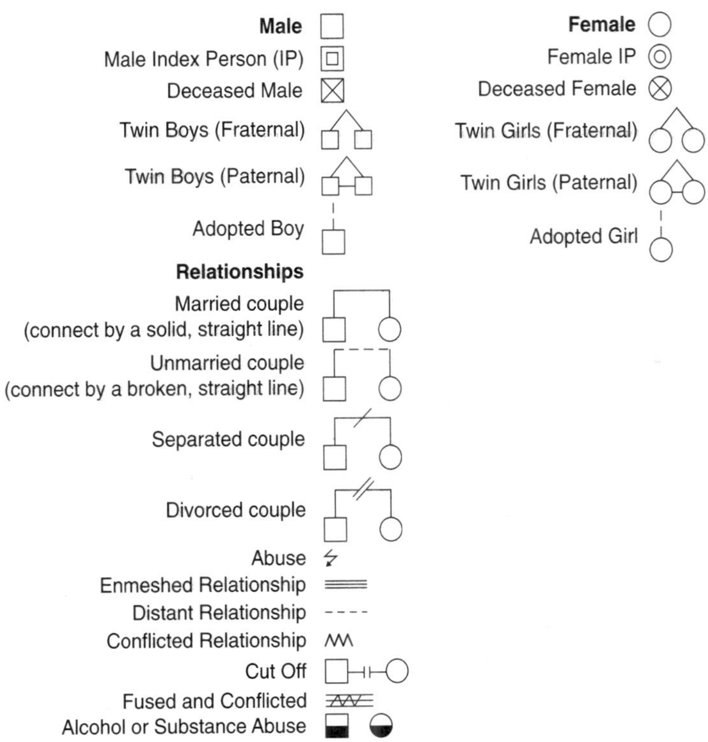

FIGURE 18.2 Symbols for Constructing a Family Genogram.

Additional genograms can be created to portray different types of information. The basic genogram may indicate the family's structure and demographics, while another may be used to show patterns of relationships between family members. Additional biographical information such as occupations, incomes, level of education, cause of death, or any other information the clinician would like to track can also be added.

According to McGoldrick and colleagues (2008), every genogram will contain some missing items. This is to be expected and may actually be the source of important information for the therapist, such as when clients do not have information about their immediate family members, or when former spouses or stepchildren have become cut off from the family.

Genograms can also be used to display a variety of interpersonal issues such as family members who are extremely close, those who are helpful, types of marital difficulties, and even the power dynamics within the family such as who is intimidated by others, who has more power, or who has no power. Genograms can illustrate culture, race, religion, socioeconomic status, and so on. Because of the wealth of information that can be collected, it often becomes necessary to create a separate genogram for these types of questions.

Sample Genogram

Figure 18.1 (on page 398) contains a genogram of the Diaz family. The genogram provides a quick illustration of the demographic information we have about Roberto and Edie. Roberto comes from a large Puerto Rican–American family. He was married twice before he met Edie. Edie's background is quite different. She grew up as one of two sisters in a Jewish–American family. Her parents are divorced and her mother remarried. We can see that Edie has a history of abuse. Roberto and Edie have been married 14 years and their 10-year-old daughter Ava is the index person in this genogram.

CASE ILLUSTRATION

Edie and Roberto mentioned to the family's counselor that Roberto had recently changed jobs and this had resulted in his frequent absences from home to attend weeklong business trips in another state. During Roberto's absence, Edie reported, their 10-year-old daughter Ava seemed withdrawn and had been shutting herself in her room. When Roberto returned home for the weekend, Ava continued to ignore her parents and refused to do what she was told.

The counselor had previously met with Ava in several individual sessions and together with her family. She remembered the girl's openness, and encouraged Edie and Roberto to bring Ava to their next session, during which the counselor used family sculpting techniques to help Ava and her parents understand the child's underlying feelings:

CLINICIAN: Ava, I'm so glad that you are with us today. I've noticed you've been very quiet during our session. Is there anything you'd like to talk about?

AVA: Not really.

CLINICIAN: Okay. Well, I have an idea of something you might enjoy doing that doesn't involve talking. Would you like to try it?

AVA: Okay. What do I have to do?

CLINICIAN: First, let's have everybody stand up. Roberto, Edie . . . now, Ava, I'd like for you to think a minute about this past week and what it was like at home. When you're ready, I'd like you to position your parents and yourself as if you are all statues frozen in place. As you do this, try to represent for me what it was like at home this week.

For a few minutes Ava thought about how she would like to position each of her parents. Then she took her father's hand and walked with him toward the door. She turned him to face the door, with his back to the people in the room. Then Ava moved her mother into the center of the room, turning her to face her husband's back. Ava took her mother's right hand and positioned the hand up to her ear as if her mother were talking on the telephone. Appearing satisfied with her mother's pose, Ava moved behind and away from her, so that her mother could not see her, as she slowly curled up on the couch and stared off into space.

The clinician invites Ava to tell her about her sculpture.

AVA: Well, I put Daddy by the door because he was working all week so he was never home, not even at night for dinner. It's like he wasn't even there.

CLINICIAN: That must have been very difficult for you.

AVA: I missed him. He always comes home from work at night and makes me laugh. We goof around doing silly things until dinner's ready. But Daddy doesn't come home from work anymore and I just sit in my room with nothing to do.

CLINICIAN: I see you positioned yourself on the couch.

AVA: That's because you don't have a bed in here. But at home, I just go to my bed and wrap up in my favorite blanket. I wish Daddy was there. I wish I had something to do.

CLINICIAN: But what about your mother? Explain to me what your mother is doing.

AVA: She's always on the phone whenever Daddy isn't home. She just talks, talks, talks, blah, blah, blah. She calls Grandma, my aunt, her friends, anybody she can find to talk to and just ignores me. She even calls and orders pizza over the phone and then calls someone else while she's waiting for the pizza to come. She never talks to me! When Daddy's not around, it's as if I don't exist. Like I'm in the way or something. She'd be better off without me so that she could just go and have fun with her friends.

EDIE: I never knew she felt that way! I miss Roberto terribly while he's gone and I guess I do spend a lot of time trying to keep myself busy by calling friends. And with Roberto not around, there's no reason to make a big dinner. But I didn't realize Ava felt that way, too! Is that why you go in your room? Because there's nothing to do?

ROBERTO: I can't believe how much has changed in our family in just a few short weeks. I don't like going away either, but I have to travel for my new job. I guess both of my girls are feeling lost without me. It's nice to be missed, but this has got to change.

CLINICIAN: What do you think you could do differently?

EDIE: Well, Ava and I can do something together. Maybe we can start making dinner together when Daddy's not home. Would you like to do that?

AVA: Can we make spaghetti?

EXERCISES

Large-Group Exercises

1. Review the discussion of family sculpting in the preceding Case Illustration. Ask for a volunteer to assume the role of the client. This person should select other classmates to represent his or her family members and pose the family to represent the relationships between either real family members or a fictitious family. As always, clients should take care of themselves. Discuss the meaning behind the family sculpture.
2. Discuss the general systems theory concept that all problems are related to interactions within a larger family system. Do you agree? Does this remove personal responsibility for actions and behavior? Can you think of any situations in which a person's problems seemed unrelated to the larger family system? Consider several problems (e.g., depression, anxiety, substance abuse) from both a systemic and an individual perspective.
3. Several of the innovations developed by the Milan School included "long" brief therapy and positioning other therapists behind a one-way mirror to provide suggestions and feedback throughout the session. Because of the distances families traveled to reach the therapists, sessions were scheduled once each month, for a 12-month period. Discuss the drawbacks and the positive aspects of long brief therapy and the benefits and drawbacks of having other therapists behind a one-way mirror.

Small-Group Exercises

1. Research indicates that family therapy is equally as successful as individual therapy. What might be some situations in which you would recommend an individual client seek marital or family counseling? What are some of the benefits of family therapy over individual? What are some of the drawbacks? Would you recommend specific family therapies for specific problems? Explain. Discuss your answers in a large group discussion of the benefits and drawbacks of family therapy.
2. Divide into your groups of four students. Each dyad should have an opportunity to role-play a couple in emotionally focused couples therapy. Allow 15 to 20 minutes for each role-play. One of the partners should open the session by describing an upsetting experience in which they felt their partner let them down. The task of the clinician is to guide the dissatisfied partner through the use of the following interventions:
   - Reflecting emotional responses
   - Asking evocative questions
   - Validating and normalizing responses
   - Getting behind secondary emotions to tap the client's primary emotions (e.g., fear, sadness, disgust, happiness, anger)
   - Reframing patterns in terms of attachment and negative cycles
   - Tracking and replaying key moments to enhance the impact
   - Asking the client to look at his or her partner and reenact or repeat attachment wounds or feelings of vulnerability
   - Slowly encouraging new ways of connecting.

   Allow time for group members to share feedback after each role-play has finished. Feedback should look at both general counseling skills and the process of taking the couple through the previous steps and should focus on both strengths and suggestions for improvement.
3. The founders of emotionally focused couples therapy recommend that this treatment modality is not appropriate for couples in which violence, abuse, or extreme anger is a problem. Why

would this be so? Discuss how you would screen couples to determine their suitability for this mode of treatment. Develop a list of 5 to 10 questions you would use to help you decide whether this approach is suitable for a particular couple. Then develop a list of 5 to 10 criteria that suggest a couple's suitability for emotionally focused couples therapy.

Individual Exercises

1. Using the symbols and genogram example illustrated in the Skill Development section, construct a three-generation genogram of your family. Begin at the bottom. Use the appropriate symbols for yourself and your siblings in chronological birth order. Move up to the previous generation and include your parents and their siblings if there is room. Complete the genogram with your grandparents at the top of the page. Add as much information as possible including birth dates, dates of marriages and divorces, and dates of deaths. Use appropriate lines to connect relationships. Include themes and family patterns (drug/alcohol abuse, violence, any mental illnesses). Also indicate strengths (education, cultural ties, professional success). Put ages inside the symbols and write names and birth dates on the side. You might want to consult with your parents or grandparents for specific details and dates, but that is not necessary. Every person's genogram looks different. In your journal, write about your experience completing your genogram. Were there any challenges or difficulties? How might the use of genograms impact your effectiveness as a counselor?
2. Write a family snapshot. In 100 words or fewer, capture a poignant moment in the life of your family. Describe a memorable event or a time that was particularly important to your family. The snapshot may be of an event, a celebration, or a spontaneous occurrence in the daily life of your family. The purpose of the exercise is to capture a poignant moment, describe it in an engaging way, and color in the emotions, thoughts, and feelings. Record this family snapshot in your weekly journal.
3. Think for a few minutes about what constitutes a family. In your family what roles, if any, are traditionally assigned to the men? To the women? Now think about your cultural and religious or spiritual background. How do they influence your own attitudes? Will your attitudes make it hard for you to be objective in working with families? What types of issues, populations, or families would be difficult for you to work with? Write about this in your journal.

Summary

This chapter has provided an overview of family systems theories, beginning with von Bertalanffy's innovative development of general systems theory. Highlights of each of the major family systems theories were included. Although each of these theories is very different, they are all united in their focus on systems and relationships rather than on the individual. The chapter concluded with a Skill Development section on creating genograms followed by a Case Illustration using Virginia Satir's family sculpting technique with the Diaz family.

Recommended Readings

Goldenberg, H., & Goldenberg, I. (2012). *Family therapy: An overview* (8th ed.). Pacific Grove, CA: Brooks/Cole.

Contemporary Family Therapy Journal. (2002). Special Issue on Virginia Satir, *24*.

Johnson, S. M. (2004). *The practice of emotionally focused couple therapy: Creating connection*. New York, NY: Brunner-Routledge.

Journal of Individual Psychology. (2007, Fall). Special Issue on Couples Therapy, Relationship Education, and Individual Psychology, *63*(3).

McGoldrick, M., Gerson, R., & Petry, S. (2008). *Genograms: Assessment and intervention* (3rd ed.). New York, NY: W. W. Norton.

Walsh, F. (Ed.). (2012). *Normal family processes: Growing diversity and complexity* (4th ed.). New York, NY: Guilford.

Additional Sources of Information

http://www.aamft.org—The American Association for Marriage and Family Therapy provides resources for marriage and family therapists including clinical updates on treatment approaches, effectiveness research, and the *Journal of Marital and Family Therapy*.

http://www.AlfredAdler.org—The North American Society of Adlerian Psychology promotes research, knowledge, and application of Adlerian family therapy.

http://http:www.steppublishers.com—The website for information on Systematic Training for Effective Parenting based on Adlerian family therapy.

http://www.thebowencenter.org—Bowen Center for the Study of the Family at Georgetown Family Center. This center provides information on Bowenian family therapy including research, training, publications, and clinical services.

http://www.ifta-familytherapy.org—An international association devoted to improving the quality of family therapy. IFTA conducts an annual convention and educational programs, and publishes the *Journal of Family Psychotherapy* and the newsletter *International Connection*.

http://www.minuchincenter.org—The Minuchin Family Therapy Center is located in New York City and offers training, workshops, and an externship program in structural family therapy.

http://www.mri.org—Home of the Mental Research Institute (MRI) in Palo Alto, California. Offers training, workshops, and research in strategic family therapy in the tradition of Jay Haley.

http://www.satirglobal.org—The Virginia Satir Global Network (formerly known as Avanta). Established in 1977 by Virginia Satir, this international network offers educational programs, annual conferences, and historical and research materials based on Virginia Satir's theory and practice.

http://satirpacific.org—Website of the Satir Institute of the Pacific, which offers worldwide training, workshops, and accreditation in Satir Transformational System Therapy (STST).

http://www.iceeft.com—Website for the International Center for Excellence in Emotionally Focused Therapy, which promotes research and training for emotionally focused therapy particularly as it relates to couples and family counseling. Founded in 1998 by Susan Johnson, the site offers educational programs, certification, workshops, and publications on EFT.

Glossary of Terms

Family systems theory has a language all its own. Following is a short glossary of terms frequently used in family systems theory.

- ***Alliance*** Connection with another person in the family subsystem.
- ***Attachment*** The innate need to connect with another person.
- ***Attachment wound or injury*** A wound that occurs when one partner fails to respond to the other in a critical time of need. This incident then becomes a clinically recurring theme and creates a barrier to relationship repair (Johnson, Makinen, & Millikin, 2001, p. 155).
- ***Boundaries*** Emotional or physical barriers between people.
- ***Coalition*** An alliance formed between two family members against a third.
- ***Conjoint therapy*** Therapy in which two or more people are treated together.
- ***Cross-generational coalition or alliance*** A parent and child who develop an inappropriate alliance against another family member.
- ***Cybernetics*** The study of processes that occur in systems.
- ***Differentiation of self*** A balance between emotions and cognitions that leaves one with healthy

boundaries that are not too rigid and not too permeable. A person who is differentiated will resist participation in dysfunctional family patterns.

- ***Disengagement*** The process, found in rigid family systems, in which one or more members withdraw and feel unconnected from the day-to-day family transactions.
- ***Dyad*** A two-person relationship.
- ***Emotional cutoff*** The establishment of rigid boundaries that disconnect or cut off from contact problematic family members.
- ***Enactments*** Therapist-choreographed interventions in which clients are directed to repeat or expand on interactions, so that the therapist can observe, and then help to change, dysfunctional family interactions.
- ***Enmeshed*** A family system in which members are overly concerned or involved in each other's lives, preventing individual autonomy.
- ***Family constellation*** The overall structure of the family; in Adlerian family therapy, particular attention is paid to birth order.
- ***Family maps*** A technique used in structural family therapy to identify the structural outline of the family, including boundaries and subsystems; the map provides a hypothesis and direction for change.
- ***Family sculpting*** A physical arrangement of family members to represent one person's symbolic view of relationships within the family.
- ***Feedback loops*** Information about how a system is functioning is fed back into the system in order to correct or govern the system's functioning.
- ***First-order change*** A change in behavior on the part of one person in a family unit that does not result in change to the overall organization of the system. Considered to be superficial.
- ***Fusion*** Term applied to a family that lacks individuation or appropriate interpersonal boundaries. See also *enmeshed*.
- ***General systems theory*** Developed by Ludwig von Bertalanffy, general systems theory is the study of the parts of an interactional system, emphasizing organizational hierarchy and interactions within subunits of the system.
- ***Genogram*** A multigenerational diagram of a family's relationship system that includes all members and relevant information about them.
- ***Identified patient*** The person identified by the family as having the problem.
- ***Joining*** A therapeutic tactic in which the therapist becomes part of a family system in order to understand and ultimately improve aspects of the system.
- ***Multigenerational transmission process*** The process whereby dysfunctional family patterns are passed down from one generation to the next generation.
- ***Multinuclear family*** Two separate families who live in the same house. The number of multinuclear families has been increasing since 2008, largely as a result of financial considerations.
- ***Paradoxical intervention*** A therapeutic technique in which the therapist prescribes an action that he or she wants resisted. Change occurs when the client defies the directive.
- ***Process/content*** Distinction between how people relate in the moment and what they talk about.
- ***Relabeling/reframing*** Verbally redefining an event in order to elicit more positive responses to the behavior.
- ***Scapegoat*** A member of the family, likely to be the identified patient, who is the object of criticism, blame, or scorn.
- ***Second-order change*** Changes in the fundamental organization of a system.
- ***Stuck*** Repeating the same behavior that isn't working.
- ***Subsystem*** Any subunit of a family having its own autonomous functions as well as a role within the larger family system (e.g., siblings, parents, children).
- ***Symbiotic*** An intense relationship between two people in which the boundaries are blurred and they respond as one (often occurs between mother and child).
- ***Tracking*** A therapeutic tactic in structural family therapy in which the therapist attends to the language, style, tone, and values of the family and uses this to influence the family's patterns of interaction.
- ***Triad*** A relationship of three people.
- ***Triangulation*** An interactional pattern in which a third person becomes involved in conflict between two individuals.

CHAPTER 19

Integrative Therapies

The most popular treatment methodologies of most mental health professionals are integrated or eclectic methods. In fact, nearly 34% of counseling psychologists, 26% of social workers, and 23% of counselors describe their primary theoretical orientation as eclectic or integrative (Prochaska & Norcross, 2009). These percentages have been increasing over the years, and the trend seems likely to continue. Even clinicians who adhere to one theoretical orientation commonly incorporate into their work interventions from other treatment approaches. However, it should be stressed that before a clinician can integrate treatment approaches, they must first be grounded in a theory and knowledgeable about the different approaches to treatment overall.

Parts 2 through 5 of this book focused on theories of counseling and psychotherapy reflecting four major emphases—background, emotions, thoughts, and actions—and reviewed treatment strategies and skills associated with each. Knowledge of an array of theoretical approaches is necessary so that clinicians can determine which treatment approach is best for them and for each of their clients and to afford clinicians an array of useful interventions. Although this knowledge is integral to the professional development of every effective clinician, many counselors and psychologists today do not align themselves strongly with one particular approach. Instead, they draw on a variety of theories and interventions in developing a treatment plan that seems likely to help a given person.

REASONS FOR THE GROWTH OF ECLECTIC AND INTEGRATED APPROACHES

Many factors account for this trend toward integrative and eclectic treatment. Chief among them is the fact that no single theory has yet been found that can clearly capture the entire range of human experiences across the life span. In light of the diversity of people seeking treatment—who vary according to many dimensions including culture, ethnicity, gender, sexual orientation, intelligence, abilities, interpersonal skills, life experiences, self-awareness, support systems, and symptoms—strictly adhering to one specific model of counseling or psychotherapy may greatly reduce therapeutic options. At the same time, evidence increasingly indicates that matching clients who have a preferred treatment modality or type of therapist with that preference reduces the dropout rate and is more likely to result in improvements in therapeutic outcomes (Swift, Callahan, & Vollmer, 2011).

Not so surprisingly, Miller, Duncan, and Hubble (2002) found that as a therapist's years of experience increased, they were less likely to strictly follow just one theoretical approach. Perhaps this is because clinical expertise has been found to be necessary for finding and combining the best research-based practices that match specific client needs (APA Presidential Task Force on Evidence-Based Practice, 2006).

In addition, no one theoretical model has proven itself superior to the rest despite efforts to identify such a theory. Luborsky, Singer, and Luborsky (1975) reviewed the comparative literature on psychotherapy and concluded that the result was a dodo bird verdict. (The dodo bird, in *Alice's Adventures in Wonderland,* stated that since everyone had won the race, all must have prizes.) Despite extensive research since 1975, the dodo bird verdict still stands. According to Hansen (2002), ". . . meta-analysis of counseling outcome studies clearly shows that no one approach has emerged as the correct or most helpful . . . it seems that all well-established approaches promote healing" (p. 315). In fact, research suggests that what the therapist does is as empirically validated as the type of treatment that is used (Duncan, Miller, Wampold, & Hubble, 2010).

At the same time, research has demonstrated that some treatment approaches are more effective than others with particular problems, diagnoses, or types of people. For example, cognitive therapy and interpersonal psychotherapy are particularly powerful in the treatment of major depressive disorder (Nathan & Gorman, 2002), whereas reality therapy has been widely used in treating conduct disorders. In addition, recent research indicates that psychotherapy is more enduring than medication management (Hollon, Stewart, & Strunk, 2006).

The following 12 factors have combined during the past 30 years to move clinicians in the direction of preferring integrative and eclectic approaches over adherence to one specific treatment system (Prochaska & Norcross, 2009):

1. The large and growing number of approaches to treatment; more than 500 treatment systems have been identified
2. The increasing diversity and complexity of clients and their concerns
3. The inability of any one treatment system to successfully address all clients and all problems
4. The growing importance of solution-focused brief approaches that encourage clinicians to draw on and combine interventions from various systems of therapy to find the most effective and efficient strategy for each treatment situation
5. The availability of training opportunities, as well as case studies and other informative literature, that give clinicians the opportunity to study, observe, and gain experience in a wide variety of treatment approaches
6. The requirement of some state and national credentialing bodies that clinicians obtain post-graduate continuing education units; this encourages continued professional growth and development of new skills and ideas
7. Increasing pressure from managed care organizations, governmental agencies, consumers, and others for clinicians to determine the most effective and efficient treatment approach for each client, to plan and document their work, and to maintain accountability
8. The growing body of compelling research demonstrating which treatment approaches are most likely to be successful in the treatment of particular people, disorders, or problems (Seligman & Reichenberg, 2012)
9. The increasing availability of manuals, providing detailed and empirically validated treatment plans for specific mental disorders
10. The development of organizations such as the Society for the Exploration of Psychotherapy Integration that focus on studying and promoting treatment integration
11. The emergence of models providing blueprints or guidelines for logical and therapeutically sound integration of treatment approaches
12. Clinicians' increasing awareness that common factors among treatment approaches, such as the nature of the therapeutic alliance, are at least as important in determining treatment success as are specific strategies.

This array of factors nudges many clinicians toward an eclectic or integrative model as their preferred orientation toward treatment.

THE CHALLENGES OF ECLECTIC AND INTEGRATED APPROACHES

Choosing to adopt an eclectic or integrated theoretical orientation is challenging and probably demands more of clinicians than does adherence to one specific theory. If clinicians decide, for example, that they will specialize in cognitive therapy, they should develop expertise in that approach and know when it is and is not likely to be helpful so that they can refer to others those clients who are unlikely to benefit from cognitive therapy. Because they have limited the scope of their work, these clinicians do not have to develop expertise in other treatment approaches, although they should be familiar with other approaches.

However, clinicians who view their primary theoretical orientation as eclectic or integrated need expertise in a range of treatment systems so they can draw on those approaches in creating effective treatment plans. Of course, clinicians who have an eclectic or integrated orientation also set limits on the scope of their practice; no clinician could have sufficient knowledge and expertise in the entire range of therapeutic approaches to treat all clients and all problems. Clinicians should define the scope of their practice according to the nature of their clientele, the problems or mental disorders they treat, and the strategies they employ. Nevertheless, clinicians who prefer eclectic or integrated treatment approaches still have a professional role that is more comprehensive and challenging than that of clinicians with a specific theoretical orientation.

In addition, clinicians advocating an eclectic or integrated treatment approach must carefully think through their treatment of each client to ensure that the disparate parts of treatment comprise a seamless whole in which each intervention is chosen deliberately to accomplish a purpose. Treatment must not just be an amalgam of "tricks of the trade" but, rather, should reflect coherence, relevance, and planning and be solidly grounded in both theory and empirical research. As Schwartz and Waldo (2003) stated, "The danger of creating a 'hodge-podge' of apples and oranges can be avoided if the theories are compatible, carefully integrated, and if they reflect the basic characteristics of mental health counseling" (pp. 101–102).

THE BENEFITS OF ECLECTIC AND INTEGRATED APPROACHES

Integrated and eclectic theoretical approaches have benefits as well as challenges. They bring flexibility to the treatment process, enabling clinicians to tailor their work to specific clients and concerns in an effort to find a good fit between treatment and client.

This is especially important when clinicians treat people from diverse cultural backgrounds who may respond better to modified or integrated approaches than they do to standardized ones. For example, people from Asian backgrounds may respond best to treatment approaches that are structured in nature but that also recognize the importance of the family and society. Clinicians can demonstrate multicultural competence by creating integrated treatment plans that reflect sensitivity to clients' culture and context.

Because they have greater flexibility in their work, clinicians espousing an integrated or eclectic approach probably can work with a broader range of people and problems than those who affiliate themselves with a single treatment system. Of course, all clinicians must practice within their areas of expertise or obtain supervision or training to expand their skills.

In addition, integrated and eclectic approaches allow clinicians to adapt standard treatment approaches to their own beliefs about human growth and development as well as to their natural style and personality.

Finally, integrated and eclectic approaches facilitate clinician efforts to assume a scientist-practitioner role and to combine theoretical information, empirical research, and practical experience. Basing their work on treatment approaches that have proven their value through research, clinicians can expand on that foundation by incorporating into their work ideas that have face validity as well as strategies that they have used successfully with other clients.

THE NATURE OF ECLECTIC AND INTEGRATED APPROACHES

When clinicians first began to describe their theoretical orientations as *eclectic,* the term lacked a clear meaning; it simply suggested that clinicians drew on more than one approach to treatment. Although some clinicians who characterized their work as eclectic were gifted therapists and astute theoreticians with a clear rationale for combining interventions in their work, others lacked a thoughtful and systematic approach to treatment. Eysenck (1970) denounced what he referred to as "lazy eclecticism" (p. 140), the use of a grab bag of interventions combined without an overriding logic. Without a logic or structure, eclecticism can lead to treatment that is haphazard and inconsistent, lacking in direction and coherence. This has been referred to as *syncretism*. Such an approach reflects a lack of knowledge and professionalism and is incompatible with current emphases on accountability and treatment planning in counseling and psychotherapy.

Types of Eclectic and Integrated Approaches

Four types of eclecticism have been identified:

1. ***Atheoretical eclecticism*** is characterized by combining interventions without an overriding theory of change or development. Unless an intuitive or underlying logic prevails, clinicians whose work reflects atheoretical eclecticism run the risk of syncretism—providing treatment that is without direction, including elements that are disparate and perhaps incompatible. Such an approach probably will be confusing to clients, may lead them to question the clinician's competence (as well as their own), can interfere with client cooperation and motivation, and may well lead to treatment failure.
2. ***Common factors eclecticism*** hypothesizes that certain elements of treatment, notably a therapeutic alliance that communicates support, empathy, and unconditional positive regard, are primarily responsible for promoting client growth and change (Norcross & Wampold, 2011). Specific interventions are linked to these common factors rather than to a specific theory. In Part 1 you learned about commonalities in successful treatment.
3. ***Technical eclecticism*** provides a framework for combining interventions from different treatment systems without necessarily subscribing to the theories or philosophies associated with those interventions. In general, counselors who practice technical eclecticism seek out the most effective techniques available for their client's specific problems. Technical eclecticism can be thought of as an organized collection of interventions, rather than an integration of ideas. The selection of interventions should have an empirical basis, reflecting research on the effectiveness of various interventions in successfully addressing clients' concerns. However, technical eclecticism lacks a coherent model for human development and growth. Lazarus's multimodal therapy exemplifies this type of eclecticism.
4. ***Theoretical integration*** offers conceptual guidelines for combining two or more treatment approaches to provide a clearer understanding of clients and more effective ways to help them. A theoretical integration usually provides clinicians with a framework for understanding how people grow and change and guidelines for developing treatment plans that reflect that understanding. Integrated treatment approaches often include a multistage, systematic approach to treatment as well as information on assessing client strengths and difficulties and matching treatment to client. Clinicians have guidelines to help them answer the seminal question "*What* treatment, by *whom,* is the most effective for *this* individual with *that* specific problem, and under what set of circumstances?" (Paul, 1967, p. 109). In a true theoretical integration, the whole is greater than the sum of its parts. The combination of approaches blends well and forms a new theory or treatment system that builds on and improves each of the individual approaches to form a better product. Treatment is theory focused rather than technique driven. Hill's three-stage integration model, discussed later in this chapter, is an example of theoretical integration.

INTEGRATING TREATMENT SYSTEMS

Although most clinicians do not adhere to a systematic approach to theoretical integration, they probably have formulated their own logic for combining compatible theories. The most common combinations of theories, in descending order of frequency, include (1) cognitive and behavioral treatment systems, (2) humanistic and cognitive approaches, and (3) psychoanalytic and cognitive approaches (Prochaska & Norcross, 2009). The presence of cognitive therapy in all three combinations is noteworthy, suggesting the flexibility of that approach and its importance in treatment.

Characteristics of Sound Eclectic and Integrated Approaches

Certain hallmarks distinguish conceptually sound integrated and eclectic approaches from eclecticism that is haphazard and ill conceived. Sound eclecticism has the following characteristics:

- Evidence of building on the strengths of existing theories
- A coherent combination of theories that creates a unified whole
- An underlying theory of human behavior and development
- A philosophy or theory of change
- Logic, guidelines, and procedures for adapting the approach to a particular person or problem
- Strategies and interventions, related to the underlying theories, that facilitate change
- Inclusion of the commonalities of effective treatment, such as support, positive regard, empathy, and client–clinician collaboration.

FORMULATING AN INTEGRATIVE TREATMENT SYSTEM

When clinicians formulate an integrative treatment system, they must address many questions, including the following:

1. What model of human development underlies the theory?
2. How does this treatment approach suggest that change is best facilitated?
3. What information should be obtained in an intake interview?
4. What conception does this approach have of the influence of the past on the present, and how should past experiences and difficulties be addressed in treatment?
5. How important is insight in promoting change, and how much attention should be paid in treatment to improving insight?
6. How important is exploration of emotions in promoting change, and how much attention should be paid in treatment to helping people identify, express, and modify their emotions?
7. How important is identification and modification of dysfunctional cognitions in promoting change, and how much attention should be paid in treatment to helping people alter their cognitions?
8. How important is identification and modification of self-destructive and unhelpful behaviors in promoting change, and how much attention should be paid in treatment to helping people alter their behaviors?
9. What sorts of people and problems are likely to respond well to this approach?
10. In what treatment settings and contexts is this approach likely to be successful?
11. How well does this approach address issues of diversity, and what is the appropriate use of this approach with people from multicultural backgrounds?
12. What is the place of diagnosis and treatment planning in this approach?
13. What are the overall goals of treatment?
14. What types of therapeutic alliances and client–clinician interactions are most likely to be productive?
15. What clinical skills are especially important for those who adopt this approach?
16. What interventions and strategies are compatible with this treatment system?

17. How should this approach be adapted for use with individuals? Families? Groups?
18. How long is treatment likely to last?
19. How is effectiveness measured, and what determines when treatment is finished?
20. Has this treatment system been adequately substantiated by empirical research? If not, what information is needed to support the value of this approach?

Some of the shortcomings of eclectic and integrated approaches can be overcome by adopting a sound and systematic rationale for developing treatment plans. As Lazarus and Beutler (1993) stated, "Procedures are not selected haphazardly, but their selection is specifically dependent on a logical decisional process that takes into account the client, setting, problem, and the nature of the counselor's skills" (p. 384).

This chapter reviews some established or promising approaches that demonstrate ways to provide integrated treatment by design rather than default. Two models receive particular attention: cyclical psychodynamic–behavior therapy developed by Paul Wachtel, and multimodal therapy developed by Arnold Lazarus. These two approaches differ considerably, although both are well-developed treatment systems with demonstrated success. We also give some attention to other integrated and eclectic treatment systems, including the transtheoretical model of change developed by Prochaska and his colleagues, Hill's three-stage integrated model of helping, and common factors models.

INTEGRATIVE PSYCHODYNAMIC–BEHAVIOR THERAPY

The first person to truly integrate two separate theoretical orientations was Paul Wachtel (1977), who combined psychodynamic therapy with behavioral therapy to create cyclical psychodynamic–behavior therapy. As its name implies, the treatment approach integrates the insight achieved through psychodynamic therapy with applied behavioral interventions, with the goal of providing a more powerful intervention than either treatment modality alone.

Wachtel's groundbreaking work, is considered to be an example of technical eclecticism (Sharf, 2012). It broadened the field by providing a primary and secondary approach to treatment while also emphasizing the need to adapt treatment to the client's worldview, to consider both social and psychological dimensions, and to empower the client (Wachtel, 2008; Wachtel, Kruk, & McKinney, 2005).

Stricker and Gold (2011) consider Wachtel's theory to be "the most comprehensive and influential integrative theory of personality" (p. 343). Wachtel and others found much support for the theory of a cyclical nature of personality dynamics. The term "vicious cycles" comes to mind, in which people continue to repeat patterns of behavior, or even make reality consistent with their expectations of what will happen. Research has shown that people induce in others the behavior they expect from them (Gilbert & Jones, 1986). Such self-fulfilling prophesies, also known as fundamental attribution errors or expectancy biases, can keep a person stuck in a continuing pattern despite his or her greatest efforts to overcome them.

Wachtel suggests that early experiences trigger cycles or patterns of behavior that are maintained by present attitudes or inclinations. He believes that an integration of psychodynamic and behavioral approaches provides a dynamic treatment in which insight leads to behavioral change and behavioral change leads to insight in a cyclical pattern.

The opposite is also true. For example, a person who leans toward depression may actually elicit and contribute to relationships that maintain that negativity. Even while protesting that they want to change, they may actually surround themselves with people who reinforce negative behaviors and increase the sense of victimization. A similar dynamic occurs when we solicit an opinion from a friend or colleague—we are seeking out the person who will give us the answer we want to hear. Alternatively, we avoid those who do not act in accordance with our needs (Wachtel, 1997). Cyclical psychodynamic–behavior therapy emphasizes the contextual nature of psychological processes and circular causation—how people mutually shape each other's experience (Stricker & Gold, 2011).

When assessing clients, therapists who use cyclical psychodynamic–behavioral therapy look at areas such as conflict, character, resistance, and object representations. After initial assessments, ongoing evaluations and adjustments occur throughout the treatment process to integrate behavioral or psychodynamic interventions, as the need arises.

For example, Mark, a 35-year old government employee, came for therapy because he had had an affair. He noted in the first session that he didn't know why he did it, but recalled "doing stupid things" when he was a teenager and thinks that might somehow be related to his current behavior. During the session he reveals that sometimes he also participates in self-defeating behaviors (smokes pot, drinks alcohol), but he doesn't know why he does this. He recognizes the potential risks involved (job loss, relationship loss, arrest), but also is feeling "stuck" in his job and a sense of insecurity that he is not good enough for promotion.

Using Wachtel's cyclical dynamics and an interpersonal perspective, the therapist first focused on Mark's externalization of his feelings, to help him become aware of, and recognize, the anger and resentment that he suppressed and then tried to avoid by reaching for drugs, alcohol, or sex. Encouraging both insight and action gradually exposes people to their frightening images and fantasies so that they can learn to cope with them more effectively. Mark was able to identify a pattern of behavior that had been with him since childhood, of not wanting to recognize or express difficult feelings that made him uncomfortable. Over the years, Mark had externalized his feelings, and would turn to drugs or sex to make himself feel better and reaffirm his self-worth. He recognized the cyclical nature of the pattern, and the fact that it was self-defeating, but he felt helpless to do anything about it. Consider the following excerpt from a therapy session with Mark:

THERAPIST: So, you said a woman approached you in a bar, made overtures, and you went home with her, but you don't know why.

MARK: Yes, exactly. She came on to me. She was beautiful.

THERAPIST: How did you feel about that?

MARK: I feel stupid now. I told my girlfriend about it and she wants to break up with me.

THERAPIST: But what did you feel back in the bar, when this was happening?

MARK: I guess I thought here's this great opportunity that doesn't come around very often.

THERAPIST: Mmmm. How do you feel right now, talking to me about this?

MARK: What do you mean?

THERAPIST: What do you feel here, telling me this? What are your feelings?

MARK: I don't know. It was difficult to come here today.

THERAPIST: Okay, so here we are, two people having an interaction, and you don't know what you are feeling?

MARK: No.

THERAPIST: What would you like to do about that?

MARK: About what?

THERAPIST: About recognizing your feelings.

MARK: Ummm. That's why I'm here. I don't seem to know what I'm feeling or even that I'm feeling something, I just want to go off and do something else, and . . .

THERAPIST: And avoid the uncomfortable feelings?

MARK: Exactly. I just want to put the feelings out of my mind and go have fun. Why do I do that?

THERAPIST: Mark, I'd like to help you, and part of that is getting to know you better, staying connected and being honest, and exploring in the session how this feels—how this interaction between us feels to you as you try to explore your feelings more deeply.

MARK: Does it matter?

THERAPIST: It matters a great deal. If you are willing to do that, to be more open with me and to try to express what you're going through as feelings come up, I will understand you better, and feel more connected to you.

MARK: But it's hard for me. I get frustrated when I can't put it in words.

THERAPIST: Let's see if we can slow it down a bit. I wonder if this is similar to what happens in your relationships. You feel something, and those feelings quickly become overwhelming and all jumbled together, and then you become frustrated or angry and start to feel overwhelmed and . . . .

MARK: Exactly! And then I just want to DO something to make those feelings go away. Can you help me?

THERAPIST: I think you've taken a good first step. You said that you have problems recognizing feelings, and why you act on them. I'm here to help you figure that out. I think if you can slow down, try to explain what you feel in the moment, and when you get overwhelmed or frustrated just sit with those feelings for a moment. There's no need to escape or act on the feelings. You can also start trying to do this with other relationships in your life. With your girlfriend. You can try to feel what you feel, and ask her to help out. That's how we connect with each other, right? Do you think you can try that this week?

MARK: It won't be easy, but I'll try.

In a departure from the usual stance of psychoanalytical therapy, the therapist is active and affirming, working from a relational psychodynamic perspective. The therapist helped Mark to identify that his feelings become overwhelming, and he acts out to escape from the discomfort. By providing an opportunity in the session for Mark to try to express his feelings, the therapist is helping Mark to recognize the pattern of disengagement that seems to be causing him problems in relationships, and substituting another more effective behavior of attempting to express himself to others. Practicing this new type of behavior will raise more feelings and at times Mark may feel overwhelmed and be tempted to disengage. Prior to this session the therapist had helped Mark to identify alternative, healthy behaviors he enjoys, such as exercise, playing music, and reading, which he can substitute for the self-defeating behaviors (substance use, sex) when he starts to feel overwhelmed.

As we can see from this short vignette, the cyclical psychodynamic–behavior therapist is supportive and directive and provides a safe environment within the session for Mark to explore his feelings and attempt to change his interactional patterns. With continued practice, Mark's goal will be to recognize his feelings and share them in the moment, reduce his anxiety, and eliminate the behaviors that continue to cause problems in his life.

Integrative therapies that are client centered or interpersonal tend to focus on empathy, unconditional positive regard, and re-creating the client's problems in the therapy session with the therapist. The relationship becomes the "vehicle of change" (Stricker & Gold, 2011, p. 442). Most CBT-focused integrative therapies do not dismiss the importance of the therapeutic alliance, but view the alliance as only one of many factors in the change process.

Wachtel's cyclical psychodynamic therapy is just one of many forms of integrative therapy that provides a dynamic source of behavioral change. Now, we turn to a discussion of multimodal therapy.

MULTIMODAL THERAPY

Multimodal therapy (MMT) is one of the best known of the technical eclectic approaches (Harwood, Beutler, & Charvat, 2010, p. 99). MMT is a system for integrating theories and interventions, rather than a self-contained treatment approach. Grounded in behaviorism and emphasizing outcomes, multimodal therapy also draws heavily on cognitive therapy as well as social learning theory. In addition, multimodal therapy has a humanistic component and values the uniqueness and self-determination of each individual. This approach also pays attention to context, looking at the individual as well as the person's culture, society, politics, and environment (Lazarus, 1996).

Multimodal therapy was developed by Arnold Lazarus, a pioneer in technical eclecticism. Lazarus was trained in behavior therapy, although he soon recognized the limitations of that approach and began to incorporate cognitive and other strategies into his work. Suggesting that clinicians take a broad view of people and ways to help, Lazarus advocates technical eclecticism, which draws on many theories and strategies to match a treatment to a client and problem.

Theory and Practice of Multimodal Therapy

Lazarus and other therapists who take a multimodal approach look at the client holistically; consequently, treatment needs to be flexible and versatile, drawing on a variety of approaches. For Lazarus, technical eclecticism, in which therapists select procedures from different treatment modalities based on what works best for the client's needs but without necessarily subscribing to the overall theories, is the ideal way to plan such a treatment (Lazarus, 1989). The ability to address client concerns from multiple vantage points simultaneously gives multimodal therapists considerable power and leverage, and results in more effective outcomes.

Treatment that reflects technical eclecticism, as described by Lazarus, has the following characteristics. It is:

1. Grounded in a theory of the clinician's choice
2. Enhanced by interventions associated with compatible approaches to treatment
3. Focused on interventions that have had their value substantiated by research.

Selection of specific treatment strategies is guided by a systematic framework for matching intervention to client, problem, and situation (Lazarus, 2006).

BASIC I.D. In multimodal therapy, a careful assessment of clients and their concerns is an essential precursor to treatment planning. One of Lazarus's most important contributions to the growing movement toward integrative treatment was the development of an assessment model that delineates seven basic categories of client functioning, represented by the acronym BASIC I.D.:

1. *Behavior:* Observable actions, responses, and habits
2. *Affect:* Moods and emotions
3. *Sensations:* Physical concerns, sensory experiences (touch, taste, smell, sight, hearing)
4. *Images:* Fantasies, dreams, memories, mental pictures, and people's views of themselves, their lives, and their futures
5. *Cognitions:* Thoughts, beliefs, philosophies, values, plans, opinions, insights, self-talk
6. *Interpersonal relations:* Friendships and intimate relationships, interactions with others
7. *Drugs, biology:* Broadly defined as biological functioning, including overall health, nutrition, exercise, self-care.

ASSESSMENT INSTRUMENTS Treatment via multimodal therapy typically begins with a comprehensive assessment of these seven areas, using questions and scales to identify both strengths and problem areas. This helps clinicians identify interventions that might be helpful in the specific area of concern. For example, let's create a BASIC I.D. for Edie. Imagine that Edie came in for the first session. Our initial goal is to assess her functioning in each area of the BASIC I.D. During the intake interview, we elicit information from Edie about her history, her family life, her relationship with Roberto and with her daughter Ava. Based on Edie's responses, we develop the following chart:

B: *Behavior:* Edie is arguing with Roberto more than usual. She is having trouble sleeping, and her relationship with her daughter is tense.

A: *Affect:* She feels taken for granted and angry.

S: *Sensations:* She is starting to get headaches.

I: *Images:* Edie imagines that all of the stress she is under is causing her cancer to come back. She visualizes the cancer cells growing inside of her.

C: *Cognitions:* Normally very compassionate with herself, she has started to criticize herself and engage in negative self-talk that she is a poor wife and mother.

I: *Interpersonal relations:* Edie has distanced herself from her friends and from her mother.

D: *Drugs:* Edie denies any problems with substance abuse.

Now that we have elicited this information from Edie, the question becomes one of where to begin and how to use the information to create an effective treatment plan that takes the client's needs into account. Lazarus (2006) found that each person favors some BASIC I.D. modalities over others. For example, a person might be characterized as a sensory reactor, an affective reactor, or an imagery reactor depending on which modality is preferred.

The *Structural Profile Inventory* helps identify a person's preferred modalities. This form asks people to indicate on a scale of 1 to 7 how important each of the seven areas of functioning is in their lives. Listing the seven areas in descending order of a person's ratings yields a structural profile for that person. Constructing a diagram or bar graph of the relative strengths of a person's seven areas of functioning is useful in clarifying patterns (Lazarus, 1976).

As an example, we asked Edie to rank order the list of seven modalities. Following are her results.

- Interpersonal relations: 7
- Affect: 6
- Cognitions: 5

- Behavior: 4
- Sensations: 3
- Images: 2
- Drugs, biology: 1

Completing this profile helped Edie realize that she sometimes lets her strong emotions and need for approval and closeness cloud her judgment so that her feelings control her decisions. Changes she saw as desirable included moderating these two areas and improving her self-care and health habits.

Another way to use the BASIC I.D. is to look at a person's modality firing order. Lazarus suggests that each person has a characteristic sequence of reactions to stressors and that this sequence usually mirrors that person's structural profile. For example, when Edie was under stress, she usually first felt rejected and unloved (interpersonal relations), while becoming angry and scared (affect). Then she began a dialogue with herself, focused on how unlovable she felt and how many mistakes she had made in her relationships. This often caused her difficulty because she would erroneously accuse others of not caring about her, would overreact with anger and fear, and would then blame herself for the conflict. None of these reactions afforded her a way to discuss and dispel conflict with others. Consciously making some changes—in particular, moderating her emotions, considering new cognitions, and developing behaviors that promoted dialogue and resolution—helped Edie handle stress more effectively.

The Multimodal Life History (1991, 1998), developed by Arnold Lazarus and his son Clifford, facilitates the assessment process. This is an extensive written questionnaire that asks clients about their backgrounds, personal and social histories, presenting problems, and details about the seven areas of functioning.

People seem to respond best to interventions that target their preferred modalities. For example, a person who emphasizes imagery is likely to benefit from visualization, whereas a person who focuses on thinking and analyzing probably will respond well to interventions that help identify and modify cognitive distortions. The resulting chart can then be discussed with the client, along with recommended treatment approaches that have been found to be effective for his or her specific problems.

Structural profiles are useful in couples counseling as well as individual therapy. Comparing two people's structural profiles can shed light on their similarities and differences and help to explain and normalize some of their conflicts. An explanation of each person's preferred firing order is also helpful (Lazarus, 2006).

ANALYZING THE BASIC I.D. The BASIC I.D. is a rich source of information about a person and can be processed in several ways. In addition to rating and rank-ordering the seven modalities, clients can identify changes they would like to make in each modality. Lazarus (1976) refers to this process as a second-order analysis of the BASIC I.D. A second-order analysis also can focus on identifying symptoms in each of the seven areas. This can also be a useful step for relieving a treatment impasse.

BRIDGING AND TRACKING Bridging and tracking are two useful techniques associated with multimodal therapy. In bridging, clinicians initially relate to clients through the clients' dominant modality to build connection and rapport and then branch off into other dimensions that are likely to promote new skills and ways of responding. Tracking is the process of using interventions in the same sequence as a person's preferred firing order. In Edie's case, the clinician would choose interventions that addressed interpersonal relations and affect regulation first. This seems to maximize receptivity to the interventions.

Therapeutic Alliance

Lazarus (1993) considers that therapists should become "authentic chameleons" (p. 404) as they consider the client's needs and preferences. Therapists must decide how reflective, directive, or supportive they will be with a client; whether they will be formal or informal, business-like or relaxed, reflective or more confrontational. Lazarus suggests therapists adjust their therapeutic style to fit the expectations or preferences of the client.

Although collaboration between clients and clinicians is valued in multimodal therapy, clinicians assume the primary role in assessment and treatment planning and remain active and in charge of treatment throughout the process. The multimodal therapist should constantly ask "What works, for whom, and under which particular circumstances?" in an effort to select the type of interventions that are most likely to be helpful for the particular client and his or her specific problem (Miller, Hubble, Duncan, & Wampold, 2010).

Application and Current Status

The importance of assessment in multimodal therapy requires that clients have some self-awareness; be motivated and reasonably reliable informants; and be capable of at least a moderate level of planning, organizing, and self-monitoring. Despite these constraints, multimodal therapy is a flexible and adaptable approach that can be used with a broad range of people and problems. It can be combined with medication for people who would benefit from its use, integrate several treatment systems that are likely to be helpful, and be adapted to the needs of people from diverse cultural backgrounds. People who present a combination of different concerns (e.g., anxiety, time management, and poor social skills) might be particularly responsive to multimodal therapy. Interventions can be developed in each relevant modality, providing a systematic approach to both addressing specific concerns and relieving feelings of being overwhelmed and discouraged, both of which are usually seen in multiproblem clients.

Recognizing the current trend toward short-term therapy, Lazarus (2006) has described ways to adapt multimodal therapy to a brief framework. He suggests a four-step process:

1. Use the BASIC I.D. format to screen for the presence of significant problems.
2. In collaboration with the client, identify three or four focal concerns.
3. If indicated, refer for a medication evaluation as well as a physical examination.
4. Use empirically validated treatment modalities and interventions to address the client's focal concerns.

Multimodal therapy seems to be appropriate for a variety of disorders and populations. MMT has been implemented in the treatment of anxiety and mood disorders, sexual disorders, serious mental illnesses such as bipolar disorder and schizophrenia, and eating disorders, among others. Additionally, case studies in the literature illustrate the application of MMT to agoraphobia, posttraumatic stress disorder, somatization (Lazarus, 1985), and substance misuse (Lazarus, 2006). Multimodal therapy has been used with children, couples, and families; in inpatient and outpatient settings; and in therapy groups (Lazarus, 1989, 2006).

Evaluation

Multimodal therapy has some shortcomings and limitations. Some clinicians are concerned about the lack of a cohesive theory to unify this model. In the hands of an unskilled clinician, MMT could become a poorly organized array of techniques not much different from syncretism (discussed earlier). MMT also lacks some of the strengths of a sound treatment system, including a concept of human development, a theory of change, and an explanation of why people develop problems. Another shortcoming is the inherent need for organization, structure, detail, and planning, as well as the demands the approach places on clinicians who must be familiar with and skilled in a broad array of theoretical approaches and interventions.

Nevertheless, MMT has many strengths, the most important of which is flexibility. It also can be powerful, systematically addressing client concerns on many fronts, using interventions that make a difference. In addition, the BASIC I.D. framework provides a useful and accessible way to gather client information and is interesting and appealing to most people. MMT is holistic, comprehensive, individualized, and goal directed. It offers structure and a clear direction to treatment, which can reassure clients and help make problems manageable.

Additional research is needed, but initial studies report that 75% of people treated via multimodal therapy achieved major treatment goals (Lazarus, 1976). At the same time, the significance of research on multimodal therapy is unclear because each person is treated differently, prohibiting replication. Even so, clinicians who use this approach are solidly grounded in cognitive–behavioral methods while also drawing from empirically supported treatments in other therapeutic models.

MMT facilitates treatment planning, provides an essential tool for conducting assessments, and also demonstrates accountability and meeting the requirements of third-party payers. It is also compatible with a short-term treatment model and, consequently, with much of the treatment that is provided today (Lazarus, 2006).

More than 20 years ago Lazarus predicted that a "systematic, prescriptive, technically eclectic orientation" would eventually become "the psychotherapeutic Zeitgeist" (Lazarus & Beutler, 1993, p. 384). Indeed, the use of multimodal and other technically integrative therapies are the most popular types of therapy offered today, with their use seeming to appeal to clients, clinicians, and managed care providers alike.

EMERGING INTEGRATED AND ECLECTIC TREATMENT SYSTEMS

Since upwards of two-thirds of therapists in the United States consider themselves to be either eclectic or integrative (Schottenbauer, Glass, & Arnkoff, 2007, p. 225), most clinicians probably would benefit from having a framework or theory to guide them in organizing and applying a diverse array of treatment strategies, so that they can successfully treat a broad range of clients and concerns. Not only is this desirable from a clinical point of view, but a systematic approach to eclecticism would facilitate clinicians' efforts to demonstrate accountability and present treatment plans to third-party payers and clients in persuasive and powerful ways.

Clinicians and theoreticians today have developed an array of approaches to eclectic and integrated treatment. These can be categorized as follows:

- *Approaches that match treatment to client level of readiness for change and/or client personal characteristics:* multimodal therapy, transtheoretical model, adaptive counseling and therapy, the thinking-feeling-adapting (TFA) model, the three-dimensional model of multicultural counseling
- *Approaches that feature a planned integration of specific theories:* Hill's three-stage integrated model of helping, Wachtel's cyclical psychodynamic therapy
- *Common factors models*

We have already reviewed multimodal therapy and cyclical psychodynamic therapy. We briefly review some of the emerging integrated or eclectic approaches here, touching on the more important of these at greater length than on those with less development, application, or use. Readers are encouraged to read further about these approaches, most of which are in a relatively early stage of development.

Transtheoretical Model of Change

The *transtheoretical model* (TTM), developed by Prochaska and others (Prochaska & DiClemente, 1986; Prochaska & Norcross, 2009), provides a theory of behavior change that incorporates elements from many different theoretical perspectives (hence the name, *transtheoretical*). Inherent in the theory is recognition of the uniqueness and diversity of other models, as well as their commonalities. Also known as the stage-of-change model, TTM reflects the scientist-practitioner approach to developing theories and is based on both empirical research and practice.

The transtheoretical model is intended to apply to mental health and behavioral health problems and has been used successfully to reduce smoking, stress, violence, and bullying behaviors. It is a stage model that links interventions (*processes of change*) and the target of change efforts (*levels of change*) to the person's *stage of change*. Assessment and matching are essential ingredients in this approach, as they are in many eclectic and integrated treatment models.

TTM provides an organized and methodical approach to planning and integrating treatment strategies based on the following:

- ***Five stages of change:*** Clients go through predictable stages as they engage in treatment and that treatment must be matched to a person's level of readiness for change. Although progression through these phases may be direct and linear, it is more likely to reflect a spiral, with relapses and other factors causing people to cycle back through previous phases in the change process. The five stages include (Petrocelli, 2002):
  - ***Precontemplation:*** People in this stage see no need to change. They may be involuntary clients, seeking help because of a court order or family pressure.
  - ***Contemplation:*** People in this stage recognize that they have difficulties but have not made a commitment to take action needed for change.
  - ***Preparation:*** At this stage, people have decided to change and have even taken some small steps toward change.
  - ***Action:*** Now people are motivated and committed to make changes. They exert effort over time to accomplish those changes.
  - ***Maintenance:*** People act in ways that are likely to maintain and continue their positive changes and avoid relapse.
- ***Ten processes of change:*** Determination of a person's stage of change is used to identify strategies and interventions that are likely to be successful and to help that person progress to the next stage of change. The developers of TTM identified 10 change processes that demonstrated their value in both research and practice: consciousness raising, catharsis/dramatic relief, self-reevaluation, environmental reevaluation, self-liberation, social liberation, counterconditioning, stimulus control, contingency management, and helping relationships (Prochaska & Norcross, 2009, p. 17). Strategies that promote awareness such as consciousness raising and evaluation of self and environment are particularly helpful and well received during the early precontemplation and contemplation stages, whereas action-oriented interventions such as contingency management and conditioning are more useful in the later action and maintenance stages.

- ***Five levels of change:*** The transtheoretical model considers a hierarchical organization of five levels of psychological problems that are likely to be addressed in psychotherapy (Prochaska & Norcross, 2009, p. 502). The five levels include:

  1. Symptom/situational problems
  2. Maladaptive cognitions
  3. Current interpersonal conflicts
  4. Family/systems conflicts
  5. Intrapersonal conflicts.

TTM recognizes the importance of the therapeutic alliance, which Prochaska and Norcross (2009) view as the most robust common factor in therapy. They also see the value of a healing setting and a confiding relationship. The clinician is viewed as an expert on change who has the task of tailoring the therapeutic relationship, as well as the treatment plan, to each client's stage of change.

TTM shows considerable promise. It provides a conceptual scheme to explain how people change and how to facilitate that change. It generalizes to a broad range of problems, it encourages innovation, and advocates both empirical research and experience to determine the value of this approach. Overall, Prochaska and Norcross (2009) report that 25 years of controlled research on the transtheoretical treatment model indicates that "TTM is an evidence-based self-help treatment for addictions and habits" (p. 511) and that it shows promise as a psychotherapy for depression and other disorders, but more research is needed. Even so, behavioral health programs that have tailored treatment to match the client's stage of change and the processes of change have been found to be more effective. Specific programs have increased abstinence rates for smokers, improved stress management in an at-risk population, and reduced bullying and violence among high school and middle school students at 25 selected schools in the United States (Prochaska & Norcross, 2009). This, and the TTM program for stress reduction, have both achieved evidence-based status from the Substance Abuse and Mental Health Services Administration. Additional controlled research trials are ongoing.

Other Stages-of-Change and Matching Models

TTM probably is the best developed of the stages-of-change and matching models. Others are briefly reviewed here.

THE THREE-DIMENSIONAL MODEL OF MULTICULTURAL COUNSELING In a similar model, Atkinson, Kim, and Caldwell (1998) suggest adapting treatment to the special needs of multicultural clients by looking at three dimensions:

1. ***Level of acculturation:*** high or low
2. ***Location of problem:*** internal or external
3. ***Intervention needed:*** remediation or prevention.

Once a client has been described according to these three dimensions, the approach suggests clinician roles and strategies that are likely to be helpful. For example, people with a low level of acculturation and internal problems needing remediation would probably benefit from healers from their own culture. On the other hand, people who are high in acculturation, that is, focused on external concerns requiring prevention, are more likely to benefit from a helper in a consultant role.

Hill's Three-Stage Integrated Model

Clara Hill's (2009) three-stage integrated model is solidly grounded in the work of a diverse group of important theorists: Freud, Rogers, Erikson, Mahler, Skinner, Ellis, Beck, and others. This approach takes the position that early experiences, especially those that are integral to the development of attachment and self-esteem, lay the groundwork for personality development and must be explored and understood in order for people to make positive changes.

This approach includes the following three stages:

1. ***Exploration.*** With Rogers's person-centered approach as the foundation, clinicians build rapport and a positive therapeutic alliance while exploring clients' thoughts, feelings, and actions. As clients tell their stories, clinicians develop hypotheses to facilitate understanding and also examine their own reactions to the clients.
2. ***Insight and understanding.*** With psychoanalysis and the ideas of Freud, Erikson, Mahler (individuation), Bowlby (attachment), and Teyber (interpersonal) as the underlying theoretical framework in this stage, clinicians and clients seek insight and understanding into clients' thoughts, feelings, and actions. Strategies such as interpretation, self-disclosure, and immediacy help people see themselves in new ways and make sense of their lives. Clinicians also attend to conflicts and attachments in the therapeutic relationship.
3. ***Action.*** Based on what they have learned through the exploration and insight stages, clients now take constructive action including learning new skills, addressing barriers to growth, and experimenting with and evaluating changes in thoughts, feelings, and actions. The cognitive and behavioral theories of Skinner, Bandura, Ellis, and Beck are the basis for this stage. Important interventions include teaching and reinforcing new behaviors, providing feedback, and creating action plans.

Empathic collaboration is an important part of each stage of the treatment process. Therapists are not experts on how clients should live their lives, but rather provide support, coaching, and encouragement. Hill (2009) stresses that empathic attunement and collaboration are ways of being with a client, not techniques to be used or skills to be learned, but rather an attitude that flows out of respect, knowledge, self-awareness, and a genuine desire to be of help.

Also integral to Hill's three-stage model, as it should be to all theoretical orientations, is cultural competence. Each of us belongs to many cultures (gender, race, sexual orientation, socioeconomic status, ability status, spiritual or religious persuasion). In the exploration stage of the three-stage model, it is important for clinicians to ask about culture to understand the client in the context of her or his current functioning. In the insight and action stages, it is important to note that not all cultures value insight and action to the same degree. Culturally sensitive clinicians are aware of their own values, but do not impose those values on their clients.

Common Factors Models

Some approaches to eclectic treatment have, as their unifying basis, a grounding in the common factors that make treatment effective (discussed in Chapter 1). These approaches reflect the finding that, overall, "despite the theoretical and technical diversity among models of therapy, they share important similarities that are responsible for the equivalent therapeutic outcomes" (Lampropoulos, 2000, p. 416). These similarities are known by many terms including common change elements, universal healing factors, shared therapeutic components, therapeutic common factors, and others.

Norcross and Beutler (2011) present a series of client factors that are routinely used in integrative treatment systems—stages of change, diagnosis, reactance level, client preferences, and coping styles. With the exception of stages of change, which was discussed earlier, each is reviewed individually below.

DIAGNOSIS The *Diagnostic and Statistical Manual of Mental Disorders,* Fifth Edition (American Psychiatric Association, in press), is the "bible" on which all mental health professionals rely for their diagnosis and treatment planning. Norcross and Beutler (2011) note, however, that diagnosis is not enough for the development of successful treatment plans. Client strengths should also be included, as should a complete multi-axial diagnosis with medical history, and current GAF score to indicate the client's present level of functioning.

REACTANCE (OR LEVEL OF RESISTANCE) Research indicates that high levels of reactance on the part of the client require less directiveness on the part of the therapist, if therapy is to be successful. Opposition, rejection of therapists' suggestions, and not taking advice are all typical of highly reactant clients. Conversely, clients who are nonreactive are more likely to work effectively with cognitive–behavioral therapy, homework assignments, and behavioral contracting (Norcross & Beutler, 2011).

CLIENT PREFERENCES Client matching has not been shown to be effective or efficient, but therapists who take into consideration client preferences whenever ethically possible are far more likely to meet with success than those who do not attend to client's needs (Swift & Callahan, 2010). Especially in the areas of therapist gender, ethnicity, cultural background, or sexual preference, clinicians who recognize, discuss, and help clients express any preferences or problems in these areas can "decrease misunderstandings, facilitate the alliance, and establish collaboration—which are all qualities connected to treatment success" (Norcross & Beutler, 2011, p. 515).

CLIENT COPING STYLES Coping style is another important variable in treatment planning. How the client responds to new or problematic situations becomes a behavior and then the behavior becomes a habit. Recognizing which type of coping pattern the client uses (externalizing or internalizing) is important for treatment success. People who use an externalizing coping style are more likely to act out, be impulsive, or seek stimulation. They benefit most from skill-oriented interventions. People with an internalizing coping style tend to be self-critical and introverted. They are more likely to benefit from insight and awareness (Norcross & Beutler, 2011).

In planning treatment, they suggest that clinicians look at four variables: client characteristics, treatment context, client–clinician relationship variables, and specific strategies and techniques. Beutler, Consoli, and Lane (2005) assume that certain universal clinician qualities, including respect, a receptive attitude, and flexibility, are associated with positive outcomes and suggest that these traits should underlie all treatment. Beyond that, systematic eclectic psychotherapy provides guidelines for fitting the treatment approach to the person. Clinicians pay particular attention to the client's level of motivation and coping style when determining the treatment plan.

The research literature indicates a great deal of empirical support for integrated theories. Specific integrative therapies that have been deemed effective based on randomized controlled trials include DBT, ACT, MBCT, and EMDR, which are integrated cognitive–behavioral therapies (discussed in Chapter 16), emotionally focused couples therapy (discussed in Chapter 18), and transtheoretical psychotherapy (discussed earlier in this chapter).

In general, integrative therapy models are available for work with individuals, couples, families, and all age groups, including children and high-risk adolescents. An excellent summary of the research can be found in Schottenbauer, Glass, and Arnkoff (2005). Clearly, development and study of integrative and eclectic treatment approaches is a growing area in counseling and psychotherapy because it reflects what most mental health professionals already do. Clinicians now have an ever-growing number of diverse treatment options from which to choose.

SKILL DEVELOPMENT: TERMINATION OF TREATMENT

The final skill presented in this book is the process of terminating psychotherapy or counseling with a client. Done well, that process can solidify gains, promote further growth, leave clients with positive feelings about their efforts and successes, and give clinicians a sense of pride and accomplishment. On the other hand, negative terminations can leave both clients and clinicians with unanswered questions and unfinished business, as well as feelings of anger, frustration, and disappointment.

Termination typically occurs in one of three ways:

1. ***Clinician's choice.*** Clinicians may be leaving the agency, retiring from practice, or making other changes that necessitate ending treatment with their clients.
2. ***Client's choice.*** Clients, too, may be relocating and so must end treatment. They may also decide to leave treatment because of its cost or because they do not view the process as beneficial. They may discuss their intent to end treatment with the clinician or may simply cancel an appointment and decide not to reply to telephone messages from the clinician.
3. ***Mutual agreement.*** Usually, termination by mutual agreement occurs when clients and clinicians both believe that the client has made good progress toward his or her goals and is ready to stop treatment, at least temporarily. Occasionally, clients and clinicians agree that treatment is not working and that the client would benefit more from another clinician or approach to treatment.

When termination occurs before clients have made satisfactory progress toward their goals, termination may be difficult for both client and clinician. The following guidelines can facilitate the process of premature termination:

- If possible, *allow time to process the termination of treatment.* How much time is needed depends on many factors including the duration of the treatment thus far, the clinician's theoretical orientation, the nature of the client's concerns, and the client's strengths and resilience. As a general guideline, clinicians who are ending treatment should allow their clients a minimum of three sessions to talk about their reactions to termination. Clients who unilaterally stop treatment may be reluctant to return for additional sessions, but often are willing to come in for one wrap-up session. If that cannot be arranged, they should have an opportunity to discuss their decision over the telephone.
- *Expect a variety of surprising client reactions.* Clients often show little emotion when initially informed that a clinician must end treatment. Over time, however, anger at the clinician may emerge as well as feelings of sadness and loss, perhaps accompanied by relief that they can avoid addressing their concerns further. Clients who initiate termination early may feel disappointed and angry because they perceive the treatment as a failure. However, sometimes they are contented with what they have gained from treatment and simply do not realize that a planned and gradual termination can be beneficial. Clinicians should allow space and time for clients to talk about their reactions to ending treatment, perhaps mentioning common reactions if clients have difficulty expressing or identifying their feelings.
- *Expect a variety of surprising clinician reactions.* Clinicians are human and may feel annoyed or angry with clients who terminate treatment suddenly and without explanation. Clinicians also may feel sad at the end of treatment, regret not being able to continue helping their clients, or feel sorry at the end of contact with people with whom they have developed a rewarding

therapeutic alliance. Clinicians may feel guilty about leaving their clients or failing to meet the needs of clients who have ended treatment prematurely. Clinicians also may feel relief that they will no longer have to work with particularly contentious and difficult clients. Clinicians need time to become aware of their own feelings about termination, perhaps discussing them with a colleague or supervisor, and trying to use them as a learning experience. Of course, expression of these feelings to clients should be done with care and thought, if at all.

- *Ask clients for feedback about their treatment,* especially if they have initiated the termination. Many clients have difficulty criticizing their therapists, so clinicians may have to work hard to obtain meaningful suggestions for change. Sometimes asking clients to identify both the most beneficial aspect of treatment and one change they would have made in the treatment can help them overcome their reluctance to express any reservations. Clinicians should try to keep an open mind, listening for suggestions that may be helpful to future clients, but also not overreacting to the complaints of one unhappy client.
- *Leave clients with positive feelings about the treatment process and themselves.* Review clients' accomplishments with them, being sure to underscore gains and help clients take credit for those gains. Remind them that although they might currently feel finished with treatment, you and your agency are available to help in the future. Offer referrals if clients need other sources of help.

Many of these guidelines also are relevant for mutually agreed-on terminations, although some changes and additions are likely. Pay attention to both clients' and your reactions to the end of treatment; again, expect surprises. Clients sometimes feel angry or abandoned as may clinicians, even though both agree that treatment has been beneficial and the time has come to end treatment.

Clinicians should request feedback, eliciting clients' thoughts about both the strengths and weaknesses of treatment. Identifying and solidifying gains that clients have made in treatment can be particularly rewarding for both clients and clinicians. Writing down clients' accomplishments is reinforcing and provides them with a record of their successes. Clients should direct the process of listing achievements as much as possible. The clinician might write down the items on the list as the client mentions them. Clinicians also can help clients identify their gains by reminding them of their initial treatment goals and facilitating clients' efforts to describe their successes in specific terms.

Clients rarely recall or think of all the successes they have had in treatment; so once they have run out of items to add to the list, clinicians can suggest other gains that they believe clients have made. Before writing down an item, the clinician should be sure the client does perceive it as a gain and that it is presented in language that is meaningful to the client.

Clinicians also might help clients formulate a list of goals they have for themselves now that treatment has ended. Identifying initial steps toward accomplishing those goals can help clients maintain the forward momentum they have developed through treatment.

CASE ILLUSTRATION

This is the concluding case study in this book. It illustrates termination with Edie.

CLINICIAN: Edie, we agreed that next week would be our last session, although, of course, you can contact me in the future if you believe that some additional sessions might be useful to you.

EDIE: I'm glad to know that; but as we discussed, I feel I have really made progress through my work with you, and I am ready to be launched . . . to try to put into practice all I have learned here.

CLINICIAN: I agree that you have made good progress. Last week I suggested that we spend this session listing the accomplishments you have made through treatment. I encouraged you to think about what you might put on that list. How did that go?

EDIE: I didn't actually write anything down, but I have been thinking about it. The more I think, the more I come up with for the list.

CLINICIAN: How about if I write them down while you tell me what you've come up with?

EDIE: Fine. My mood is certainly much better. We saw the numbers come down on that depression inventory you gave me, and I can tell the difference. I feel more cheerful and optimistic, I certainly don't have thoughts of suicide, I'm sleeping better, and I don't feel so guilty about any little thing that I don't do perfectly.

CLINICIAN: Sounds like you are seeing many signs of the change in your mood.

EDIE: Yes, it feels great! You know, sometimes I got so bogged down in depression, I didn't even know I was depressed; but I can really tell the difference now. Another important change is in my relationship with Roberto. I see lots of improvement.

CLINICIAN: What are the signs of improvement?

EDIE: I look forward to seeing him, we go out together and enjoy ourselves . . . we've even resumed a sexual relationship. I used to blow up at him all the time. I can't say he never ticks me off, but now I can just tell him and he seems to listen to me and be concerned. And Ava and I are doing better too.

CLINICIAN: What are you doing to make that happen?

EDIE: Before, I was always after her about something. . . . Remember to do your homework; don't forget your lunch money; be sure to get home for dinner. What I thought was expressing my love was really driving her away and giving her the message that I didn't have any confidence in her. Now I can see that she's pretty responsible. Of course, she still needs my help; but now, instead of nagging, I can put some of that energy into doing something fun with her. Last week she and I went to a place where you paint unfinished pottery; together we painted a coffee cup and a snack plate for Roberto's birthday. We both enjoyed making a special gift for him.

CLINICIAN: So things at home are better in many ways. How about the way you relate to your mother and stepfather?

EDIE: I've seen some changes there too. Now I usually can tell my mother what's on my mind in a way that she can hear without getting angry. We don't see eye to eye about my stepfather, but at least we can listen to each other and agree to disagree. Mom is spending more time with Ava, taking her out for lunch or ice cream, and that seems good for both of them.

CLINICIAN: Let's look back at our initial goals to see if that reminds you of any other gains. One of your goals was to blame yourself less for the abuse you experienced and to distance yourself more from that experience. You rated your level of self-blame as an eight out of ten. Any changes in this area?

EDIE: Yes. I didn't remember that I had rated that so high. I still have twinges of guilt about the abuse, but I'd say the rating is down to three or four. I can see that it wasn't my fault; I did the best I could.

CLINICIAN: So you've made real progress there. How about in distancing yourself from the abuse?

EDIE: That eye movement work we did seemed to make a difference. I remember what happened to me, and I'll never forget it; but it doesn't seem like a raw wound anymore. . . .

CLINICIAN: So your perceptions of that experience have really changed, and it does seem more distant for you. Are there other changes you can think of?

EDIE: My reactions to having been diagnosed with cancer also have changed. I know I had cancer and it was awful, but it seems like a long time ago. I don't worry much about a recurrence, at least not like I used to, and I don't worry so much that every little thing I do is going to cause the cancer to return. Another area that's better is work. I'm managing work better, feeling less overwhelmed, but I still don't have as much balance in my life as I would like.

CLINICIAN: How about starting another list? This one would include goals that you would like to work on after we finish our sessions.

EDIE: Yes, that sounds good. More balance is one.

CLINICIAN: How would you start to work toward that goal?

EDIE: I bring work home too often. And I don't allow enough time for exercise. Those are two changes I could make.

CLINICIAN: I'll jot those down for you. You might think about other future goals, and we can talk further about those in our last session, which will be next week. Let's take another look at your current list of achievements. One possible accomplishment I've heard you talk about is developing friendships. I remember you talking about feeling very isolated and lonely when you began treatment, and now you have two women friends you really like. What do you think about adding that to the list of accomplishments?

EDIE: Yes, definitely. I forgot about that. I'll never be the life of the party, but I do feel better about my social skills; and I have been spending time with Bettie and Sandy, who both seem to enjoy my company.

CLINICIAN: So that is another area of accomplishment. I'll give you a copy of this list so you can review it and make any other additions you might think about. Before we wrap up for today, I wanted to ask you for some feedback about our work together. What has been helpful?

EDIE: I don't know. It's all been useful.

CLINICIAN: Can you pinpoint a few aspects of our work that stand out in your mind?

EDIE: Teaching me how to change my thoughts when they didn't make any sense was helpful. I use that a lot. And the work on developing my social skills. Also the Myers-Briggs helped me understand myself and Roberto better and be more accepting of our differences. Also I felt you never gave up on me; you always had a plan to help me, and you really seemed to care about me.

CLINICIAN: I'm glad to hear that so many aspects of our work together were helpful. I would also like to hear about any weaknesses. Perhaps you can identify one or two ways in which our work could have been improved.

EDIE: I didn't like that book you gave me to read on assertiveness. It made me feel that I should turn into some other person. It's just not who I am.

CLINICIAN: So that book wasn't right for you. I'm glad you could tell me that. What other changes would you suggest?

EDIE: Once I called you when I was very upset. I guess I didn't tell you how upset I was when I left a message, but it took you three hours to return my call. I felt angry about that.

This session illustrates three of the important procedures in the termination process: listing and reinforcing the client's accomplishments during treatment, identifying future goals and initial steps toward them, and eliciting both positive and negative feedback on the treatment process. Although the clinician gives direction and structure to the process, the client takes an active role as she prepares to leave treatment. As this dialogue shows, termination is an important part of the treatment process. It can be rewarding to both client and clinician and continues the process of positive change.

EXERCISES

Large-Group Exercises

1. Discuss and list the benefits and shortcomings of eclectic and integrated approaches to treatment. Discuss and list the benefits and shortcomings of adhering to a single treatment approach. Which would you prefer at this stage in your career? Which do you think will be right for you after you have 10 more years of experience as a clinician?
2. Using the BASIC I.D. format, develop a hypothetical structural profile for Roberto, as well as appropriate goals and interventions for helping Roberto in each area.
3. This chapter introduced you to many integrated and eclectic treatment approaches. Discuss the common elements found in all or most of these approaches. Then discuss what makes each approach unique. Although your understanding of these approaches is limited, discuss which treatment approaches seem most likely to make an important contribution and why.
4. Integrating disparate treatment approaches can be challenging; some theories mesh well, while others seem incompatible. Discuss whether and how the following combinations could be successfully integrated:
    - Person-centered and psychodynamic approaches
    - Reality therapy and Adler's individual psychology
    - Existentialism and cognitive psychotherapy
    - Gestalt therapy and behavior therapy.

Small-Group Exercises

1. Divide into your groups of four, composed of two dyads. Each dyad should engage in a 15-minute, role-played interview in which the clinician helps the client develop his or her structural profile using the BASIC I.D. format as was done with Edie earlier in this chapter. Briefly discuss the person's strengths and desired changes in each of the seven areas. Focus feedback following the role-play on the process of developing the profile, considering both strengths and areas that need improvement.
2. Each dyad should role-play another interview, approximately 10 minutes long, focused on exploring the most important function in the client's structural profile. Clinicians should try

to be intentional and deliberate in their interventions, having a purpose in mind each time they speak. Record the interview and then play it back, stopping at each intervention to discuss the clinician's goal and whether it was accomplished.

3. Assume that your small group is going to develop an integrated approach to treatment. List the choices and decisions you need to make in developing your approach. Then make some of these choices and decisions as a group.

Individual Exercises

1. Using the BASIC I.D. format of multimodal therapy, develop your own structural profile. Rate the importance in your life of each of the seven areas. List those ratings in your journal, along with a list of your strengths and any changes you would like to make in each of the seven areas.
2. Identify the firing order of your first three preferred reactions to stressors. How well does that pattern of responses work for you? Do your characteristic responses to stress mirror your structural profile? Consider what changes, if any, you would like to make in the pattern of your responses to stress. Write about this in your journal.
3. According to developmental counseling and therapy, people can be described in terms of four cognitive developmental orientations: sensorimotor, concrete-operational/situational, formal-operational/reflective, and dialectic/systemic. Write about your own cognitive developmental orientations, responding to the following questions:

   - Which of these orientations best characterizes your current primary mode of functioning?
   - Identify a time in your life when another orientation was primary for you. What was that orientation?
   - How much flexibility do you have in your ability to move from one orientation to another?
   - Which orientation is most difficult for you to access?
   - Do you rely too heavily on one or two orientations?
   - Do your responses to these questions suggest any desirable changes?

Summary

A majority of clinicians report that their primary theoretical orientation is an integrative or eclectic approach. Integrated approaches are grounded in theory and seek to combine and blend multiple treatment strategies into a unique whole that is more than the sum of its parts. Eclecticism, on the other hand, lacks a unifying theory but is practical, providing a prototype or structure for selecting and applying interventions drawn from many approaches to counseling and psychotherapy. An increase in research on the common factors that exist in therapies across all theoretical orientations has provided additional support for the development of systems that allow therapists to create tailored experiences for clients that address the seminal question of what works best for whom, in the here and now of the therapy session.

This chapter described cyclical psychodynamics, a treatment system developed by Paul Wachtel; multimodal therapy, developed by Arnold Lazarus; and Clara Hill's three-stage theory. It also introduced you to some emerging integrative models.

As Lazarus predicted more than 20 years ago, technical integration of different modes of therapy is becoming the new worldview in psychotherapy. We expect to see the development of even newer integrated approaches in the areas of religion and spirituality, multicultural psychotherapy, and common factors approaches to treatment in the not too distant future.

Recommended Readings

Hill, C. E. (2009). *Helping skills: Facilitating exploration, insight, and action* (3rd ed.). Washington, DC: American Psychological Association.

Lazarus, A. A. (2008). Technical eclecticism and multimodal therapy. In J. L. Lebow (Ed.), *Twenty-first century psychotherapies: Contemporary approaches to theory and practice* (pp. 424–452). Hoboken, NJ: John Wiley & Sons.

Lazarus, A. A. (2006). *Brief but comprehensive psychotherapy: The multimodal way*. New York, NY: Springer.

Schneider, K. (2008). *Existential-integrative psychotherapy: Guideposts to the core of practice*. New York, NY: Routledge.

Teyber, E., & McClure, F. H. (2011). *Interpersonal process in therapy: An integrative model* (6th ed.). Belmont, CA: Thomson/Brooks Cole.

Wachtel, P. L. (2011). *Inside the session: What really happens in psychotherapy*. Washington, DC: American Psychological Association.

Also recommended is the *Journal of Psychotherapy Integration*.

Additional Sources of Information

http://www.sepiweb.org—Society for the Exploration of Psychotherapy Integration website and publishers of the *Journal of Psychotherapy Integration*.

http://www.newtherapist.com—The New Therapist website provides articles and information on integrative and eclectic therapy.

http://www.meaning.ca—The International Network on Personal Meaning website describes an integrative model of meaning-centered counseling that draws heavily on Alfred Adler's ideas, existential therapy, and cognitive–behavioral therapy, and also incorporates ideas from other treatment approaches.

CHAPTER 20

Solidifying Understanding of Treatment Systems

Finally! You have reached the concluding chapter in this book and probably the end of a course or training program. Your mind is full of theories and theorists, strategies and skills. While you may be eager to apply what you have learned, you may also feel overwhelmed by all this information. This chapter should help. It provides a structured review of the important treatment approaches we have considered, organizing information on each one into categories to facilitate your understanding of major concepts as well as of differences and similarities.

In addition, this chapter will help you choose a treatment approach that reflects your strengths and beliefs as a clinician and is likely to be effective with your clients. Combining this information with what you already have learned about systems, strategies, and skills of counseling and psychotherapy should help you answer the critical question: "*What* treatment, by *whom,* is most effective for *this* individual with *that* specific problem under *which* set of circumstances?" (Paul, 1967, p. 111).

An additional section on future directions in counseling and psychotherapy brings closure to this chapter and this book. Anticipating changes in our field can help you meet your professional goals, provide effective treatment, and contribute to your profession.

COMMON FACTORS IN EFFECTIVE TREATMENT

A great deal of attention has been paid during the past 20 years to identifying important commonalities in successful treatment. Research and clinical experience increasingly confirm the existence of common factors in counseling and psychotherapy, overriding characteristics associated with successful treatment, regardless of a clinician's theoretical orientation. Chapter 1 considered desirable characteristics of the clinician and the client, as well as of the treatment context. Now that you know about a broad range of treatment systems and strategies, you probably have realized that beneficial commonalities in treatment approaches also play an important part in determining treatment outcome. In fact, as much as 70% of the outcome variance between different types of therapy can be attributed to common factors shared by all successful therapies (Wampold, 2010). The factors most commonly found across all therapeutic types and orientations are:

- A positive therapeutic alliance that is collaborative
- A credible treatment approach that addresses the client's problems
- Factors related to the client, such as self-efficacy, problem-solving, motivation for change, and hopefulness that therapy will work (Norcross & Lambert, 2011).

Historically, the research on common factors accounting for client improvement can be divided into three broad categories (Lambert, 1992; Lambert & Bergin, 1994):

1. ***Support factors,*** including a positive, reassuring, and trusting therapeutic alliance and a clinician who communicates warmth, respect, empathy, genuineness, and acceptance
2. ***Learning factors,*** including changes in clients' thinking and perceptions, receiving advice, acquisition of insight, corrective emotional experiences, and increased self-acceptance and expectations for personal effectiveness
3. ***Action factors,*** including an expectation for positive change, improved behavioral regulation, reality testing, modeling, practicing, completing homework tasks, receiving suggestions, confronting fears and problems, processing, working through, and having success experiences.

Does this mean that theoretical orientation is not important? Absolutely not! Treatment factors account for between 8% and 15% of the variance. Treatment needs to be tailored to the needs of the specific client, and regardless of which modality is used, therapists must also attend to the relationship between client and clinician (Norcross & Lambert, 2011).

Another useful resource is Norcross's (2011) book *Psychotherapy Relationships That Work,* now in its second edition. This book is sponsored by the American Psychological Association (APA) Division of Clinical Psychology and the APA Division of Psychotherapy and spells out, chapter by chapter, the effective elements of the therapeutic relationship—what we might call Carl Rogers's *plus*. As Rogers emphasized in the 1940s and 1950s, and empirical research in the past 20 years now supports, the alliance, empathy, congruence, and positive regard are the building blocks of effective therapy. In addition (the "plus" in our essential conditions), therapists must manage the countertransference, repair any ruptures that occur in the therapeutic alliance, request and listen to feedback from clients, and work collaboratively with them. Serious students of effective psychotherapy practice should have this book in their reference libraries.

In summary, many writers have succinctly synthesized the research on commonalities in treatment. Clinicians now can have a clear vision of the kind of therapeutic contexts, relationships, and processes that are most likely to lead to a positive outcome.

OVERVIEW OF TREATMENT SYSTEMS

Although the literature gives some guidance on the treatment interventions most likely to be facilitative (for example, those that encourage people to confront difficulties and increase their empowerment), it has not yet identified the specific strategies or treatment systems most likely to succeed. Clinicians still have the challenging task of identifying which treatment approaches are most compatible with their own conceptions of effective treatment and most appropriate for use with their clients. The following sections of this chapter are designed to help clinicians make those choices.

Hundreds of approaches to counseling and psychotherapy have been identified. Of course, this book has not tried to review all of them. Rather, it has focused primarily on treatment systems that meet all or most of the following 10 criteria of sound theories:

1. The theories are clear, coherent, and easily communicated.
2. They are compatible with or can be adapted to include the therapeutic commonalities just discussed.
3. They encompass a concept of positive emotional development and health that can be used in setting goals and assessing progress.
4. They help clinicians organize and make sense of information.
5. They are comprehensive, explaining and addressing a broad range of concerns and disorders.
6. They give clinicians direction, steps, and guidelines for facilitating positive change.
7. They encompass strategies and interventions that grow out of and are consistent with the underlying theory.
8. They provide clinicians with a common language that facilitates treatment and collaboration.
9. They are widely used in practice and generate research. Even if these approaches have not been conclusively validated by empirical research, the research is promising and their widespread use or growing popularity suggests that clinicians find these approaches beneficial to their clients.
10. They focus on individual counseling and psychotherapy. (This book primarily addresses treatment of individuals with the exception of one chapter on family systems.)

The following four sections summarize the major treatment systems covered in this book. They can help readers learn more about these approaches, review their important concepts, clarify the differences among approaches, and develop treatment plans. Many of the emerging, eclectic, and integrated approaches are not included here because they are not yet comprehensive and well-developed treatment systems. Family systems theories are not included because the chapter itself is a summarization.

TREATMENT SYSTEMS EMPHASIZING BACKGROUND

Classic Psychoanalysis

Founder/major contributor: Sigmund Freud.

Area of focus: Background.

Underlying theory/view of change: Biology, drives, and early childhood experiences largely determine development. Making the unconscious conscious through analysis and interpretation promotes insight, reduces the influence of the past, lessens internal conflict, and facilitates healthier choices.

Other important concepts:

- Id, ego, and superego comprise the personality.
- Psychosexual stages characterize development: oral, anal, phallic, latency, genital.
- Three levels of consciousness exist: conscious, preconscious, unconscious.
- Dreams, mistakes, and symptoms reflect unconscious wishes.
- Defense mechanisms are important in understanding personality.

Treatment of background: Understanding the first 5 years of life is essential.

Treatment of emotions and sensations: Affect must accompany recall of unconscious material. Abreaction is important in effecting change.

Treatment of thoughts: The ego is the thinking part of people and is important in the process of working through issues.

Treatment of actions and behavior: Actions are important largely as reflections of the unconscious.

Important strategies, techniques: Analysis and interpretation, transference, free association, working through.

Therapeutic alliance: Therapist remains relatively anonymous. Transference is encouraged and is integral to treatment.

Level of directiveness: Direction comes largely from the client, although the clinician keeps sessions on track.

Growth- versus problem-focused: Treatment of problems is the focus, but successful treatment leads to growth.

Client profile: Approach is primarily for people with "neurotic" disorders, not those in crisis.

Attention to environment, diversity: Approach pays some attention to context, but little attention to diversity.

Emphasis on goals, treatment planning: Overall goal is improving ego functioning. Little attention is paid to goal setting and treatment planning.

Duration: Very lengthy.

Use of homework, tasks between sessions: Not important.

Extent of research validation: Limited.

Individual Psychology

Founder/major contributors: Alfred Adler, Rudolf Dreikurs.

Area of focus: Background.

Underlying theory/view of change: Heredity and upbringing are important, but people's own efforts to find meaning and success can be more powerful.

Other important concepts: Social interest is an essential part of healthy development.

Treatment of background: Treatment involves extensive analysis of early recollections, family constellation, birth order, roles in family, childhood experiences.

Treatment of emotions and sensations: Particular attention is paid to feelings of encouragement/discouragement, superiority/inferiority.

Treatment of thoughts: Individual perceptions and private logic are important.

Treatment of actions and behavior: Behavior is viewed as purposeful, reflecting goals and lifestyle.

Important strategies, techniques: Education; encouragement; discussion and analysis of dreams, early recollections, lifestyle; acting as if, interpretation, and use of hunches to promote insight.

Therapeutic alliance: Clinicians are educators and role models as well as therapists; they encourage cooperation, mutual trust, and respect.

Level of directiveness: Collaboration with client is important.

Growth- versus problem-focused: Can be both, but Adler emphasized growth.

Client profile: Appropriate for a broad range of clients, including children, adults, couples, and people with most of the common mental disorders.

Attention to environment, diversity: Social interest and social context receive considerable attention, as do people with disabilities.

Emphasis on goals, treatment planning: Shared goal setting is important.

Duration: Traditionally lengthy, but flexible.

Use of homework, tasks between sessions: Important for learning.

Extent of research validation: Limited, more needed.

Analytical Psychology

Founder/major contributor: Carl Jung.

Area of focus: Background.

Underlying theory/view of change: Development is determined not only by our early experiences, but also by innate unconscious archetypes. Through analysis of dreams, symbols, and other material, as well as through regression, the unconscious can be brought into the conscious to promote balance, growth, and integration.

Other important concepts:

- The unconscious is a source of creativity and emotional growth as well as of psychological difficulties.
- The elements of the psyche, including the persona, ego, anima/animus, archetypes, shadow, and personal and collective unconscious, are important.

Treatment of background: Individual background, as well as archetypes and ancestral background, are very important.

Treatment of emotions and sensations: Catharsis is encouraged, especially early in the treatment process.

Treatment of thoughts: Thoughts receive attention, and education is an important treatment component.

Treatment of actions and behavior: Actions receive attention when they reflect imbalance and lack of integration.

Important strategies, techniques: Catharsis, clarification of meaning of symptoms and symbols, associations, analysis of dreams, education, use of myths and fairy tales.

Therapeutic alliance: Support, encouragement, and establishment of a collaborative therapeutic alliance are essential. Transference and countertransference are inevitable and should be used therapeutically.

Level of directiveness: The clinician is active and provides education and information, but collaboration is emphasized.

Growth- versus problem-focused: Growth-oriented.

Client profile: People experiencing an imbalance in their functioning, spiritual concerns, or lack of integration. This approach is largely directed toward people not in crisis who have mild to moderate concerns and a great interest in personal growth.

Attention to environment, diversity: Social values and relationships are important. Little attention is paid to diversity, but emphasis on spirituality facilitates individuation of approach.

Emphasis on goals, treatment planning: Not important.

Duration: Lengthy.

Use of homework, tasks between sessions: Dreams and other material should be brought to sessions. Otherwise, not specified.

Extent of research validation: Very limited.

Other important information: Jung viewed the second half of life as a time of particular growth and creativity.

Post- and Neo-Freudian Psychotherapy

Founder/major contributors: Karen Horney, Harry Stack Sullivan, Anna Freud, John Bowlby, object relations theorists, Heinz Kohut.

Area of focus: Background.

Underlying theory/view of change: Early relationships are more important than drives; they provide the foundation for current relationships. Analysis and interpretation, in which past relationships are linked to present ones, facilitate essential change and development of the ego.

Other important concepts:

- Internalization of an image of the childhood caregiver influences the self-image.
- The ego and relationships throughout life are important in development.
- Developmental patterns and defense mechanisms receive considerable attention.
- Several of these approaches provide perspectives on women's development.

Treatment of background: Relationships and interactions during the very early years play a key role in development.

Treatment of emotions and sensations: Feelings about the self are important. Particular attention is paid to symptoms of depression and anxiety.

Treatment of thoughts: Some theorists are phenomenological, stressing the importance of people's ideas and perceptions.

Treatment of actions and behavior: Focus on behavior is limited, although some attention is paid to styles of relating to others.

Important strategies, techniques: Analysis and interpretation are paramount.

Therapeutic alliance: Transference is emphasized, but so is collaboration. Clinicians strive to communicate acceptance, support, and empathy.

Level of directiveness: Client and clinician collaborate whenever possible, although the clinician guides the sessions.

Growth- versus problem-focused: Concerned with both alleviation of symptoms and personal and interpersonal growth.

Client profile: People with mood, anxiety, and personality disorders seem well suited for these approaches. Motivation, commitment, and psychological-mindedness are likely to facilitate treatment.

Attention to environment, diversity: Approach pays little attention to diversity, but family and society are viewed as important.

Emphasis on goals, treatment planning: Overriding goals include building ego strength, self-concept, and sound interpersonal relationships.

Duration: Lengthy.

Use of homework, tasks between sessions: Little specific mention, but not excluded.

Extent of research validation: Research on attachment theory has lent some support to this treatment system, but otherwise relevant research is limited.

Brief Psychodynamic Psychotherapy

Founder/major contributors: Alexander and French, Davanloo, Klerman, Levenson, Malan, Mann, Sifneos, Strupp.

Area of focus: Background.

Underlying theory/view of change: Problems stem from inability of the ego to suppress or moderate drives of the id. Change comes from awareness of the connection of the past to present patterns.

Other important concepts: Careful screening and selection of clients is essential.

Treatment of background: The past is important, especially attachment to and separation from primary caregivers.

Treatment of emotions and sensations: Emotional release is important in treatment.

Treatment of thoughts: Some attention is paid to thoughts that are related to the focal concern.

Treatment of actions and behavior: Behaviors are believed to reflect underlying conflicts.

Important strategies, techniques: Identification of a focal concern, strengthening the ego, making the unconscious conscious, promoting awareness and insight, resolving conflicts, providing education on skill development.

Therapeutic alliance: Treatment should provide a corrective emotional experience. Some attention is paid to transference. Collaboration, support, and empathy are valued.

Level of directiveness: Relatively directive.

Growth- versus problem-focused: Both are emphasized.

Client profile: Relatively healthy and well-functioning people with identifiable focal concern and history of at least one successful relationship.

Attention to environment, diversity: Limited. May not be appropriate for many people from non-Western cultures.

Emphasis on goals, treatment planning: Identification of focal concern and written statement of goals is essential. Overall goals include understanding and changing inner experience as well as developing improved relationships.

Duration: Medium length, usually 3 to 6 months.

Use of homework, tasks between sessions: Not essential.

Extent of research validation: Some strong evidence of effectiveness, especially the use of interpersonal psychotherapy (IPT) in treatment of depression.

TREATMENT SYSTEMS EMPHASIZING EMOTIONS AND SENSATIONS

Person-Centered Counseling

Founder/major contributor: Carl Rogers.

Area of focus: Emotions.

Underlying theory/view of change: A climate of acceptance and unconditional positive regard promotes self-actualization and facilitates growth.

Other important concepts: Theory is phenomenological and humanistic.

Treatment of background: Approach recognizes that childhood messages shape attitudes, emotions, and behavior, but believes that the negative impact of those messages can be overcome through the therapeutic alliance and unconditional positive regard.

Treatment of emotions and sensations: Great importance is placed on eliciting and exploring emotions as well as communicating empathy.

Treatment of thoughts: Thoughts are viewed as resulting from past experiences and perceptions.

Treatment of actions and behavior: Behaviors are viewed as resulting from past experiences and perceptions.

Important strategies, techniques: Techniques are de-emphasized, but the approach does make considerable use of acceptance, reflection, and empathy.

Therapeutic alliance: Clinicians should communicate genuineness, congruence, acceptance, caring, and empathy to establish treatment conditions that facilitate growth.

Level of directiveness: Low; client direction of sessions is encouraged as long as the direction is therapeutically sound.

Growth- versus problem-focused: Growth-oriented.

Client profile: Ideal candidates are relatively healthy people who have difficulties finding fulfillment, self-actualization, and relationships.

Attention to environment, diversity: Approach emphasizes people's differences and commonalities, as well as the importance of respecting their perceptions and values.

Emphasis on goals, treatment planning: Overriding goals include promoting feelings of empowerment and competence, encouraging people to become fully functioning and actualized, respect themselves and others. Treatment planning is de-emphasized.

Duration: Flexible, depending on the needs of the client. Typically medium length.

Use of homework, tasks between sessions: Rarely used.

Extent of research validation: Core conditions of the therapeutic alliance have received considerable support.

Existential Therapy

Founder/major contributors: Viktor Frankl, Rollo May, Irvin Yalom, Abraham Maslow, and others.

Area of focus: Emotions.

Underlying theory/view of change: Through treatment and a positive therapeutic alliance, clinicians help people to face the uncertainties of life, gain awareness, and make responsible choices that create meaning and fulfillment in their lives.

Other important concepts:

- People always have choices.
- People need to accept the inevitability of death, and existential aloneness.
- People give meaning to their own lives.

Treatment of background: The early years are recognized as formative and usually are discussed, but in relation to existential concerns.

Treatment of emotions and sensations: Depression and existential guilt and anxiety are common symptoms addressed through this approach.

Treatment of thoughts: Thoughts about meaning and values are explored.

Treatment of actions and behavior: Behaviors are looked at in relation to the meaning in people's lives to determine whether the behavior is helping or hindering people's efforts to find fulfillment.

Important strategies, techniques: Symbolic growth experiences, paradoxical intention, dereflection, and discussion are designed to promote awareness.

Therapeutic alliance: This is an essential ingredient of this approach, which is viewed as a collaborative journey. Clinicians play an active role in sharing themselves and encouraging clients to value freedom, responsibility, authenticity, positive relationships, and actualization.

Level of directiveness: Collaboration is advocated, but clinicians do take a stance about what values are important.

Growth- versus problem-focused: Strongly growth-oriented.

Client profile: Suitable for people who are open to new ideas and seeking greater meaning in their lives. This approach is especially appropriate for people at a crossroads; those who are dealing with losses, life-threatening illnesses, and limitations and disabilities; or those who have long-standing underlying depression or anxiety.

Attention to environment, diversity: Social responsibility and the importance of the individual are emphasized.

Emphasis on goals, treatment planning: Goals include becoming actualized, clarifying values and meaning, and establishing a deep connection with other people and the world. Treatment planning is not important.

Duration: Varies but often lengthy.

Use of homework, tasks between sessions: Not specifically addressed; up to the client.

Extent of research validation: Some research suggests the value of this model in helping people clarify their values and deal with adversity.

Gestalt Therapy

Founder/major contributors: Frederick (Fritz) Perls, Laura Perls.

Area of focus: Emotions and sensations.

Underlying theory/view of change: People need awareness and an inner sense of balance and wholeness to deal with the constant flux around them. Treatment enables them to bring needed closure, integrate polarities, and function more fully. The whole is greater than the sum of its parts.

Other important concepts:

- Figure-ground
- Ego boundary
- Unity of the mind and the body.

Treatment of background: Little attention is paid to background; here and now is emphasized. Past issues are brought into the present to effect change.

Treatment of emotions and sensations: Emotions and sensations are the focus of treatment, especially bodily sensations.

Treatment of thoughts: Little attention is paid to cognitions, although the importance of awareness of all aspects of the self is stressed.

Treatment of actions and behavior: Awareness of and taking responsibility for one's actions are important.

Important strategies, techniques: Promoting awareness and balance, use of language, experiments, dreamwork, integration of polarities, role-play, empty chair, hot seat, fantasy trip.

Therapeutic alliance: Clinician creates a climate conducive to hope, trust, and awareness. Treatment alliance is a partnership in which client takes the lead.

Level of directiveness: This varies; clinician does not interrupt as long as client is aware and fully present. Clinician may become directive when client is not working productively.

Growth- versus problem-focused: Both important, although growth is emphasized.

Client profile: Not for people who are severely disturbed. Suitable for people with depression and anxiety, somatoform disorders, eating disorders, mild personality disorders and traits, physical disabilities.

Attention to environment, diversity: Interdependence and connection of people and environment are important. Individualizing the treatment to the person is emphasized.

Emphasis on goals, treatment planning: Goals include helping people to live in the present, use their resources, bring closure to unfinished business, achieve integration and wholeness, develop self-esteem, become more actualized, and achieve meaningful contact with self and others. Experiments (exercises or strategies) are developed for each person.

Duration: Varies, usually medium length.

Use of homework, tasks between sessions: Experiments and homework are an essential component of treatment.

Extent of research validation: Limited.

Other important information: Treatment system is humanistic and phenomenological and is useful in group therapy.

Narrative Therapy

Founder/major contributors: Michael White and David Epston (influenced by French philosopher Michel Foucault).

Area of focus: Emotions.

Underlying theory/view of change: People socially construct meaning and are capable of reauthoring the narrative stories of their lives. The person is not the problem, the problem is the problem.

Other important concepts:

- Postmodern, constructivist thought; there is no objective reality.
- Underlying assumptions must be deconstructed.

Treatment of background: The person can only be understood in the context of the larger society.

Treatment of emotions and sensations: Emotions and sensations are the focus of treatment.

Treatment of thoughts: Words and language choice are important. Thoughts are deconstructed to identify underlying presuppositions.

Treatment of actions and behavior: Actions and behaviors are understood within the broader context of social, economic, and political influences on the person.

Important strategies, techniques: Deconstruction and rewriting of stories, externalization of problems, use of metaphors.

Therapeutic alliance: Counselors are not experts, but collaborate to help clients tell their stories, understand relevant social constructs, and form new plots.

Level of directiveness: Very directive in externalizing problems, extensive use of questions to explore meaning

Growth- versus problem-focused: Both important, although growth is emphasized.

Client profile: Not for people who are severely disturbed. Suitable for people going through life transitions and those with personality disorders and traits or physical disabilities.

Attention to environment, diversity: Emphasis is on how culture, society, gender, socioeconomic status, and age affect the client's narrative.

Emphasis on goals, treatment planning: Goals include helping the client rewrite his or her story in a more acceptable manner, encouraging a wider perspective; use of metaphor.

Duration: Varies; can be practiced with few sessions.

Use of homework, tasks between sessions: Sometimes assigned; more likely to use therapeutic writing or documents

Extent of research validation: Limited.

Other important information: Treatment system is humanistic and phenomenological; can be integrated with other treatment modalities.

Solution-Focused Brief Therapy

Founder/major contributors: Insoo Kim Berg, Steve de Shazer.

Area of focus: Actions.

Underlying theory/view of change: Small behavioral changes lead to larger changes that have ripple effects on the whole system.

Other important concepts:

- People's worldviews lead to their problems.
- People have the resources they need to solve their problems.

Treatment of background: Generally, little attention is paid to background and history.

Treatment of emotions and sensations: Actions are the route to changing emotions. Little direct attention is paid to emotions.

Treatment of thoughts: This approach is phenomenological, giving thoughts and perceptions some importance in the treatment process.

Treatment of actions and behavior: Behaviors are the focus of treatment. Changes in actions lead to changes in thinking, understanding, and emotions.

Important strategies, techniques: Scaling questions, exceptions, the miracle question, presuppositional and other solution-focused language, reinforcement, viewing problems as outside the person.

Therapeutic alliance: Collaboration is essential.

Level of directiveness: Clinician is responsible for suggesting tasks and determining interventions as well as for providing support and encouragement and maximizing client involvement in the treatment process.

Growth- versus problem-focused: Both are important. The focus is on current problems, but treatment helps people become more confident and capable of solving future problems.

Client profile: This approach is ideal for people who are motivated, have solved past problems, and have some supportive relationships. It is best for treatment of mild to moderately severe disorders and problems, but success also has been reported in treatment of abuse and chronic and severe mental disorders.

Attention to environment, diversity: Clients' social systems are viewed as important. Although the approach does not specifically address client diversity, it is respectful, nonintrusive, and empowering.

Emphasis on goals, treatment planning: Co-constructing specific, realistic, and measurable goals is important. Careful selection of interventions also is essential.

Duration: Usually fewer than 10 sessions, but takes as long as needed for people to reach their goals. Schedule is flexible, often including long intervals between sessions, as well as extended follow-up.

Use of homework, tasks between sessions: Tasks are important and are carefully planned and geared to client's level of motivation and readiness for change.

Extent of research validation: More case studies and descriptions of application are available than empirical research, but strong support for this treatment system is emerging.

TREATMENT SYSTEMS EMPHASIZING THOUGHTS

Rational Emotive Behavior Therapy (REBT)

Founder/major contributor: Albert Ellis.

Area of focus: Thoughts.

Underlying theory/view of change: Irrational beliefs are the source of people's disturbances. Changing those thoughts to rational beliefs effects positive changes in emotions and behaviors.

Other important concepts:

- People have inborn drives toward both actualization and irrational thinking.
- Helping people take responsibility for their thoughts is important in treatment.

Treatment of background: Although life experiences are believed to combine with innate predispositions to determine how people think and act, treatment generally pays little attention to a client's history.

Treatment of emotions and sensations: Awareness of emotions, especially the underlying anxiety that usually accompanies disturbances, is important. However, emotions are believed to result from thoughts, viewed as the route to changing emotions.

Treatment of thoughts: Thoughts are the focus of treatment.

Treatment of actions and behavior: Actions are a secondary focus. They are used as targets of change and task assignments. They provide a useful gauge of progress.

Important strategies, techniques: *ABCDE* model for identifying, disputing, and modifying irrational beliefs; strategies for disputing beliefs; a wide variety of other cognitive, behavioral, and affective strategies.

Therapeutic alliance: Collaboration and client responsibility are emphasized.

Level of directiveness: Clinicians are relatively directive and use persuasion, self-disclosure, and humor to facilitate client change.

Growth- versus problem-focused: Short-term REBT seeks to alleviate symptoms, whereas longer-term REBT aims toward growth.

Client profile: People who are intelligent, articulate, pragmatic, logical, and tough minded are likely to respond well to REBT. This approach probably is useful in treating people with disabilities and those with a range of mild to moderately severe mental disorders.

Attention to environment, diversity: Social interest is viewed as an important aspect of mental health. However, caution should be exercised when using this sometimes forceful approach with people from culturally diverse backgrounds, especially those from non-Western countries.

Emphasis on goals, treatment planning: Overall goals include helping people think rationally, become more actualized, and enjoy their lives. Attention to treatment planning and establishment of specific goals is limited.

Duration: Relatively brief but flexible. Extended follow-up often used.

Use of homework, tasks between sessions: Task assignments are essential.

Extent of research validation: Considerable research validation demonstrates that, in general, REBT is superior to no treatment.

Other important information: Useful in individual, group, and family counseling; with children and adults; and for psychoeducation as well as treatment.

Cognitive Therapy

Founder/major contributor: Aaron Beck.

Area of focus: Thoughts.

Underlying theory/view of change: Distorted thinking causes people's difficulties. Analysis and modification of dysfunctional cognitions lead to changes in emotions and behavior.

Other important concepts: People have levels of distorted cognitions, including automatic thoughts, intermediate beliefs, core beliefs, and schemas.

Treatment of background: Attention is paid as needed, especially in people with long-standing disorders. Enough information is gathered to make an accurate diagnosis.

Treatment of emotions and sensations: Emotions and sensations are explored and their intensity is rated. However, they are considered primarily in relation to thoughts.

Treatment of thoughts: Thoughts are the focus and the vehicle for effecting change.

Treatment of actions and behavior: Some attention is paid to behaviors to understand clients fully. However, behaviors are considered primarily in relation to thoughts.

Important strategies, techniques: This treatment system includes a wide variety of useful strategies including questioning, identification and reality testing of thoughts, categorization of distorted cognitions, modification of thoughts, guided discovery, experiments, affirmations, cognitive rehearsal, and thought-stopping.

Therapeutic alliance: A collaborative therapeutic alliance is essential to treatment, with clinicians providing the core conditions, including empathy, concern, and congruence.

Level of directiveness: This is a structured approach; clinicians take an active role in planning and implementing treatment.

Growth- versus problem-focused: Treatment of symptoms is emphasized, but growth is also important and stems from learning skills that people can use after treatment.

Client profile: Suitable for a broad range of clients, particularly people coping with depression and anxiety.

Attention to environment, diversity: Little specific attention is paid to environment and diversity, but the respectful nature of this approach makes it suitable for a wide range of clients.

Emphasis on goals, treatment planning: Both are viewed as important. The overriding goals are helping people think clearly and cope effectively with their lives.

Duration: Short, usually 4 to 14 sessions, with extended follow-up.

Use of homework, tasks between sessions: Task assignments are essential.

Extent of research validation: Extensive validation is available, especially on the approach's effectiveness in treating depression and anxiety.

TREATMENT SYSTEMS EMPHASIZING ACTIONS

Behavior Therapy and Cognitive–Behavioral Therapy

Founder/major contributors: Early contributors include Pavlov, Skinner, Watson, Wolpe, Dollard and Miller, and Bandura. Donald Meichenbaum developed stress inoculation training and Francine Shapiro created eye movement desensitization and reprocessing.

Area of focus: Actions in behavior therapy; actions and thoughts in cognitive–behavioral therapy.

Underlying theory/view of change: All behavior is learned. Negative behaviors therefore can be unlearned, and new and more effective behaviors can be learned. Thoughts and behaviors are intertwined; focusing on both can enhance the impact of treatment.

Other important concepts: Thoughts and emotions stem primarily from behaviors.

Treatment of background: Actions should be viewed in context. Consequently, some exploration of background is important.

Treatment of emotions and sensations: Depression and anxiety are common targets of behavior therapy and cognitive–behavioral therapy. Assessment of subjective units of distress is important in measuring progress.

Treatment of thoughts: In cognitive–behavioral therapy, thoughts receive considerable attention. They are less important in behavior therapy.

Treatment of actions: Actions are a major focus of treatment. Identification, assessment, and modification of dysfunctional behaviors, as well as the learning of new behaviors and skills, are the essence of these treatment systems.

Important strategies, techniques: A broad range of strategies is used, including education, skill development, systematic desensitization, activity scheduling, relaxation, modeling, hypnosis, acting as if, and reinforcement.

Therapeutic alliance: Collaboration and active involvement of both client and clinician are essential.

Level of directiveness: The clinician suggests tasks and interventions, but the client has primary responsibility.

Growth- versus problem-focused: Primarily problem-focused; but education and skill development, as well as generalization of learning, contribute to growth.

Client profile: Useful in treating almost any person or problem, although the approach may need to be combined with medication or another treatment system. These approaches are especially useful for people presenting problems of depression, anxiety, and dysfunctional behaviors.

Attention to environment, diversity: Behavior therapy and cognitive–behavioral therapy recognize the importance of context but pay little specific attention to client diversity. However, these treatment approaches usually are not intrusive or threatening, so they may be good choices for people from a wide variety of backgrounds.

Emphasis on goals, treatment planning: Establishing specific and measurable goals and a clear treatment plan is an integral part of these approaches.

Duration: Usually relatively brief (12 to 15 sessions), although extended follow-up is common and treatment length is flexible.

Use of homework, tasks between sessions: Homework and practice of new skills are important elements in treatment.

Extent of research validation: Extensive research validation is available, demonstrating a wide variety of positive benefits. Symptom substitution is uncommon.

Other important information: These treatment systems are effective with children, adolescents, and adults and can be used in group and family settings.

Reality Therapy

Founder/major contributors: William Glasser, Robert Wubbolding.

Area of focus: Actions.

Underlying theory/view of change: People are self-determining and choose their thoughts, actions, and emotions. Treatment helps people make responsible and realistic choices and responses that are likely to meet their basic needs.

Other important concepts:

- Five basic needs: belonging, power/achievement, fun/enjoyment, freedom/independence, survival
- Quality world
- No excuses
- Total behavior
- Importance of awareness
- Emphasis on respecting the rights of other people to pursue fulfillment of their needs.

Treatment of background: Problems are believed to originate in childhood, but are best resolved by focusing on the present.

Treatment of emotions and sensations: Emotions are not targeted directly. Change in emotions results from changes in thoughts and actions.

Treatment of thoughts: This approach is phenomenological; people's beliefs, perceptions, and ideas are important and are considered in treatment.

Treatment of actions and behavior: Behaviors are usually the focus of treatment and are perceived as more amenable to change than are thoughts and emotions.

Important strategies, techniques: WDEP, $SAMI^2C^3$, paradoxical intention, positive addiction, questions, metaphors, caring confrontation, natural consequences, evaluation of own total behavior, other creative interventions.

Therapeutic alliance: Establishing a collaborative alliance is very important. Clinicians are encouraged to get involved with clients, become their ally, and never give up.

Level of directiveness: Clinician has considerable responsibility for the direction and success of the treatment.

Growth- versus problem-focused: Growth and process are more important than remediation and results, although all receive attention.

Client profile: This approach is useful for people with mild to moderate concerns, especially conduct disorders, oppositional defiant disorders, substance use disorders, and mood and anxiety disorders. It also is likely to help people coping with physical disabilities and those from non-Western cultural backgrounds.

Attention to environment, diversity: Treatment system emphasizes the importance of people having a role in society. Clinicians seek to understand people's worldviews and adapt treatment to the individual.

Emphasis on goals, treatment planning: Identification of goals is important in treatment planning. However, process is more important than product.

Duration: Flexible, typically medium length.

Use of homework, tasks between sessions: Homework is an important component.

Extent of research validation: A substantial body of research supporting reality therapy is accumulating. Its use in school settings is particularly well substantiated.

Other important information: Useful for individual, group, and family treatment.

TREATMENT EFFICACY

The American Psychological Association, the American Psychiatric Association, and the American Counseling Association all promote research to determine which treatments succeed in ameliorating the symptoms of which mental disorders. An important effort toward identifying evidence-based treatments has been conducted by the Task Force on Promotion and Dissemination of Psychological Procedures of the Division of Clinical Psychology of the American Psychological Association (Division 12 Task Force, 1996). An extensive review of the literature led the task force to identify 18 treatments whose efficacy had been well established and another 7 that were probably efficacious.

Treatments viewed as particularly effective include the following:

- Interpersonal therapy for treating depression and bulimia
- Cognitive–behavioral therapy for treating chronic pain, panic disorder, generalized anxiety disorder, and social phobia
- Beck's cognitive therapy for treating depression
- Behavior modification or therapy for treating developmental disabilities, enuresis and encopresis, headaches, irritable bowel syndrome, female orgasmic dysfunction, male erectile dysfunction, and marital difficulties
- Exposure treatment for phobias and obsessive-compulsive disorders
- Family education programs to help people diagnosed with schizophrenia
- Parent training to effect positive change in children with oppositional behavior
- Systematic desensitization for treating specific phobias
- Token economy programs for treating a wide variety of undesirable behaviors.

Many treatment systems, including person-centered therapy, psychoanalysis, and existential therapy, do not appear on this list. This does not mean that they are ineffective. Rather, because their application varies so widely, making replication difficult, and because they use few specific intervention strategies, conducting research on their effectiveness is extremely difficult.

These findings about treatment efficacy have made an important contribution to counseling and psychotherapy, not only in identifying successful treatment approaches, but in clarifying how little clinicians know with any certainty. Both novice and experienced clinicians are encouraged to keep up to date on the rapidly growing body of literature on treatment effectiveness to maximize the quality of their work.

FINDING YOUR PREFERRED CLINICAL STYLE

Readers who are relatively new to counseling and psychotherapy may view it as presumptuous or unrealistic to consider which clinical approach is best for them. However, choosing and emulating a style of the masters is a good way to learn almost any skill. Even Picasso, generally regarded as one of the most creative and innovative artists of the 20th century, began his career as a representational artist, painting in the traditional styles of the masters and only moving on to seek his own style after he had developed skill in established approaches to painting. In counseling and psychotherapy, acquiring expertise in treatment systems that have established their value can provide a solid foundation for eventually developing your own eclectic or integrated approach or deciding to specialize in one or two established treatment systems.

Determinants of Theoretical Orientation

Although surveys suggest that as many as half of all clinicians align themselves primarily with eclectic or integrated approaches to treatment, the other half are affiliated with specific treatment systems. Many determinants, including the five factors that follow, contribute to a clinician's choice of theoretical orientation:

1. Clinicians who are encouraged, through course work and professional experiences, to adopt a particular approach to treatment are more likely to embrace a specific treatment system than an integrated or eclectic approach (Robertson, 1979). This is especially true if they are exposed to a charismatic proponent of that theory.
2. Beginning clinicians are more likely to embrace a specific theoretical approach. They have not yet determined which treatment system best fits them and their clients, nor have most beginning clinicians acquired enough understanding of the entire spectrum of treatment approaches to allow thoughtful integration of a variety of approaches. In addition, adherence to a single theory can provide new clinicians with reassuring structure and guidelines.
3. Similarly, length of clinical experience bears a positive relationship to the likelihood that a clinician will have adopted an integrated or eclectic orientation (Prochaska & Norcross, 2009). Exposure to a diverse and complex array of clients and concerns, as well as to clinicians who practice a range of treatment approaches, leads many counselors and psychologists to conclude that any one theory is too limited to meet their needs. Even theories that seem comprehensive and well supported in the literature may have gaps and shortcomings in practice.
4. Clinicians' perceptions of their work are another relevant factor. Robertson (1979) suggested that clinicians who view their work as a reflection of their philosophy of life are more likely to assume an integrated or eclectic stance than are clinicians who view their work in practical terms, seeing it primarily as a way to earn a living.
5. Clinicians' personalities and worldviews are other important factors. Finding a theoretical approach that is compatible with who they are and how they conceive of the process of helping people seems likely to enhance clinicians' effectiveness as well as their enjoyment of their work. Clinicians who are more cognitively oriented tend to gravitate toward behavioral approaches (reality therapy, behavior therapy). Those who score higher on intuition preference on the MBTI are more likely to choose a humanistic theoretical orientation such as Gestalt, person centered, or existential, whereas clinicians who score higher on the thinking preference tend to prefer cognitive and cognitive–behavioral therapies such as REBT or CBT (Coan, 1979; Hart, 1982; Topolinski & Hertel, 2007). Among students, however, more recent research has found no correlation between personality type and choice of theoretical orientation (Freeman, Hayes, Kuch, & Taub, 2007). There do, however, seem to be some similarities in the personalities of people who choose to become therapists. Tremblay and colleagues (1986) found that regardless of their theoretical orientation, therapists tend to exhibit strong self-acceptance and self-regard, to focus on the present moment, and to have a positive view of human nature.

For many clinicians, their early years in the profession give them the opportunity to experiment with many approaches; determine what is and is not successful for them; and find a treatment system that is compatible with their professional roles, their self-images, their personalities, and their worldviews. Robertson (1979), for example, found that people who were skeptical and innovative were more likely to gravitate toward developing their own integrated approaches; this probably contributed to their feelings of ownership, genuineness, and congruence in their work. On the other hand, people who craved security, order, and structure were more likely to embrace a specific theoretical model. Most clinicians find that their professional interests and ideas evolve with experience, enabling them to refine their treatment approaches as they hone their skills. Later in their careers, therapists who are self-employed and who are able to practice a theoretical orientation that is congruent with their personalities report greater job satisfaction (Topolinski & Hertel, 2007).

QUESTIONS TO HELP YOU IDENTIFY YOUR TREATMENT STYLE

Having studied many systems of counseling and psychotherapy, you may already have a preferred approach in mind. On the other hand, you may feel overwhelmed by the vast array of appealing choices. Responding to the following questions will help you determine the theoretical approach that currently seems right for you.

Background Questions

1. What theoretical approaches have been emphasized in your training and modeled by your professors?
2. If you have been employed as a clinician, what treatment approaches were advocated at your place(s) of employment? Which ones seemed most effective and compatible with your personal style?
3. If you received counseling or psychotherapy yourself, what approaches did your clinician emphasize? How successful were those approaches in helping you?

Multiple-Choice Questions

The following questions are linked to the previous comparative analysis of the major treatment approaches reviewed in this book. For each item, circle all responses that are compatible with your beliefs. Do not think of this as a test but, rather, as a way to explore and better understand your thoughts and preferences about counseling and psychotherapy.

1. Positive change can best be facilitated by
   - **a.** Promoting insight, making the unconscious conscious
   - **b.** Promoting awareness and expression of emotions
   - **c.** Eliciting and modifying dysfunctional cognitions
   - **d.** Facilitating change in self-destructive behaviors
2. The following strategies are very likely to make a difference in treatment:
   - **a.** Analysis of transference, interpretation of dreams
   - **b.** Reflection of feelings, focusing on sensations, experiential learning
   - **c.** *ABCDE* technique of rational emotive behavior therapy, visual imagery
   - **d.** Systematic desensitization, reinforcement
3. Clinicians should
   - **a.** Be relatively anonymous to facilitate transference
   - **b.** Be genuine, warm, caring, and empathic, letting clients take the lead
   - **c.** Build a positive therapeutic alliance, but take an active role in structuring sessions, planning treatment, and identifying dysfunctional thoughts

   d. Build a positive therapeutic alliance, but set clear goals and limits, use caring confrontations, and point out consequences

4. Direction of treatment sessions
   a. Is unpredictable and determined largely by important unconscious factors
   b. Should be primarily up to the clients
   c. Should follow a clear plan for eliciting and modifying thoughts
   d. Should be determined by the establishment of clear, specific, and measurable goals

5. The primary goal(s) of treatment should be
   a. Eliciting unconscious material, promoting the working-through of past experiences, and developing insight
   b. Promoting expression of feelings and building self-awareness, self-confidence, and self-actualization
   c. Replacing dysfunctional thoughts and attitudes with ones that are more realistic and empowering of the self
   d. Replacing dysfunctional actions with new and healthier behaviors and skills

6. Problems and disorders I am most interested in treating include
   a. Long-standing, underlying depression and anxiety, the milder personality disorders
   b. Low self-esteem, confusion about goals and direction, lack of meaning in life
   c. Depression and anxiety, pessimism and hopelessness
   d. Drug and alcohol problems, eating disorders, conduct disorders, other problems of impulse control

7. The clinical setting(s) where I am most interested in working include
   a. Private practice, psychoanalytic psychotherapy training programs
   b. Programs designed to promote personal growth and self-esteem
   c. Mental health centers, private practice
   d. Drug and alcohol rehabilitation programs, schools

8. Understanding and addressing a person's environment and socioeconomic, ethnic, and cultural background are
   a. Not essential for successful treatment
   b. Important if they are important to the client
   c. Important in order to understand a person's worldview
   d. Important in understanding behavioral reinforcers and ways to effect change

9. Development of specific goals and treatment plans is
   a. Only important in short-term focused treatment
   b. Up to the client
   c. Essential for giving direction to treatment and empowering the client
   d. Essential for tracking progress and determining whether treatment is effective

10. Duration of treatment should be
   a. Lengthy in most cases to facilitate exploration of the past
   b. As long as needed to provide holistic treatment
   c. Relatively brief, but depends on diagnosis
   d. Relatively brief, with booster sessions used to prevent relapse

11. Use of homework assignments and between-session tasks is
   a. Not generally part of treatment
   b. Largely left up to the client
   c. Essential; treatment is unlikely to succeed unless people are willing to formulate plans and help themselves
   d. Very important and likely to enhance treatment

12. I view empirical research validating any treatment approaches I use as
a. or **b.** Not as important as case studies and my own experiences
c. or **d.** Essential

Evaluating the Questionnaire

Now that you have completed this questionnaire, go back and add up the numbers of *a*'s, *b*'s, *c*'s, and *d*'s you selected. As you probably have realized, the letters are associated with the four groups of treatment systems presented in this book:

***a*'s:** theories emphasizing background (psychodynamic approaches)

***b*'s:** theories emphasizing emotions and sensation (person-centered, existential, and Gestalt approaches)

***c*'s:** theories emphasizing thoughts (rational emotive behavior therapy, cognitive therapy)

***d*'s:** theories emphasizing actions (behavior, cognitive–behavioral, reality, and solution-focused therapy)

If your choices reflect a clear preference for one letter and one treatment system, especially if that preference is compatible with your responses to the background questions, you should pay particular attention to the theories in that section of the book as you continue your training and professional experience. You probably will find your preferred theoretical orientation there.

If no clear pattern emerges from your responses to the questionnaire or the background questions, you still may be sorting out your perceptions of yourself as a clinician and your beliefs about how to provide effective treatment. On the other hand, your preferred style might be an eclectic or integrated one that combines two or more treatment approaches. Asking people who have observed you in the clinician role which theory they think best characterizes your style might be a place to start finding your way as a clinician. Additional reading, especially case studies reflecting the application of a variety of treatment approaches, also might be helpful.

Clinical Orientation and Clinician Personality

Whether or not you have honed in on your current theory of choice, be sure to pay attention to the influence of your personality. Clinicians tend to prefer approaches that are compatible with their personality styles. Erickson (1993), for example, studied the relationship between clinicians' preferred theoretical orientations and their personality types as reflected on the Myers-Briggs Type Indicator (MBTI). Findings suggested that "thinking types are disproportionately likely to choose predominately cognitive techniques (Adlerian, behavioral, rational-emotive, and reality therapy), whereas feeling types are more likely to choose predominantly affective approaches (Gestalt and client-centered therapy)" (p. 39).

Using your self-knowledge, feedback you have received from others, and the results of the MBTI or any personality inventories you might have taken, think about your personality and the treatment systems with which it seems most compatible. Again, further reading on and exposure to those treatment approaches might help you choose a theoretical approach that is best for you at this point in your career. Keep in mind that you are not making an irrevocable commitment, but merely choosing a starting point that will help you continue the development of your clinical skills in a comfortable and focused way. With experience, you will become increasingly clear about the best approach for you and your clients, and you will find your treatment style changing, evolving, and improving.

FUTURE DIRECTIONS IN COUNSELING AND PSYCHOTHERAPY

The following trends and issues are likely to impact the direction of systems and strategies of counseling and psychotherapy in the 21st century (Prochaska & Norcross, 2009; Seligman & Reichenberg, 2012):

- Cultural competence will become the norm as therapists attend to their own, as well as their clients', worldviews. Background, culture, religion and philosophy, ability, age, and gender are important aspects of each person's social location and must be integrated into any efforts to tailor therapy to meet the needs of each person.
- Attention to the contributions of biology and neurophysiology to emotional health and development will increase. Assessments such as MRIs and fMRIs will be used more frequently in diagnosis. Increased use of medications, as well as more medication "cocktails" will be developed to provide more effective treatment.
- Combination treatment approaches that integrate medication management with behavioral interventions will be developed. These approaches will be solidly based on research on effectiveness.
- Legal and ethical guidelines will continue to be developed to regulate the use of technology in the counseling profession. Therapists who use online counseling, Skype, virtual reality, e-mail, text messaging, and social media will need to stay current with federal, state, and local laws regarding insurance reimbursement, confidentiality, and privacy requirements.
- Assessment will play an increasingly important role in treatment because of its contributions to diagnosis, clarification of the nature and severity of problems, goal setting, and monitoring of treatment effectiveness.
- Recognition of childhood antecedents to adult mental disorders will lead to the development of earlier prevention programs, but financial constraints will continue to limit the availability of preventive treatment for mental health problems.
- With the forthcoming publication of the American Psychiatric Association's fifth edition of the *Diagnostic and Statistical Manual of Mental Disorders* (*DSM-5*), our understanding of diagnostic criteria is expected to take on a more developmental flavor. Reliability of diagnosis is expected to improve, and much-needed clarification is expected for disorders that currently experience overlapping symptoms (e.g., personality disorders).
- Managed care will continue to focus on accountability. Many federal, state, and military funding agencies already require the use of empirically supported treatments as a prerequisite of reimbursement for services. The medical model will continue to become the norm, and clinicians will be expected to use evidence-based practices if they want to be eligible for third-party reimbursement.
- In the future, an increasing number of therapists will elect not to participate in insurance plans, as managed care systems continue to exert influence over therapeutic decision making, require manualized care, set clinical guidelines, and track therapist effectiveness.
- Research will continue to focus on and clarify the common elements across treatment approaches that are linked to treatment success.
- Not only will a positive and collaborative therapeutic alliance continue to be one of the most important elements of successful therapy, but research into the specific factors that foster an effective and collaborative alliance will increase.
- Transdiagnostic treatment approaches will continue to evolve in response to the increasing need for effective, practical, and cost-effective treatments.
- New models of psychotherapy will be proposed, theoretical integration will expand, and the existing models will be further refined.

- With the increasing recognition of the negative lifelong effects of childhood trauma, neglect, and abuse, attachment-related and trauma-based therapies will grow in importance and use.
- Brief psychodynamic psychotherapies, especially those related to attachment and interpersonal dynamics, will be especially influential in directing clinical attention to understanding and resolving internal conflicts.
- Narrative, constructivist, feminist, and other nonlinear treatment approaches will continue to influence conceptions of counseling and psychotherapy and are increasingly likely to be integrated into other treatment systems.
- Spirituality and religion will be integrated into the assessment, conceptualization, and practice of all different types of treatment approaches, as clients seek to find holistic therapies that focus on mind, body, and spirit.
- The use of self-help groups and homework tasks as adjuncts to treatment will increase because of the contributions they make to outcome.
- Eastern influenced philosophies and the tools of mindfulness meditation, acceptance, and compassion (loving kindness) will be integrated into most treatment modalities as a way to reduce stress and provide a holistic approach to treatment. Treatment will increasingly be used to help people deal with chronic and life-threatening illnesses, chronic pain, and to assist with end-of-life issues.
- Collaborations between school counselors and mental health clinicians will increase in an effort to address problems of bullying, school violence, suicide, and crisis management.
- Counseling and psychotherapy will continue to be important in helping people cope with problems and emotional difficulties, in part because the value of mental health treatment has been so well established and in part because research and holistic thinking will extend the breadth of its reach.

EXERCISES

Large-Group Exercises

1. Review the pages in this chapter that summarize the highlights of the major treatment approaches. Look particularly at the information about the therapeutic alliance advocated by each approach. Discuss differences and similarities in the ways in which the various approaches view the therapeutic alliance. Do you see more similarities or more differences? What differences seem particularly important? Do the older theories reflect a different conception of the therapeutic alliance than do the newer theories?
2. Discuss the following questions in relation to the following four cases:
   - What treatment systems and strategies seem most likely to be effective in treating each person? Why?
   - What treatment systems and strategies seem least likely to be effective in treating each person? Why?
   - What sort of therapeutic alliance would be best for each client?
   - What possible obstacles to successful treatment are presented by each person? What interventions or approaches might you use to overcome these obstacles?

   Case A. Seneesha, age 15, was brought to counseling by her mother. Seneesha's mother is African American; her father is white. Six months ago, her father left the family to move in with a woman with whom he had been having a long affair. Since then, Seneesha has seemed very sad, lost weight, and has been sleeping at least 10 hours a day. She has withdrawn from most of her friends, especially her white friends, and has been talking about how different she feels from her friends. She blames herself for her father's departure and stated that if she were prettier or smarter, he might not have left. She has avoided contact with her father and has little interest in her schoolwork.

Case B. Brian, age 33, has been married for 9 years and has two children, ages 5 and 7. He sought treatment reluctantly at the urging of his wife. According to Brian, his wife believes his use of drugs and alcohol is a problem. Brian stated that he does consume 8 to 12 cans of beer each night and smokes marijuana on the weekends, but also runs a successful business, earns a good income, and "doesn't run around." He agrees that maybe he should spend some more time with the children when he comes home from work, but otherwise sees no need for change.

Case C. Lea, age 42 and single, was recently diagnosed with breast cancer. With treatment, her prognosis is excellent. However, she is terrified of surgery and is endangering her life by postponing her treatment. She explains her reactions by stating that she feels all alone with no one to help her and doesn't know how she can handle her recovery from surgery and her subsequent chemotherapy. Throughout the session, Lea makes poor eye contact, speaks in a low voice, and appears very shy and fearful. She tells you that she is lesbian, but has not dated since a long-term relationship ended 6 years ago.

Case D. Carmen, age 25 and recently married, sought treatment after one of the teachers in the elementary school where she is employed was found guilty of child abuse. This brought back to Carmen vivid memories of her own childhood sexual abuse by her brother. These memories have made it difficult for her to be intimate with her husband and led her to feel considerable discomfort at work.

3. Review the section on future directions in counseling and psychotherapy. Discuss whether you agree that each of these trends is likely and provide a rationale for your response. What future directions would you add to this list? What trends seem unlikely to happen but would be helpful to the mental health fields?

Small-Group Exercises

1. If you have not already completed and assessed your responses to the questionnaire included in this chapter, do so now. Then share your results with the other members of your group, discussing what those results mean to you. Drawing on what you know about the personalities and clinical style of the group members, give each person in the group feedback about what treatment system might be best as his or her preferred approach. Be sure to discuss the rationale behind your recommendations.
2. Each member of the group should serve as an advocate of one of the four categories of treatment systems (background, emotions, thoughts, actions) discussed in this book. Then discuss the following questions, with each spokesperson presenting an informed view of his or her chosen group of treatment approaches:
   - Which treatment system best addresses issues of culture and diversity?
   - Which can be used with the broadest range of clients and problems?
   - Which is most likely to grow in use and importance in the coming years?
3. Form into your groups of four participants. You have probably been working together for many weeks and have learned a great deal about each other. Collaborate in developing a list of at least three clinical strengths for each member of the group. To make the feedback particularly meaningful, identify experiences in your group in which each of those strengths was evident.

Individual Exercises

1. By now, you probably have learned a great deal about yourself as a clinician. In your journal, list three clinical strengths that you believe you have. List three areas in which you think you need to improve your clinical skills. List three topics in this book that you would like to study further. Identify the first steps you could take in improving your skills and continuing your learning.
2. Identify the exercise or learning experience in this book that has been most interesting or enlightening for you. Write briefly in your journal about what made that experience so meaningful.

Summary

This chapter synthesized information about a broad range of approaches to counseling and psychotherapy, summarizing them in the lists in this chapter. The questionnaire in this chapter can help clinicians identify their preferred approaches to mental health treatment, as can the exercises designed to facilitate professional growth. This chapter also reviewed trends expected to have an impact on counseling and psychotherapy in the future.

Counseling and psychotherapy are vital and exciting professions that help many people and provide a rewarding career to many clinicians. Our hope is that this book has helped you to learn many important treatment approaches, skills, and strategies you can use to help others. However, like any book on theories and strategies of counseling and psychotherapy, it can give you only an introduction to these approaches. Our field is constantly changing and we strongly encourage you to continue to study and practice these treatment approaches through additional reading, continuing education, supervised experience, peer feedback, and research on your own practice.

As clinicians, we do very important work, work that can make a great difference in the lives of individuals, groups, families, and even societies. We hope you will treasure and honor the trust that people put in you and will do your best to use your skills to do good for others. We also hope that this book will help you to keep the energy and spirit of the mental health professions alive in your work.

REFERENCES

Abdel-Tawab, N., & Roter, D. (2002). The relevance of client-centered communication to family planning settings in developing countries: Lessons from the Egyptian experience. *Social Science and Medicine, 54,* 1357–1368.

Abramson, Z. (2007). Adlerian family and couples therapy. *Journal of Individual Psychology, 63,* 371–386.

Ackerman, S. J., & Hilsenroth, M. J. (2003). A review of therapist characteristics and techniques positively impacting the therapeutic alliance. *Clinical Psychology Review, 23,* 1–33.

Acosta, F. X., Yamamoto, J., Evans, L. A., & Skilbeck, W. M. (1983). Preparing low-income Hispanic, black, and white patients for psychotherapy: Evaluation of a new orientation program. *Journal of Clinical Psychology, 39,* 872–877.

Adams, A. N., Adams, A. N., & Miltenberger, R. G. (2008). Habit reversal training. In W. T. O'Donohue & J. E. Fisher (Eds.), *Cognitive behavior therapy: Applying empirically supported techniques in your practice* (2nd ed., pp. 245–252). Hoboken, NJ: John Wiley & Sons.

Adler, A. (1931). *What life should mean to you.* Boston, MA: Little, Brown.

Adler, A. (1938). *Social interest: A challenge to mankind* (J. Linton & R. Vaughan, Trans.). London, UK: Faber and Faber.

Adler, A. (1956). (1) The neurotic disposition; (2) Psychology of use; (3) Social interest. In H. L. Ansbacher & R. R. Ansbacher (Eds.), *The individual psychology of Alfred Adler* (pp. 126–162, 205–262). New York, NY: Basic Books.

Adler, A. (1963a). *The practice and theory of individual psychology.* Paterson, NJ: Littlefield, Adams.

Adler, A. (1963b). *The problem child.* New York, NY: Putnam.

Adler, A. (1979). *Superiority and social interest.* New York, NY: W. W. Norton.

Adler, A. (1998). *Social interest: Adler's key to the meaning of life.* Boston, MA: One World Publications.

Adler, J. (2006, March 27). Freud in our midst. *Newsweek,* pp. 43–51.

Adler, J. (2011). Epistemological tension in the future of personality disorder diagnosis. *American Journal of Psychiatry, 168,* 1221–1222.

Adler, J. (2012). Living into the story: Agency and coherence in a longitudinal study of narrative identity development and mental health over the course of psychotherapy, *Journal of Personality and Social Psychology, 102,* 367–389.

Ainsworth, M. D. S., Blehar, M. C., Waters, E., & Walls, S. (1978). *Patterns of attachment: A psychological study of the strange situation.* Hillsdale, NJ: Erlbaum.

Alexander, F., & French, T. M. (1946). *Psychoanalytic therapy: Principles and application.* New York, NY: Ronald Press.

Alexander, J., & Harman, R. (1988). One counselor's intervention in the aftermath of a middle school student's suicide: A case study. *Journal of Counseling and Development, 66,* 283–285.

Al-Krenawi, A. (1999). An overview of rituals in Western therapies and intervention: Argument for their use in cross-cultural therapy. *International Journal for the Advancement of Counseling, 21,* 3–17.

Allen, J. R., & Allen, B. A. (2002). Redecision therapy. In K. Tudor (Ed.), *Transactional analysis approaches to brief therapy: What do you say between saying hello and goodbye?* (pp. 83–98). Thousand Oaks, CA: Sage.

Almagor, M. (2011). *The functional dialectic system approach for therapy with individuals, couples, and families.* Minneapolis, MN: University of Minnesota Press.

Alonzo, D. (2005). Working with same-sex couples. In M. Harway (Ed.), *Handbook of couples therapy* (pp. 370–385). Hoboken, NJ: John Wiley & Sons.

Altman, A. N., Inman, A. G., Fine, S. G., Ritter, H. A., & Howard, E. E. (2010). Exploration of Jewish ethnic identity. *Journal of Counseling & Development, 88,* 163–173.

Altman, N. (2008). Psychoanalytic therapy. In J. Frew & M. D. Spiegler (Eds.), *Contemporary psychotherapies for a diverse world* (pp. 41–92). Boston, MA: Houghton Mifflin.

American Counseling Association. (2005). *ACA code of ethics and standards of practice.* Alexandria, VA: Author.

American Psychiatric Association. (2000). *The diagnostic and statistical manual of mental disorders* (4th ed., rev. ed.). Arlington, VA: Author.

American Psychiatric Association. (2004). *Practice guideline for the treatment of patients with acute stress disorder and posttraumatic stress disorder.* Arlington, VA: Author.

American Psychiatric Association. (in press). *The diagnostic and statistical manual of mental disorders* (5th ed.). Arlington, VA: Author.

American Psychological Association. (2002). *Ethical principles of psychologists and code of conduct.* Washington, DC: Author.

American Psychological Association. (2003). Guidelines on multicultural education, training, research, practice, and organizational change for psychologists. *American Psychologist, 58*, 377–402.

American Psychological Association. (2006). Special issue: The relevance of Sigmund Freud for the 21st century. *Psychoanalytic Psychology, 23*(2).

American Psychological Association. (2007). *Guidelines for psychological practice with girls and women.* Washington, DC: Author. Retrieved from http://www.apa.org/practice/guidelines/girls-and-women.pdf

American Psychological Association. (2012). Guidelines for psychological practice with lesbian, gay, and bisexual clients, *American Psychologist,* 67, 10–42.

American Psychologist. (1989, July). On the politics of psychological constructs, *44*(7), 1118–1123.

Anderson, B., & Anderson, W. (1989). Counselors' reports of their use of self-disclosure with clients. *Journal of Clinical Psychology, 45,* 404–415.

Anderson, H. (2001). Postmodern collaborative and person-centered therapies: What would Carl Rogers say? *Journal of Family Therapy*, 23, 339–360.

Anderson, T., Lunnen, K. M., & Ogles, B. M. (2010). Putting models and techniques in context. In B. L. Duncan, S. D. Miller, B. E. Wampold, & M. A. Hubble (Eds.), *Heart and soul of change in psychotherapy* (2nd ed., pp. 143–166). Washington, DC: American Psychological Association.

Anderson, T., Ogles, B. M., Patterson, C. L., Lambert, M. J., & Vermeersch, D. A. (2009). Therapist effects: Facilitative interpersonal skills as a predictor of therapist success. *Journal of Clinical Psychology, 65*, 755–768.

Andreas, S. (1991). *Virginia Satir: The patterns of her magic.* Moab, UT: Real People Press.

Andreas, S. (2012). The true genius of Virginia Satir. *The Satir Journal: Transformational Systemic Therapy, 5*, 1.

Angermann, D. (1998). Gestalt therapy for eating disorders: An illustration. *Gestalt Journal, 21,* 19–47.

Ansbacher, H. L., & Ansbacher, R. R. (Eds.). (1956). *The individual psychology of Alfred Adler: A systematic presentation in selections from his writings.* New York, NY: Basic Books.

Antony, M. M., & Roemer, L. (2011). *Behavior therapy.* Washington, DC: American Psychological Association.

APA Presidential Task Force on Evidence-Based Practice. (2006). Evidence-based practice in psychology. *American Psychologist, 61,* 271–285.

Arkowiz, H., Westra, H. A., Miller, W. R., & Rollnick, S. (Eds.). (2008). *Motivational interviewing in the treatment of psychological problems.* New York, NY: Guilford Press.

Arntz, A., & Van Den Hout, M. (1996). Psychological treatments of panic disorders without agoraphobia: Cognitive therapy versus applied relaxation. *Behavior Research and Therapy, 34*(2), 113–122.

Asagba, R. B., Alarape, A., & Chowen, C. O. (2009). Cross-cultural validation of selected logotherapy tests among undergraduate students at the University of Ibadan. *International Forum for Logotherapy, 32*, 78–83.

Asay, T. P., & Lambert, M. J. (1999). The empirical case for the common factors in therapy: Quantitative findings. In M. A. Hubble, B. L. Duncan, & S. D. Miller (Eds.), *The heart and soul of change: What works in therapy* (pp. 33–55). Washington, DC: American Psychological Association.

Ashby, J. S., LoCicero, K. A., & Kenny, M. C. (2003). The relationship of multidimensional perfectionism to psychological birth order. *Journal of Individual Psychology, 59,* 42–51.

Atkinson, D. R., Kim, B. S. K., & Caldwell, R. (1998). Ratings of helper roles by multicultural psychologists and Asian American students: Initial support for the three-dimensional models of multicultural counseling. *Journal of Counseling Psychology, 25*(4), 414–423.

Austad, C. (2009). *Counseling and psychotherapy today.* New York, NY: McGraw Hill.

Axline, V. M. (1969). *Play therapy* (rev. ed.). New York, NY: Ballantine Books.

Bachar, E. (1998). The contributions of self-psychology to the treatment of anorexia and bulimia. *American Journal of Psychotherapy, 52*(2), 147–165.

Baddeley, J., & Singer, A. A. (2010). A loss in the family: Silence, memory and narrative identity after bereavement. *Memory, 18*, 198–207.

Baer, R. A., & Huss, D. B. (2008). Mindfulness- and acceptance-based therapy. In J. L. Lebow (Ed.), *Twenty-first century psychotherapies: Contemporary approaches to theory and practice* (pp. 123–166). Hoboken, NJ: John Wiley & Sons.

Baker, E. L. (1985). Psychoanalysis and psychoanalytic psychotherapy. In S. J. Lynn & J. P. Garske (Eds.), *Contemporary psychotherapies: Models and methods* (pp. 19–68). Upper Saddle River, NJ: Merrill/Prentice Hall.

Baker, R., Baker, E., Allen, H., Thomas, P., Newth, J., Hollingbery, T., . . . Gibson, S. (2002). A naturalistic longitudinal evaluation of counselling in primary care. *Counselling Psychology Quarterly, 15,* 359–373.

Baldwin, S. A., Walpold, B. E., & Imel, Z. E. (2007). Untangling the alliance-outcome correlation: Exploring the relative importance of therapist and patient variability in the alliance. *Journal of Consulting and Clinical Psychology, 75,* 842–852.

Ballou, M., Hill, M., & West, C. (Eds.). (2008). *Feminist therapy theory and practice: A contemporary perspective.* New York, NY: Springer.

Bandura, A. (1969). *Principles of behavior modification.* New York, NY: Holt, Rinehart, & Winston.

Bandura, A. (1973). *Aggression: A social learning analysis*. Upper Saddle River, NJ: Prentice Hall.

Bandura, A. (1977). *Social learning theory*. Upper Saddle River, NJ: Prentice Hall.

Bandura, A. (1982). Self-efficacy mechanism in human agency. *American Psychologist, 37,* 122–147.

Bandura, A. (1986). *Social foundations of thought and action: A social cognitive theory.* Upper Saddle River, NJ: Prentice Hall.

Bandura, A. (2006). Toward a psychology of human agency. *Perspectives on Psychological Science, 1,* 164–180.

Banks, M. E. (2010). 2009 Division 35 presidential address: Feminist psychology and women with disabilities: An emerging alliance. *Psychology of Women Quarterly, 34*, 431–442.

Banks, T., & Zionts, P. (2009), REBT used with children and adolescents who have emotional and behavioral disorders in educational settings: A review of the literature. *Journal of Rational-Emotive and Cognitive–Behavior Therapy, 27*, 51–65.

Banmen, A., & Banmen, E. (Eds.). (1991). *Meditations of Virginia Satir: Peace between, peace within, peace among*. Palo Alto, CA: Science and Behavior Books.

Banmen, E. (Ed.). (2008). *In her own words. . . Virginia Satir: Selected papers 1963–1983*. Phoenix, AZ: Zeig, Tucker, and Theisen.

Bannick, F. (2007). Solution-focused brief therapy. *Journal of Contemporary Psychotherapy, 37*, 87–94.

Barbanell, L. (2006). *Removing the mask of kindness: Diagnosis and treatment of the caretaker personality disorder.* Lanham, MD: Jason Aronson.

Barber, C. (2008). *Comfortably numb: How psychiatry is medicating a nation.* New York, NY: Pantheon.

Barbieri, J. L. (2008). The URGES approach: Urge reduction by growing ego strength (URGES) for trauma/addiction treatment using alternate bilateral stimulation, hypnotherapy, ego state therapy and energy psychology, *Sexual Addiction & Compulsivity: The Journal of Treatment & Prevention, 15,* 116–138.

Barnard, L. K., & Curry, J. F. (2012). Self-compassion: Conceptualizations, correlates, & interventions. *Review of General Psychology, 15*, 289–303.

Barnett, L., & Madison, G. (2012). *Existential psychotherapy: Legacy, vibrancy, and dialogue*. New York, NY: Routledge.

Barr, Y. (2009). Reality therapy and the Talmud. *International Journal of Reality Therapy, 29*, 31–35.

Barrett, M., & Berman, J. (2001). Is psychotherapy more effective when therapists disclose information about themselves? *Journal of Consulting and Clinical Psychology, 69,* 597–603.

Barrett-Leonard, G. T. (1981). The empathy cycle: Refinement of a nuclear concept. *Journal of Counseling Psychology, 28,* 91–100.

Bartholomew, K., & Horowitz, L. M. (1991). Attachment styles among young adults: A test of a four-category model. *Journal of Personality and Social Psychology, 6,* 226–244.

Barton, A. (1992). Humanistic contributions to the field of psychotherapy: Appreciating the human and liberating the therapist. *Humanist Psychologist, 20,* 332–348.

Bateman, A., & Fonagy, P. (2012). *Handbook of mentalizing in mental health practice*. Washington, DC: American Psychiatric Publishing.

Bauman, S., & Waldo, M. (1998). Existential theory and mental health counseling: If it were a snake, it would have bitten! *Journal of Mental Health Counseling, 20,* 13–27.

Beal, D., Kopec, A. M., & DiGiuseppe, R. (1996). Disputing clients' irrational beliefs. *Journal of Rational-Emotive & Cognitive–Behavior Therapy, 14*(4), 215–229.

Beck, A. T. (1976). *Cognitive therapy and the emotional disorders.* Madison, CT: International Universities Press.

Beck, A. T., Freeman, A., & Davis, D. D. (2006). *Cognitive therapy of personality disorders* (2nd ed.). New York, NY: Guilford Press.

Beck, A. T., & Greenberg, R. L. (1995). *Coping with depression.* Bala Cynwyd, PA: The Beck Institute.

Beck, A. T., Rector, N. A., Stolar, N., & Grant, P. (2008). *Schizophrenia: Cognitive theory, research, and therapy.* New York, NY: Guilford Press.

Beck, A. T., Rush, A. J., Shaw, B. F., & Emery, G. (1979). *Cognitive therapy of depression.* New York, NY: Guilford Press.

Beck, J. S. (2005). *Cognitive therapy for challenging problems: What to do when the basics don't work.* New York, NY: Guilford Press.

Beck, J. S. (2011). *Cognitive behavioral therapy: Basics and beyond* (2nd ed.). New York, NY: Guilford Press.

Becvar, D. S., & Becvar, R. J. (2006). *Family therapy: A systemic integration* (6th ed.). Upper Saddle River, NJ: Pearson.

Beisser, A. (1970). The paradoxical theory of change. In J. Fagan & I. Sheperd (Eds.), *Gestalt therapy now* (pp. 77–80). Palo Alto, CA: Science and Behavior Books.

Benedek, D. M., & Wynn, G. H. (2011). Clinical manual for management of PTSD. Arlington, VA: American Psychiatric Publishing.

Benish, S., Imel, Z. E., & Wampold, B. E. (2008). The relative efficacy of bona fide psychotherapies of post-traumatic stress disorder: A meta-analysis of direct comparisons. *Clinical Psychology Review, 28,* 746–758.

Benner, D. G. (2005). Intensive soul care: Integrating psychotherapy and spiritual direction. In L. Sperry & E. P. Shafranske (Eds.), *Spiritually oriented psychotherapy* (pp. 287–306). Washington, DC: American Psychological Association.

Berg, I. K., & Miller, S. D. (1992). Working with Asian American clients one person at a time. *Families in Society: The Journal of Contemporary Human Services, 73,* 356–363.

Berg, I. K., & Szabo, P. (2005). *Brief coaching for lasting solutions.* New York, NY: W. W. Norton.

Bernard, M. E. (2009). Dispute irrational beliefs and teach rational beliefs: An interview with Albert Ellis. *Journal of Rational-Emotive and Cognitive–Behavioral Therapy, 27,* 66–76.

Bernard, M. E. (2011). *Rationality and the pursuit of happiness: The legacy of Albert Ellis.* New York, NY: Wiley.

Bernard, M. E., Froh, J. J., DiGiuseppe, R., Joyce, M. R., & Dryden, W. (2010). Albert Ellis: Unsung hero of positive psychology. *The Journal of Positive Psychology, 5,* 302–310.

Berne, E. (1961). *Transactional analysis in psychotherapy.* New York, NY: Grove.

Berne, E. (1964). *Games people play.* New York, NY: Grove.

Bernier, A., & Dozier, M. (2002). The client–counselor match and the corrective emotional experience: Evidence from interpersonal and attachment research. *Psychotherapy: Theory, Research, Practice, Training, 39,* 32–43.

Bertolino, B. (2010). *Strengths-based engagement and practice: Creating effective helping relationships.* New York, NY: Pearson.

Berzoff, J., Flanagan, L. M., Hertz, P., & Basham, K. (2011). *Inside out and outside in: Psychodynamic clinical theory and psychopathology in contemporary multicultural contexts* (3rd ed.). Lanham, MD: Rowman & Littlefield.

Beutler, L. E., Consoli, A. J., & Lane, G. (2005). Systematic treatment selection and prescriptive psychotherapy: An integrative eclectic approach. In J. C. Norcross & M. R. Goldfried (Eds.), *Handbook of psychotherapy integration* (2nd ed., pp. 121–143). New York, NY: Oxford.

Bezanson, B. (2004). The application of solution-focused work in employment counseling. *Journal of Employment Counselling, 41,* 183–191.

Binder, J. L. (2004). *Key competencies in brief dynamic psychotherapy: Clinical practice beyond the manual.* New York, NY: Guilford Press.

Binswanger, L. (1963). *Being-in-the-world: Selected papers of Ludwig Binswanger.* London, UK: Condor Books.

Bisson, J., & Andrew, M. (2007). Psychological treatment of post-traumatic stress disorder (PTSD). *Cochrane Database of Systematic Reviews,* 2007(3). doi:10.1002/14651858.CD003388.pub3

Black, T. G. (2004). Psychotherapy and outcome research in PTSD: Understanding the challenges and complexities in the literature. *Canadian Journal of Counseling, 38,* 277–288.

Blom, R. (2006). *Handbook of Gestalt play therapy.* Philadelphia: Jessica Kingsley.

Bloom, D., & Brownell, P. (2011). *Gestalt therapy now.* Newcastle upon Tyne, UK: Cambridge Scholastic.

Bohart, A. C., & Tallman, K. (2010). Clients: The neglected common factor in psychotherapy. In B. L. Duncan, S. D. Miller, B. E. Wampold, & M. A. Hubble (Eds.), *Heart and soul of change in psychotherapy* (2nd ed., pp. 83–111). Washington, DC: American Psychological Association.

Bojuwoye, O., & Sodi, T. (2010). Challenges and opportunities to integrating traditional healing into counselling and psychotherapy. *Counselling Psychology Quarterly, 23,* 283–296.

Bond, F. W., & Bunce, D. (2000). Mediators of change in emotion-focused and problem-focused work site stress management interventions. *Journal of Occupational Health Psychology, 5,* 156–163.

Boss, M. (1963). *Psychoanalysis and Daseinsanalysis.* New York, NY: Basic Books.

Bowen, M. C. (1976). Principles and techniques of multi-family therapy. In M. P. H. Guerin Jr. (Ed.), *Family therapy: Theory and practice* (pp. 388–404). New York, NY: Gardner Press.

Bowen, M. C. (1978). *Family therapy in clinical practice.* New York, NY: Aronson.

Bowlby, J. (1978). Attachment theory and its therapeutic implications. *Adolescent Psychiatry, 6,* 5–33.

Bowlby, J. (1988). *A secure base: Parent–child attachment and healthy human development.* New York, NY: Basic Books.

Bowman, C. E. (2005). The history and development of Gestalt therapy. In A. L. Woldt and S. M. Toman (Eds.), *Gestalt therapy: History, theory, and practice* (pp. 3–20). Thousand Oaks, CA: Sage.

Bowman, C. E. (2012). Reconsidering holism in Gestalt therapy: A bridge too far. In T. B. Levine (Ed.), *Gestalt therapy: Advances in theory and practice* (pp. 27–38). New York, NY: Routledge.

Bowman, D., Scogin, F., Floyd, M., & McKendree-Smith, N. (2001). Psychotherapy length of stay and outcome: A meta-analysis of the effect of therapist sex. *Psychotherapy, 38,* 142–148.

Bozarth, J. D., Zimring, F. M., & Tausch, R. (2001). Client-centered therapy: The evolution of a revolution. In D. J. Cain & J. Seeman (Eds.), *Humanistic psychotherapies: Handbook of research and practice* (pp. 147–188). Washington DC: American Psychological Association.

Brach, T. (2003). *Radical acceptance: Embracing your life with the heart of a Buddha.* New York, NY: Bantam Books.

Bradley, H. (2007). *Gender.* Hoboken, NJ: Wiley.

Bradley, R., Greene, J., Russ, E., Dutra, L., & Westen, D. (2005). A multidimensional meta-analysis of psychotherapy for PTSD. *American Journal of Psychiatry, 162,* 214–227.

Bratter, T. E. (2010). Rejection of psychotropic medicine and DSM-IV nomenclature produce positive outcomes for gifted, alienated, and dually diagnosed John Dewey Academy students who were self-destructive: Part I. *Journal of Ethical Human Psychology and Psychiatry, 11,* 16–28.

Bratter, T. E., Esparat, D., Kaufman, A., & Sinsheimer, L. (2008). Confrontational psychotherapy: A compassionate and potent therapeutic orientation for gifted adolescents who are self-destructive and engage in dangerous behavior. *International Journal of Reality Therapy, 27,* 13–25.

Breitbart, W., & Heller, K. S. (2003). Reframing hope: Meaning-centered care for patients near the end of life. *Journal of Palliative Medicine, 6,* 979–988.

Brown, C. (2007). Situating knowledge and power in the therapeutic alliance. In C. Brown and T. Augusta-Scott (Eds.), *Narrative therapy: Making meaning, making lives* (pp. 3–22). Thousand Oaks, CA: Sage.

Brown, C., & Augusta-Scott, T. (Eds.). (2007). *Narrative therapy: Making meaning, making lives.* Thousand Oaks, CA: Sage.

Brown, D., & Brooks, L. (1991). The genogram as an assessment device. In D. Brown & L. Brooks (Eds.), Career counseling techniques (pp. 126–137). Needham Heights, MA: Allyn & Bacon.

Brown, L. S. (2001). Feelings in context: Countertransference and the real world in feminist therapy. *Journal of Clinical Psychology, 57,* 1005–1012.

Brown, L. S. (2008). *Cultural competence in trauma therapy: Beyond the flashback.* Washington, DC: American Psychological Association.

Brown, L. S. (2010). *Feminist therapy.* Washington, DC: American Psychological Association.

Bruner, J. (1986). *Actual minds, possible worlds*. Cambridge, MA: Harvard University Press.

Bruner, J. (2002). *Making stories*. New York, NY: Farrar, Strauss, and Giroux.

Brunner, J. (1998). Oedipus politicus. In M. S. Roth (Ed.), *Freud: Conflict and culture* (pp. 80–93). New York, NY: Knopf.

Bruns, C. M., & Trimble, C. (2001). Rising tide: Taking our place as young feminist psychologists. *Women & Therapy, 23,* 19–36.

Buber, M. (1970). *I and thou*. New York, NY: Scribner.

Budman, S. H., & Gurman, A. S. (1988). *Theory and practice of brief therapy*. New York, NY: Guilford Press.

Bugental, J. F. T. (1965). *The search for authenticity: An existential-analytic approach to psychotherapy*. New York, NY: Holt, Reinhart, & Winston.

Bugental, J. F. T. (1978). *Psychotherapy and process: The fundamentals of an existential humanistic approach*. Reading, MA: Addison-Wesley.

Bugental, J. F. T. (1987). *The art of the psychotherapist*. New York, NY: W. W. Norton.

Bugental, J. F. T. (1990). *Intimate journeys*. San Francisco, CA: Jossey-Bass.

Bugental, J. F. T. (1996). Rollo May (1909–1994). *American Psychologist, 51,* 418–419.

Bugental, J. F. T. (2008). Preliminary sketches for a short-term existential-humanistic therapy. In K. Schneider (Ed.), *Existential integrative therapy* (pp. 165–167). New York, NY: Routledge.

Buhle, M. J. (1998). *Feminism and its discontents: A century of struggle with psychoanalysis*. Cambridge, MA: Harvard University Press.

Burdenski, T. K., & Wubbolding, R. E. (2011). Extending reality therapy with focusing: A humanistic road for the choice theory total behavior car. *International Journal of Reality Therapy, 31,* 14–30.

Bureau of Labor Statistics, U.S. Department of Labor. (2012). *Households and families: 2010*. Retrieved from http://www.census.gov/prod/cen2010/briefs/c2010br-14.pdf

Burnett, L. (2009). *When death enters the therapeutic space: Existential perspective in psychotherapy and counseling*. New York, NY: Schneider Routledge.

Burns, D. D. (1999). *The feeling good handbook*. San Francisco, CA: HarperCollins.

Burns, M. K., Vance, D., Szadokierski, I., & Stockwell, C. (2006). Student Needs Survey: A psychometrically sound measure of the five basic needs. *International Journal of Reality Therapy, 25,* 4–8.

Busch, F. N., & Milrod, B. (2012). Psychodynamic treatment for panic disorder. In R. A. Levy, J. S. Ablon, and H. Kachele (Eds.), *Psychodynamic psychotherapy research* (pp. 29–44). New York, NY: Humana Press.

Butler, A. C., Chapman, J. E., Forman, E. M., & Beck, A. T. (2006). The empirical status of cognitive–behavioral therapy: A review of meta-analyses. *Clinical Psychology Review, 26,* 17–31.

Butler, G., Fennell, M., & Hackmann, A. (2008). *Cognitive–behavioral therapy for anxiety disorders: Mastering clinical challenges*. New York, NY: Guilford Press.

Cain, D. J. (1987). Carl R. Rogers: The man, his vision, his impact. *Person-Centered Review, 2,* 283–288.

Cain, D. J. (2008). Person-centered therapy. In J. Frew & M. D. Spiegler (Eds.), *Contemporary psychotherapies for a diverse world* (pp. 177–227). Boston, MA: Houghton Mifflin.

Cain, D. J., & Seeman, J. (Eds.). (2001). *Humanistic psychotherapies: Handbook of research and practice* (pp. 147–188). Washington, DC: American Psychological Association.

Cambray, J. (2009). *Synchronicity: Nature and psyche in an interconnected universe*. College Station: Texas A&M University Press.

Capuzzi, D., & Gross, D. (2011). *Counseling and psychotherapy: Theories and interventions* (5th ed.). Alexandria, VA: American Counseling Association.

Carey, T. A. (2003). Improving the success of anti-bullying intervention programs: A tool for matching programs with purposes. *International Journal of Reality Therapy, 22*(2), 16–24.

Carlson, J. D., & Dinkmeyer, D. (2003). *Time for a better marriage*. Atascadero, CA: Impact Publishers.

Carlson, J. D., & Englar-Carlson, M. (2008). Adlerian therapy. In J. Frew & M. D. Spiegler (Eds.), *Contemporary psychotherapies for a diverse world* (pp. 93–140). Boston, MA: Houghton Mifflin.

Carlson, J., & Maniacci, M. P. (2011). *Alfred Adler revisited*. New York, NY: Routledge.

Carlson, J. D., & Robey, P. A. (2011). An integrative Adlerian approach to family counseling, *Journal of Individual Psychotherapy, 67,* 232–244.

Carlson, J., & Sperry, L. (2000). *Brief therapy with individuals and couples.* Phoenix, AZ: Zeig, Tucker & Theisen.

Carlson, J., Watts, R. E., & Maniacci, M. (2006). *Adlerian therapy: Theory and practice.* Washington, DC: American Psychological Association.

Carney, J. V., & Hazler, R. J. (1998). Suicide and cognitive–behavioral counseling: Implications for mental health counselors. *Journal of Mental Health Counseling, 20*(1), 28–41.

Carr, A. (1998). Michael White's narrative therapy. *Contemporary Family Therapy, 20,* 485–503.

Carrick, L. (2007). Person-centered approach to crisis intervention. In M. Cooper, M. O'Hara, P. F. Schmid, & G. Wyatt (Eds.), *The handbook of person-centered psychotherapy* (pp. 293–304). New York, NY: Palgrave MacMillan.

Carroll, J. (1999). Compatibility of Adlerian theory and practice with the philosophy and practices of Alcoholics Anonymous. *Journal of Addictions & Offender Counseling, 19*(2), 50–61.

Carroll, J. S., & Doherty, W. J. (2003). Evaluating the effectiveness of premarital prevention programs: A meta-analytic review of outcome research. *Family Relations, 52,* 105–118.

Caselman, T. (2007). *Teaching children empathy, the social emotion.* Chapin, SC: Youthlight.

Cashdan, S. (1988). *Object relations therapy: Using the relationship.* New York, NY: W. W. Norton.

Cashwell, C. S., & Young, J. S. (Eds.). (2005). *Integrating spirituality and religion into counseling: A guide to competent practice.* Alexandria, VA: American Counseling Association.

Cedar, B., & Levant, R. F. (1990) A meta-analysis of the effects of parent effectiveness training. *American Journal of Family Therapy, 18,* 373–384.

Celani, D. P. (2010). *Fairbairn's object relations theory in the clinical setting.* New York, NY: Columbia University Press.

Chae, M., & Foley, P. (2010). Relationship of ethnic identity, acculturation, and psychological well-being among Chinese, Japanese, and Korean Americans. *Journal of Counseling & Development, 88*, 466–476.

Chambless, D. L., Baker, M. J., Baucom, D. H., Beutler, L. E., Calhoun, K. S., Crits-Cristoph, P., . . . Woody, S. R. (1998). Update on empirically validated therapies, II. *Clinical Psychologist, 51,* 3–16.

Chambless, D. L., & Hollon, S. D. (1998). Defining empirically supported therapies. *Journal of Consulting and Clinical Psychology, 66,* 7–18.

Chang, R., & Page, R. C. (1991). Characteristics of the self-actualized person: Visions from the East and West. *Counseling and Values, 36,* 2–11.

Chapman, A. H. (1978). *The treatment techniques of Harry Stack Sullivan.* New York, NY: Brunner/Mazel.

Charles, S. T., Mather, M., & Carstensen, L. L. (2003). Aging and emotional memory: The forgettable nature of negative images for older adults. *Journal of Experimental Psychology: General, 132,* 310–324.

Chodron, P. (1991). *The wisdom of no escape and the path of loving-kindness.* Boston, MA: Shambhala.

Claessens, M. (2009). Mindfulness and existential therapy. *Existential Analysis, 20,* 109–119.

Clark, D., & Beck, A. T. (2011). *Cognitive therapy of anxiety disorders: Science and practice.* New York, NY: Guilford Press.

Clark, D. A., Hollifield, M., Leahy, R., and Beck, J. S. (2009). Theory of cognitive therapy. In G. O. Gabbard (Ed.), *Textbook of psychotherapeutic treatments in psychiatry* (pp. 165–200). Arlington, VA: American Psychiatric Publishing.

Clarkin, J. F., Yeoman, F. E., & Kernberg, O. E. (2006). *Psychotherapy for borderline personality: Focusing on object relationships.* Washington, DC: American Psychiatric Publishing.

Clarkson, P. (1990). A multiplicity of psychotherapeutic relationships. *British Journal of Psychotherapy, 7*(2), 148–161.

Clarkson, P., & Mackewn, J. (1993). *Fritz Perls.* London, UK: Sage.

Clemmens, M. C. (2005). Gestalt approaches to substance use/abuse/dependency: Theory and practice. In A. L. Woldt & S. M. Toman (Eds.), *Gestalt therapy: History, theory, and practice* (pp. 279–300). Thousand Oaks, CA: Sage.

Coan, R. W. (1979). *Psychologists: Personal and theoretical pathways.* New York, NY: Irvington.

Cocks, G. (Ed.). (1994). *The curve of life: Correspondence of Heinz Kohut.* Chicago, IL: University of Chicago Press.

Coelho, H. F., Canter, P. H., & Ernst, E. (2007). Mindfulness-based cognitive therapy: Evaluating current evidence and informing future research. *Journal of Consulting and Clinical Psychology, 75*, 1000–1005.

Cogan, R. (2007). Therapeutic aims and outcomes of psychoanalysis. *Psychoanalytic Psychology, 24,* 193–207.

Cohen, K. H. (2010). On becoming meta. *American Journal of Psychology, 70,* 53–60.

Coleman, H. K. L., Wampold, B. E., & Casali, S. L. (1995). Ethnic minorities' ratings of ethnically similar and European American counselors: A meta-analysis. *Journal of Counseling Psychology, 42,* 55–64.

Coles, R. (1992). *Anna Freud: The dream of psychoanalysis.* New York, NY: Addison-Wesley.

Colman, W. (2011). Synchronicity and the meaning-making psyche. *Journal of Analytical Psychology, 56,* 471–491.

Comstock, D. L. (2004). Reflections on life, loss, and resilience. In M. Walker & W. B. Rosen (Eds.), *How connections heal: Stories from relational-cultural therapy* (pp. 83–102). New York, NY: Guilford Press.

Connell, G. M. (1996). Carl Whitaker: In memoriam. *Journal of Marital and Family Therapy, 22,* 3–8.

Conoley, C. W., & Garber, R. A. (1985). Effects of reframing and self-control directives on loneliness, depression and controllability. *Journal of Counseling Psychology, 32,* 139–142.

Conradi, H. J., & de Jonge, P. (2009). Recurrent depression and the role of adult attachment: A prospective and a retrospective study. *Journal of Affective Disorders, 116,* 93–99.

Constantino, M. J., & Wilson, K. R. (2007). Commentary: Negotiating cultural difference and the therapeutic alliance. In C. Muran (Ed.), *Dialogues on difference: Studies of diversity in the therapeutic relationship* (pp. 236–242). Washington, DC: American Psychological Association.

Conway, C. E. (2007). Using the crucial C's to explore gender roles with couples. *Journal of Individual Psychology, 56,* 495–501.

Cooper, M. (2008). Existential psychotherapy. In J. L. LeBow (Ed.), *Twenty-first century psychotherapies: Contemporary approaches to theory and practice.* New York, NY: Wiley.

Cooper, M., Schmid, P. F., O'Hara, M., & Wyatt, G. (2007). *The handbook of person-centered psychotherapy and counselling.* Basingstoke, UK: Palgrave.

Cooper, M., Watson, J. C., & Bolldampt, D. (Eds.). (2010). *Person-centered and experiential therapies work: A review of the research on counseling, psychotherapy, and related practices.* Ross-on-Wye, UK: PCCS Books.

Cooper, S. J. (2012). Contributors. In T. Malinen, S. J. Cooper, & F. N. Thomas (Eds.), *Masters of narrative and collaborative therapies: The voices of Andersen, Anderson, and White.* New York, NY: Routledge.

Corcoran, J., & Stephenson, M. (2000). The effectiveness of solution-focused therapy with child behavior problems: A preliminary report. *Families in Society: The Journal of Contemporary Human Services, 81*(5), 548–562.

Corey, G., Corey, M. S., & Callanan, P. (2011). *Issues and ethics in the helping professions.* Belmont, CA: Thompson Brooks/Cole.

Cornelius-White, J. H. D. (2005). Teaching person-centered multicultural counseling. *The Journal of Humanistic Counseling, Education, and Development, 44,* 225–239.

Cornelius-White, J. H. D. (2007). Learner-centered teacher-student relationships are effective: A meta-analysis, *Review of Educational Research, 77,* 113–143.

Cosby, B. (2009). *Little Bill: Young readers series.* New York, NY: Scholastic.

Cottone, J., Drucker, P., & Javier, R. A. (2003). Gender differences in psychotherapy dyads: Changes in psychological symptoms and responsiveness to treatment during three months of therapy. *Psychotherapy, 40,* 297–308.

Crane, N. (2009). *Mindfulness-based cognitive therapy.* New York, NY: Routledge.

Crane, R. (2012). *Mindfulness-based cognitive therapy: Distinctive features.* New York, NY: Routledge.

Crane, R. S., Kuyken, W., Hastings, R. P., Rothwell, N., & Williams, M. G. (2010). Training teachers to deliver mindfulness-based interventions: Learning from the UK experience. *Mindfulness, 1,* 74–86.

Crawley, S. A., Podell, J. L., Beidas, R. S., Braswell, L., & Kendall, P. C. (2010). Cognitive–behavioral therapy with youth. In K. S. Dobson (Ed.), *Handbook of cognitive behavioral therapies* (3rd ed., pp. 375–410). New York, NY: Guilford Press.

Crocker, S. F. (2005). Phenomenology, existentialism, and Eastern thought in Gestalt therapy. In A. L. Woldt & S. M. Toman (Eds.), *Gestalt therapy: History, theory, and practice* (pp. 65–80). Thousand Oaks, CA: Sage.

Crocket, K. (2008). Narrative therapy. In J. Frew & M. D. Spiegler (Eds.), *Contemporary psychotherapy for a diverse world* (pp. 489–533). Boston, MA: Houghton Mifflin.

Cuje, B. B. (2010). *Be the person you were meant to be: The choice cube method, step-by-step to choice and change*. Arlington, VA: Booksurge.

Curlette, W. L., & Kern, R. M. (2010). Ethics, research, and applications. *Journal of Individual Psychology, 66*, 133–134.

Curran, J., Ekers, D., McMillan, D., & Houghton, S. (2012). Behavioural activation. In W. Dryden (Ed.), *Cognitive behaviour therapies* (pp. 236–260). Thousand Oaks, CA: Sage.

Dallos, R. (2006). *Attachment narrative therapy: Integrating systemic, narrative and attachment approaches*. Maidenhead, Berkshire, UK: Open University Press.

Dalrymple, K. I., Fiorentino, L., Politi, M. C., & Posner, D. (2010). Incorporating principles from acceptance and commitment therapy into cognitive–behavioral therapy for insomnia: A case example. *Journal of Contemporary Psychotherapy, 40*, 209–217.

Damasio, A. R. (1994). *Descartes' error: Emotion, reason, and the human brain*. New York, NY: Putnam.

Damasio, A. R. (1999). *The feeling of what happens: Body and emotion in the making of consciousness*. Orlando, FL: Harcourt.

Danielian, J. (2010). Meta-realization in Horney and the teaching of psychoanalysis. *American Journal of Psychoanalysis, 70*, 10–22.

Dattilio, F. M. (2005). Restructuring family schemas: A cognitive–behavioral perspective. *Journal of Marital and Family Therapy, 31*, 15–30.

Dattilio, F. M., & Freeman, A. (2007). *Cognitive behavioral strategies in crisis intervention* (3rd ed.). New York, NY: Guilford Press.

Davanloo, H. (1979). Techniques of short-term psychotherapy. *Psychiatric Clinics of North America, 2*, 11–22.

Davanloo, H. (1980). A method of short-term dynamic psychotherapy. In H. Davanloo (Ed.), *Short-term dynamic psychotherapy*. Northvale, NJ: Aronson.

Davidson, P. R., & Parker, K. C. H. (2001). Eye movement desensitization and reprocessing (EMDR): A meta-analysis. *Journal of Consulting and Clinical Psychology, 69*, 305–316.

Day, S. X. (2008). *Theory and design in counseling and psychotherapy* (2nd ed.). Boston, MA: Houghton Mifflin.

Decker, H. S. (1998). Freud's "Dora" case. In M. S. Roth (Ed.), *Freud: Conflict and culture* (pp. 105–114). New York, NY: Knopf.

Deckersbach, T., Rauch, S., Buhlmann, U., & Wilhem, S. (2006). Habit reversal versus supportive psychotherapy in the treatment of Tourette's disorder: A randomized controlled trial and predictors of treatment response. *Behaviour, Research, and Therapy, 44*, 1079–1090.

Dehing, J. (1992). The therapist's interventions in Jungian analysis. *Journal of Analytical Psychology, 37*, 29–47.

De Jong, P., & Berg, I. K. (2012). *Interviewing for solutions* (4th ed.). Pacific Grove, CA: Brooks/Cole.

Demos, V. C., & Prout, M. F. (1993). A comparison of seven approaches to brief psychotherapy. *International Journal of Short-Term Psychotherapy, 8*, 3–22.

Department of Veterans Affairs & Department of Defense. (2004). *VA/DoD clinical practice guideline for the management of posttraumatic stress* (Publication10Q-CPG/PTSD-04). Washington, DC: Veterans Health Administration, Department of Veterans Affairs and Health Affairs, Department of Defense, Office of Quality and Performance.

DeRobertis, E. M. (2010). Winnicott, Kohut, and the developmental context of well-being. *The Humanistic Psychologist, 38*, 336–354.

DeRubeis, R. J., Hollon, S. D., Amsterdam, J. D., Shelton, R. C., Young, P. R., Salomon, R. M., . . . Gallop, R. (2005). Cognitive therapy vs. medication in the treatment of moderate to severe depression. *Archives of General Psychiatry, 62*, 409–416.

de Shazer, S. (1982). *Patterns of brief family therapy: An ecosystem approach*. New York, NY: Guilford Press.

de Shazer, S. (1985). *Keys to solutions in brief therapy*. New York, NY: W. W. Norton.

de Shazer, S. (1988). *Clues: Investigating solutions in brief therapy*. New York, NY: W. W. Norton.

de Shazer, S. (1991). *Putting difference to work*. New York, NY: W. W. Norton.

de Shazer, S., & Dolan, Y. (2007). *More than miracles: The state of the art of solution-focused brief therapy*. Binghamton, NY: Haworth Press.

DeYoung, P. A. (2003). *Relational psychotherapy: A primer*. New York, NY: Brunner-Routledge.

Diamond, G. S., & Stern, R. (2003). Attachment-based family therapy for depressed adolescents: Repairing attachment failures. In S. M. Johnson & V. Whiffen (Eds.), *Attachment processes in couple and family therapy* (pp. 191–214). New York, NY: Guilford Press.

Diamond, S. A. (2007). *Anger, madness, and the daimonic: The psychological genesis of violence, evil, and creativity.* Albany, NY: State University of New York Press.

Diamond, S. A. (2009). What is existential psychotherapy? In D. A. Leeming, K. Madden, & S. Marlan (Eds.), *Encyclopedia of psychology and religion* (pp. 304–305). New York, NY: Springer Verlag.

DiGiuseppe, R. (1996). The nature of irrational and rational beliefs: Progress in rational emotive behavior therapy. *Journal of Rational-Emotive & Cognitive–Behavior Therapy, 14*(1), 5–28.

DiGiuseppe, R., & Bernard, M. (2006). REBT assessment and treatment with children. In A. Ellis & M. Bernard (Eds.), *Rational emotive behavior therapy application to childhood disorders* (Sec. 1, pp. 85–114). New York, NY: Springer

Dimeff, L. A., Koerner, K., & Linehan, M. (2007). *Dialectical behavior therapy in clinical practice: Applications across disorders and settings.* New York, NY: Guilford Press.

Dimidjian, S., Hollon, S. D., Dobson, K. S., Schmaling, K. B., Kohlenberg, R. J., Addis, M. E., . . . Jacobson, N. S. (2006). Randomized trial of behavioral activation, cognitive therapy, and antidepressant medication in the acute treatment of adults with major depression. *Journal of Consulting and Clinical Psychology, 74,* 658–670.

Dinkmeyer, D. C., & McKay, K. (1997). *Systematic training for effective parenting.* Circle Pines, MN: American Guidance Services.

Division 12 Task Force. (1996). An update on empirically validated therapies. *Clinical Psychologist, 49,* 5–18.

Dobson, K. S. (Ed.). (2010). *Handbook of cognitive behavioral therapies.* New York, NY: Guilford Press.

Dobson, K. S., & Dozois, D. J. A. (2010). Historical and philosophical bases of the cognitive–behavioral therapies. In K. S. Dobson (Ed.), *Handbook of cognitive behavioral therapies* (p. 38). New York, NY: Guilford Press.

Dollard, J., & Miller, N. E. (1950). *Personality and psychotherapy: An analysis in terms of learning, thinking and culture.* New York, NY: McGraw-Hill.

Dolliver, R. H. (1995). Carl Rogers's emphasis on his own direct experience. *Journal of Humanistic Psychology, 35,* 129–139.

Douglas, C. J. (2008). Teaching supportive psychotherapy to psychiatric residents. *American Journal of Psychiatry, 165,* 445–452.

Dourley, J. P. (2008). *Paul Tillich, Carl Jung, and the recovery of religion.* New York, NY: Routledge.

Drauker, C. B. (1998). Narrative therapy for women who have lived with violence. *Archives of Psychiatric Nursing, 7,* 162–168.

Dreikurs, R. (1973). Private logic. In H. H. Mosak (Ed.), *Alfred Adler: His influence on psychology today* (pp. 19–32). Park Ridge, NJ: Noyes.

Dreikurs, R., Cassel, P., & Ferguson, E. D. (2004). *Discipline without tears* (rev. ed.). Toronto, Canada: Wiley.

Dreikurs, R., & Soltz, V. (1991). *Children: The challenge.* New York, NY: Plume Books.

Dryden, W. (2011). *Dealing with emotional problems using rational emotive cognitive behavior therapy.* New York, NY: Routledge.

Dryden, W., & Branch, R. (2008). *The fundamentals of rational emotive behavior therapy: A training handbook* (2nd ed.). Chichester, UK: Wiley.

Dryden, W., DiGiuseppe, R., & Neenan, M. (2010). *A primer of rational emotive behavior therapy* (3rd ed.). Champaign, IL: Research Press.

Dryden, W., & Ellis, A. (2001). Rational emotive behavior therapy. In K. S. Dobson (Ed.), *Handbook of cognitive–behavioral therapy* (pp. 295–348). New York, NY: Guilford Press.

Duncan, B. L. (2010). Prologue: Saul Rosenzweig: The founder of the common factors. In: B. L. Duncan, S. D. Miller, B. E. Wampold, & M. A. Hubble (Eds.), *Heart and soul of change in psychotherapy* (2nd ed., pp. 3–22). Washington, DC: American Psychological Association.

Duncan, B. L., Miller, S. D., Wampold, B. E., & Hubble, M. A. (Eds.). (2010). *Heart and soul of change in psychotherapy* (2nd ed.). Washington, DC: American Psychological Association.

Dunkley, D. M., Blankstein, K. R., & Segal, Z. V. (2010). Cognitive assessment: Issues and methods. In K. S. Dobson (Ed.), *Handbook of cognitive behavioral therapies* (3rd ed., pp. 133–171). New York, NY: Guilford Press.

Duran, E. (2006). *Healing the soul wound*. New York, NY: Teachers College Press.

D'Zurilla, T. J., & Goldfried, M. R. (1971). Problem-solving and behavior modification, *Journal of Abnormal Psychology, 78*, 107–126.

D'Zurilla, T. J., & Nezu, A. M. (2007). *Problem-solving therapy: A positive approach to clinical intervention* (3rd ed.). New York, NY: Springer.

D'Zurilla, T. J., & Nezu, A. M. (2010). Problem-solving therapy. In K. S. Dobson (Ed.), *Handbook of cognitive behavioral therapies* (3rd ed., pp. 197–225). New York, NY: Guilford Press.

Eckardt, M. H. (2005). Karen Horney: A portrait. The 120th anniversary, Karen Horney, September 16, 1885. *American Journal of Psychoanalysis, 65*, 95–101.

Ecker, B., & Hulley, L. (2008). Coherence therapy: Swift change at the core of emotional truth. In J. D. Raskin & S. K. Bridges (Eds.), *Studies in meaning 3: Constructivist psychotherapy in the real world* (pp. 57–84). New York, NY: Pace University Press.

Eckstein, D. J., & Kern, R. M. (2002). *Psychological fingerprints: Lifestyle assessment and interventions*. Dubuque, IA: Kendall-Hunt.

Edwards, D., & Arntz, A. (2012). Schema therapy in historical perspective. In M. van Vreeswijk, J. Broersen, & M. Nadort (Eds.), *The Wiley-Blackwell handbook of schema therapy: Theory, research, and practice*. Malden, MA: Wiley.

Eifert, G. H., & Forsyth, J. P. (2005). *Acceptance and commitment therapy for anxiety disorders*. Oakland, CA: New Harbinger.

Eisenberg, M. (1989). Exposing prisoners to logotherapy. *International Forum for Logotherapy, 12*, 89–94.

Elliott, R., Bohart, A. C., Watson, J. C., & Greenberg, L. S. (2011). Empathy. In J. C. Norcross (Ed.), *Psychotherapy relationships that work: Evidence-based responsiveness* (2nd ed. pp. 132–152). New York, NY: Oxford.

Elliott, R., Watson, J., Goldman, R., & Greenberg, L. (2004). *Learning emotion-focused therapy: The process-experiential approach to change*. Washington, DC: American Psychological Association.

Elliott, T. R., Uswatte, G., Lewis, L., & Palmatier, A. (2000). Goal instability and adjustment to physical disability. *Journal of Counseling Psychology, 47*, 251–265.

Ellis, A. (1957). *How to live with a neurotic*. Oxford, UK: Crown Publishers.

Ellis, A. E. (1984). Foreword. In W. Dryden, *Rational-emotive therapy: Fundamentals and innovations* (pp. i–xv). London, UK: Croom Helm.

Ellis, A. E. (1986). An emotional control card for inappropriate and appropriate emotions using rational-emotive imagery. *Journal of Counseling and Development, 65*, 205–206.

Ellis, A. E. (1988). *How to stubbornly refuse to make yourself miserable about anything—Yes, anything!* Secaucus, NJ: Lyle Stuart.

Ellis, A. E. (1992). Secular humanism and rational-emotive therapy. *Humanistic Psychologist, 20*(2/3), 349–358.

Ellis, A. E. (1995). Changing rational-emotive therapy (RET) to rational emotive behavior therapy (REBT). *Journal of Rational-Emotive & Cognitive–Behavior Therapy, 13*(2), 85–89.

Ellis, A. E. (1996). The treatment of morbid jealousy: A rational emotive behavior approach. *Journal of Cognitive Psychotherapy, 10*(1), 23–33.

Ellis, A. E. (1997). Using rational emotive behavior therapy techniques to cope with disability. *Professional Psychology: Research and Practice, 28*, 17–22.

Ellis, A. E. (2001). *Overcoming destructive beliefs, feelings, and behaviors: New directions for rational emotive behavior therapy*. New York, NY: Brunner/Mazel.

Ellis, A. E. (2002). *Overcoming resistance: A rational emotive behavior therapy integrated approach*. New York, NY: Springer.

Ellis, A. E. (2003). Early theories and practices of rational emotive behavior therapy and how they have been augmented and revised during the last three decades. *Journal of Rational-Emotive & Cognitive–Behavior Therapy, 21*, 219–243.

Ellis, A. (2007). *Overcoming resistance: A rational emotive behavior therapy integrative approach* (2nd ed.). New York, NY: Springer.

Ellis, A. (2009). *All out! An autobiography*. New York, NY: Prometheus Books.

Ellis, A., & Dryden, W. (2007). *The practice of rational emotive behavior therapy* (2nd ed.). New York, NY: Springer.

Ellis, A., & Ellis, D. J. (2011). *Rational emotive behavior therapy*. Washington, DC: American Psychological Association.

Ellis, A., & MacLaren, C. (2005). *Rational emotive behavior therapy: A therapist's guide* (2nd ed.). Atascadero, CA: Impact Publishers.

Ellis, A., & Velten, E. (1998). *Optimal aging: Getting over getting older*. Chicago, IL: Open Court Books.

Ellison, J. A., Greenberg, L. S., Goldman, R. N., & Angus, L. (2009). Maintenance of gains following experiential therapies for depression. *Journal of Consulting and Clinical Psychology, 77,* 103–112.

Ellsworth, L. (2007). *Choosing to heal: Using reality therapy in treatment with sexually abused children.* New York, NY: Routledge.

Ellwood, R. (1999). *The politics of myth: A study of C. G. Jung, Mircea Eliade, and Joseph Campbell.* New York: State University of New York Press.

Emmelkamp, P. M. G. (2004). Behavior therapy with adults. In M. Lambert (Ed.), *Bergin and Garfield's handbook of psychotherapy and behavior change* (5th ed., pp. 393–446). New York, NY: Wiley.

Emmelkamp, P. M. G., Ehring, T., & Powers, M. B. (2010). Philosophy, psychology, cases, and treatments of mental disorders. In N. Kazantzis, M. A. Reinecke, & A. Freeman. *Cognitive and behavioral theories in clinical practice* (pp. 1–27). New York, NY: Guilford Press.

Enns, C. (1987). Gestalt therapy and feminist therapy: A proposed integration. *Journal of Counseling and Development, 66,* 93–95.

Enns, C. Z. (1993). Twenty years of feminist counseling and psychotherapy: From naming biases to implementing multifaceted practice. *The Counseling Psychologist, 21,* 3–87.

Enns, C. Z. (2004). *Feminist theories and feminist psychotherapies: Origins, themes, and diversity* (2nd ed.). Binghamton, NY: Haworth Press.

Epp, L. R. (1998). The courage to be an existential counselor: An interview of Clemmont E. Vontress. *Journal of Mental Health Counseling, 20,* 1–12.

Epston, D. (2008). Saying hullo again: Remembering Michael White. *Journal of Systemic Therapies, 27,* 1–15.

Erford, B. T., Eaves, S. H., Bryant, E. M., & Young, K. A. (2010). *35 techniques every counselor should know*. Upper Saddle River, NJ: Pearson.

Erickson, D. B. (1993). The relationship between personality types and preferred counseling model. *Journal of Psychological Type, 27,* 39–41.

Erikson, E. H. (1982). *The life cycle completed.* New York, NY: W. W. Norton.

Erskine, R. G., Moursund, J., & Trautmann, R. L. (1999). *Beyond empathy: A theory of contact-in-relationship.* London, UK: Routledge.

Erwin, J. C. (2004). *The classroom of choice: Giving students what they need and getting what you want.* Alexandria, VA: Association for Supervision and Curriculum Development.

Esposito, M. A. (2009). *REBT with children and adolescents: A meta-analytic review of efficacy studies.* New York, NY: St John's University.

Evans, D. B. (1982). What are you doing? An interview with William Glasser. *Personnel and Guidance Journal, 60*(8), 460–466.

Evans, K., & Gilbert, M. C. (2005). *An introduction to integration psychotherapy*. London, UK: Palgrave.

Ewen, R. B. (1993). *An introduction to theories of personality* (4th ed.). Hillsdale, NJ: Erlbaum.

Eysenck, H. J. (1970). A mish-mash of theories. *International Journal of Psychiatry, 9,* 140–146.

Fabry, D. (2010). Evidence base for paradoxical intention: Reviewing clinical outcome studies. *International Forum for Logotherapy, 33,* 21–29.

Fagan, J., & Shepherd, I. L. (1970). *Gestalt therapy now.* Palo Alto, CA: Science and Behavior Books.

Farber, B. A., & Doolin, E. M. (2011). Positive regard and affirmation. In J. C. Norcross (Ed.), *Psychotherapy relationships that work: Evidence-based responsiveness* (2nd ed., pp. 168–186). New York, NY: Oxford.

Farber, B. A., & Metzger, J. A. (2009). Attachment theory. In. J. H. Obegi & E. Berant (Eds.), *Attachment theory and research in clinical work with adults* (pp. 46–70). New York, NY: Guilford Press.

Farrell, J. M., Shaw, I. A., & Webber, M. A. (2009). A schema-focused approach to group psychotherapy for outpatients with borderline personality disorder: A randomized controlled trial. *Journal of Behavior Therapy and Experimental Psychiatry, 40,* 317–328.

Fenell, D., & Weinhold, B. (2003). *Counseling families: An introduction to marriage and family therapy* (3rd ed.). Denver, CO: Love.

Ferenczi, S. (1980). Technical difficulties in the analysis of a case of hysteria: Including observations of larval forms of onanism and onanistic equivalents. In J. Rickman (Ed.), *Further contributions to the theory and technique of psychoanalysis* (pp. 291–294). New York, NY: Bruner/Mazel.

Fernald, P. S. (2000). Carl Rogers: Body-centered counselor. *Journal of Counseling and Development, 78,* 172–180.

Fernando, D. M. (2007). Existential theory and solution-focused strategies: Integration and application. *Journal of Mental Health Counseling, 29,* 226–241.

Finlay, L., & Evans, K. (2009). *Relational-centered research for psychotherapists.* Malden, MA: Wiley-Blackwell.

Finlay, S. W. (2000). Influence of Carl Jung and William James on the origin of Alcoholics Anonymous. *Review of General Psychology, 4,* 3–12.

Finn, A. (2011). Jungian analytical theory. In D. Capuzzi & D. R. Gross (Eds.), *Theories of counseling and psychotherapy* (pp. 77–94). Washington, DC: American Counseling Association.

Fisher, S. K., & Fisher, R. (2002). Chemical dependence lifestyle assessment interview, *Counselor Magazine, 3.*

Fleuridas, C., Nelson, T. S., & Rosenthal, D. M. (1986). The evolution of circular questions: Training family therapists. *Journal of Marital and Family Therapy, 12,* 113–127.

Foa, E. B., Keane, T. M., & Friedman, M. J. (2000). *Effective treatments of PTSD: Guidelines from the International Society for Traumatic Stress Studies.* New York, NY: Guilford Press.

Foley, E., Baillie, A., Huxter, M., Price, M., & Sinclair, E. (2010). Mindfulness-based cognitive therapy for individuals whose lives have been affected by cancer. *Journal of Consulting and Clinical Psychology, 78,* 72–79.

Fonagy, P., & Luyten, P. (2009). A developmental, mentalization-based approach to the understanding and treatment of borderline personality disorder. *Developmental Psychopathology, 21,* 1355–1381.

Fonagy, P., & Target, M. (2009). Theoretical models of psychodynamic psychotherapy. In G. O. Gabbard, Ed., *Textbook of psychotherapeutic treatments* (pp. 3–42). Washington, DC: American Psychiatric Publishing.

Forcehimes, A. A. (2004). *De profundis*: Spiritual transformations in Alcoholics Anonymous. *Journal of Clinical Psychology, 60,* 503–517.

Forsyth, J. P., Fuse, T., & Acheson, D. T. (2009). Interoceptive exposure for panic disorder. In W. T. O. Donohue & J. E. Fisher (Eds.), *Cognitive behavioral therapy: Applying empirically supported techniques in your practice* (pp. 296–308). New York, NY: John Wiley & Sons.

Fox, A. P., & Leung, N. (2009). Existential well-being in younger and older adults with anorexia nervosa—A preliminary investigation. *European Eating Disorders Review, 17,* 24–30.

Frank, E. (2005). *Treating bipolar disorder: A clinician's guide to interpersonal and social rhythm therapy.* New York, NY: Guilford Press.

Frank, M. L. B. (2007). Existential theory. In D. Capuzzi & D. Gross (Eds.), *Counseling and psychotherapy: Theories and interventions* (4th ed., pp. 164–188). Upper Saddle River, NJ: Pearson/Prentice Hall.

Frankl, V. E. (1963). *Man's search for meaning.* Boston, MA: Beacon.

Frankl, V. E. (1967). *Psychotherapy and existentialism.* New York, NY: Washington Square Press.

Frankl, V. E. (1969). *The will to meaning: Foundations and applications of logotherapy.* New York, NY: Penguin Books.

Frankl, V. E. (1978). *The unheard cry for meaning.* New York, NY: Simon & Schuster.

Frankl, V. E. (1987). On the meaning of love. *International Forum for Logotherapy, 10,* 5–8.

Frankl, V. E. (1992). Meaning in industrial society. *International Forum for Logotherapy, 15,* 66–70.

Frankl, V. E. (2000). *Man's search for ultimate meaning.* New York, NY: Perseus.

Fransella, F., & Neimeyer, R. A. (2005). George Alexander Kelly: The man and his theory. In F. Fransella (Ed.), *The essential practitioner's handbook of personal construct psychology* (pp. 3–13). New York, NY: Wiley.

Freeman, J., Epston, D., & Lebovitz, D. (1997). *Playful approaches to serious problems: Narrative therapy with children and their families.* New York, NY: W. W. Norton.

Freeman, M. S., Hayes, B. G., Kuch, T. A., & Taub, G. (2007). Personality: A predictor of theoretical orientation of students enrolled in a counseling theories course. *Counseling Education and Supervision, 46,* 254–265.

Freud, S. (1938). *The basic writings of Sigmund Freud* (A. A. Brill, Trans.). New York, NY: Modern Library.

Freud, A. (1946). *The ego and the mechanisms of defense.* New York, NY: International Universities Press.

Freud, S. (1957). Mourning and melancholia. In J. Strachey (Ed.), *The standard edition of the complete psychological works of Sigmund Freud, Volume XIV (1914–1916): On the history of the psycho-analytic movement, papers on metapsychology and other works* (pp. 237–258). London, UK: Hogarth Press and Institute of Psycho-Analysis.

Freud, A. (1965). *Normality and pathology in childhood.* New York, NY: International Universities Press.

Freud, A. (1983). Excerpts from seminars and meetings. *Bulletin of the Hampstead Clinic, 6,* 115–128.

Freud, A., & Burlingham, D. T. (1943). *War and children.* New York, NY: Medical War Books, International Universities Press.

Freud, A., & Burlingham, D. T. (1944). *Infants without families: The case for and against residential nurseries.* New York, NY: Medical War Books, International Universities Press.

Freud, S. (1930/2005). *Civilization and its discontents.* New York, NY: W. W. Norton.

Freud, S. (1936). *The problem of anxiety* (H. A. Bunker, Trans.). New York, NY: W. W. Norton.

Freud, S. (1938). *The basic writings of Sigmund Freud* (A. A. Brill, Trans.). New York, NY: Modern Library.

Frick, W. B. (1987). The symbolic growth experience and creation of meaning. *International Forum for Logotherapy, 10,* 35–41.

Fruzzetti, A. E., & Erikson, K. R. (2010). Mindfulness and acceptance interventions in cognitive–behavioral therapy. In K. S. Dobson (Ed.), *Handbook of cognitive behavioral therapies* (3rd ed., pp. 340–372). New York, NY: Guilford Press.

Fulkerson, M. (2003). Integrating the Karpman drama triangle with choice theory and reality therapy. *International Journal of Reality Therapy, 23*(1), 17–20.

Funderburk, J. R., & Fukuyama, M. A. (2001). Feminism, multiculturalism, and spirituality: Convergent and divergent forces in psychotherapy. *Women & Therapy, 24,* 1–18.

Gabbard, G. O. (2005). *Psychodynamic psychiatry in clinical practice* (4th ed.). Washington, DC: American Psychiatric Publishing.

Gabbard, G. O. (Ed.). (2009). *Textbook of psychotherapeutic treatments.* Washington, DC: American Psychiatric Publishing.

Gabbard, G. O. (2010). *Long-term psychodynamic psychotherapy: A basic text* (2nd ed.). Washington, DC: American Psychiatric Publishing.

Gaffney, S. (2008). Gestalt group supervision in a divided society. Theory, practice, perspective, and reflections. *British Gestalt Journal, 17,* 27–40.

Gaffney, S. (2012). A neo-Lewinian perspective on Gestalt group facilitation. In T. B. Levine (Ed.), *Gestalt therapy: Advances in theory and practice* (pp. 149–160). New York, NY: Routledge

Galanter, M., & Kaskutas, L. A. (Eds.). (2008). *Recent developments in alcoholism, Vol. 18: Research on Alcoholics Anonymous and spirituality in addiction recovery.* New York, NY: Humana Press.

Gallagher-Thompson, D., Steffen, A. M., & Thompson, L. W. (Eds.). (2008). *Handbook of behavioral and cognitive therapies with other adults.* New York, NY: Springer.

Gallup, G. (2006). *The Gallup Poll: Public opinion 2006.* Wilmington, DE: Scholarly Resources.

Ganley, A. L. (1988). Feminist therapy with male clients. In M. A. Dutton-Douglas & L. E. Walker (Eds.), *Feminist psychotherapies: Integration of therapeutic and feminist systems* (pp. 186–205). Norwood, NJ: Ablex.

Garrow, S., & Walker, J. A. (2001). Existential group therapy and death anxiety. *Adultspan Journal, 3,* 77–87.

Gauvreau, P., & Bouchard, S. (2008). Preliminary evidence for the efficacy of EMDR in treating generalized anxiety disorder. *Journal of EMDR Practice and Research, 2,* 26–40.

Geller, J. D., Norcross, J. C., & Orlinsky, D. E. (Eds.). (2005). *The psychotherapist's own psychotherapy: Patient and clinician perspectives.* New York, NY: Oxford University Press.

Gendlin, E. T. (1996). *Focusing-oriented psychotherapy: A manual of the experiential method.* New York, NY: Guilford Press.

George, C., Kaplan, N., & Main, M. (1996). *Adult attachment interview.* Berkeley: University of California–Berkeley.

Gergen, K. J. (1991). *The saturated self: Dilemmas of identity in contemporary life.* New York, NY: Basic Books.

Gergen, K. J. (1995). The social constructionist movement in modern psychology, *American Psychologist, 40,* 266–275.

Gerson, M. J. (1996). *The embedded self: A psychoanalytic guide to family therapy.* London, UK: Routledge.

Gfroerer, K. P., Gfroerer, C. A., & Curlette, W. L. (2003). Psychological birth order and the Basis-A Inventory. *Journal of Individual Psychology, 59,* 30–41.

Giesen-Bloo, J., van Dyck, R., Spinhoven, P., van Tilburg, W., Dirksen, C., van Asselt, T., . . . Arntz, A. (2006). Outpatient psychotherapy for borderline personality disorder: A randomized trial of schema-focused therapy versus transference-focused therapy. *Archives of General Psychiatry, 63,* 649–658.

Gilbert, D. T, & Jones, E. E. (1986). Perceiver-induced constraint: Interpretations of self-generated reality. *Journal of Personality and Social Psychology, 50,* 269–280.

Gilligan, C. (1977). In a different voice: Women's conception of self and morality. *Harvard Educational Review, 47,* 481–517.

Gilligan, C. (1982). *In a different voice: Psychological theory and women's development.* Cambridge, MA: Harvard University Press.

Gilligan, C. (1993). *In a different voice: Psychological theory and women's development.* Cambridge, MA: Harvard University Press.

Gilligan, C. (1996). The centrality of relationship in human development: A puzzle, some evidence, and a theory. In G. G. Noam and K. W. Fischer (Eds.), *Development and vulnerability in close relationships* (pp. 237–261). Mahwah, NJ: Lawrence Erlbaum Associates.

Gilligan, C. (2008). *Exit-voice dilemmas in adolescent development.* New York, NY: Analytic Press.

Gilman, S. L. (2001). Karen Horney, M.D., 1885–1952. *American Journal of Psychiatry, 158,* 1205.

Gladding, S. T. (2007). *Family therapy: History, theory, and practice* (4th ed.). Upper Saddle River, NJ: Pearson/Prentice Hall.

Gladding, S. T. (2010). *Family therapy: History, theory, and practice* (5th ed.). Upper Saddle River, NJ: Pearson/Prentice Hall.

Glasser, W. (1961). *Mental health or mental illness?* New York, NY: Harper & Row.

Glasser, W. (1965). *Reality therapy: A new approach to psychiatry.* New York, NY: Harper & Row.

Glasser, W. (1975). *Reality therapy.* New York, NY: Harper & Row.

Glasser, W. (1976). *Positive addiction.* New York, NY: Harper & Row.

Glasser, W. (1984). *Control theory.* New York, NY: Harper & Row.

Glasser, W. (1986). *Control theory in the classroom.* New York, NY: Harper & Row.

Glasser, W. (1998a). *Choice theory.* New York, NY: HarperCollins.

Glasser, W. (1998b). *The quality school.* New York, NY: HarperCollins.

Glasser, W. (2000). *Counseling with choice theory.* New York, NY: HarperCollins.

Glasser, W. (2001). *Fibromyalgia: Hope from a completely new perspective.* Chatsworth, CA: William Glasser, Inc.

Glasser, W. (2003). *Warning: Psychiatry can be hazardous to your mental health.* New York, NY: HarperCollins.

Glasser, W., & Glasser, C. (1999). *The language of control theory.* New York, NY: HarperCollins.

Glasser, W., & Glasser, C. (2000). *Getting together and staying together: Solving the mystery of marriage.* New York, NY: HarperCollins.

Glasser, W., & Glasser, C. (2007). *Eight lessons for a happier marriage.* New York, NY: HarperCollins.

Glauser, A. S., & Bozarth, J. D. (2001). Person-centered counseling: The culture within. *Journal of Counseling and Development, 79,* 142–147.

Goldenberg, H., & Goldenberg, I. (2008). *Family therapy: An overview* (7th ed.). Pacific Grove, CA: Thomson-Brooks/Cole.

Goldenberg, H., & Goldenberg, I. (2012). *Family therapy: An overview* (8th ed.). Pacific Grove, CA: Thomson-Brooks/Cole.

Goldfried, M. R. (2004). Integrating integratively-oriented brief psychotherapy. *Journal of Psychotherapy Integration, 14,* 93–100.

Goldman, R., Greenberg, L., & Angus, L. (2006). The effects of adding emotion-focused interventions to the therapeutic relationship in the treatment of depression. *Psychotherapy Research, 16,* 537–549.

Goldner-Vukov, M., Moore, L., & Cupina, D. (2007). Bi-polar disorder from psychoeducational to existential group therapy. *Australasian Psychiatry, 15,* 30–34.

Goldstein, E. G. (2001). *Self-psychology and object relations theory in social work practice.* New York, NY: Free Press.

Goldstein, J., Freud, A., & Solnit, A. J. (1973). *Beyond the best interests of the child.* New York, NY: Free Press.

Goldstein, J., Freud, A., & Solnit, A. J. (1979). *Before the best interests of the child.* New York, NY: Free Press.

Goodman, G. (2010). *Therapeutic attachment relationships: Interaction structures and the processes of therapeutic change.* Lanham, MD: Jason Aronson.

Gordon, M. (2005). *Roots of empathy: Changing the world child by child.* Toronto: Thomas Allen.

Gordon, T. (1970). *Parent effectiveness training: The no-lose program for raising responsible children.* New York, NY: Wyden.

Gottlieb, D. T., & Gottlieb, C. D. (1996). The narrative/collaborative process in couples therapy: A postmodern perspective. *Women and Therapy, 19,* 37–47.

Graber, A. (2003). *Viktor Frankl's logotherapy: Method of choice in ecumenical pastoral psychology* (2nd ed.). Lima. OH: Wyndham Hall Press.

Green, J. G., McLaughlin, K. A., Berglund, P. A., Gruber, M. J., Sampson, N. A., Zaslavsky, A. M., & Kessler, R. C. (2010). Childhood adversities and adult psychiatric disorders in the national comorbidity survey replication I: Associations with first onset of DSM-IV disorders, *Archives of General Psychiatry, 67,* 113–123.

Greenberg, J. R., & Mitchell, S. A. (1983). *Object relations in psychoanalytic therapy.* Cambridge, MA: Harvard University Press.

Greenberg, L. S. (2002). *Emotion-focused therapy.* Washington, DC: American Psychological Association.

Greenberg, L. S. (2010). *Emotion-focused therapy.* Washington, DC: American Psychological Association.

Greenberg, L. S., & Elliott, R. (2002). Emotion-focused therapy. In F. W. Kaslow (Ed.), *Comprehensive handbook of psychotherapy: Integrative/eclectic* (pp. 213–240). New York, NY: John Wiley & Sons.

Greenberg, L., Elliott, R., & Lietaer, G. (1994). Research on experiential psychotherapies. In A. E. Bergin & S. L. Garfield (Eds.), *Handbook of psychotherapy and behavior change* (4th ed., pp. 509–539). New York, NY: Wiley.

Greenberg, L. S., & Goldman, R. N. (2008). *Emotion-focused couples therapy: The dynamics of emotion, love, and power.* Washington, DC: American Psychological Association Press.

Greenberg, L. S., & Johnson, S. (1988). Emotion in systemic therapies, *Journal of Systemic Therapies, 17,* 1–17.

Greenberg, L. S., Rice, L., & Elliott, R. (1993). *Facilitating emotional change: The moment-by-moment process.* New York, NY: Guilford Press.

Greenberg, L. S., & Safran, J. D. (1987). *Emotion in psychotherapy.* London, UK: Guilford Press.

Greenman, P. S., & Johnson, S. M. (2012). United we stand: Emotionally focused therapy in the treatment of couples with posttraumatic stress disorder. *Journal of Clinical Psychology, 68,* 561–569.

Greenman, P., Young, M., & Johnson, S. M. (2009). Emotionally focused therapy with intercultural couples. In M. Rastogi & V. Thomas (Eds.), *Multicultural Couple Therapy,* pp. 143–166. Thousand Oaks, CA: Sage.

Grey, A. L. (1988). Sullivan's contributions to psychoanalysis: An overview. *Contemporary Psychoanalysis, 24,* 548–576.

Grey, L. (1998). *Alfred Adler, forgotten prophet: A vision for the 21st century.* Westport, CT: Praeger.

Grotstein, J. S., & Rinsley, D. B. (1994). *Fairbairn and the origins of object relations.* New York, NY: Guilford Press.

Gruber, J., & Kring, A. M. (2008). Narrating emotional events in schizophrenia. *Journal of Abnormal Psychology, 117,* 520–533.

Haberstroh, S., Duffey, T., Evans, M., Gee, R., & Trepal, H. (2007). The experience of online counseling. *Journal of Mental Health Counseling, 29,* 269–282.

Haley, J. (1963). *Strategies in psychotherapy.* New York, NY: Grune-Stratton.

Haley, J. (1984). *Ordeal therapy: Unusual ways to change behavior.* San Francisco, CA: Jossey-Bass.

Haley, J., & Richeport-Haley, M. (2007). *Directive family therapy.* Binghamton, NY: Haworth Press.

Hall, G. C. N. (2010). *Multicultural psychology* (2nd ed.). Upper Saddle River, NJ: Prentice-Hall.

Hall, N. G., & Okazaki, S. (Eds.). (2002). *Asian American psychology: The science of lives in context.* Washington, DC: American Psychological Association.

Hansen, J. T. (2002). Postmodern implications for theoretical integration of counseling approaches. *Journal of Counseling and Development, 80*(3), 315–321.

Hansen, J., Stevic, R., & Warner, R. (1986). *Counseling: Theory and process* (4th ed.). Boston, MA: Allyn & Bacon.

Hargaden, H., & Sills, C. (2002). *Transactional analysis: A relational perspective.* New York, NY: Taylor & Francis.

Harrington, N., & Pickles, C. (2009). Mindfulness and cognitive behavioral therapy: Are they compatible concepts? *Journal of Cognitive Psychotherapy: An International Quarterly, 23,* pp. 315–323.

Harris, M., & Brockbank, A. (2011). *An integrative approach to therapy and supervision: A practical guide for counselors and psychotherapists.* Philadelphia, PA: Jessica Kingsley.

Harris, T. A. (1967). *I'm ok—you're ok.* New York, NY: Avon.

Hart, J. J. (1982). Psychology of the scientist: XLCI: Correlation between theoretical orientation in psychology and personality type. *Psychological Reports, 50,* 795–801.

Hartling, L. M., & Ly, J. (2000). *Relational references: A selected bibliography of research, theory, and applications* (Project Report No. 7, Working Papers Series). Wellesley, MA: Stone Center Counseling Service.

Harwood, T. M., Beutler, L. E., & Charvat, M. (2010). Cognitive–behavioral therapy and psychotherapy integration. In K. S. Dobson (Ed.), *Handbook of cognitive–behavioral therapies* (3rd ed., pp. 94–130). New York, NY: Guilford Press.

Haule, J. R. (2010). *Jung in the 21st century Vol. II: Synchronicity and science.* New York, NY: Routledge.

Hayes, J. A., Gelso, C. J., & Hummel, A. M. (2011). Managing countertransference. In J. C. Norcross (Ed.), *Psychotherapy relationships that work* (2nd ed., pp. 239–260). New York, NY: Oxford University Press.

Hayes, S. C., Luoma, J. B., Bond, F. W., Masuda, A., & Lillis, J. (2006). Acceptance and commitment therapy: Models, processes and outcomes. *Behaviour Research and Therapy, 44,* 1–25.

Hayes, S. C., Strosahl, K. D., & Wilson, K. G. (1999). *Acceptance and commitment therapy: An experiential approach to behavior change.* New York, NY: Guilford Press.

Hayes, S. C., Strosahl, K. D., & Wilson, K. G. (2012). *Acceptance and commitment therapy: The process and practice of mindful change* (2nd ed.). New York, NY: Guilford Press.

Hays, P. A. (2001). *Addressing cultural complexities in practice: A framework for clinicians and counselors.* Washington, DC: American Psychological Association.

Hays, P. A. (2008). *Addressing cultural complexities in practice: Assessment, diagnosis, and therapy* (2nd ed.). Washington, DC: American Psychological Association.

Hays, P. A. (2009). Integrating evidence-based practice, cognitive–behavior therapy, and multicultural therapy: Ten steps for culturally competent practice. *Professional Psychology: Research and Practice, 40,* 354–360.

Hazan, C., & Shaver, P. (1987). Romantic love conceptualized as an attachment process. *Journal of Personality and Social Psychology, 52,* 511–524.

Heidegger, M. (1962). *Being and time.* New York, NY: Harper & Row.

Henderson, V. L., O'Hara, M., Barfield, G. L., & Rogers, N. (2007). Applications beyond the therapeutic context. In M. Cooper, M. O'Hara, P. F. Schmid, & G. Wyatt (Eds.), *The handbook of person-centered psychotherapy* (pp. 306–324). New York, NY: Palgrave Macmillan.

Hendricks, M. N. (2002). Focusing oriented/experiential psychotherapy. In D. J. Cain & J. Seeman (Eds.), *Humanistic psychotherapies: Handbook of research and practice* (pp. 221–251). Washington, DC: American Psychological Association.

Herbert, J. D., & Forman, E. M. (2011). *Acceptance and mindfulness in cognitive behavior therapy: Understanding and applying the new therapies.* Hoboken, NJ: Wiley.

Hergenhahn, B. R. (2009). *An introduction to the history of psychology* (6th ed.). Belmont, CA: Wadsworth.

Hergenhahn, B. R., & Olson, M. H. (2007). *An introduction to the theories of personality* (7th ed.). Upper Saddle River, NJ: Pearson Prentice Hall.

Herlihy, B., & Corey, G. (2006). *ACA ethical standards casebook* (6th ed.). Alexandria, VA: American Counseling Association.

Herrera, N. C., Zajonc, R. B., Weiczorkowska, G., & Cichomski, B. (2003). Beliefs about birth rank and their reflection in reality. *Journal of Personality & Social Psychology, 85,* 142–150.

Higdon, J. (2012). *Psychodynamic theory for therapeutic practice* (2nd ed.). New York, NY: Palgrave Macmillan.

Hill, C. E. (2009). *Helping skills: Facilitating exploration, insight, and action* (3rd ed.). Washington, DC: American Psychological Association.

Hill, C., Schottenbauer, M., Lui, J., Spangler, P., & Sim, W. (2008). Working with dreams in psychotherapy. What do psychoanalytic therapists report that they do? *Psychoanalytic Psychology, 25,* 565–573.

Hill, K. A. (1987). Meta-analysis of paradoxical interventions, *Psychotherapy: Theory, Research, Practice, Training, 24,* 266–270.

Hill, P., & Pargament, K. I. (2003). Advances in the conceptualization and measurement of religion and spirituality: Implications for physical and mental health research. *American Psychologist, 58,* 64–74.

Hillman, J. (1996). *The soul's code: In search of character and calling*. New York, NY: Random House.

Hinrichsen, G. A., & Clougherty, K. F. (2006). *Interpersonal psychotherapy for depressed older adults.* Washington, DC: American Psychological Association.

Hinterkopf, E. (2005). The experiential focusing approach. In L. Sperry & E. P. Shafranske, (Eds.), *Spiritually oriented psychotherapy* (pp. 207–234). Washington, DC: American Psychological Association.

Hinton, D. E., Rivera, E. I., Hofmann, S. G., Barlow, D. H., & Otto, M. W. (2012). Adapting CBT for traumatized refugees and ethnic minority patients: Examples from culturally adapted CBT (CA-CBT). *Transcultural Psychiatry, 49,* 340–365.

Hirschman, L. (1997). Restoring complexity to the subjective worlds of profound abuse survivors. In A. Goldberg (Ed.), *Conversations in self-psychology: Progress in self-psychology* (Vol. 13, pp. 307–323). Hillsdale, NJ: Analytic Press.

Hoch, A. L. (2009). Trauma-focused cognitive behavioral therapy for children. In A. Rubin & D. W. Springer (Eds.), *Treatment of traumatized adults and children: Clinician's guide to evidence-based practice* (pp. 179–253). Hoboken, NJ: John Wiley & Sons.

Hoffman, E. (1994). *The drive for self: Alfred Adler and the founding of individual psychology.* Reading, MA: Addison-Wesley.

Hoffman, L. (2009). Introduction to existential psychology in a cross-cultural context: East-West dialogue. In L. Hoffman, M. Yang, F. Kaklauskas, & A. Chan (Eds.), *Existential psychology East-West* (pp. 1–67). Colorado Springs, CO: University of the Rockies Press.

Hoffman, L., Yang, M., Kaklauskas, F., & Chan, A. (Eds.). (2009). *Existential psychology East-West* (pp. 1–67). Colorado Springs, CO: University of the Rockies Press.

Hofmann, S. G. (2012). *An introduction to modern CBT: Psychological solutions to mental health problems.* Malden, MA: Wiley-Blackwell.

Hofmann, S. G., Sawyer, A. T., & Fang, A. (2010). The empirical status of the "new wave" of cognitive behavioral therapy. *Psychiatric Clinics of North America, 33,* 701–710.

Hoglend, P. (2003). Long-term effects of brief dynamic psychotherapy. *Psychotherapy Research, 13*(3), 271–292.

Hollon, S. D., Stewart, M. O., & Strunk, D. (2006). Enduring effects for cognitive behavioral therapy in the treatment of depression and anxiety. *Annual Review of Psychology, 57,* 285–315.

Holzel, B. K., Lazar, S. W., Gard, T., Schuman-Olivier, Z., Vago, D. R., & Ott, U. (2011). How does mindfulness meditation work? Proposing mechanisms of action from a conceptual and neural perspective, *Perspectives on Psychological Science, 6,* 537–559.

Horney, K. (1937). *The neurotic personality of our time.* New York, NY: W. W. Norton.

Horney, K. (1939). *New ways in psychoanalysis.* New York, NY: W. W. Norton.

Horney, K. (1945). *Our inner conflicts.* New York, NY: W. W. Norton.

Horney, K. (1950). *Neurosis and human growth: The struggle toward self-realization.* New York, NY: W. W. Norton.

Hornyak, M., Grossmann, C., Kohnen, R., Schlatterer, M., Richter, H. Voderholzer, U., . . . Berger, M. (2008). Cognitive behavioral group therapy to improve patients' strategies for coping with restless legs syndrome: A proof-of-concept trial. *Journal of Neurological Neurosurgical Psychiatry, 79,* 823–825.

Horowitz, M., Marmar, C., Krupnick, J., Wilner, N., Kaltreider, N., & Wallerstein, R. (2001). *Personality styles and brief psychotherapy.* New York, NY: Basic Books.

Horvath, A. O., & Symonds, B. D. (1991). Relation between working alliance and outcome in psychotherapy: A meta-analysis. *Journal of Consulting and Clinical Psychology, 38,* 139–149.

Houston, G. (2003). *Brief Gestalt therapy.* Thousand Oaks, CA: Sage.

Howatt, W. A. (2003). Choice theory: A core addiction recovery tool. *International Journal of Reality Therapy, 22*(2), 12–15.

Hubble, M. A., Duncan, B. L., Miller, S. D., & Wampold, B. E. (2010). Introduction. In B. L. Duncan, S. D. Miller, B. E. Wampold, & M. A. Hubble (Eds.), *The heart and soul of change* (2nd ed., pp. 23–46). Washington, DC: American Psychological Association.

Hughes, D., Rodriguez, Smith, E. P., Johnson, D. J., Stevenson, H. C., & Spicer, P. (2006). Parents' ethnic-racial socialization processes: A review of research and directions for future study. *Developmental Psychology, 42*, 747–770.

Hutson-Comeaux, S. L., & Kelly, J. R. (2002). Gender stereotypes of emotional reactions: How we judge an emotion as valid. *Sex Roles, 48,* 1–10.

Indelicato, N. A., & Springer, S. H. (2007). Feminist therapy. In J. Archer & C. J. McCarthy (Eds.), *Theories of counseling and psychotherapy: Contemporary applications* (pp. 310–339). Columbus, OH: Pearson Merrill Prentice Hall.

Jakupcak, M., Salters, K., Gratz, K. L., & Roemer, L. (2003). Masculinity and emotionality: An investigation of men's primary and secondary emotional responding. *Sex Roles, 49,* 111–120.

James, M. (1996). *Born to win: Transactional analysis with Gestalt experiments.* Reading, MA: Addison Wesley.

Jencius, M., & West, J. (2003). Traditional counseling theories and cross-cultural implications. In F. D. Harder & J. McFadden (Eds.), *Culture and counseling: New approaches* (pp. 339–349). Boston, MA: Pearson Education.

Johnson, S. M. (2002). *Emotionally focused couple therapy with trauma survivors: Strengthening attachment bonds*. New York, NY: Guilford Press.

Johnson, S. M. (2004). *The practice of emotionally focused couple therapy: Creating connection.* New York, NY: Brunner-Routledge.

Johnson, S. M. (2007). A new era for couple therapy: Theory, research, and practice in concert. *Journal of Systemic Therapies, 26,* 5–16.

Johnson, S. M. (2008). *Hold me tight: Seven conversations for a lifetime of love.* New York, NY: Little, Brown and Company.

Johnson, S. M., Bradley, B., Furrow, J., Lee, A., Palmer, G., Tilley, D., & Woolley, S. (2005). *Becoming an emotionally focused couple therapist: The workbook.* New York, NY: Routledge.

Johnson, S. M., & Greenberg, L. S. (1985). Emotionally focused couples therapy: An outcome study. *Journal of Marital and Family Therapy, 11,* 313–317.

Johnson, S. M., & Greenberg, L. S. (1987). Emotionally focused marital therapy: An overview. *Psychotherapy: Theory, Research & Practice, 24,* 552–560.

Johnson, S. M., & Greenman, P. S. (2006). The path to a secure bond: Emotionally focused couple therapy. *Journal of Clinical Psychology, 62,* 597–609.

Johnson, S. M., & Lee, A. C. (2000). Emotionally focused family therapy: Children in family therapy. In C. E. Bailey (Ed.), *Working with children in family therapy* (pp. 112–116). New York, NY: W. W. Norton.

Johnson, S. M., Makinen, J. A., & Millikin, J. W. (2001). Attachment injuries in couple relationships: A new perspective on impasses in couples therapy. *Journal of Marital and Family Therapy, 27,* 145–155.

Johnson, S. M., & Whiffen, V. E. (Eds.). (2005). *Attachment processes in couple and family therapy.* New York, NY: Guilford Press.

Johnson, S. M., & Woolley, S. (2009). Emotionally focused couples therapy: An attachment based theory. *Psychotherapeutic Treatments*, 121–142.

Jones, E. (1953). *The life and work of Sigmund Freud* (Vol. 1). New York, NY: Basic Books.

Jones, E. (1955). *The life and work of Sigmund Freud: Years of maturity, 1901–1919* (Vol. 2). New York, NY: Basic Books.

Jones, E. (1957). *The life and work of Sigmund Freud: The last phase, 1919–1939* (Vol. 3). New York, NY: Basic Books.

Jordan, J. V. (1999). *Toward connection and competence* (Work in Progress No. 83, Working Papers Series). Wellesley, MA: Stone Center Counseling Service.

Jordan, J. V. (2010). *Relational-cultural therapy.* Washington, DC: American Psychological Association.

Jordan, J. V., Handel, M., Alvarez, M., & Cook-Nobles, R. (2004). Application of the relational model to time-limited therapy. In J. V. Jordan, M. Walker, & L. M. Hartling (Eds.), *The complexity of connection.* New York, NY: Guilford Press.

Jung, C. G. (1907/1960). The psychology of dementia praecox. In *The collected works of C. G. Jung* (Vol. 4). Princeton, NJ: Princeton University Press.

Jung, C. G. (1912/1956). Symbols of transformation. In *The collected works of C. G. Jung* (Vol. 5). Princeton, NJ: Princeton University Press.

Jung, C. G. (1921/1971). Psychological types. In *The collected works of C. G. Jung* (Vol. 6). Princeton, NJ: Princeton University Press.

Jung, C. G. (1953). Two essays on analytical psychology. In *The collected works of C. G. Jung* (Vol. 7). Princeton, NJ: Princeton University Press.

Jung, C. G. (1960). *Collected works 8: The structure and dynamics of the psyche.* New York, NY: Pantheon.

Jung, C. G. (1963). *Memories, dreams, reflections.* New York, NY: Pantheon.

Jung, C. G. (1964). *Man and his symbols.* Garden City, NY: Doubleday.

Jusoh, A. J., & Ahmad, R. (2009). The practice of reality therapy from the Islamic perspective in Malaysia and variety of custom in Asia. *International Journal of Reality Therapy, 28,* 3–8.

Kabat-Zinn, J. (1982). An outpatient program in behavioral medicine for chronic pain patients based on the practice of mindfulness meditation: Theoretical considerations and preliminary results. *General Hospital Psychiatry, 4,* 33–47.

Kabat-Zinn, J. (1990). *Full catastrophe living: Using the wisdom of your body and mind to face stress, pain, and illness.* New York, NY: Delacorte.

Kakar, S. (2006). Culture and psychoanalysis. *Social Analysis, 50,* 25–44.

Kandel, E. R. (2008). *In search of memory: The emergence of a new science of mind.* New York, NY: W. W. Norton.

Kaner, A., & Prelinger, E. (2005). *The craft of psychodynamic psychotherapy.* Lanham, MD: Rowman and Littlefield.

Kanter, J., Busch, A., & Rusch, L. (2009). *Behavioural activation.* London, UK: Routledge.

Kaslow, N. J., Broth, M. R., Smith, C. O., & Collins, M. H. (2012). Family-based interventions for child and adolescent disorders. *Journal of Marital and Family Therapy, 38,* 82–100.

Kaufman, M. (2007, July 25). Albert Ellis, provoker of change in psychotherapy is dead at 93. *New York Times.*

Keith, D. V., Connell , G., & Whitaker, C. A. (1992). Group supervision in symbolic experiential family therapy. *Journal of Family Psychotherapy, 3,* 93–102.

Kellogg, S. H., & Young, J. E. (2008). Cognitive therapy. In J. L. Lebow (Ed.), *Twenty-first century psychotherapies: Contemporary approaches to theory and practice* (pp. 43–79). Hoboken, NJ: John Wiley & Sons.

Kelly, G. (1955). *The psychology of personal constructs.* New York, NY: W. W. Norton.

Kelly, W. L. (1990). *Psychology of the unconscious: Mesmer, Janet, Freud, Jung, and current issues.* New York, NY: Prometheus.

Kelsch, D. M. (2002). Multiple sclerosis and choice theory: It is a disease and choice theory works! *International Journal of Reality Therapy, 22*(1), 24–30.

Kern, R. (1992). *Kern lifestyle scale.* Coral Springs, FL: CMTI Press.

Kern, R. M., Wheeler, M. S., & Curlette, W. L. (1997). *BASIS-A interpretive manual.* Coral Springs, FL: CMTI Press.

Kerr, M. E. (1981). Family systems theory and therapy. In A. S. Gurman & D. P. Kniskern (Eds.), *Handbook of family therapy* (pp. 226–264). New York, NY: Bruner-Mazel.

Kierkegaard, S. (1941). *Concluding unscientific postscript.* Princeton, NJ: Princeton University Press.

Kierkegaard, S. (1944). *The concept of dread.* Princeton, NJ: Princeton University Press.

Kim, B. H. (2002). Church as a self-object environment: A self-psychological psychoanalytic exploration of male members of two Korean immigrant congregations. *Dissertation Abstracts International, 62* (10-A) (UMI No. 3438).

Kim, J. (2005). Effectiveness of reality therapy program for schizophrenic patients. *Taehan Kanho Hakhoe Chi, 35,* 1485–1492.

Kim, J. (2007). A reality therapy group counseling program as an Internet addiction recovery method for college students in Korea. *International Journal of Reality Therapy, 26,* 3–9.

Kim, J. (2011). Structuring background by letting go of clinging and avoidance. *Gestalt!, 11.*

Kim, R. I., & Hwang, M. (2006). A meta-analysis of reality therapy and choice theory group programs for self-esteem and locus of control in Korea. *International Journal of Reality Therapy, 1,* 25–30.

Kim-Cohen, J., Caspi, A., Moffitt, T. E., Harrington, H., Milne, B. J., & Poulton, R. (2003). Prior juvenile diagnoses in adults with mental disorders: Developmental follow-back of a prospective longitudinal cohort, *Archives of General Psychiatry, 60,* 709–717.

Kingdon, D., Rathod, S., Weiden, P., & Turkington, D. (2008). Cognitive therapy for schizophrenia. *Journal of Psychiatric Practice, 14,* 55–57.

Kirk, U., Downar, J., & Montague, P. R. (2011). Interoception drives increased rational decision-making in meditators playing the ultimatum game, *Frontiers in Decision Neuroscience, 5,* 49. doi:10.3389/fnins.2011.00049

Kirschenbaum, H. (2004). Carl Rogers's life and work: An assessment on the 100th anniversary of his birth. *Journal of Counseling and Development, 82,* 116–124.

Kirschenbaum, H. (2009). *The life and work of Carl Rogers.* Alexandria, VA: American Counseling Association.

Klever, P. (2009). Goal direction and effectiveness, emotional maturity, and nuclear family functioning. *Journal of Marital and Family Therapy, 35,* 308–324.

Klingberg, H. (2001). *When life calls out to us: The love and lifework of Viktor and Elly Frankl.* New York, NY: Doubleday.

Klinger, E., Bouchard, S., Legeron, P., Roy, S., Lauer, F., Chemin, I., & Nugues, P. (2005). Virtual reality therapy versus cognitive behavior therapy for social phobia: A preliminary controlled study, *CyberPsychology & Behavior, 8,* 76–88.

Knaus, W. J. (2005). Frustration tolerance training for children. In A. Ellis & M. E. Bernard (Eds.), *Rational emotive behavioral approaches to childhood disorders: Theory, practice and research* (pp. 133–155). New York, NY: Springer.

Knox, R., & Cooper, M. (2010). Relationship qualities that are associated with moments of relational depth: The client's perspective. *Person-Centered and Experiential Psychotherapy, 9,* 236–256.

Kohlberg, L. (1981). *The philosophy of moral development: Essays on moral development* (Vols. 1–2). San Francisco, CA: Harper and Row.

Kohut, H. (1971). *The analysis of the self: A systematic approach to the psychoanalytic treatment of narcissistic personality disorders.* New York, NY: International Universities Press.

Kohut, H. (1977). *The restoration of the self.* New York, NY: International Universities Press.

Kohut, H. (1982). Introspection, empathy, and the semicircle of mental health. *International Journal of Psychoanalysis, 63,* 395–407.

Krause, N. (2004). Stressors arising in highly valued roles, meaning in life, and the physical health status of older adults. *Journal of Gerontology: Social Sciences, 59,* S287–S297.

Kubany, E. S., Owens, J. A., McCaig, M. A., Hill, E. E., Iannuce-Spencer, C., & Tremayne, K. J. (2004). Cognitive trauma therapy for battered women with PTSD. *Journal of Consulting and Clinical Psychology, 72,* 3–18.

Lachmann, F. M., & Beebe, B. (1995). Self psychology: Today. *Psychoanalysis Dialogues, 5,* 375–384.

Laird, T. G., & Shelton, A. J. (2006). From an Adlerian perspective: Birth order, dependency, and binge drinking on a historically black university campus. *Journal of Individual Psychology, 62,* 18–35.

Lambert, M. J. (1992). Psychotherapy outcome research: Implications for integrative and eclectic therapists. In J. C. Norcross & M. R. Goldfried (Eds.), *Handbook of psychotherapy integration* (pp. 94–129). New York, NY: Basic Books.

Lambert, M. J. (2010). "Yes, it is time for clinicians to routinely monitor treatment outcome." In B. L. Duncan, S. D. Miller, B. E. Wampold, & M. A. Hubble (Eds.), *Heart and soul of change in psychotherapy* (2nd ed., pp. 239–266). Washington, DC: American Psychological Association.

Lambert, M. J., & Bergin, A. E. (1994). The effectiveness of psychotherapy. In A. E. Bergin & S. L. Garfield (Eds.), *Handbook of psychotherapy and behavior change* (4th ed., pp. 143–189). New York, NY: John Wiley & Sons.

Lambert, M. J., Bergin, A. E., & Garfield, S. L. (2004). Introduction and historical overview. In M. J. Lambert (Ed.), *Bergin and Garfield's handbook of psychotherapy and behavior change* (5th ed., pp. 3–15). New York, NY: John Wiley & Sons.

Lambert, M. J., & Cattani-Thompson, K. (1996). Current findings regarding the effectiveness of counseling: Implications for practice. *Journal of Counseling and Development, 74,* 601–608.

Lampropoulos, G. K. (2000). Definitional and research issues in the common factors approach to psychotherapy integration: Misconceptions, clarifications, and proposals. *Journal of Psychotherapy Integration, 10*(4), 415–438.

Landridge, D. (2012). *Existential counseling and psychotherapy*. Thousand Oaks, CA: Sage.

Lantz, J. (2000). Phenomenological reflection and time in Viktor Frankl's existential psychotherapy. *Journal of Phenomenological Psychology, 3,* 220–228.

Lantz, J., & Gregoire, T. (2000). Existential psychotherapy with couples facing breast cancer: A twenty-year report. *Contemporary Family Therapy, 29,* 315–327.

Lanza, M. L., Anderson, J., Boisvert, C. M., LeBlanc, A., Fardy, M., & Steel, B. S. (2002). Assaultive behavior intervention in the Veterans Administration: Psychodynamic group psychotherapy compared to cognitive behavior therapy. *Perspectives in Psychiatric Care, 38,* 89–97.

Lawe, C. F., Horne, A. M., & Taylor, S. V. (1983). Effects of pretraining procedures for clients in counseling. *Psychological Reports, 53,* 327–334.

Lazar, S. G. (Ed.). (2010). *Psychotherapy, is it worth it? A comprehensive review of its cost-effectiveness.* Arlington, VA: American Psychiatric Publishing.

Lazarus, A. A. (1976). *Multimodal behavior therapy.* New York, NY: Springer.

Lazarus, A. A. (Ed.). (1985). *Casebook of multimodal therapy.* New York, NY: Guilford Press.

Lazarus, A. A. (1989). *The practice of multimodal therapy (update).* Baltimore, MD: Johns Hopkins University Press.

Lazarus, A. A. (1996). Some reflections after 40 years of trying to be an effective psychotherapist. *Psychotherapy: Theory, Research, Practice, Training, 33,* 142–145.

Lazarus, A. A. (2006). *Brief but comprehensive psychotherapy: The multimodal way.* New York, NY: Springer.

Lazarus, A. A. (2008). Technical eclecticism and multimodal therapy. In J. L. Lebow (Ed.), *Twenty-first century psychotherapies: Contemporary approaches to theory and practice* (pp. 424–452). Hoboken, NJ: John Wiley & Sons.

Lazarus, A. A., & Beutler, L. E. (1993). On technical eclecticism. *Journal of Counseling and Development, 71*(4), 381–385.

Lazarus, A. A., & Lazarus, C. N. (1991). *Multimodal life history inventory* (2nd ed.). Champaign, IL: Research Press.

Lazarus, A., & Lazarus, C. (1998). *The multimodal life history.* Champaign, IL: Research Press.

Leahy, R. L., Tirch, D., & Napolitano, L. A. (2011). *Emotion regulation in psychotherapy: A practitioner's guide.* New York, NY: Guilford Press.

Lebow, J. L. (2008). Couples and family therapy. In J. L. Lebow (Ed.), *Twenty-first century psychotherapies: Contemporary approaches to theory and practice* (pp. 307–346). Hoboken, NJ: John Wiley & Sons.

Lee, B. K., & Rovers, M. (2008). Bringing torn lives together again: Effects of the first congruence couple therapy training application to clients in pathological gambling. *International Gambling Studies, 8,* 113–129.

Lee, C. C. (2007). *Counseling for social justice* (2nd ed.). Alexandria, VA: American Counseling Association.

Lee, J. (1997). Women re-authoring their lives through feminist narrative therapy. *Women and Therapy, 20,* 1–22.

Lega, L. I., & Ellis, A. (2001). Rational emotive behavior therapy (REBT) in the new millennium: A cross-cultural approach. *Journal of Rational-Emotive & Cognitive–Behavior Therapy, 19,* 201–222.

Leichsenring, F. (2009). Psychodynamic psychotherapy: A review of efficacy and effectiveness studies. In K. N. Levy and J. S. Ablon (Eds.), *Handbook of evidence-based psychodynamic psychotherapy: Bridging the gap between science and practice, Part I* (pp. 3–28). New York, NY: Humana Press.

Lennon, B. (2003). Review: "Warning: Psychiatry can be hazardous to your mental health." *International Journal of Reality Therapy, 23*(1), 15–17.

Lerner, H. D. (2008). Psychodynamic perspectives. In M. Hersen & A. M. Gross (Eds.), *Handbook of clinical psychology* (Vol. 1, pp. 127–160). Hoboken, NJ: John Wiley & Sons.

Lesser, J. G. (2000). The group as self-object: Brief psychotherapy with women. *International Journal of Group Psychotherapy, 50,* 363–380.

Levant, R. F. (1996, Spring). What is the status of manhood today? *Bulletin of the Society for the Psychological Study of Men and Masculinity, 1*(2), 10–13.

Levant, R. F. (2001). Desperately seeking language: Understanding, assessing, and treating normative male alexithymia in men. In G. R. Brooks & G. E. Good (Eds.), *The handbook of psychotherapy and counseling with men: A comprehensive guide to settings, problems, and treatment approaches* (pp. 424–443). San Francisco, CA: Jossey-Bass.

Levant, R. F., & Wimer, D. J. (2009). The new fathering movement. In C. Z. Oren & D. C. Oren (Eds.), *Counseling fathers* (pp. 3–21). New York, NY: Routledge.

Levant, R. F., Wimer, D. J., Williams, C. M., Smalley, K. B., & Noronha, D. (2009). The relationships between masculinity variables, health risk behaviors and attitudes toward seeking psychological help. *International Journal of Men's Health, 8,* 3–21.

Levenson, E. A. (1992). Harry Stack Sullivan: From interpersonal psychiatry to interpersonal psychoanalysis. *Contemporary Psychoanalysis, 28,* 450–466.

Levenson, H. (2003). Time-limited dynamic psychotherapy: An integrationist perspective. *Journal of Psychotherapy Integration, 13,* 300–333.

Levenson, H. (2010). *Brief dynamic therapy*. Washington, DC: American Psychological Association.

Levenson, H., & Strupp, H. (1999). Recommendations for the future of training in brief dynamic psychotherapy. *Journal of Clinical Psychology, 55,* 385–391.

Levin, J., & Levine, T. B. (2012). Gestalt in the new age. In T. B. Levine (Ed.), *Gestalt therapy: Advances in theory and practice* (pp. 1–12). New York, NY: Routledge.

Levine, D. A. (2005). *Teaching empathy: A blueprint for caring, compassion, and community*. Bloomington, IN: Learning Tree.

Levine, T. B. (2012). *Gestalt therapy: Advances in theory and practice*. New York, NY: Routledge.

Levy, K. N., Ellison, W. D., Scott, L. N., & Bernecker, S. L. (2011). Attachment style. In J. C. Norcross (Ed.), *Psychotherapy relationships that work: Evidence-based responsiveness* (2nd ed.). New York, NY: Oxford University Press.

Levy, R. A., Ablon, J. S., & Kachele, H. (Eds.). (2012). *Psychodynamic psychotherapy research*. New York, NY: Humana Press.

Levy, R. A., Wasserman, R. H., Scott, L., & Yeomans, F. E. (Eds.). (2012). Empirical evidence for transference-focused psychotherapy and other psychodynamic psychotherapies for borderline personality disorder. In R. A. Levy, J. S. Ablon, and H. Kachele (Eds.), *Psychodynamic psychotherapy research* (pp. 93–120). New York, NY: Humana Press.

Lewis, B. (2011). Narrative and psychiatry. *Current Options in Psychiatry, 24,* 489–494.

Li, C. (1998). Impact of acculturation on Chinese-Americans' life and its implications for helping professionals. *International Journal of Reality Therapy, 17*(2), 7–11.

Li, Y., & Vivien, W. (2010). Applying the Satir Model of counseling in mainland China: Illustrated with case studies. *The Satir Journal: Transformational Systemic Therapy, 4*(1).

Licht, C., & Chabot, D. (2006). The Chabot Emotional Differentiation Scale: A theoretically and psychometrically sound instrument for measuring Bowen's intrapsychic aspect of differentiation. *Journal of Marital and Family Therapy, 32,* 167–180.

Lichtenberg, P. (2012). In gratitude. In T. B. Levine (Ed.), *Gestalt therapy: Advances in theory and practice* (pp. 116–122). New York, NY: Routledge.

Lieberman, J. A., & Murray, R. M. (2012). *Comprehensive care of schizophrenia: A textbook of clinical management*. New York, NY: Oxford University Press.

Linehan, M. (1993). *Cognitive–behavioral treatment of borderline personality disorder*. New York, NY: Guilford Press.

Linehan, M. M., & Kehrer, C. A. (1993). Borderline personality disorder. In D. A. Barlow (Ed.), *Clinical handbook of psychological disorders* (2nd ed., pp. 396–441). New York, NY: Guilford Press.

Linehan, M. M., McDavid, J., Brown, M. Z., Sayrs, J. H. R., & Gallop, R. J. (2008). Olanzapine plus dialectical behavior therapy for women with high irritability who meet criteria for borderline personality disorder: A double blind, placebo-controlled pilot study. *Journal of Clinical Psychiatry, 69,* 999–1005.

Livingston, M., & Livingston, L. (2000). Sustained empathic focus and the clinical application of self-psychological theory in group psychotherapy. *International Journal of Group Psychotherapy, 56,* 67–85.

Livneh, H., & Antonak, R. F. (2005). Psychosocial adaptation to chronic illness and disability: A primer for counselors. *Journal of Counseling and Development, 83,* 12–20.

Livneh, H., & Sherwood, A. (1991). Application of personality theories and counseling strategies to clients with physical disabilities. *Journal of Counseling and Development, 69*(6), 525–538.

Lombardi, D. M. (1996). Antisocial personality disorder and addictions. In L. Sperry & J. Carlson (Eds.), *Psychopathology and psychotherapy* (pp. 371–390). Washington, DC: Accelerated Development.

Looyeh, M. Y., Kamali, K., & Shafieian, R. (2012). An exploratory study of the effectiveness of group narrative therapy on the school behavior of girls with attention-deficit/hyperactivity disorder symptoms. *Archives of Psychiatric Nursing, 26,* 404–410.

Lubbe, T. (2011). *Object relations in depression: A return to theory.* New York, NY: Routledge.

Luborsky, L. (1984). *Principles of psychoanalytic psychotherapy: A manual for supportive-expressive treatment.* New York, NY: Basic Books.

Luborsky, L., & Mark, D. (1991). Short term supportive-expressive psychoanalytic psychotherapy. In P. Crits-Cristoph & J. P. Barber (Eds.), *Handbook of short-term dynamic psychotherapy* (pp. 110–136). New York, NY: Basic Books.

Luborsky, L., Singer, B., & Luborsky, L. (1975). Comparative studies of psychotherapies. *Archives of General Psychiatry, 32,* 995–1008.

Lundahl, B., & Burke, B. I. (2009). The effectiveness and applicability of motivational interviewing: A practice friendly review of four meta-analyses. *Journal of Clinical Psychology: In Session, 11,* 1232–1245.

Lundahl, B., Kunz, C., Brownell, C., Tollefson, D., & Burke, B. I. (2010). A meta-analysis of motivational interviewing: Twenty-five years of empirical studies. *Research on Social Work Practice, 22,* 137–160.

Lundin, R. W. (1977). Behaviorism: Operant reinforcement. In R. J. Corsini (Ed.), *Current personality theories* (pp. 177–202). Itasca, IL: Peacock.

Lynch, G. (1997). The role of community and narrative in the work of the therapist: A post-modern theory of the therapist's engagement in the therapeutic process. *Counseling Psychology Quarterly, 10,* 353–363.

Ma, S. H., & Teasdale, J. D. (2004). Mindfulness based cognitive therapy for depression: Replication and exploration of differential relapse prevention effects. *Journal of Consulting and Clinical Psychology, 72,* 31–40.

MacGeorge, E. L. (2003). Gender differences in attributions and emotions in helping contexts. *Sex Roles, 49,* 175–182.

MacIntosh, H. B., & Johnson, S. (2008). Emotionally focused therapy for couples and childhood sexual abuse survivors. *Journal of Marital and Family Therapy, 34,* 298–315.

Mackewn, J. (1997). *Developing Gestalt counseling: A field theoretical and relational model of contemporary Gestalt counseling and psychotherapy.* Thousand Oaks, CA: Sage.

Madanes, C. (1991). Strategic family therapy. In A. S. Gurman & D. P. Kniskern (Eds.), *Handbook of family therapy* (Vol. II). New York, NY: Brunner/Mazel.

Mahalik, J. R., Good, G. E., & Englar-Carlson, M. (2003). Masculinity scripts, presenting concerns, and help seeking: Implications for practice and training. *Professional Psychology: Research and Practice, 34,* 123–131.

Mahoney, M. J. (1988). Constructive metatheory. I: Basic features and historical foundations. *International Journal of Personal Construct Psychology, I,* 1–35.

Mahoney, M. J. (2003). *Constructive psychotherapy.* New York, NY: Guilford Press.

Mahrer, A. R. (1996/2004). *The complete guide to experiential psychotherapy.* Boulder, CO: Bull Publishing.

Malinen, T., Cooper, S. J., & Thomas, F. N. (2011). *Masters of narrative and collaborative therapies: The voices of Anderson, Anderson, and White.* New York, NY: Routledge.

Manaster, G. J. (2009). Private logic and the logic of social living. *Journal of Individual Psychology, 65,* 4–12.

Markowitz, J. C., & Weissman, M. M. (2012). *Casebook of interpersonal psychotherapy.* New York, NY: Oxford University Press.

Maroda, K. J. (2010). *Psychodynamic techniques: Working with emotion in the therapeutic relationship.* New York, NY: Guilford Press.

Marra, T. (2005). *Dialectical behavior therapy in private practice: A comprehensive and practical guide.* Oakland, CA: New Harbinger .

Martin, G., & Pear, J. (2007). *Behavior modification: What it is and how to do it* (8th ed.). Upper Saddle River, NJ: Pearson/Prentice Hall.

Mascher, J. (2002). Narrative therapy: Inviting the use of sport as metaphor. *Women and Therapy, 25,* 57–74.

Maslow, A. (1954). *Motivation and personality.* New York, NY: Harper & Row.

Maslow, A. (1968). *Toward a psychology of being* (2nd ed.). New York, NY: Van Nostrand.

Matlin, M. (1996). *The psychology of women.* Orlando, FL: Harcourt Brace.

May, R. (1950). *The meaning of anxiety.* New York, NY: Dell.

May, R. (Ed.). (1969a). *Existential psychology* (2nd ed.). New York, NY: Random House.

May, R. (1969b). *Love and will*. New York, NY: W. W. Norton.

May, R. (1975). *The courage to create*. New York, NY: W. W. Norton.

May, R. (1981). *Freedom and destiny*. New York, NY: W. W. Norton.

May, R. (1983). *The discovery of being: Writings in existential psychology*. New York, NY: W. W. Norton.

May, R. (1990a). On the phenomenological bases of therapy. *Review of Existential Psychology and Psychiatry, 20,* 49–61.

May, R. (1990b). Will, decision and responsibility. *Review of Existential Psychology and Psychiatry, 20,* 269–278.

May, R. (1996). *Psychology and the human dilemma*. New York, NY: W. W. Norton.

May, R., Angel, E., & Ellenberger, H. F. (Eds.). (1958). *Existence: A new dimension in psychiatry and psychology*. New York, NY: Simon & Schuster.

May, R., & Yalom, I. (1995). Existential psychotherapy. In R. J. Corsini & D. Wedding (Eds.), *Current psychotherapies* (5th ed., pp. 262–292). Itasca, IL: Peacock.

Mayes, L. C., & Cohen, D. J. (1996). Anna Freud and developmental psychoanalytic psychology. *Psychoanalytic Study of the Child, 51,* 117–141.

McFarlane, W. R., Dixon, L., Lukens, E., & Lucksted, A. (2003). Family psychoeducation schizophrenia: A review of the literature. *Journal of Marital and Family Therapy, 29,* 223–245.

McGoldrick, M. (1998). *You can go home again: Reconnecting with your family*. New York, NY: W. W. Norton.

McGoldrick, M., Gerson, R., & Petry, S. (2008). *Genograms: Assessment and intervention* (3rd ed.). New York, NY: W. W. Norton.

McGoldrick, M., Giordano, J., & Garcia-Preto, N. (2005). *Ethnicity and family therapy* (3rd ed.). New York, NY: Guilford Press.

McGoldrick, M., & Hardy, K. V. (2008). *Re-visioning family therapy: Race, culture, and gender in clinical practice* (2nd ed.). New York, NY: Guilford Press.

McMain, S. F., Links, P. S., Gnam, W. H., Gruimond, T., Cardish, R. J., Korman, L., & Steiner, D. L. (2009). A randomized trial of dialectical behavior therapy versus general psychiatric management for borderline personality disorder. *American Journal of Psychiatry, 166,* 1365–1374.

McMillan, M. (2004). *The person-centered approach to therapeutic change*. Thousand Oaks, CA: Sage.

Means-Christensen, A. J., Snyder, D. K., & Negy, C. (2003). Assessing nontraditional couples: Validity of the Marital Satisfaction Inventory–Revised with gay, lesbian, and co-habiting heterosexual couples. *Journal of Family and Marital Therapy, 29,* 69–83.

Mearns, D. (2003). *Developing person-centered counseling*. Thousand Oaks, CA: Sage.

Mearns, D., & Thorne, B. (1999). *Person-centered counseling in action* (3rd ed.). Thousand Oaks, CA: Sage.

Meichenbaum, D. (1969). The effects of instruction and reinforcement on thinking and language behaviors of schizophrenics. *Behaviour Research and Therapy, 7,* 101–114.

Meichenbaum, D. (1974). Self-instructional training: A cognitive prosthesis for the aged. *Human Development, 17,* 273–280.

Meichenbaum, D. (1977). *Cognitive–behavior modification: An integrative approach*. New York, NY: Springer.

Meichenbaum, D. (1985). *Stress inoculation training*. Elmsford, NY: Pergamon.

Meichenbaum, D. (1993). Changing conceptions of cognitive–behavior modification: Retrospect and prospect. *Journal of Consulting and Clinical Psychology, 61*(2), 202–204.

Meichenbaum, D. (1994). *A clinical handbook/practical therapist manual: For assessing and treating adults with post-traumatic stress disorder*. Waterloo, Canada: Institute Press.

Meichenbaum, D. (2007). Stress inoculation training: A preventative and treatment approach. In P. M. Lehrer, R. L. Woolfolk, & W. E. Sime (Eds.), *Principles and practice of stress management* (3rd ed., pp. 497–516). New York, NY: Guilford Press.

Meissner, W. W. (2007). Therapeutic alliance: Theme and variations. *Psychoanalytic Psychology, 24,* 231–254.

Melnick, J., & Nevis, S. M. (2005). Gestalt therapy methodology. In A. L. Woldt & S. M. Toman (Eds.), *Gestalt therapy: History, theory, and practice* (pp. 101–115). Thousand Oaks, CA: Sage.

Melton, A. M. A., & Schulenberg, S. E. (2008). On the measurement of meaning: Logotherapy's empirical contributions to humanistic psychology. *The Humanistic Psychologist, 36,* 31–44.

Menassa, B. M. (2009). Theoretical orientation and play therapy: Examining therapist role, session structure, and therapeutic objectives. *Journal of Professional Counseling, Practice, Theory, & Research, 37,* 13–26.

Mercadante, L. (2010). Helping addicts move beyond the spiritual wading pool: A new approach to religion and spirituality in the healing of addictions. *International Journal of Existential Psychology and Psychotherapy, 3,* 1–6.

Mesquita, B., & Walder, R. (2002). Cultural differences in emotions: A context for interpreting emotional experiences. *Behaviour Research and Therapy, 41,* 777–793.

Messer, S. B., & Warren, C. S. (1995). *Models of brief psychodynamic therapy: A comparative approach.* New York, NY: Guilford Press.

Metcalf, L. (1998). *Solution-focused group therapy: Ideas for groups in private practice, schools, agencies, and treatment programs.* New York, NY: Free Press.

Meyer, A. (1957). *Psycho-biology: A science of man.* Springfield, IL: Charles C. Thomas.

Miars, R. D. (2002). Existential authenticity: A foundational value for counseling. *Counseling and Values, 46,* 218–226.

Miklowitz, D. J. (2008). *Bi-polar disorder: A family-focused treatment approach* (2nd ed.). New York, NY: Guilford Press.

Miklowitz, D. J. (2010). A pilot study of mindfulness-based cognitive therapy for bipolar disorder. *International Journal of Cognitive Therapy, 2,* 373–382.

Miller, J. B. (1976). *Toward a new psychology of women.* Boston, MA: Beacon Press.

Miller, J. B., & Stiver, I. P. (1997). *The healing connection: How women form relationships in therapy and in life.* Boston, MA: Beacon Press.

Miller, L. (2009). Family survivors of homicide: Symptoms syndromes, and reaction patterns. *American Journal of Family Therapy, 37,* 67–79.

Miller, N. E., & Dollard, J. (1941). *Social learning and imitation.* New Haven, CT: Yale University Press.

Miller, S. D., Duncan, B. L., & Hubble, M. (1997). *Escape from Babel: Toward a unifying language for psychotherapy practice.* New York, NY: W. W. Norton.

Miller, S. D., Duncan, B. L., & Hubble, M. A. (2002). Client-directed, outcome-informed clinical work. In F. W. Kaslow & J. Lebow (Eds.), *Comprehensive handbook of psychotherapy: Vol. 4: Integrative/eclectic* (pp. 185–212). New York, NY: Wiley.

Miller, S. D., Hubble, M. A., Duncan, B. L., & Wampold, B. E. (2010). Delivering what works. In B. L. Duncan, S. D. Miller, B. E. Wampold, & M. A. Hubble (Eds.), *Heart and soul of change in psychotherapy* (2nd ed., pp. 421–430). Washington, DC: American Psychological Association.

Miller, W. R., & Rollnick, S. (2002). *Motivational interviewing: Preparing people for change* (2nd ed.). New York, NY: Guilford Press.

Mills, P. J. (2002). Spirituality, religiousness, and health from research to clinical practice. *Annals of Behavioral Medicine, 24,* 1–2.

Minuchin, S. (1974). *Families and family therapy.* Cambridge, MA: Harvard University Press.

Minuchin, S., Rosman, B. L., & Baker, L. (1978). *Psychosomatic families: Anorexia nervosa in context.* Cambridge, MA: Harvard University Press.

Miranda, J., Chung, J. Y., Green, B. L., Krupnick, J., Siddique, J., Revicki, D. A., & Belin, T. (2003). Treating depression in predominantly low-income young minority women: A randomized controlled trial. *Journal of the American Medical Association, 290,* 57–65.

Mitchell, S. A. (1986). Symposium. Interpersonal psychoanalysis: Its roots and its contemporary status. *Journal of Contemporary Psychoanalysis, 22,* 458–466.

Mitchell, S. A. (1988). *Relational concepts in psychoanalysis: An integration.* Cambridge, MA: Harvard University Press.

Mitchell, S. A. (1993). *Hope and dread in psychoanalysis.* New York, NY: HarperCollins.

Mitchell, S. A. (2000). *Relationality: From attachment to intersubjectivity.* Hillsdale, NJ: Analytic Press.

Mitchell, S. A. (2003). *Can love last? The fate of romance over time.* New York, NY: W. W. Norton.

Mitchell, S. A., & Black, M. J. (1995). *Freud and beyond: A history of modern psychoanalytic thought.* New York, NY: Basic Books.

Mobley, J. A. (2005). *An integrated existential approach to counseling theory and practice.* Lewiston, NY: Edwin Mellen Press.

Monk, G. (1997). How narrative therapy works. In G. Monk, J. Winslade, K. Crocket, & D. Epston (Eds.), *Narrative therapy in practice: The archaeology of hope* (pp. 3–31). San Francisco, CA: Jossey-Bass.

Moodley, R. (2010). In the therapist's chair is Clemmont E. Vontress: A wounded healer in cross-cultural counseling. *Journal of Multicultural Counseling and Development, 38,* 2–15.

Moodley, R., & Walcott, R. (Eds.). (2010). *Counseling across and beyond cultures: Exploring the work of Clemmont E. Vontress in clinical practice*. Toronto, Canada: University of Toronto Press.

Moon, B. L. (2009). *Existential art therapy: The canvas mirror*. Springfield, IL: Charles C. Thomas.

Moore, B. A. A. (2012). *Handbook of counseling military couples*. New York, NY: Routledge.

Moore, H. L. (2007). *The subject of anthropology: Gender, symbolism, and psychoanalysis*. Boston, MA: Polity.

Moretti, M. M., & Holland, R. (2003). The journey of adolescence: Transitions in self within the context of attachment relationships. In S. Johnson & V. Whiffen (Eds.), *Attachment processes in couple and family therapy* (pp. 234–257). New York, NY: Guilford Press.

Morgan, H. (2002). Exploring racism. *Journal of Analytical Psychology, 47,* 567–581.

Morris, E., & Oliver, J. E. (2012). Acceptance and commitment therapy. In W. Dryden (Ed.), *Cognitive behavior therapies* (pp. 70–92). Thousand Oaks, CA: Sage.

Morrison, M. O. (2009). Adlerian psychotherapy with a traumatized boy. *Journal of Individual Psychology, 65,* 57–68.

Mortberg, E., Clark, D. M., & Bergerot, S. (2011). Group cognitive therapy and individual cognitive therapy for social phobia: Sustained improvement at 5-year follow-up. *Journal of Anxiety Disorders, 25,* 994–1000.

Mosak, H. H. (1971). Lifestyle. In A. G. Nikelly (Ed.), *Techniques for behavior change* (pp. 77–84). Springfield, IL: Charles C. Thomas.

Mothersole, G. (2002). TA as a short-term cognitive therapy. In K. Tudor (Ed.), *Transactional analysis approaches to brief therapy* (pp. 54–82). London, UK: Sage.

Mottern, R. (2002). Using choice theory in coerced treatment for substance abuse. *International Journal of Reality Therapy, 22*(1), 20–24.

Mottern, R. (2003). Using the rule of six and traditional American Indian learning stories to teach choice theory. *International Journal of Reality Therapy, 23*(1), 27–34.

Moyers, T. B., Miller, W. R., & Hendrickson, S. M. L. (2005). How does motivational interviewing work? Therapist interpersonal skill predicts client involvement within motivational interviewing sessions. *Journal of Consulting and Clinical Psychology, 73,* 590–598.

Mueller, A., Mitchell, J. E., Crosby, R. D., Glaesmer, H., & de Zwaan, M. (2009). The prevalence of compulsive hoarding and its association with compulsive buying in a German population-based sample. *Behavioral Research Therapy, 47,* 705–709.

Mufson, L., Dorta, K. P., Moreau, D., & Weissman, M. M. (2011). *Interpersonal psychotherapy for depressed adolescents* (2nd ed.). New York, NY: Guilford Press.

Mulder, C. L., Emmelkamp, P. M. G., Antoni, M. H., Mulder, J. W., Sandfort, T. G. M., & de Vries, M. J. (1994). Cognitive–behavioral and experiential group psychotherapy for asymptomatic HIV-infected homosexual men: A comparative study. *Psychosomatic Medicine, 3,* 271–288.

Muller, U., & Tudor, K. (2002). Transactional analysis as brief therapy. In K. Tudor (Ed.), *Transactional analysis approaches to brief therapy* (pp. 19–44). London, UK: Sage.

Murdock, N. L. (2009). *Theories of counseling and psychotherapy: A case approach* (2nd ed.). Upper Saddle River, NJ: Pearson/Merrill.

Murphy, B. C., & Dillon, C. (2008). *Interviewing in action in a multicultural world* (3rd ed.). Pacific Grove, CA: Brooks/Cole.

Murphy, L. (1997). Efficacy of reality therapy in schools: A review of the research from 1980–1995. *Journal of Reality Therapy, 16*(2), 12–20.

Myers, I. B. (1998). *Introduction to type* (6th ed.). Palo Alto, CA: Consulting Psychologists Press.

Myers, I. B., McCaulley, M. H., Quenk, N. L., & Hammer, A. L. (1998). *MBTI manual* (3rd ed.). Palo Alto, CA: Consulting Psychologists Press.

Myers, J. E., & Young, J. S. (2012). Brain wave biofeedback: Benefits of integrating neurofeedback into counseling. *Journal of Counseling and Development, 90,* 20–29.

Nadort, M., Arntz, A., Smit, J. H., Giesen-Bloo, J., Eikelenboom, M., Spinhoven, P., . . . van Dyck, R.

(2009). Implementation of outpatient schema therapy for borderline personality disorder with versus without crisis support by the therapist outside office hours: A randomized trial. *Behavior Research and Therapy, 47,* 961–973.

Najavits, L. M., & Strupp, H. H. (1994). Differences in the effectiveness of psychodynamic therapists: A process-outcome study. *Psychotherapy, 31*(1), 114–123.

Napier, A. Y., & Whitaker, C. (1978). *The family crucible*. New York, NY: Harper Collins.

Nathan, P. E., & Gorman, J. M. (Eds.). (2002). *A guide to treatments that work* (2nd ed.). London, UK: Oxford University Press.

Neenan, M., & Dryden, W. (2011). *Rational emotive behavior therapy in a nutshell* (2nd ed.). London, UK: Sage.

Neff, K., Kirkpatrick, K., & Rude, S. (2007). Self-compassion and adaptive psychological functioning. *Journal of Research in Personality, 41,* 139–154.

Neimeyer, R. A. (1993). An appraisal of constructivist psychotherapies. *Journal of Consulting and Clinical Psychology, 61,* 221–234.

Neimeyer, R. A., & Raskin, J. D. (2001). Varieties of constructivism in psychotherapy. In K. S. Dobson (Ed.), *Handbook of cognitive–behavioral therapies* (2nd ed., pp. 393–430). New York, NY: Guilford Press.

Nelson, T. S. (Ed.). (2010). *Doing something different: Solution focused brief therapy practices*. New York, NY: Routledge.

Nezu, A. M., Nezu, C. M., & D'Zurilla, T. J. (2010). Problem-solving therapy. In N. Kazantzis, M. A. Reinecke, & A. Freeman (Eds.), *Cognitive and behavioral theories in clinical practice* (pp. 76–114). New York, NY: Guilford Press.

Nichols, M. P. (2009). *The essentials of family therapy* (4th ed.). Boston, MA: Pearson Education.

Nichols, M. P. (2010). *Family therapy concepts and methods* (9th ed.). Boston, MA: Pearson Education.

Nicoll, W. G. (1994). Developing effective classroom guidance programs: An integrative framework. *School Counselor, 41,* 360–364.

Nicoll, W. G. (2007). Resilience-focused brief family therapy: An Adlerian approach. *Journal of Individual Psychology,67,* 206.

Nielsen, S. L., & Ellis, A. E. (1994). A discussion with Albert Ellis: Reason, emotion and religion. *Journal of Psychology and Christianity, 13,* 327–341.

Nisbitt, R. (2003). *The geography of thought: How Asians and Westerners think differently, and why*. New York, NY: Free Press.

Nolen-Hoeksema, S., & Hilt, L. M. (2009). *Handbook of depression in adolescents*. New York, NY: Routledge.

Nolte, T., Guiney, J., Fonagy, P., Mayes, L. C., & Luyten, P. (2011). Interpersonal stress regulation and the development of anxiety disorders: An attachment-based developmental framework. *Frontiers in Behavioral Neuroscience, 5,* 1–21.

Norcross, J. C. (2010). The therapeutic relationship. In B. L. Duncan, S. D. Miller, B. E. Wampold, & M. A. Hubble (Eds.), *Heart and soul of change in psychotherapy* (2nd ed., pp. 113–141). Washington, DC: American Psychological Association.

Norcross, J. C. (Ed.). (2011). *Psychotherapy relationships that work: Evidence-based responsiveness* (2nd ed.). New York, NY: Oxford University Press.

Norcross, J. C., & Beutler, L. E. (2011). Integrative psychotherapies. In R. J. Corsini & D. Wedding (Eds.), *Current psychotherapies* (9th ed., pp. 502–535). Belmont, CA: Brooks/Cole.

Norcross, J. C., & Goldfried, M. R. (Eds.). (2005). *Handbook of psychotherapy integration* (2nd ed.). New York, NY: Oxford University Press.

Norcross, J. C., & Lambert, M. J. (2011). Evidence-based therapy relationships. In J. C. Norcross (Ed.), *Psychotherapy relationships that work: Evidence-based responsiveness* (2nd ed., pp. 3–21). New York, NY: Oxford.

Norcross, J. C., & Wampold, B. E. (2011). Evidence-based therapy relationships: Research conclusions and clinical practices. *Psychotherapy, 48,* 98–102.

Nutt, R. L., & Brooks, G. R. (2008). Psychology of gender. In S. D. Brown & R. W. Lent (Eds.), *Handbook of counseling psychology* (4th ed., pp. 176–193). Hoboken, NJ: John Wiley.

Nylund, D. (2002). *Treating Huckleberry Finn: A new narrative approach to working with children diagnosed with ADD/ADHD*. San Francisco, CA: Jossey-Bass.

Nystul, M. S. (2006). *Introduction to counseling: An art and science perspective*. Upper Saddle River, NJ: Pearson-Merrill.

Oaklander, V. (1994). Gestalt play therapy. In K. J. O'Connor & C. E. Schaefer (Eds.), *Handbook of play therapy* (Vol. 2, pp. 143–156). New York, NY: Wiley Interscience.

Oaklander, V. (1997). The therapeutic process with children and adolescents. *Gestalt Review, 1,* 292–317.

Oaklander, V. (2007). *Hidden treasure: A map to the child's inner self.* London, UK: Karnac Books.

Obegi, J. H., & Berant, E. (Eds.). (2009). Attachment theory and research in *clinical application with adults.* New York, NY: Guilford Press.

Oberst, D., & Stewart, A. E. (2003). *Adlerian psychotherapy: An advanced approach to individual psychology.* New York, NY: Bruner-Routledge.

O'Connell, B. (1998). *Solution-focused therapy.* London, UK: Sage.

Odell, M., & Quinn, W. H. (1998). Therapist and client behaviors in the first interview: Effects on session impact and treatment duration. *Journal of Marital and Family Therapy, 24,* 369–388.

O'Grady, K. A., & Richards, P. S. (2010). The role of inspiration in the helping professions, *Psychology of Religion and Spirituality, 2,* 57–66.

Ohanian,V., & Rashed, R. (2012). Schema therapy. In W. Dryden (Ed.), *Cognitive behavior therapies* (pp. 166–188). Thousand Oaks, CA: Sage.

O'Hanlon, B., & Weiner-Davis, M. (1989). *In search of solutions: A new direction in psychotherapy.* New York, NY: W. W. Norton.

Olatunji, B. O., & Feldman, G. (2008). Cognitive–behavioral therapy. In M. Hersen & A. M. Gross (Eds.), *Handbook of clinical psychology* (Vol. 1, pp. 551–584). New York, NY: John Wiley & Sons.

Olson, M. E. (2001). Listening to the voices of anorexia: The researcher as an "outsider witness." *Journal of Feminist Family Therapy, 11,* 25–46.

O'Neill, B. (2012). Gestalt family therapy: A field perspective. In T. B. Levine (Ed.), *Gestalt therapy: Advances in theory and practice* (pp. 137–148). New York, NY: Routledge.

O'Neill, P., & Devlin, N. J. (2010). An analysis of NICE's "restricted" (or optimized) decisions, *Pharmacoeconomics, 28,* 987–993.

Organista, K. C. (2007). Commentary: The need to explicate culturally competent approaches with Latino clients. In C. Muran (Ed.), *Dialogues on difference: Studies of diversity in the therapeutic relationship* (pp. 168–175). Washington, DC: American Psychological Association.

Orgler, H. (1963). *Alfred Adler: The man and his works.* New York, NY: Liveright.

Orlinsky, D. E., Grawe, K., & Parks, B. K. (1994). Process and outcome in psychotherapy—*noch einmal.* In B. A. Garfield & S. L. Garfield (Eds.), *Handbook of psychotherapy and behavior change* (4th ed., pp. 270–276). New York, NY: Wiley.

Osborn, C. J. (1999). Solution-focused strategies with "involuntary" clients: Practical applications for the school and clinical setting. *Journal of Humanistic Education & Development, 37*(3), 169–182.

Ost, L. G. (2008). Efficacy of the third wave of behavioral therapies: A systematic review and meta-analysis. *Behaviour Research and Therapy, 46,* 296–321.

Otis, J. (2007). *Managing chronic pain: A cognitive behavioral therapy approach.* London, UK: Oxford University Press.

Packer, G. (2008, January 28). The choice. *New Yorker.*

Paivio, S., & Greenberg, L. S. (1995). Resolving "unfinished business": Efficacy of experiential therapy using empty chair dialogue. *Journal of Consulting and Clinical Psychology, 63,* 419–425.

Pantalone, D. W., Iwamasa, G. W., & Martell, C. R. (2010). Cognitive behavioral therapy with diverse populations. In K. S. Dobson (Ed.), *Handbook of cognitive behavioral therapies* (3rd ed., pp. 445–464). New York, NY: Guilford Press.

Pargament, K. I. (2007). *Spiritually integrated psychotherapy: Understanding and addressing the sacred.* New York, NY: Guilford Press.

Pargament, K. I., & Krumrei, E. J. (2009). Clinical assessment of clients' spirituality. In J. D. Aten, & M. M. Leach (Eds.), *Spirituality and the therapeutic process: A comprehensive resource from intake to termination* (pp. 93–119). Washington, DC: American Psychological Association.

Paris, B. J. (1994). *Karen Horney: A psychoanalyst's search for self understanding.* New Haven, CT: Yale University Press.

Paris, B. J. (1996). Introduction to Karen Horney. *American Journal of Psychoanalysis, 56,* 135–140.

Parker, G., Roy, K., & Eyers, K. (2003). Cognitive behavior therapy for depression? Choose horses for courses. *American Journal of Psychiatry, 160,* 825–834.

Parker, W. D. (1998). Birth-order effects in the academically talented. *Gifted Children Quarterly, 42,* 29–38.

Parlett, M. (2005). Contemporary Gestalt therapy: Field theory. In A. L. Woldt & S. M. Toman (Eds.), *Gestalt therapy: History, theory, and practice* (pp. 41–64). Thousand Oaks, CA: Sage.

Passaro, P., Moon, M., Wiest, D., & Wong, E. (2004). A model for school psychology practice: Addressing the needs of students with emotional and behavioral challenges through the use of an in-school support room and reality therapy. *Adolescence, 39,* 503–517.

Paul, G. L. (1967). Strategy of outcome research in psychotherapy. *Journal of Consulting Psychology, 31,* 109–118.

Pavlov, I. P. (1927). *Conditioned reflexes* (G. V. Anrep, Trans.). London, UK: Oxford University Press.

Pavuluri, M. N. (2004). Child- and family-focused cognitive–behavioral therapy for pediatric bipolar disorder: Development and preliminary results. *Journal of the American Academy of Child and Adolescent Psychiatry, 43,* 528–537.

Payne, M. (2006). *Narrative therapy: An introduction for counselors* (2nd ed.). Thousand Oaks, CA: Sage.

Pedersen, P. B., Draguns, J. G., Lonner, W. J., & Trimble, J. E. (Eds.). (2007). *Counseling across cultures* (6th ed.). Alexandria, VA: American Counseling Association.

Perls, F. (1969a). *Gestalt therapy verbatim.* Lafayette, CA: Real Person Press.

Perls, F. (1969b). *In and out of the garbage pail.* Lafayette, CA: Real Person Press.

Perls, F., Hefferline, R. F., & Goodman, P. (1951). *Gestalt therapy: Excitement and growth in the human personality.* New York, NY: Julian.

Perls, F., & Philippson, P. (2012). *From planned psychology to Gestalt therapy*. Gouldsboro, ME: The Gestalt Journal Press.

Perls, L. (1992). Concepts and misconceptions of Gestalt therapy. *Journal of Humanistic Psychology, 32,* 50–56.

Persons, J. B. (1989). *Cognitive therapy in practice.* New York: W. W. Norton.

Petrocelli, J. V. (2002). Processes and stages of change: Counseling with the transtheoretical model of change. *Journal of Counseling and Development, 80*(1), 22–30.

Philippson, P. (2009). *The emergent self: An existential-Gestalt approach*. London: London, UK: Karnac Books Ltd.

Pierce, J. (2003). Mindfulness-based reality therapy. *International Journal of Reality Therapy, 23*(1), 20–24.

Piercy, K. W. (2010). *Working with aging families: therapeutic solutions for caregivers*. New York, NY: W. W. Norton.

Pike, K. M., Walsh, B. T., Vitousek, K., Wilson, G. T., & Bauer, J. (2003). Cognitive behavior therapy in the posthospitalization treatment of anorexia nervosa. *The American Journal of Psychiatry, 160,* 2046–2049.

Pinsof, W., & Wynne, L. (2000). Toward progress research: Closing the gap between family therapy practice and research. *Journal of Marital and Family Therapy, 26,* 1–8.

Polster, E. (2012). Flexibility in theory formation: Point and counterpoint. In T. B. Levine (Ed.), *Gestalt therapy: Advances in theory and practice* (pp. 15–25). New York, NY: Routledge.

Polster, E., & Polster, M. (1973). *Gestalt therapy integrated.* New York, NY: Brunner/Mazel.

Polster, E., & Polster, M. (1993). Fritz Perls: Legacy and invitation. *Gestalt Journal, 16,* 23–25.

Pos, A. E., Greenberg, L., & Elliott, R. (2008). Experiential therapy. In J. L. Lebow (Ed.), *Twenty-first century psychotherapies: Contemporary approaches to theory and practice* (pp. 80–122). Hoboken, NJ: John Wiley & Sons.

Powers, M. B., & Emmelkamp, P. M. G. (2008). Virtual reality exposure therapy for anxiety disorders: A meta-analysis. *Journal of Anxiety Disorders, 22*, 561–569.

Powers, M. B., Zum Vorde Sive Vording, M. B., & Emmelkamp, P. M. G. (2009). Acceptance and commitment therapy: A meta-analytic review. *Psychotherapy and Psychosomatics, 78,* 73–80.

Powers, R. L., & Griffith, J. (1986). *Individual psychology client workbook.* Chicago, IL: American Institute of Adlerian Studies.

Powers, R. L., & Griffith, J. (1987). *Understanding life-style: The psycho-clarity process*. Chicago, IL: American Institute of Adlerian Studies.

Powers, W. T. (1973). *Behavior: The control of perception.* Chicago, IL: Aldine.

Presbury, J. H., Echterling, L. G., & McKee, J. E. (2008). *Beyond brief counseling and therapy: An integrative approach* (2nd ed.). Upper Saddle River, NJ: Pearson Education.

Prochaska, J. O., & DiClemente, C. C. (1986). The transtheoretical approach. In J. C. Norcross (Ed.), *Handbook of eclectic psychotherapy* (pp. 163–200). New York, NY: Brunner/Mazel.

Prochaska, J. O., & DiClemente, C. C. (2002). Transtheoretical therapy. In F. W. Kaslow & J. Lebow (Eds.), *Comprehensive handbook of psychotherapy: Vol. 4. Integrative/eclectic* (pp. 165–183). New York, NY: Wiley.

Prochaska, J. O., & Norcross, J. C. (2009). *Systems of psychotherapy: A transtheoretical analysis* (7th ed.). Pacific Grove, CA: Brooks/Cole.

Psychotherapy Networker. (2007, March/April). The top ten: The most influential therapists of the last quarter century, pp. 24–37.

Quinn, W. H., Dotson, D., & Jordan, K. (1997). Dimensions of the therapeutic alliance and their associations with outcome in family therapy. *Psychotherapy Research, 74,* 429–438.

Rabung, S., & Leichsenring, F. (2012). Effectiveness of long-term psychodynamic psychotherapy: First meta-analytic evidence and its discussion. In R. A. Levy, J. S. Ablon, and H. Kachele (Eds.), *Psychodynamic psychotherapy research, Part 1* (pp. 27–49). New York, NY: Humana Press.

Rafaeli, A. K., & Markowitz, J. C. (2011). Interpersonal psychotherapy for PTSD: A case study. *American Journal of Psychotherapy, 65,* 205–223.

Rafaeli, E., Bernstein, D. P., & Young, J. (2011). *Schema therapy*. New York, NY: Routledge.

Rapport, Z. (2007). Using choice theory to assess the needs of persons who have a disability and sexual/intimacy/romantic issues. *International Journal of Reality Therapy, 27,* 22–25.

Rasheed, J. M., & Rasheed, M. N. (2011). *Family therapy: Models and techniques*. Thousand Oaks, CA: Sage.

Rasmussen, P. R. (2003). The adaptive purpose of emotional expression: A lifestyle elaboration. *Individual Psychology, 59,* 388–409.

Ratey, J. J., & Hagerman, E. (2008). *Spark: The revolutionary new science of exercise and the brain*. New York, NY: Little, Brown.

Reinecke, M. A., Dattilio, F. M., & Freeman, A. (2006). *Cognitive therapy with children and adolescents* (2nd ed.). New York, NY: Guilford Press.

Reis, B. G., & Brown, L. G. (1999). Reducing psychotherapy dropouts: Maximizing perspective convergence in the psychotherapy dyad. *Psychotherapy, 36,* 123–126.

Reker, G. T. (1994). Logotheory and logotherapy: Challenges, opportunities, and some empirical findings. *International Forum for Logotherapy, 17,* 47–55.

Remer, P. (2008). Feminist therapy. In J. Frew & M. D. Spiegler (Eds.), *Contemporary psychotherapies for a diverse world* (pp. 397–441). Boston, MA: Houghton Mifflin.

Rheem, K. D., Woolley, S. R., & Weissman, N. (2012). Using emotion focused therapy with military couples. In B. A. Moore (Ed.), *Handbook for counseling military couples* (pp. 89–112). New York, NY: Routledge.

Richards, P. S., & Bergin, A. E. (2005). *A spiritual strategy for counseling and psychotherapy* (2nd ed.). Washington, DC: American Psychological Association.

Richert, A. J. (2003). Living stories, telling stories, changing stories: Experiential use of the relationship in narrative therapy. *Journal of Psychotherapy Integration, 13,* 188–210.

Richert, A. J. (2010). *Integrating existential and narrative therapy: A theoretical base for eclectic practice.* Pittsburgh, PA: Duquesne University Press.

Ridge, D., & Zeibland, S. (2006). "The old me could never have done that": How people give meaning to recovery following depression. *Qualitative Healthcare Resolutions, 16,* 1038–1053.

Rigazio-DiGilio, S. A., & McDowell, T. (2008). Family therapy. In J. Frew & M. D. Spiegler (Eds.), *Contemporary psychotherapies for a diverse world* (pp. 442–488). Boston, MA: Houghton Mifflin.

Robb, C. (2006). *This changes everything*. New York, NY: Picador.

Robbins, M. S., Feaster, D. J., Horigian, V. E., Rohrbaugh, M., Shoham, B., Backrach, . . . Szapocznik, J. (2011). Brief strategic family therapy versus treatment as usual: Results of a multi-site randomized trial for drug abusing adolescents. *Journal of Consulting and Clinical Psychology, 79,* 713–727.

Roberts, R. L., Harper, R., Caldwell, R., & Decora, M. (2003). Adlerian lifestyle analysis of Lakota women: Implications for counseling. *Journal of Individual Psychology, 59,* 15–29.

Robertson, M. (1979). Some observations from an eclectic therapy. *Psychotherapy, 16,* 18–21.

Robey, P. (Ed.). (2011a). *Contemporary issues in couples counseling: A choice theory and reality therapy approach.* Portland, OR: Book News.

Robey, P. (2011b). Reality therapy and choice theory: An interview with Robert Wubbolding. *Family Journal, 19,* 231–237.

Robey, P., Burdenski, T. K., Britzman, M., & Crowell, J. (2011). Systematic application of choice theory and reality therapy: An interview with Glasser scholars. *Family Journal, 19,* 421–433.

Robinson, L. A., Berman, J. S., & Neimeyer, R. A. (1990). Psychotherapy for the treatment of depression: A comprehensive review of controlled outcome research. *Psychological Bulletin, 108,* 35.

Rochland, A. B., Zack, J. S., & Speyer, C. (2004). Online therapy: Review of relevant definitions, debates, and current empirical support. *Journal of Clinical Psychology, 60,* 269–283.

Rochlen, A., Beretvas, S., & Zack, J. (2004). The online and face-to-face counseling attitudes scales: A validation study. *Measurement & Evaluation in Counseling & Development, 37,* 95–111.

Rogers, C. R. (1942). *Counseling and psychotherapy.* Boston, MA: Houghton Mifflin.

Rogers, C. R. (1946). Significant aspects of client-centered therapy. *American Psychologist, 1,* 415–422.

Rogers, C. R. (1951). *Client-centered therapy: Its current practice, implications and theory.* Boston, MA: Houghton Mifflin.

Rogers, C. R. (1955). Person or science? A philosophical question. *American Psychology, 10,* 267–278.

Rogers, C. R. (1959). A theory of therapy, personality, and individual relationships as developed in the client-centered framework. In S. Koch (Ed.), *Psychology: A study of a science* (pp. 184–256). New York, NY: McGraw-Hill.

Rogers, C. R. (1961). *On becoming a person.* Boston, MA: Houghton Mifflin.

Rogers, C. R. (1967). The conditions of change from a client-centered viewpoint. In B. Berenson & R. Carkhuff (Eds.), *Sources of gain in counseling and psychotherapy.* New York, NY: Holt, Rinehart, & Winston.

Rogers, C. R. (1970). *Carl Rogers on encounter groups.* New York, NY: Harper & Row.

Rogers, C. R. (1975). Empathic: An unappreciated way of being. *The Counseling Psychologist, 5,* 2–10.

Rogers, C. R. (1980). *A way of being.* Boston, MA: Houghton Mifflin.

Rogers, C. R. (1987). Our international family. *Person-Centered Review, 2,* 139–149.

Rollnick, S., Miller, W. R., & Butler, C. C. (2008). *Motivational interviewing in health care: Helping patients change behavior.* New York, NY: Guilford Press.

Rosner, R. I., Lyddon, W. J., & Freeman, A. (Eds.). (2004). *Cognitive therapy and dreams.* New York, NY: Springer.

Rossano, F. (1996). Psychoanalysis and psychiatric institutions: Theoretical and clinical spaces of the Horney approach. *American Journal of Psychoanalysis, 56,* 203–212.

Roth, B., & Creaser, T. (1997). Mindfulness meditation-based stress reduction: Experience with a bilingual inner-city program. *Nurse Practitioner, 22,* 150–152, 154, 157.

Roth, M. S. (Ed.) (1998). *Freud: Conflict and culture.* New York, NY: Alfred A. Knopf.

Rothbaum, B. O. (2005). Commentary on Riva, G., Virtual reality in psychotherapy: Review. *Cyber Psychology & Behavior, 8,* 239–240.

Rowan, J. (1998). *The reality game* (2nd ed.). London, UK: Routledge.

Rowe, C. (2005). A brief treatment with a posttraumatic stress disordered patient—A self-psychological perspective. *Clinical Social Work Journal, 33,* 473–484.

Rowen, T., & O'Hanlon, B. (1999). *Solution-oriented therapy for chronic and severe mental illness.* New York, NY: Wiley.

Rule, M. L., & Bishop, W. R. (Eds.). (2005). *Adlerian lifestyle counseling: Practice and research.* New York, NY: Routledge.

Rule, W. R., & Comer, A. T. (2006). Family constellation and birth order: Variables related to vocational choice of dentistry. In W. R. Rule & M. Bishop (Eds.), *Adlerian lifestyle counseling practice and research* (pp. 255–263). New York, NY: Routledge.

Ryback, D. (2011). Humanistic psychology's impact and accomplishments, *Journal of Humanistic Psychology, 51,* 413–418.

Sabourin, S., Gendreau, P., & Frenette, L. (1987). The satisfaction level of drop-out cases in a university psychology service. *Canadian Journal of Behavioral Science, 19,* 314–323.

Sachse, R. (1993). The effect of intervention phrasing on therapist–client communication. *Psychotherapy Research, 3,* 260–277.

Safran, J. D., Muran, J. C., & Eubanks-Carter, C. (2011). Repairing alliance ruptures. In J. C. Norcross (Ed.), *Psychotherapy relationships that work: Evidence-based responsiveness* (2nd ed.). New York, NY: Oxford.

Salande, J. D., & Perkins, G. R. (2011). An object relations approach to cult membership. *American Journal of Psychotherapy, 66,* 381–391.

Saltzburg, S. (2007). Narrative therapy pathways for re-authoring with parents of adolescents coming-out as lesbian, gay, and bisexual. *Contemporary Family Therapy, 29,* 57–69.

Saltzman, N. (1989). Integrating intensely emotional methods with psychodynamic, Gestalt, cognitive and behavioral therapeutic elements: I. Emotional freedom versus emotional control. *Psychotherapy in Private Practice, 7,* 57–67.

Samai, S., & Almagor, A. (2011). *The dialectical approach as a tool for changing perception and level of anxiety symptoms.* Unpublished manuscript, University of Haifa, Israel.

Sanchez, W., & Garriga, O. (1996). Control theory, reality therapy and cultural fatalism: Toward an integration. *Journal of Reality Therapy, 15*(2), 30–38.

Sanders, C. J. (2007). A poetics of resistance: Compassionate practice in substance misuse therapy. In C. Brown & T. Augusta-Scott (Eds.), *Narrative therapy: Making meaning, making lives* (pp. 59–76). Thousand Oaks, CA: Sage.

Sandler, A. (1996). The psychoanalytic legacy of Anna Freud. *Psychoanalytic Study of the Child, 51,* 270–284.

Sandler, J., & Freud, A. (1985). *The analysis of defense: The ego and the mechanisms of defense revisited.* New York, NY: International Universities Press.

Sands, T. (1998). Feminist counseling and female adolescents: Treatment strategies for depression. *Journal of Mental Health Counseling, 20,* 42–54.

Sapp, M. (2006). The strength-based model for counseling at-risk youths. *The Counseling Psychologist, 34,* 108–117.

Sapp, M., & Farrell. W. (1994). Cognitive–behavioral interventions: Applications for academically at-risk and special education students. *Preventing School Failure, 38*(2), 19–24.

Sapriel, L. (2012). Creating an embodied, authentic self: Integrating mindfulness with psychotherapy when working with trauma. In T. B. Levine (Ed.), *Gestalt therapy: Advances in theory and practice* (pp. 107–122). New York, NY: Routledge.

Saroglou, V. (2012). Are we born to be religious? *Scientific American Mind, 23,* 52–57.

Sartre, J. P. (1956). *Being and nothingness.* New York, NY: Philosophical Library.

Satir, V. (1975). *Conjoint family therapy.* Palo Alto, CA: Science and Behavior Books.

Sava, F. A., Yates, B. T., Lupu, V., Szentagotai, A., & David, D. (2009). Cost-effectiveness and cost-utility of cognitive therapy, rational emotive behavioral therapy, and fluoxetine (Prozac) in treating depression: A randomized clinical trial. *Journal of Clinical Psychology, 65,* 36–52.

Sayers, J. (1991). *Mothers of psychoanalysis: Helene Deutsch, Karen Horney, Anna Freud, Melanie Klein.* New York, NY: W. W. Norton.

Scharff, J. S., & Scharff, D. E. (2005). *The primer of object relations* (2nd ed.). Northvale, NJ: Aronson.

Scharwachter, P. (2008). Abortion decision making by focusing. *European Journal of Contraception & Reproductive Health Care, 13,* 191–197.

Schlosser, L. Z., & Safran, D. A. (2009). Implementing treatments that incorporate clients' spirituality. In J. D. Aten & M. M. Leach (Eds.), *Spirituality and the therapeutic process: A comprehensive resource from intake to termination* (pp. 193–216). Washington, DC: American Psychological Association.

Schneider, K. (2004). *Rediscovery of awe: Splendor, mystery, and the fluid center of life.* St. Paul, MN: Paragon House.

Schneider, K. (2008). *Existential-integrative psychotherapy: Guideposts to the core of practice.* New York, NY: Routledge.

Schnyder, U. (2009). Future perspectives in psychotherapy, *European Archives of Psychiatry and Clinical Neuroscience, 259,* Suppl. 2, S123–S128.

Schoen, D. E. (2009). *The war of the gods in addiction: C. G. Jung, Alcoholics Anonymous, and archetypal evil.* New Orleans, LA: Spring Journal.

Schoo, A. (2008). Motivational interviewing in the prevention and management of chronic disease: Improving physical activity and exercise in line with choice theory. *International Journal of Reality Therapy, 27,* 26–29.

Schottenbauer, M. A., Glass, C. R., & Arnkoff, D. B. (2005). Outcome research on psychotherapy integration. In J. C. Norcross & M. R. Goldfried (Eds.),

Handbook of psychotherapy integration (pp. 459–493). New York, NY: Oxford University Press.

Schottenbauer, M. A., Glass, C. R., & Arnkoff, D. B. (2007). Decision making and psychotherapy integration: Theoretical considerations, preliminary data, and implications for future research. *Journal of Psychotherapy Integration, 17,* 225–250.

Schulenberg, S. E., Schnetzer, L. W., Winters, M. R., & Hutzell, R. R. (2010). Meaning-centered couples therapy: Logotherapy and intimate relationships. *Journal of Contemporary Psychotherapy, 40,* 95–102.

Schwartz, A. M. (1995). School reform and restructuring through the use of "quality school" philosophy. *Journal of Reality Therapy, 14*(2), 23–28.

Schwartz, J. P., & Waldo, M. (2003). Interpersonal manifestations of lifestyle: Individual psychology integrated with interpersonal theory. *Journal of Mental Health Counseling, 25*(2), 101–108.

Schwartz, S. E. (2007). Jungian analytical theory. In D. Capuzzi & D. Gross (Eds.), *Counseling and psychotherapy: Theories and interventions* (4th ed., pp. 98–122). Upper Saddle River, NJ: Pearson/ Prentice Hall.

Scott, C. (2010). Solution focused assessment. In T. S. Nelson (Ed.), *Doing something different: Solution focused brief therapy practices* (pp. 23–24). New York, NY: Routledge.

Scott, J., & Freeman, A. (2010). Beck's cognitive therapy. In N. Kazantzis, M. A. Reinecke, & A. Freeman (Eds.), *Cognitive and behavioral theories in clinical practice* (pp. 28–75). New York, NY: Guilford Press.

Sedgwick, D. (2001). *Introduction to Jungian therapy.* New York, NY: Brunner-Routledge.

Seeman, J. (2008). *Psychotherapy and the fully functioning person.* Bloomington, IN: AuthorHouse.

Seibel, C. A., & Dowd, E. T. (1999). Reactance and therapeutic noncompliance. *Cognitive Therapy and Research, 23,* 373–379.

Seiler, L. (2008). *Cool connections with cognitive behavioral therapy: Encouraging self-esteem, resilience and well-being in children and young people using CBT approaches.* London, UK: Jessica Kingsley.

Seligman, L. (1994). *Developmental career counseling and assessment.* Thousand Oaks, CA: Sage.

Seligman, L. (1996). *Promoting a fighting spirit: Psychotherapy for cancer patients, survivors, and their families.* San Francisco, CA: Jossey-Bass.

Seligman, L. (2004). *Diagnosis and treatment planning in counseling* (3rd ed.). New York, NY: Kluwer/Plenum.

Seligman, L. (2009). *Fundamental skills for mental health professionals.* Upper Saddle River, NJ: Pearson.

Seligman, L., & Reichenberg, L. W. (2012). *Selecting effective treatments: A comprehensive, systematic guide to treating mental disorders* (4th ed.). Hoboken, NJ: Wiley.

Seligman, M. E. P. (1995). The effectiveness of psychotherapy. *American Psychologist, 50*(12), 965–974.

Serlin, I. (1992). Tribute to Laura Perls. *Journal of Humanistic Psychology, 32,* 57–66.

Sexton, T. L. (1995). Competency survey results. In M. K. Altekruse & T. L. Sexton (Eds.), *Mental health counseling in the '90s* (pp. 25–44). Tampa, FL: National Commission for Mental Health Counseling.

Sexton, T. L., & Whiston, S. C. (1991). A review of the empirical basis for counseling: Implications for practice and training. *Counselor Education and Supervision, 30,* 330–354.

Shafranske, E. P. (2001). The religious dimensions of patient care within rehabilitation medicine: The role of religious attitudes, beliefs, and professional practices. In T. G. Plante & A. C. Sherman (Eds.), *Faith and health: Psychological perspectives* (pp. 311–338). New York, NY: Guilford Press.

Shafranske, E. P. (2005). A psychoanalytic approach to spiritually oriented psychotherapy. In L. Sperry & E. P. Shafranske, (Eds.). *Spiritually oriented psychotherapy* (pp. 105–131). Washington, DC: American Psychological Association.

Shainess, M. (1978). Reflections on the contributions of Harry Stack Sullivan. *American Journal of Psychoanalysis, 38,* 301–315.

Shamdasani, S. (Ed.). (2009). *Liber novus: The "red book" of C. G. Jung* (Philemon Series). New York, NY: W. W. Norton.

Shamdasani, S. (2011). *C.G. Jung: A biography in books.* New York, NY: W. W. Norton.

Shapiro, R. (2005). *EMDR solutions: Pathways to healing.* New York, NY: W. W. Norton.

Sharf, R. S. (2012). *Theories of psychotherapy and counseling.* Belmont, CA: Brooks/Cole.

Shea, M., Cachelin, F., Uribe, L., Striegel, R., Thompson, D., & Wilson, T. (2012). Cultural adaptation of a cognitive behavior therapy guided self-help program for

Mexican American women with binge eating disorders. *Journal of Counseling & Development, 90,* 308–318.

Shedler, J. (2010). The efficacy of psychodynamic psychotherapy. *American Psychologist, 65,* 98–109.

Shedler, J. (2012). The efficacy of psychodynamic psychotherapy. In R. A. Levy, J. S. Ablon, & H. Kachele (Eds.), *Psychodynamic psychotherapy research* (pp. 9–26). New York, NY: Humana Press.

Sheldon, K. M., Arndt, J., & Houser-Marko, L. (2003). In search of the organismic valuing process: The human tendency to move towards beneficial goal choices. *Journal of Personality, 71,* 835–869.

Sherman, R., & Nwaorgu, A. (2002). Adlerian therapy: A century of tradition and research. In F. W. Kaslow (Ed.), *Comprehensive handbook of psychotherapy: Interpersonal/humanistic/existential.* New York, NY: John Wiley & Sons.

Shifron, R. (2010). Adler's need to belong as the key to mental health. *Journal of Individual Psychotherapy, 66,* 10–29.

Shilts, L. (2010). Using scaling questions to assess couples readiness for therapy. In T. S. Nelson (Ed.), *Doing something different: Solution focused brief therapy practices* (pp. 17–21). New York, NY: Routledge.

Shulman, B. H., & Mosak, H. H. (1988). *Manual for life style assessment.* Muncie, IN: Accelerated Development.

Siegel, D. J. (2009). Mindful awareness, mindsight, and neural integration. *The Humanistic Psychologist, 37,* 137–158.

Sifneos, P. E. (1979a). *Short-term dynamic psychotherapy: Evaluation and technique.* New York, NY: Plenum.

Sifneos, P. E. (1979b). *Short-term psychotherapy and emotional crisis.* Cambridge, MA: Harvard University Press.

Sifneos, P. E. (1984). The current status of individual short-term dynamic psychotherapy and its future: An overview. *American Journal of Psychotherapy, 38*(4), 472–483.

Simkin, J. S. (1975). An introduction to Gestalt therapy. In F. C. Stephenson (Ed.), *Gestalt therapy primer: Introductory readings in Gestalt therapy* (pp. 3–12). Springfield, IL: C. C. Thomas.

Simmonds, L. (2006). The oceanic feeling and a sea change: Historical challenges to reductionist attitudes to religion and spirit from within psychoanalysis. *Psychoanalytic Psychology, 23,* 128–142.

Singh, J., & Tudor, K. (1997). Cultural considerations of therapy, *The Person-Centered Journal, 4,* 32–46.

Skinner, B. F. (1938). *The behavior of organisms.* New York, NY: Appleton-Century.

Skinner, B. F. (1948/2005). *Walden II.* Indianapolis, IN: Hackett.

Skinner, B. F. (1957). *Verbal behavior.* New York, NY: Appleton-Century-Crofts.

Skinner, B. F. (1969). *Contingencies of reinforcement: A theoretical analysis.* New York, NY: Appleton-Century-Crofts.

Skinner, B. F. (1971). *Beyond freedom and dignity.* New York, NY: Knopf.

Skinner, B. F. (1974). *About behaviorism.* New York, NY: Knopf.

Sklare, G. (2000). Solution-focused brief counseling strategies. In J. Carlson & L. Sperry (Eds.), *Brief therapy with individuals and couples* (pp. 437–468). Phoenix, AZ: Zeig, Tucker & Theisen.

Smith, L. D., & Peck, P. L. (2004). Dialectical behavior therapy: A review and call to research. *Journal of Mental Health Counseling, 26,* 25–39.

Smith, M. L., Glass, G. V., & Miller, T. I. (1980). *The benefits of psychotherapy.* Baltimore, MD: Johns Hopkins University Press.

Smith, T. B., Rodriquez, M. M. D., & Bernal, G. (2011). Culture. In J. C. Norcross (Ed.), *Psychotherapy relationships that work: Evidence-based responsiveness* (2nd ed., pp. 316–335). New York, NY: Oxford.

Solnit, S. J. (1997). A legacy: Anna Freud's views on childhood and development. *Child Psychiatry and Human Development, 28,* 5–14.

Sommerbeck, L. (2011). An introduction to pre-therapy. *Psychosis, 3,* 235–241.

Spaulding, W., & Nolting, J. (2006). Psychotherapy for schizophrenia in the year 2030: Prognosis and prognostication. *Schizophrenia Bulletin, 32* (Suppl. 1), S94–S105.

Speca, M., Carlson, L. E., Mackenzie, M. J., & Angen, M. (2006). Mindfulness-based stress reduction (MBSR) as an intervention for cancer patients. In R. A. Baer (Ed.), *Mindfulness-based treatment approaches: Clinician's guide to evidence base and applications* (pp. 239–261). Burlington, MA: Elsevier.

Spencer, B., & Brown, J. (2007). Fusion or internalized homophobia? A pilot study of Bowen's differentiation of self hypothesis with lesbian couples. *Family Process, 46,* 257–268.

Sperry, L. (2006). *Cognitive behavior therapy of DSM-IV-TR personality disorders* (2nd ed.). New York, NY: Routledge.

Sperry, L. (2012). *Spirituality in clinical practice: Theory and practice of spiritually oriented psychotherapy* (2nd ed.). New York, NY: Routledge.

Sperry, L., & Shafranske, E. P. (Eds.). (2005). *Spiritually oriented psychotherapy*. Washington, DC: American Psychological Association.

Spiegler, M. (2008). Behavior therapy II: Cognitive behavior therapy. In J. Frew & M. D. Spiegler (Eds.), *Contemporary psychotherapies for a diverse world* (pp. 320–359). Boston, MA: Houghton Mifflin.

Spinelli, E. (2007). *Practising existential psychotherapy: The relational world*. London, UK: Sage.

Spinelli, M. G. (1997). *Interpersonal psychotherapy for depressed antepartum women*. New York, NY: College of Physicians and Surgeons, Columbia University Press.

Springer, P. R., & Wheeler, M. A. (2012). The relational self-esteem pot. A Satir intervention in family therapy. *The Satir Journal: Transformational Systemic Therapy, 5*(1).

Stafford-Clark, D. (1965). *What Freud really said*. New York, NY: Schocken.

Stasiewicz, P., Herrman, D., Nochajski, T., & Dermen, K. (2006). Motivational interviewing: Engaging highly resistant clients in treatment. *Counselor, 7*.

Stehno, J. T. (1995). Classroom consulting with reality therapy. *Journal of Reality Therapy, 15*(1), 81–86.

Stein, B. C., Jaycox, L. H., Kataoka, S. H., Wong, M., Tu, W., Elliott, M. N., & Fink, A. (2003). A mental health intervention for school children exposed to violence. *Journal of the American Medical Association, 290*, 603–611.

Stein, H. T. (2007). Adler's legacy: Past, present and future. *Journal of Individual Psychology, 63*, 205–213.

Stein, M. (Ed.). (2010). *Jungian psychoanalysis: Working the spirit of C. G. Jung*. Chicago, IL: Carus.

Steketee, G. (Ed.). (2011). *Handbook of obsessive compulsive and spectrum disorders*. New York, NY: Oxford University Press.

Steketee, G., Frost, R. O., Tolin, D. F., Rasmussen, J., & Brown, T. A. (2010). Waitlist-controlled trial of cognitive behavior therapy for hoarding disorder. *Depression and Anxiety, 27*, 476–484.

Stewart, R. E., & Chambless, D. L. (2007). Does psychotherapy research inform treatment decisions in private practice? *Journal of Clinical Psychology, 63*, 267–281.

Stifler, K., Greer, J., Sneck, W., & Dovenmuehle, R. (1993). An empirical investigation of the discriminability of reported mystical experiences among religious contemplatives, psychotic inpatients, and normal adults. *Journal for the Scientific Study of Religion, 32*, 366–372.

Stoehr, T. (2009). Perls, Hefferline, and Goodman: Gestalt therapy—An afterword. *Gestalt Review, 13*, 82–95.

Strasser, F., & Strasser, A. (1997). *Existential time-limited therapy: The wheel of existence*. New York, NY: Wiley.

Strean, H. S. (1994). *Essentials of psychoanalysis*. New York, NY: Brunner/Mazel.

Strean, H. S. (2001). *Controversies on countertransference*. Lanham, MD: Jason Aronson.

Stricker, G., & Gold, J. (2006). *A casebook of psychotherapy integration*. Washington, DC: American Psychological Association.

Stricker, G., & Gold, J. (2011). Integrative approaches to psychotherapy. In S. Messer & A. Gurman (Eds.), *Essential psychotherapies* (3rd ed., pp. 425–459). New York, NY: Guilford Press.

Strozier, C. B. (2001). *Heinz Kohut: The making of a psychoanalyst*. New York, NY: Farrar, Strauss and Giroux.

Strumpfel, U. (2006). *Therapie der Gefuehle: Forschungsbefunde zur Gestalttherapie*. Cologne, Germany: Edition Humansistiche Psychologie. Summary available at http://therapie-der-gefuehle.de/summary.html

Strumpfel, U., & Goldman, R. (2002). Contacting Gestalt therapy. In D. J. Cain & J. Seeman (Eds.), *Humanistic psychotherapies: Handbook of research and practice* (pp. 189–219). Washington, DC: American Psychological Association.

Strumpfel, U., & Martin, C. (2004). Research on Gestalt therapy. *International Gestalt Journal, 27*, 9–54.

Strupp, H. H. (1992). The future of psychodynamic psychotherapy. *Psychotherapy, 29*(1), 21–27.

Stuart, R. B. (1998). Updating behavior therapy with couples. *Family Journal, 6*(1), 6–12.

Sue, D. W., & Sue, D. (2008). *Counseling the culturally diverse: Theory and practice* (5th ed.). New York, NY: John Wiley & Sons.

Sullivan, H. S. (1947). *Conceptions of modern psychiatry*. Washington, DC: William Alanson White Institute.

Sullivan, H. S. (1953). *The interpersonal theory of psychiatry*. New York, NY: W. W. Norton.

Sullivan, H. S. (1970). *The psychiatric interview*. New York, NY: W. W. Norton.

Sulloway, F. J. (1995). Birth order and evolutionary psychology: A meta-analytic overview. *Psychological Inquiry, 6,* 75–80.

Sulloway, F. J., & Zweigenhaft, R. L. (2010). Birth order and risk taking in athletics: A meta-analysis and study of major league baseball players. *Personality and Social Psychology Review, 14,* 402–416.

Summers, R. F., & Barber, J. P. (2009). *Psychodynamic therapy: A guide to evidence-based practice*. New York, NY: Guilford Press.

Surcinelli, P., Rossi, N., Montebarocci, O., & Baldaro, B. (2010). Adult attachment styles and psychological disease: Examining the mediating role of personality traits. *Journal of Psychology Interpersonal and Applied, 144,* 523–534.

Surrey, J. L. (1991). The "self-in-relation": A new theory of women's development. In J. V. Jordon, A. G. Kaplan, J. B. Miller, I. P. Stiver, & J. L. Surrey (Eds.), *Women's growth in connection: Writings from the Stone Center*. New York, NY: Guilford Press.

Swales, M. (2012). Dialectical behavior therapy. In W. Dryden (Ed.), *Cognitive behavioral therapies* (pp. 93–114). Thousand Oaks, CA: Sage.

Sweeney, D. S., & Homeyer, L. E. (2010). Sandtray therapy. In A. A. Drewes (Ed.), *Blending play therapy with cognitive behavioral therapy* (pp. 297–318). Hoboken, NJ: John Wiley & Sons.

Sweeney, T. J. (2009). *Adlerian counseling: A practitioner's approach* (5th ed.). Philadelphia, PA: Taylor & Francis.

Sweet, A. D. (2010). Paranoia and psychotic process: Some clinical applications of projective identification in psychoanalytic psychotherapy. *American Journal of Psychotherapy, 64,* 339–358.

Swift, J. K., & Callahan, J. L. (2010). A comparison of client preferences for intervention empirical support versus common therapy variables, *Journal of Clinical Psychology, 66,* 1217–1231.

Swift, J. K., Callahan, J. L., & Vollmer, B. M. (2011). Preferences. In J. C. Norcross (Ed.), *Psychotherapy relationships that work: Evidence-based responsiveness*. New York, NY: Oxford University Press.

Symonds, D., & Horvath, A. O. (2004). Optimizing the alliance in couples therapy. *Family Process, 43,* 443–455.

Tacey, D. (2009). *Edge of the sacred: Jung, psyche, and earth*. Einsiedein, Switzerland: Daimon Verlag.

Tarragona, M. (2008). Postmodern/poststructuralist therapies. In J. L. Lebow (Ed.), *Twenty-first century psychotherapies: Contemporary approaches to theory and practice* (pp. 167– 205). Hoboken, NJ: John Wiley & Sons.

Tavernese, S. (2012, May 17). Whites account for under half of births in U.S. *New York Times,* p. A-1.

Teasdale, J., Williams, J., Soulsby, J. M., Segal, Z. V., Ridgeway, V. A., & Lau, M. A. (2000). Prevention of relapse/recurrence in major depression by mindfulness-based cognitive therapy. *Journal of Consulting and Clinical Psychology, 68,* 623–625.

Teyber, E., & McClure, F. H. (2011). *Interpersonal process in therapy: An integrative model* (6th ed.). Belmont, CA: Thomson/Brooks Cole.

Thomas, F. (2010a). 7-Eleven. In T. S. Nelson (Ed.), *Doing something different: Solution focused brief therapy practices* (pp. 5–6). New York, NY: Routledge.

Thomas, F. (2010b). Scaling agency with clients when they begin taking anti-depressants. In T. S. Nelson (Ed.), *Doing something different: Solution focused brief therapy practices* (pp. 11–15). New York, NY: Routledge.

Thompson, C. (2011). A meaning-centered therapy for addictions. *Journal of Mental Health and Addiction,* 9367–9411.

Thompson, R. A. (2003). *Counseling techniques*. Washington, DC: Accelerated Development.

Thorne, B. (1991). *Person-centred counseling: Therapeutic and spiritual dimensions*. London, UK: Whurr.

Thorne, B. (2002). *The mystical power of person-centred therapy: Hope beyond despair*. London, UK: Whurr.

Tillich, P. (1952). *The courage to be*. New Haven, CT: Yale University Press.

Tinker, R., & Wilson, W. (1999). *Through the eyes of a child.* New York, NY: W. W. Norton.

Toman, S. M., & Bauer, A. (2005). Adolescents: Development & practice from a Gestalt perspective. In A. L. Woldt & S. M. Toman (Eds.), *Gestalt therapy: History, theory, and practice* (pp. 179–200). Thousand Oaks, CA: Sage.

Tomm, K. (1984). Interventive interviewing: Part I. Strategizing as a fourth guideline for the therapist. *Family Process, 26,* 3–13.

Topolinski, S., & Hertel, G. (2007). The role of personality in psychotherapists' careers: Relationships between personality traits, therapeutic schools, and job satisfaction. *Psychotherapy Research, 17,* 378–390.

Tori, C. D., & Bilmes, M. (2002). Multiculturalism and psychoanalytic psychology: The validation of a defense mechanisms measure in an Asian population. *Psychoanalytic Psychology, 19,* 701–721.

Totton, N. (2010). *The problem with the humanistic therapies*. London, UK: Karnac Books.

Tremblay, J., Herron, W., & Schultz, C. (1986). Relation between therapeutic orientation and personality in psychotherapists. *Professional Psychology: Research and Practice, 17,* 106–110.

Truax, C., & Carkhuff, R. (2007). *Toward effective counseling and psychotherapy*. Chicago, IL: Transaction Publishers.

Tuckey, M. R., & Brewer, N. (2003). The influence of schemas, stimulus ambiguity, and interview schedule on eyewitness memory over time. *Journal of Experimental Psychology: Applied, 9,* 101–118.

Tudor, K. (2002). *Transactional analysis approaches to brief therapy: What do you say between saying hello and goodbye?* London, UK: Sage.

Tudor, K. (2008). *The adult is parent to the child: Transactional analysis with children and young people*. Dorset, UK: Russell House Publishers.

Tudor, K., & Worrall, M. (2006). *Person-centered therapy: A clinical philosophy*. New York, NY: Routledge.

Tummala-Narra, P. (2009). The relevance of a psychoanalytic perspective in exploring religious and spiritual identity in psychotherapy. *Psychoanalytic Psychology, 26,* 83–95.

Turkington, D., Kingdon, D., & Weiden, P. (2008). Cognitive behavior therapy for schizophrenia. *Focus, 6,* 266. Arlington, VA: American Psychiatric Association.

Tursi, M. M., & Cochran, J. L. (2006). Cognitive behavioral tasks accomplished in a person-centered relational framework. *Journal of Counseling and Development, 84,* 387–396.

Uhlmann, E., Pizarro, D., & Bloom, P. (2008). Varieties of social cognition. *Journal for the Theory of Social Behavior, 38,* 293–322.

Vachon, M., Fillion, L., Achille, M., Duval, S., & Leung, D. (2011). An awakening experience: An interpretative phenomenological analysis of the effects of a meaning-centered intervention shared among palliative care nurses. *Qualitative Research in Psychology, 8,* 39–54.

Vallejo, Z., & Amaro, H. (2009). Adaptation of mindfulness-based stress reduction program for addiction relapse prevention. *The Humanistic Psychologist, 37,* 192–206.

van Deurzen, E. (2002). *Existential counseling and psychotherapy in practice* (2nd ed.). London, UK: Sage.

van Deurzen, E. (2010). *Everyday mysteries: A handbook of existential psychotherapy* (2nd ed.). New York, NY: Routledge.

van Deurzen, E., & Adams, M. (2011). *Skills in existential counseling and psychotherapy*. Thousand Oaks, CA: Sage.

Van Etten, M. L., & Taylor, S. (1998). Comparative efficacy of treatments for posttraumatic stress disorder: A meta-analysis. *Clinical Psychology and Psychotherapy, 5,* 126–144.

Van Wagoner, S. L., Gelso, C. J., Hayes, J. A., & Diemer, R. A. (1991). Countertransference and the reputedly excellent therapist. *Psychotherapy, 28,* 411–421.

Veale, D., & Neziroglu, F. (2010). *Body dysmorphic disorder: A treatment manual*. Hoboken, NJ: John Wiley & Sons.

Veltro, F., Vendittelli, N., Oricchio, I., Addona, F., Avino, C., Figliolia, G., & Morosini, P. (2008). Effectiveness and efficiency of cognitive–behavioral group therapy for inpatients: 4-year follow-up study. *Journal of Psychiatric Practice, 14,* 281–288.

Verdeli, H., & Weissman, M. M. (2011). Interpersonal therapy. In R. J. Corsini & D. Wedding (Eds.), Current psychotherapies (9th ed., pp. 383–416). Belmont, CA: Brooks/Cole.

Vernon, A. (2006a). *Thinking, feeling, behaving: An emotional education curriculum for adolescents: Grades 7–12*. Champaign, IL: Research Press.

Vernon, A. (2006b). *Thinking, feeling, behaving: An emotional education curriculum for children: Grades 1–6.* Champaign, IL: Research Press.

Vernon, A. (2009). Rational emotive behavior therapy. In A. Vernon & T. Kottman (Eds.), *Counseling theories: Practical applications with children and adolescents in school settings* (pp. 154–184). Denver, CO: Love.

von Bertalanffy, L. (1968/1976). *General system theory: Foundations, development, application.* New York, NY: George Braziller.

Von Glasersfeld, E. (1996). *Radical constructivism: A way of knowing and learning.* Psychology Press.

Vontress, C. E. (1996). A personal retrospective on cross-cultural counseling. *Journal of Counseling and Development, 24,* 156–166.

Vontress, C. E. (2008a). Existential therapy. In J. Frew and M. D. Spiegler (Eds.), *Contemporary psychotherapy for a diverse world* (pp. 141–176). Boston, MA: Houghton Mifflin.

Vontress, C. E. (2008b). Preface. In P. B. Pedersen, J. G. Draguns, W. J. Lonner, & J. E. Trimble (Eds.), *Counseling across cultures* (6th ed., p. ix–xii). Alexandria, VA: American Counseling Association.

Vontress, C. E., & Epp, L. R. (1997). Historical hostility in the African American client: Implications for counseling. *Journal of Multicultural Counseling and Development, 25,* 170–184.

Vontress, C. E., Johnson, J. A., & Epp, L. R. (1999). *Cross-cultural counseling: A casebook.* Alexandria, VA: American Counseling Association.

Vromans, L., & Schweitzer, R. (2011). Narrative therapy for adults with major depressive disorder: Improved symptom and interpersonal outcomes. *Psychotherapy Resolutions, 21,* 4–15.

Vygotsky, L. (1967). Play and its role in the mental development of the child. *Journal of Russian and East European Psychology, 5,* 6–18.

Vygotsky, L. (1986). *Thought and language.* Cambridge, MA: MIT Press.

Wachtel, P. L. (1977). *Psychoanalysis and behavior therapy: Toward an integration.* New York, NY: Basic Books.

Wachtel, P. L. (1997). *Psychoanalysis, behavior therapy, and the relational world.* Washington, DC: American Psychological Association.

Wachtel, P. L. (2008). *Relational psychotherapy.* New York, NY: Guilford Press.

Wachtel, P. L. (2010). *Relational theory and the practice of psychotherapy.* New York, NY: Guilford Press.

Wachtel, P. L. (2011). *Inside the session: What really happens in psychotherapy.* Washington, DC: American Psychological Association.

Wachtel, P. L. (2012). *Therapeutic communication: Knowing what to say and when* (2nd ed.), New York, NY: Guilford Press.

Wachtel, P. L., Kruk, J., & McKinney, M. K. (2005). Cyclical psychodynamics and integrative relational therapy. In J. C. Norcross & M. R. Goldfried (Eds.), *Handbook of psychotherapy integration* (2nd ed., pp. 172–195). New York, NY: Oxford University Press.

Wagner-Moore, L. E. (2004). Gestalt therapy: Past, present, and future research. *Psychotherapy: Theory, Research, Practice, Training, 41,* 180–189.

Waites, C. (2009). Building on strengths: Intergenerational practice with African American families. *Social Work, 54,* 278–287.

Walborn, F. S. (1996). *Process variables.* Pacific Grove, CA: Brooks/Cole.

Walen, S. R., DiGiuseppe, R., & Dryden, W. (1992). *A practitioner's guide to rational-emotive therapy.* New York, NY: Oxford University Press.

Wallach, H. S., Safir, M. P., & Bar-Zvi, M. (2009). Virtual reality cognitive behavior therapy for public speaking anxiety: A randomized clinical trial. *Behavior Modification, 33,* 314–338.

Walsh, F. (1998). *Strengthening family resilience.* New York, NY: Guilford Press.

Walsh, F. (Ed.). (2012). *Normal family processes: Growing diversity and complexity* (4th ed.). New York, NY: Guilford Press.

Wampold, B. E. (2010). The research evidence for the common factors models: A historically situated perspective. In B. L. Duncan, S. D. Miller, B. E. Wampold, & M. A. Hubble. (Eds.), *Heart and soul of change in psychotherapy* (2nd ed., pp. 49–81). Washington, DC: American Psychological Association.

Wampold, B. E., Minami, T., Baskin, T. W., & Callen Tierney, S. (2002). A meta-(re)analysis of the effects of cognitive therapy versus "other therapies" for depression. *Journal of Affective Disorders, 68,* 159–165.

Warren, J. M. (2012). Mobile mind mapping: Using mobile technology to enhance rational emotive behavior therapy. *Journal of Mental Health Counseling, 34,* 72–81.

Waska, R. (2010). Moments of uncertainty in psychoanalytic practice: Interpreting within the matrix of projective identification, counter-transference, and enactment. New York, NY: Columbia University Press.

Watson, J. B. (1925). *Behaviorism.* New York, NY: W. W. Norton.

Watson, J. C., Gordon, L. B., Stermac, L., Kalogerakos, F., & Steckley, P. (2003). Comparing the effectiveness of process-experiential with cognitive–behavioral psychotherapy in the treatment of depression. *Journal of Consulting and Clinical Psychology, 71,* 773–781.

Watts, A. (1951). *The wisdom of insecurity: A message for an age of anxiety.* New York, NY: Pantheon Books.

Watts, A. (1957). *The way of Zen.* New York, NY: Pantheon Books.

Watts, R. E. (2000). Entering the new millennium: Is individual psychology still relevant? *Journal of Individual Psychology, 56,* 21–30.

Watts, R. E. (Ed.). (2003). *Adlerian, cognitive, and constructivist therapies: An integrative dialogue.* New York, NY: Springer.

Weakland, J., Fisch, R., Watzlawick, P., & Bodin, A. (1974). Brief therapy: Focused problem resolution. *Family Process, 13,* 141–168.

Weishaar, M. E. (1993). *Aaron T. Beck.* London, UK: Sage.

Weisler, S. (2006). Cancer as a turning point in life. *International Journal of Reality Therapy, 26,* 38–39.

Weiss, P. A. (2010). Time-limited dynamic psychotherapy as a model for short-term inpatient groups. *Journal of Contemporary Psychotherapy, 40,* 41–49.

Weissman, M. M., Markowitz, J., & Klerman, G. L. (2007). *Clinician's quick guide to interpersonal therapy.* New York, NY: Oxford University Press.

Wheeler, G. (1991). *Gestalt reconsidered: A new approach to contact and resistances.* New York, NY: Gardner.

Whitaker, C. A., & Napier, A. Y. (1977). Process techniques of family therapy. *Interaction, 1,* 4–19.

Whitaker, C., Warkentin, J., & Malone, T. (2011). The involvement of the professional therapist. In C. Whitaker, J. Warkentin, T. Malone, & A. Burton (Eds.), *Case studies in counseling and psychotherapy* (pp. 218–256). Englewood Cliffs, NJ: Prentice Hall.

White, J., Campbell, L., & Steward, A. (1995). Associations of scores on the White-Campbell Psychological Birth Order Inventory and the Kern Lifestyle Scale. *Psychological Reports, 77,* 1187–1196.

White, K. J., Wagener, L. M., & Furrow, J. L. (2010). What am I here for? A qualitative examination on the expression, development and integration of purpose in at-risk and thriving male adolescents. *International Journal of Existential Psychology and Psychotherapy, 3,* 1–16.

White, M. (1986). Negative explanation, restraint, and double description: A template for family. *Family Process, 25,* 169–184.

White, M. (1988–1989, Summer). The externalization of the problem and the re-authoring of lives and relationships. *Dulwich Centre Newsletter,* pp. 3–20.

White, M. (1989). *Selected papers.* Adelaide, Australia: Dulwich Centre.

White, M. (1995). *Re-authoring lives.* Adelaide, Australia: Dulwich Centre.

White, M. (2007). *Maps of narrative practice.* New York, NY: W. W. Norton.

White, M. (2011). *Narrative practice: Continuing the conversation.* New York, NY: W. W. Norton.

White, M., & Epston, D. (1989). *Literate means to therapeutic ends.* Adelaide, Australia: Dulwich Centre.

White, M., & Epston, D. (1990). *Narrative means to therapeutic ends.* New York, NY: W. W. Norton.

White, M., & Morgan, A. (2006). *Narrative therapy with children and their families.* Adelaide, Australia: Dulwich Centre.

White, W. L., & Kurtz, E. (2008). Twelve defining moments in the history of Alcoholics Anonymous. In M. Galanter & L. A. Kaskutas (Eds.). *Recent developments in alcoholism, Vol. 18: Research on Alcoholics Anonymous and spirituality in addiction recovery* (pp. 37–58). New York, NY: Humana Press.

Wickers, F. (1988). The misbehavior reaction checklist. *Elementary School Guidance and Counseling, 23,* 70–73.

Wilcoxon, S. A., Remley, T. P., Gladding, S. T., & Huber, C. H. (2007). *Ethical, legal, and professional issues in the practice of marriage and family therapy* (4th ed.). Upper Saddle River, NJ: Pearson.

Williams, M. (2006). Mindfulness-based stress reduction (MBSR) in a worksite wellness program. In R. A. Baer (Ed.), *Mindfulness-based treatment approaches: Clinician's guide to evidence base and applications* (pp. 361–376). Burlington, MA: Elsevier.

Williams, M. (2010). Mindfulness and psychological process, *Emotion, 10,* 1–7.

Williams, M., Alato, Y., Crane, C., Bernhofer, T., Fennell, M. J. V., Duggan, D. S., . . . Goodwin, G. M. (2008). Mindfulness-based cognitive therapy (MBCT) in bipolar disorder: Preliminary evaluation of immediate effects on between-episode functioning. *Journal of Affective Disorders, 107,* 275–279.

Williams, M., Teasdale, J., Segal, Z., & Kabat-Zinn, J. (2007). *The mindful way through depression.* New York, NY: Guilford Press.

Williams, P. S. (1994). Harry Stack Sullivan: Opening the door for a transpersonal vision? *Humanistic Psychologist, 22,* 62–73.

Willock, B. (2001). Stephen A. Mitchell (1946–2000). *American Psychologist, 56,* 820.

Wilson, G. T. (1995). Behavior therapy. In R. J. Corsini & D. Wedding (Eds.), *Current psychotherapies* (5th ed., pp. 127–228). Itasca, IL: Peacock.

Wilson, W. P. (2009). Psychiatric treatments involving religion: Psychotherapy from a Christian perspective. In P. Huguelet & H. P. Koenig (Eds.), *Religion and spirituality in psychiatry* (pp. 283–300). New York, NY: Cambridge University Press.

Winbolt, B. (2011). *Solution focused therapy for the helping professions.* Philadelphia, PA: Jessica Kingsley.

Wingerson, D., Sullivan, M., Dager, S., Flick, S., Dunner, D., & Roy-Byrne, P. (1993). Personality traits and early discontinuation from clinical trials in anxious patients. *Journal of Clinical Psychopharmacology, 13,* 194–197.

Winslade, J., & Monk, G. (2000). *Narrative mediation: A new approach to conflict resolution.* San Francisco, CA: Jossey-Bass.

Winslade, J., & Smith, L. (1997). Countering alcoholic narratives. In G. Monk, J. Winslade, K. Crocket, & D. Epston (Eds.), *Narrative therapy in practice: The archaeology of hope* (pp. 158–193). San Francisco, CA: Jossey-Bass.

Wintersteen, M. B., Mensinger, J. L., & Diamond, G. S. (2005). Do gender and racial differences between patient and therapist affect therapeutic alliance and treatment retention in adolescents? *Professional Psychology: Research and Practice, 36,* 400–408.

Witmer, J. M., & Sweeney, T. J. (1992). A holistic model for wellness and prevention over the lifespan. *Journal of Counseling and Development, 71,* 140–148.

Witt-Browder, A. S. (2000). Clients in partial hospitalization settings. In J. R. White & A. S. Freeman (Eds.), *Cognitive–behavioral group therapy for specific problems and populations* (pp. 361–384). Washington, DC: American Psychological Association.

Woldt, A. L., & Toman, S. M. (2005). *Gestalt therapy: History, theory, and practice.* Thousand Oaks, CA: Sage.

Wolf, E. S. (1994). Varieties of disorders of the self. *British Journal of Psychotherapy, 11,* 198–208.

Wolpe, J. (1969). *The practice of behavior therapy.* New York, NY: Pergamon.

Wong, E. C., Kim, B. S., Zane, N. W. S., Kim, I. J., & Huang, J. S. (2003). Examining culturally based variables associated with ethnicity: Influences on credibility perceptions of empirically supported interventions. *Cultural Diversity & Ethnic Minority Psychology, 9,* 88–96.

Wong, P. (2010). Meaning therapy: An integrative and positive existential psychology. *Journal of Contemporary Psychology, 40,* 85–93.

Wubbolding, R. E. (1988). *Using reality therapy.* New York, NY: Perennial.

Wubbolding, R. E. (1991). *Understanding reality therapy.* New York, NY: HarperCollins.

Wubbolding, R. E. (1995). Integrating theory and practice: Expanding the theory and use of the higher level of perception. *Journal of Reality Therapy, 15*(1), 91–94.

Wubbolding, R. E. (2000). *Reality therapy for the 21st century.* Bristol, PA: Accelerated Development.

Wubbolding, R. E. (2007a). Glasser quality school. *Group Dynamics: Theory, Research and Practice, 11,* 253–261.

Wubbolding, R. E. (2007b). Reality therapy theory. In D. Capuzzi & D. Gross (Eds.), *Counseling and psychotherapy: Theories and interventions* (4th ed., pp. 289–312). Upper Saddle River, NJ: Pearson/Prentice Hall.

Wubbolding, R. E. (2009). *Reality therapy training manual* (15th rev.). Cincinnati, OH: Center for Reality Therapy.

Wubbolding, R. E. (2011). *Reality therapy: Theories of counseling series.* Washington, DC: American Psychological Association.

Wubbolding, R. E., & Brickell, J. (2008). Frequently asked questions and not so brief answers: Part II. *International Journal of Reality Therapy, 27,* 46–49.

Wulf, R. (1998). The historical roots of Gestalt therapy theory. *Gestalt Journal, 21,* 81–92.

Xu, J. (2010). Logotherapy: A balm of Gilead for aging? *Journal of Religion, Spirituality & Aging, 22,* 180–195.

Yalom, I. D. (1980). *Existential psychotherapy.* New York, NY: Basic Books.

Yalom, I. D. (1989). *Love's executioner and other tales of psychotherapy.* New York, NY: Basic Books.

Yalom, I. (1998). *The Yalom reader: Selections from the work of a master therapist and master storyteller.* New York, NY: Basic Books.

Yalom, I. D. (2008). *Staring at the sun: Overcoming the terror of death.* San Francisco, CA: Jossey-Bass.

Yalom, I. (2009). *The gift of therapy: An open letter to a new generation of therapists.* New York, NY: Harper Collins.

Yalom, I., & Leszcz, M. (2005). *Theory and practice of group psychotherapy* (5th ed.). New York, NY: Basic Books.

Yontef, G. (1993). *Awareness, dialogue, and process: Essays on Gestalt therapy.* Highland, NY: The Gestalt Journal Press.

Yontef, G. (1998). Dialogic Gestalt therapy. In L. Greenberg, J. C. Watson, & G. Lietaer (Eds.), *Handbook of experiential psychotherapy* (pp. 82–102). New York, NY: Guilford Press.

Yontef, G. M. (2012). The four relationships of Gestalt therapy couples work. In T. B. Levine (Ed.), *Gestalt therapy: Advances in theory and practice* (pp. 123–137). New York, NY: Routledge.

Young, J. E. (1990/1999). *Cognitive therapy for personality disorders: A schema-focused approach.* Sarasota, FL: Professional Resource Exchange.

Young, J. E. (2003a). *Young Compensation Inventory.* New York, NY: Schema Therapy Institute.

Young, J. E. (2003b). *Young Parenting Inventory.* New York, NY: Cognitive Therapy Center of New York.

Young, J. E. (2005). *Young Schema Questionnaire.* New York, NY: Schema Therapy Institute.

Young, J. E., Arntz, A., Atkinson, T., Lobbastael, J., Weishear, M. E., vanVoleeswijk, M. F., & Klokman, J. (2007). *The Schema Mode Inventory.* New York, NY: Schema Therapy Institute.

Young, J. E., Klosko, J. S., & Weishaar, M. E. (2006). *Schema therapy: A practitioner's guide.* New York, NY: Guilford Press.

Young, S. (2010). Responding to bullying in primary schools. In T. S. Nelson (Ed.), *Doing something different: Solution focused brief therapy practices* (pp. 99–101). New York, NY: Routledge.

Young-Bruehl, E. (2008). *Anna Freud: A biography.* New Haven, CT: Yale University Press.

Zadeh, Z. H., Jenkins, J., & Pepler, D. (2010). A transactional analysis of maternal negativity and child externalizing behavior. *International Journal of Behavioral Development, 34,* 218–228.

Zarb, J. M. (2007). *Developmental cognitive behavioral therapy with adults.* New York, NY: Routledge.

Ziegler, D. J. (1999). The construct of personality in rational emotive behavior therapy (REBT) theory. *Journal of Rational-Emotive & Cognitive–Behavior Therapy, 17,* 19–32.

Zinbarg, R. E., & Griffith, J. W. (2008). Behavior therapy. In J. L. Lebow (Ed.), *Twenty-first century psychotherapies: Contemporary approaches to theory and practice* (pp. 8–42). Hoboken, NJ: John Wiley & Sons.

Zuroff, D. C., Kelly, A. C., Leybman, M. J., Blatt, S. J., & Wampold, B. E. (2010). Between-therapist and within-therapist differences in the quality of the therapeutic relationship: Effects on maladjustment and self-critical perfectionism. *Journal of Clinical Psychology, 66,* 681–697.

INDEX

N

Wubbolding, R. E. (2009). *Reality therapy training manual* (15th rev.). Cincinnati, OH: Center for Reality Therapy.

Wubbolding, R. E. (2011). *Reality therapy: Theories of psychotherapy series*. Washington, DC: American Psychological Association.

Wubbolding, R. E., & Brickell, J. (1998). Frequently asked questions and not so brief answers: Part II. *International Journal of Reality Therapy, 17*, 46–[illegible].

Wulf, R. (1998). The historical roots of Gestalt therapy theory. *Gestalt Journal, 21*, [illegible].

[illegible] (2011). Psychotherapy [illegible] for aging. *[illegible] Religion* [illegible].

Yalom, I. D. (1980). *Existential psychotherapy*. New York, NY: Basic Books.

Yalom, I. D. (1989). *Love's executioner and other tales of psychotherapy*. New York, NY: Basic Books.

Yalom, I. (1998). *The Yalom reader: Selections from the work of a master therapist and storyteller*. New York, NY: Basic Books.

Yalom, I. D. (2008). *Staring at the sun: Overcoming the terror of death*. San Francisco, CA: Jossey-Bass.

Yalom, I. (2009). *The gift of therapy: An open letter to a new generation of therapists*. New York, NY: Harper Collins.

Yalom, I., & Leszcz, M. (2005). *The theory and practice of group psychotherapy* (5th ed.). New York, NY: Basic Books.

Yontef, G. (1993). *Awareness, dialogue, and process: Essays on Gestalt therapy*. Highland, NY: The Gestalt Journal Press.

Yontef, G. [illegible]

Young, J. [illegible] *Advances* [illegible] York, NY: Routledge.

Young, J. E. (1990/1999). *Cognitive therapy for personality disorders: A schema-focused approach*. Sarasota, FL: Professional Resource Exchange.

Young, J. E. (2005). *Young Compensation Inventory*. New York, NY: Schema Therapy Institute.

Young, J. E. (2003). *Young Parenting Inventory*. New York, NY: Cognitive Therapy Center of New York.

Young, J. E. (2005). *Young Schema Questionnaire*. New York, NY: Schema Therapy Institute.

Young, J. E., Arntz, A., Atkinson, T., Lobbestael, J., Weishaar, M. E., van Vreeswijk, M. F., & Klokman, J. (2007). *The Schema Mode Inventory*. New York, NY: Schema Therapy Institute.

Young, J. E., Klosko, J. S., & Weishaar, M. E. (2006). *Schema therapy: A practitioner's guide*. New York, NY: Guilford Press.

Young, S. (2010). Responding to bullying in primary schools. In T. S. Nelson (Ed.), *Doing something different: Solution-focused brief therapy practices* (pp. [illegible]). New York, NY: Routledge.

Young-Bruehl, E. (2008). *Anna Freud: A biography*. New Haven, CT: Yale University Press.

Zalewski, M., [illegible] (2011). A naturalistic study of maternal negativity and child externalizing behavior. *International Journal of Behavioral Development, 35*, 218–228.

Zarb, J. M. (2007). *Developmental cognitive behavioral therapy with adults*. New York, NY: Routledge.

Ziegler, D. J. (1999). The construct of personality in rational emotive behavior therapy (REBT) theory. *Journal of Rational-Emotive & Cognitive-Behavior Therapy, 17*, 19–32.

Zinbarg, R. E., & Griffith, J. W. (2008). Behavior therapy. In J. L. Lebow (Ed.), *Twenty-first century psychotherapies: Contemporary approaches to theory and practice* (pp. 8–42). Hoboken, NJ: John Wiley & Sons.

Zuroff, D. C., Kelly, A. C., Leybman, M. J., Blatt, S. J., & Wampold, B. E. (2010). Between-therapist and within-therapist differences in the quality of the therapeutic relationship: Effects on maladjustment and self-critical perfectionism. *Journal of Clinical Psychology, 66*, 681–697.